Stochastic Processes for Adaptive Healthcare Systems

Anastasius S. Moumtzoglou
https://orcid.org/0000-0002-5899-1033
P&A Kyriakou Children's Hospital, Greece

IGI Global
Scientific Publishing
Publishing Tomorrow's Research Today

VP of Publishing Ethics & Research Integrity	Melissa Wagner
Director of Acquisitions	Mikaela Felty
Director of Book Development	Jocelynn Hessler
Production Manager	Mike Brehm
Cover Design	Jose Rosado

Published in the United States of America by
IGI Global Scientific Publishing
701 East Chocolate Avenue
Hershey, PA, 17033, USA
Tel: 717-533-8845 | Fax: 717-533-7115
Website: https://www.igi-global.com E-mail: cust@igi-global.com

Library of Congress Cataloging-in-Publication Data

LCCN: 2026019874 (CIP Data Pending)
ISBN13: 9798337397054
EISBN13: 9798337397078
British Cataloguing in Publication Data
A Cataloguing in Publication record for this book is available from the British Library.

To Lina — A.M.

Table of Contents

Detailed Table of Contents

Healthcare systems operate under persistent uncertainty arising from stochastic demand, limited resources, and delayed operational adaptation. While classical queueing and Markovian models provide a mathematical basis for analysing patient flow and service capacity, they often rely on stationarity assumptions that weaken under emergency overcrowding, demand surges, and staffing disruptions. This chapter introduces an event-driven stochastic regime framework for modelling transitions between normal operation, congestion, overload, and recovery in adaptive healthcare setting. The approach extends an M/M/c queue with regime-dependent dynamics and delayed capacity adjustment and is evaluated through discrete-event simulation using synthetic demand scenarios. Results show that policy lag amplifies backlog accumulation, prolongs overload duration, and increases recovery time, while adaptive surge staffing mitigates these effects. The chapter highlights implications for emergency department operations and identifies early-warning indicators for resilient, data-informed service design.

The healthcare trilemma, which involves balancing quantity, quality, and cost, is often treated as if these factors operate independently. This chapter demonstrates their significant interdependence and identifies technology as a pivotal factor. Using a four-dimensional production model (Quantity, Quality, Technology, Cost) evaluated across more than 60 scenarios, the analysis yields five principal findings. First, optimal technology investment increases smoothly as technological capability matures, with allocation rising from approximately 10% at low capability to about 35% at full maturity. Second, technology reduces costs ($r = -0.956$) and increases efficiency by 59% as technology levels increase from the lowest to the highest. Third, technology level is the primary driver of gradual strategic reallocation, with optimal strategies evolving smoothly rather than abruptly. Fourth, investment in quality alone is comparatively less effective. Fifth, the Continuous Strategic Adjustment Framework offers a rigorous foundation for future models that incorporate uncertainty.

Healthcare involves complex processes where patients move through multiple stages of care. Understanding these pathways is essential for improving outcomes. This chapter presents a pedagogical, worked-example application of Markov chain modeling to patient care pathways using the MIMIC-III Clinical Database Demo. The methodology represents each stage as a discrete state—Admission, ICU, Home, and Expired—and estimates transition probabilities empirically. By analyzing these transitions, the framework demonstrates how outcomes can be predicted, trajectories simulated, and resource planning informed by probabilistic estimates. The transparent Markov structure ensures interpretability. The chapter also discusses extensions toward adaptive systems, including Bayesian updating and reinforcement

Preface

OVERVIEW OF THE SUBJECT MATTER

Stochastic Processes for Adaptive Healthcare Systems addresses the growing need for probabilistic and adaptive methodologies in healthcare. Healthcare systems are inherently complex and dynamic, with uncertainty stemming from patient heterogeneity, variable treatment responses, resource limitations, and unpredictable demand. Deterministic models frequently fail to represent this complexity. In contrast, stochastic processes offer a robust mathematical framework for capturing randomness and temporal variability. This volume integrates theoretical foundations, methodological tutorials, artificial intelligence applications, and governance frameworks, serving as a comprehensive resource for understanding and implementing adaptive healthcare systems.

WHERE THE TOPIC FITS IN THE WORLD TODAY

Healthcare systems worldwide face mounting pressure to improve quality, reduce costs, and promote equity. The COVID-19 pandemic highlighted the limitations of static planning and underscored the necessity for adaptive, data-driven strategies. While artificial intelligence and real-time data present significant opportunities, they also introduce additional uncertainties and ethical considerations. Probabilistic models, including Markov processes, partially observable Markov decision processes, queueing theory, and stochastic differential equations, have become increasingly pertinent. This book sits at the intersection of applied mathematics, healthcare operations, artificial intelligence, law, and ethics, addressing the need for adaptive systems that learn from data and respond in real time while maintaining accountability and equity.

TARGET AUDIENCE

The intended audience comprises researchers, graduate students, healthcare administrators, clinical decision-makers, data scientists, artificial intelligence practitioners, legal scholars, policymakers, and regulators. This book suits courses in health informatics, operations research, stochastic modelling, artificial intelligence in healthcare, and health law. It also functions as a reference for professionals implementing adaptive systems in hospitals, clinics, public health agencies, and health technology companies. Readers should possess a foundational understanding of probability and statistics; however, the tutorials are designed to be accessible.

STRUCTURE OF THE BOOK

The sixteen chapters in this volume are organised into four sections, each addressing a distinct phase from mathematical foundations to ethical governance. This structure is intentional. Adaptive healthcare systems require more than theoretical understanding; effective implementation also depends on appropriate methods, practical applications, and governance. Accordingly, the sections follow a logical progression: defining healthcare systems, modelling them, applying those models, and governing them responsibly.

Section 1: Foundations and Theoretical Perspectives (Chapters 1–4) establishes the mathematical and conceptual architecture of adaptive healthcare systems. Chapter 1 provides the unifying synthesis, integrating continuous-time Markov processes, hidden Markov models, semi-Markov decision processes, and stochastic differential equations into a single framework. Chapter 2 challenges classical network science by introducing the Hybrid Complexity Model, showing that healthcare systems exhibit hyper-hierarchical and chaotic properties that canonical scale-free models cannot capture. Chapter 3 extends this systems perspective into operational dynamics, modelling regime shifts between normal operation, congestion, overload, and recovery under delayed policy response. Chapter 4 closes the section by examining strategic resource allocation across quantity, quality, and technology, demonstrating that technology investment should increase gradually with digital maturity rather than in discontinuous jumps. Together, these four chapters answer a single question: what kind of system is a healthcare system, and how can we represent its uncertainty mathematically?

Section 2: Methodological and Tutorial Approaches (Chapters 5–8) equips readers with practical and analytical tools. Chapters 5 and 6 form a paired tutorial sequence using the MIMIC-III Clinical Database. Chapter 5 introduces Markov chain modelling of patient care pathways, while Chapter 6 applies queueing theory and Poisson processes to patient flow. Both chapters are designed as step-by-step, reproducible demonstrations that readers can adapt to their own data. Chapter 7 introduces martingale-based monitoring and stopping-time intervention, showing how to distinguish routine variability from meaningful system drift. Chapter 8 develops potential theory and hitting probabilities for measuring access, equity, and risk, with particular attention to structural inequities between rural and urban populations. This section answers the question: how do we model adaptive healthcare systems in practice?

Section 3: AI and Stochastic Applications (Chapters 9–12) shows how the theoretical and methodological foundations apply to real-world clinical problems. Chapter 9 presents a stochastic–AI framework for real-time clinical decision support that integrates deep learning, wearables, and explainable AI. Chapter 10 develops the partially observable Markov decision process (POMDP) as a formal framework for remote patient monitoring, including belief-state representations and solution methods. Chapter 11 introduces the AI-DAR framework for robust multimodal medical imaging diagnosis, addressing stochastic variability in X-ray, CT, and MRI. Chapter 12 proposes the Autonomous Healthcare Control System (AHCS), a digital twin framework for predictive hospital resilience that integrates Markov decision processes, queueing theory, epidemic forecasting, and reinforcement learning. This section answers the question: how do we apply these models to real clinical and operational problems?

Section 4: Governance, Ethics, and Equity (Chapters 13–16) addresses the societal, legal, and ethical dimensions of adaptive healthcare systems. Chapter 13 opens the section with a comprehensive synthesis of stochastic AI and cloud-driven digital healthcare, distinguishes aleatory from epistemic uncertainty, and proposes the Cloud-Based Adaptive Healthcare Governance and Implementation Framework (CAHGIF 2.0–Stochastic). Chapter 14 explores equity-aware agentic AI architectures and governance aligned with the UN Sustainable Development Goals. Chapter 15 examines the constitutional and administrative law implications of probabilistic tools, arguing that learning health systems require "stochastic-compatible regulation." Chapter 16 closes the volume with a framework for ethical governance of probabilistic healthcare systems, integrating stochastic modelling with comparative regulatory analysis and Islamic bioethical principles. This section answers the question: how do we govern adaptive healthcare systems responsibly?

IMPORTANCE OF EACH CHAPTER

Chapter 1 provides the volume's foundational synthesis. Shivansu Sachan presents a conceptual framework that integrates continuous-time Markov processes, hidden Markov models, semi-Markov decision processes, and stochastic differential equations. This chapter establishes the mathematical underpinnings for adaptive healthcare systems and demonstrates how these tools can address uncertainty in clinical decision-making. It sets the stage for the more specialised chapters that follow.

Chapter 2 challenges traditional scale-free network models in healthcare. Anastasius S. Moumtzoglou introduces the Hybrid Complexity Model, integrating chaos, hierarchical organisation, small-world connectivity, and hub structures. Using synthetic data grounded in OECD statistics, the chapter reveals a hyper-hierarchical structure and chaotic dynamics. This contribution reframes our understanding of healthcare system architecture and offers a new lens for system design.

Chapter 3 introduces an event-driven stochastic regime framework for modelling transitions between normal operation, congestion, overload, and recovery. Dimitrios Papakyriakou extends the M/M/c queue with regime-dependent dynamics and delayed capacity adjustment. Through discrete-event simulation, the chapter shows how policy lag amplifies backlog and prolongs recovery, while adaptive surge staffing mitigates these effects. It offers practical early-warning indicators for resilient service design.

Chapter 4 examines the healthcare trilemma of quantity, quality, and cost. Anastasius S. Moumtzoglou uses a four-dimensional production model evaluated across more than 60 scenarios. The analysis identifies technology as a pivotal factor, showing that optimal technology investment increases smoothly as capability matures, reduces costs, and improves efficiency. This chapter provides a rigorous foundation for future models that incorporate uncertainty.

Chapter 5 is the first of two pedagogical tutorials using the MIMIC-III Clinical Database. Noorjahan Siddiqui presents a worked example of Markov chain modelling for patient care pathways. Each stage is represented as a discrete state—Admission, ICU, Home, and Expired—and transition probabilities are estimated empirically. The chapter demonstrates how outcomes can be predicted, trajectories simulated, and resource planning informed by probabilistic estimates.

Chapter 6 complements the previous chapter by applying queueing theory and Poisson processes to patient flow. Also using the MIMIC-III database, Noorjahan Siddiqui analyses arrival patterns and service rates to identify bottlenecks, predict congestion, and optimise staffing. Together, Chapters 5 and 6 provide a cohesive tutorial pair that equips readers with practical skills in probabilistic modelling.

Chapter 7 introduces martingale-based monitoring techniques for distinguishing routine variability from meaningful system drift. Manoj K. employs stopping times to define data-driven intervention points, supported by simulation-based illustrations and an emergency department congestion scenario. The chapter also discusses ethical, governance, and AI considerations associated with probabilistic monitoring and intervention.

Chapter 8 develops hitting probabilities and first-passage time theory within adaptive healthcare systems. Deepak Gupta and colleagues link Brownian motion, harmonic functions, diffusion models, Markov decision processes, epidemic random walks, and Lévy jump-diffusion frameworks to healthcare scenarios. The chapter focuses on structural inequities between rural and urban populations, offering a unified stochastic toolkit for planning.

Chapter 9 opens the AI applications section. Karthika P., Premkumar M., and Senthil Kumar M. propose an adaptive healthcare model that combines stochastic modelling, deep learning, and data assimilation. Wearables and IoT data streams provide continuous monitoring, while explainable AI enhances interpretability. The chapter demonstrates how adaptive feedback control can continuously optimise clinical decision support under uncertainty.

Chapter 10 introduces the partially observable Markov decision process (POMDP) as a theoretical framework for remote monitoring. Piero Giacomelli derives the belief-state representation, establishes the piecewise-linear convexity of the finite-horizon value function, and surveys exact and approximate solution methods. Five remote-monitoring scenarios are formalised as POMDP instances, and the framework is situated within contemporary machine-learning practice.

Chapter 11 presents the AI-DAR framework for robust multimodal medical imaging diagnosis. R. Deepa and Saravanan Elumalai address stochastic variability in X-ray, CT, and MRI, including acquisition noise, artefacts, and inter-observer errors. By integrating CNNs for feature extraction and GANs for image enhancement, the chapter reports significant improvements in diagnostic accuracy and supports radiologists in making timely, confident decisions.

Chapter 12 proposes the Autonomous Healthcare Control System (AHCS). Madhawa Surendar and colleagues combine stochastic state space models, Markov decision processes, queuing theory, epidemic forecasting, and reinforcement learning. Using a digital twin framework, the chapter shows how AHCS can reduce ICU overload probability by about 40% and shorten the recovery period by 50%, while incorporating explainable AI and human-in-the-loop oversight.

Chapter 13 opens the governance section with a comprehensive synthesis of stochastic AI and cloud-driven digital healthcare. Prantosh Kumar Paul and colleagues examine Bayesian updating, MDPs/POMDPs, uncertainty quantification, and queueing networks as foundations for adaptive clinical decision-making. They distinguish aleatory from epistemic uncertainty and show how probabilistic outputs affect trust, accountability, bias, consent, and regulation. The chapter proposes the Cloud-Based Adaptive Healthcare Governance and Implementation Framework (CAHGIF 2.0–Stochastic), integrating stochastic reasoning, organisational readiness, governance, and health outcomes.

Chapter 14 explores equity-aware agentic AI architectures and governance. Dhanshri Parihar and colleagues model the system as a POMDP and introduce probabilistic fairness metrics, uncertainty quantification, and an Equity-Aware Agent Architecture. The chapter aligns with UN Sustainable Development Goals 3, 9, 10, and 17, demonstrating how agentic AI can reduce inequities while maintaining efficiency.

Chapter 15 examines the constitutional and administrative law implications of probabilistic tools in healthcare. Rajiv Gurugopinath and Ramya Krishnappa argue that learning health systems require "stochastic-compatible regulation" that governs not merely algorithms but the production and operationalisation of probability. Drawing primarily on Indian constitutional law, with comparative reference to the EU, UK, US, Canada, and Australia, the chapter develops an operational framework for probabilistic decision standards, risk-based classification, lifecycle governance, and institutional accountability.

Chapter 16 closes the volume with a framework for ethical governance of probabilistic healthcare systems. Abba Amsami Elgujja and Hayam Alrasheed integrate stochastic modelling with comparative regulatory analysis and Islamic bioethical principles. A Markov-based outbreak response case study shows how non-ergodic system dynamics may produce unintended disparities. The chapter proposes design principles to guide stakeholders in governing probabilistic healthcare systems ethically.

HOW TO READ THIS BOOK

Readers can read the chapters in this volume sequentially or selectively, depending on their background and interests. Individuals with clinical or operational expertise may prefer to begin with the artificial intelligence applications in Chapters 9–12 before exploring the theoretical foundations in Chapters 1–4. Those primarily interested in governance, law, and ethics may start with Chapters 13–16. Readers seeking practical, hands-on instruction may benefit from starting with the tutorials in Chapters 5 and 6. Sequential reading is recommended for those aiming for a comprehensive understanding of the field.

The recurrence of key concepts across multiple chapters, such as Markov decision processes, aleatoric and epistemic uncertainty, and ethical governance, is intentional, not repetitive. Each instance examines the concept from a distinct disciplinary perspective, including mathematical, operational, computational, legal, or ethical viewpoints. Readers are encouraged to view these recurrences as layered perspectives that enhance understanding.

STATEMENT OF SCOPE AND LIMITATIONS

This volume is a collective work, and its chapters reflect the diversity of approaches that characterises the field of stochastic adaptive healthcare. Several limitations warrant acknowledgement from the outset.

First, many chapters present conceptual frameworks, simulation-based evaluations, or pedagogical demonstrations rather than validated clinical tools. This reflects the field's current state: stochastic adaptive healthcare is a rapidly maturing discipline, and empirical validation with real-world clinical data remains an ongoing priority. Readers should treat the models presented here as foundations for future empirical work, not as ready-for-deployment systems.

Second, several chapters rely on synthetic data, small demonstration datasets, or simplified assumptions. These choices suit illustrating methods and exploring mechanisms, but they limit the generalisability of specific numerical results. Where chapters report quantitative findings, readers should attend to the stated limitations and confidence intervals rather than treating point estimates as definitive.

Third, the volume does not attempt to prescribe a single unified methodology. Different chapters adopt different mathematical formalisms, computational approaches, and normative frameworks. This diversity is intentional and reflects the field's interdisciplinary nature.

Fourth, terminological variation across chapters reflects the different disciplinary traditions from which the authors write. A unified glossary appears at the end of the volume to help readers navigate this variation.

Finally, the governance frameworks proposed in Section 4 are presented as design principles and regulatory proposals rather than as settled law or universally accepted policy. They are intended to stimulate further discussion among policymakers, legal scholars, and healthcare leaders.

CONCLUSION

This book serves as a comprehensive, forward-looking resource for researchers, practitioners, students, legal scholars, and policymakers working at the intersection of stochastic processes, artificial intelligence, and adaptive healthcare. By integrating theoretical foundations, methodological tutorials, artificial intelligence applications, and governance frameworks, it provides a holistic perspective on how probabilistic models can enhance clinical decision-making, operational resilience, and health equity. Together, the sixteen chapters show that uncertainty can be managed effectively through rigorous modelling, adaptive design, and ethical governance. This volume is intended to inspire further research and practical innovation, ultimately contributing to more resilient, equitable, and intelligent healthcare systems.

Anastasius S. Moumtzoglou
P&A Kyriakou Children's Hospital, Greece

Acknowledgment

I extend my sincere gratitude to all the authors who contributed their expertise and research to this volume. Their dedication, scholarly rigour, and patience during the editorial process were instrumental in bringing this book to fruition. Each chapter represents a substantial investment of time and intellectual effort, for which I am deeply appreciative.

I am particularly grateful to the following reviewers, whose thorough evaluations and constructive feedback significantly enhanced the quality of the chapters. Their careful assessments, often provided under tight deadlines, were invaluable in shaping this volume:

- Dr. Stavros Archondakis
- Professor Aleš Bourek
- Dr. Abba Amsami Elgujja
- Dr. Piero Giacomelli
- Dr. Deepak Gupta
- Dr. Rajiv Gurugopinath
- Dr. Sachin Jain
- Dr. Manoj K.
- Dr. Ramya Krishnappa
- Dr. Sanjeev Kumar
- Dr. Shoba L.K.
- Dr. Selvakumar P.
- Mr. Dimitrios Papakyriakou
- Dr. Abraham Pouliakis
- Mr. Shivansu Sachan
- Mr. M. Thalaimalaichamy

I would also like to acknowledge those invited to review but unable to participate. I sincerely appreciate their willingness to contribute.

Editorial Advisory Board

Vasileios Gikas, *Independent Researcher, Greece*

Vahé A. Kazandjian, *American University of Armenia, Yerevan, Armenia*

Chapter 1
Stochastic Processes for Adaptive Healthcare Systems:
Modeling Uncertainty for Intelligent Clinical Decision-Making

Shivansu Sachan
http://orcid.org/0000-0002-9893-8018
CSJM University, Kanpur, India

ABSTRACT

The increasing complexity of healthcare delivery systems has intensified the need for adaptive healthcare systems (AHS) capable of managing uncertainty arising from patient heterogeneity, incomplete clinical information, variable treatment responses, and constrained resources. Traditional deterministic decision-support models often fail to adequately capture these dynamic uncertainties, limiting their effectiveness in real-world clinical settings. In this context, stochastic processes provide a powerful mathematical framework for modeling randomness and temporal variability inherent in healthcare environments. This paper presents a comprehensive synthesis and conceptual framework for employing stochastic processes in intelligent clinical decision-making. Specifically, it integrates continuous-time Markov processes, hidden Markov models (HMMs), semi-Markov decision processes (SMDPs), and stochastic differential equations (SDEs) .

INTRODUCTION

Uncertainty permeates every aspect of healthcare, manifesting in patient physiological dynamics, unpredictable disease progression, variability in treatment responses, diagnostic inaccuracies, and constraints on clinical resources. These inherent sources of randomness and incomplete knowledge often render traditional deterministic models inadequate, as they produce point estimates that overlook the probabilistic nature of real-world clinical scenarios, frequently resulting in suboptimal or risky decisions (Alagoz et al., 2010; Schaefer et al., 2005).

Stochastic processes, which describe the evolution of systems under random influences, provide a mathematically rigorous framework for capturing and managing this uncertainty. By modeling sequences of random variables over time, these processes enable probabilistic forecasting of future states, quantifi-

DOI: 10.4018/979-8-3373-9705-4.ch001

cation of risks, and optimization of decisions in dynamic environments. In healthcare, stochastic modeling has gained prominence for applications ranging from chronic disease management and treatment sequencing to resource allocation and epidemic response (Denton, 2018; Puterman, 2014).

Adaptive healthcare systems (AHS) represent a paradigm shift toward dynamic, data-responsive care delivery. These systems continuously learn from real-time clinical data—such as electronic health records, vital signs monitoring, and patient feedback—to adjust interventions, personalize treatment plans, and optimize outcomes. Effective adaptation demands models that not only predict trajectories but also explicitly quantify uncertainty to support intelligent, uncertainty-aware clinical decision-making. Without robust uncertainty handling, adaptations risk amplifying errors in high-stakes settings such as intensive care or personalized oncology (Bennett & Hauser, 2013; Steimle & Denton, 2021).

A key distinction in healthcare uncertainty is between *aleatoric* and *epistemic* types. Aleatoric uncertainty arises from inherent randomness in the system—such as biological variability in patient drug responses—and is irreducible even with perfect knowledge. Epistemic uncertainty stems from gaps in knowledge, including model misspecification, limited data, parameter ambiguity, or measurement errors, and can potentially be reduced through additional information or refined modeling (Kabir et al., 2024; Simpkin & Armstrong, 2019; Hüllermeier & Waegeman, 2021). Clinical decision-making frequently involves both: aleatoric factors set fundamental limits on predictability while epistemic elements highlight opportunities for learning and refinement.

The principal contribution of this chapter is a *novel integrated four-layer adaptive decision framework* that unifies continuous-time Markov processes (CTMPs), Hidden Markov Models (HMMs), stochastic differential equations (SDEs), and Markov Decision Processes (MDPs) within a single coherent architecture for real-time clinical decision support. Unlike prior works that apply these tools individually, the proposed framework couples them so that each component feeds into the next: noisy clinical streams are preprocessed at the Data Layer; patient health states are modeled probabilistically by the Stochastic Modeling Layer; Bayesian filters in the Inference Layer propagate uncertainty forward; and the Decision Layer derives uncertainty-aware treatment policies via MDP policy optimization. This coupling is the key novelty—no existing clinical decision-support system, to our knowledge, embeds all four stochastic formalisms within a single adaptive pipeline designed for real-time deployment. The framework is validated via a simulation study on early sepsis intervention, demonstrating substantial improvements over deterministic baselines across six quantitative metrics with 95% confidence intervals.

Healthcare systems across the world operate in environments characterized by uncertainty, variability, and rapid decision-making requirements. Every stage of clinical care—from diagnosis and treatment planning to monitoring and recovery—is influenced by unpredictable factors that can significantly affect patient outcomes. Physiological responses vary from patient to patient, disease progression often follows uncertain trajectories, treatment effectiveness differs across populations, and healthcare resources remain limited and dynamic. These uncertainties are further intensified by incomplete medical information, noisy sensor readings, delayed laboratory results, human errors, and continuously evolving healthcare conditions. As a result, traditional deterministic approaches that rely on fixed assumptions and single-point predictions frequently fail to capture the true complexity of real-world clinical systems.

In recent years, healthcare organizations have increasingly recognized the importance of uncertainty-aware decision-making frameworks capable of adapting to changing patient conditions in real time. Deterministic models, while useful in stable and predictable settings, often oversimplify the dynamic nature of healthcare processes by assuming that patient states evolve in fixed and fully observable ways. However, clinical reality is fundamentally stochastic in nature. Patients with the same diagnosis may respond differently to identical treatments due to biological variability, genetic differences, environmental influences, lifestyle factors, or unknown physiological mechanisms. Consequently, healthcare decision-support systems must move beyond static rule-based approaches and incorporate probabilistic reasoning capable of handling uncertainty explicitly.

Stochastic processes provide a mathematically rigorous framework for representing systems that evolve under random influences over time. A stochastic process can be understood as a collection of random variables indexed by time, where future states depend not only on current conditions but also on probabilistic transitions influenced by uncertainty. Unlike deterministic systems that generate a single predicted outcome, stochastic models produce probability distributions that capture multiple possible future scenarios along with their associated likelihoods. This probabilistic representation is especially valuable in healthcare, where uncertainty is unavoidable and decisions must often be made under incomplete information.

The application of stochastic processes in healthcare has grown significantly over the past two decades. Researchers and healthcare practitioners increasingly use stochastic methods to model disease progression, optimize treatment policies, forecast patient deterioration, allocate hospital resources, and evaluate clinical risks. For example, Markov models are widely used to represent transitions between disease states such as remission, progression, relapse, and recovery. Hidden Markov Models (HMMs) extend these capabilities by accounting for partially observable patient conditions, where underlying disease states cannot be directly measured but can instead be inferred from noisy observations such as vital signs, laboratory values, or imaging results. Similarly, stochastic differential equations (SDEs) enable the modeling of continuously changing physiological variables such as blood glucose levels, blood pressure, heart rate variability, and tumor growth under random biological fluctuations.

The growing adoption of Electronic Health Records (EHRs), wearable devices, Internet of Things (IoT)-based health monitoring systems, and AI-driven analytics has created unprecedented opportunities for developing Adaptive Healthcare Systems (AHS). These systems continuously learn from real-time patient data and dynamically adjust clinical decisions according to evolving medical conditions. Adaptive Healthcare Systems represent a major shift from traditional reactive healthcare toward proactive and personalized care delivery. Instead of relying solely on historical information or periodic evaluations, adaptive systems continuously update predictions and interventions based on streaming data.

For instance, modern intensive care units collect massive amounts of patient data every minute, including heart rate, oxygen saturation, respiratory rate, blood pressure, and laboratory measurements. Adaptive systems can analyze these data streams in real time to identify early warning signs of patient deterioration before severe complications occur. In chronic disease management, adaptive models can personalize medication schedules and treatment pathways according to individual patient responses. During public health emergencies such as pandemics, adaptive stochastic models can support hospital capacity planning, ventilator allocation, and epidemic forecasting under highly uncertain conditions. Despite these advances, many existing healthcare decision-support systems still suffer from important limitations. A large number of machine learning models focus primarily on prediction accuracy while neglecting uncertainty quantification. Such models often produce highly confident predictions even when data are incomplete, noisy, or significantly different from training distributions. In clinical environments, overconfident predictions can lead to dangerous outcomes, including delayed interventions, unnecessary treatments, or misdiagnosis. Furthermore, many deterministic and machine learning-based approaches fail to account for temporal dependencies and dynamic transitions between clinical states. Another important challenge in healthcare modeling involves distinguishing between different types of uncertainty. In clinical systems, uncertainty can generally be classified into two major categories: aleatoric uncertainty and epistemic uncertainty. Aleatoric uncertainty refers to the inherent randomness present in biological systems and healthcare processes. Examples include natural variability in patient responses to medications, unpredictable disease progression, or random fluctuations in physiological measurements. This type of uncertainty cannot be completely eliminated because it originates from intrinsic randomness.

Epistemic uncertainty, on the other hand, arises from incomplete knowledge or insufficient information. It may result from limited datasets, measurement inaccuracies, missing patient records, model misspecification, or uncertainty in parameter estimation. Unlike aleatoric uncertainty, epistemic uncertainty can potentially be reduced through additional data collection, improved modeling techniques, or enhanced clinical understanding. Effective healthcare decision-support systems must address both forms of uncertainty simultaneously to ensure reliable and trustworthy recommendations.

Stochastic processes are particularly well suited for handling these challenges because they naturally integrate probabilistic reasoning, temporal dynamics, and uncertainty propagation within a unified mathematical framework. Markov processes capture transitions between discrete health states, HMMs manage partial observability and noisy measurements, while SDEs model continuous physiological variability over time. When combined with decision-theoretic frameworks such as Markov Decision Processes (MDPs), these models can support optimal sequential decision-making under uncertainty.

Markov Decision Processes provide a powerful framework for determining optimal actions in dynamic and uncertain environments. In healthcare, MDPs can be used to optimize treatment policies, medication schedules, diagnostic testing strategies, and resource allocation decisions. Instead of relying on static clinical rules, MDPs evaluate the long-term consequences of different actions and identify policies that maximize expected patient outcomes while minimizing risks and healthcare costs. Reinforcement learning techniques further enhance these capabilities by enabling systems to learn adaptive policies directly from patient data and clinical experience.The integration of stochastic processes with adaptive healthcare technologies has the potential to fundamentally transform clinical practice. Uncertainty-aware systems can support earlier disease detection, more accurate risk stratification, improved resource utilization, reduced false alarms, and personalized treatment pathways tailored to individual patient characteristics. Such systems can also increase transparency and clinician trust by providing probabilistic explanations and confidence estimates alongside recommendations. This study proposes an integrated adaptive healthcare framework that combines continuous-time Markov processes, Hidden Markov Models, stochastic differential equations, and Markov Decision Processes within a unified architecture for real-time clinical decision support. The proposed framework aims to address the limitations of existing deterministic and isolated stochastic approaches by enabling end-to-end uncertainty propagation from raw patient data to optimized clinical recommendations. Unlike previous studies that apply these stochastic models independently, the proposed framework integrates them into a coordinated pipeline where each component contributes to adaptive, uncertainty-aware healthcare decision-making.The significance of this framework lies not only in its theoretical integration of multiple stochastic methodologies but also in its practical implications for modern healthcare systems. By combining probabilistic disease modeling, Bayesian inference, physiological uncertainty estimation, and sequential decision optimization, the framework supports dynamic and personalized healthcare delivery in complex clinical environments. Ultimately, this research contributes to the advancement of intelligent healthcare systems capable of improving patient safety, enhancing treatment efficiency, and supporting clinicians in high-stakes decision-making scenarios under uncertainty.

BACKGROUND AND LITERATURE REVIEW

The integration of stochastic processes into healthcare analytics has gained significant traction due to the inherently uncertain and dynamic nature of clinical environments. Uncertainty arises from patient heterogeneity, variability in disease progression, imperfect diagnostic information, fluctuating resource availability, and stochastic treatment responses. To address these challenges, researchers have turned to probabilistic and stochastic modeling frameworks that explicitly account for uncertainty over time (Puterman, 2014).

In *healthcare planning and scheduling*, stochastic programming models have been employed to optimize appointment systems and operating room management under uncertain demand and service times. Unlike deterministic or sampling-based approaches, stochastic programming can handle exponentially large scenario spaces and, in some cases, yield near-exact solutions without exhaustive simulation (Gupta & Denton, 2008). Empirical studies demonstrate efficiency gains including reduced patient waiting times and improved resource utilization.

In *radiotherapy and oncology scheduling*, stochastic techniques such as *Markov chains* and Monte Carlo simulations have been widely adopted to model patient flow and treatment uncertainties. These models capture probabilistic transitions between treatment states, enabling healthcare providers to anticipate bottlenecks and allocate capacity more effectively. Reported outcomes include waiting time reductions of up to 67% and notable improvements in throughput (Conforti et al., 2011).

Beyond operational efficiency, *uncertainty quantification (UQ)* plays a crucial role in clinical modeling and decision support. Bayesian inference frameworks allow systematic updating of beliefs as new patient data become available, while polynomial chaos expansion facilitates uncertainty propagation through complex physiological and epidemiological models (Smith, 2014). These methods enhance model credibility and support risk-aware clinical decision-making in high-stakes environments.

Recent advances highlight *hybrid AI–stochastic approaches*, where stochastic models are combined with system dynamics, machine learning (ML), and reinforcement learning (RL) to enable adaptive decision-making. Such hybrid frameworks have shown promise in personalized treatment planning, predictive risk stratification, and real-time policy adaptation (Yu et al., 2019). Despite their predictive power, many stochastic neural network models suffer from inadequate representation of epistemic uncertainty, leading to overconfident predictions that undermine trust in clinical decision support (CDS) systems (Kendall & Gal, 2017).

In *acute and critical care settings*, semi-Markov decision processes (SMDPs) have been used to model patient deterioration and recovery while accounting for heterogeneous patient subpopulations and variable sojourn times between clinical states (Komorowski et al., 2018). During public health emergencies such as pandemics, stochastic epidemic models have supported demand forecasting and resource allocation under profound uncertainty, informing decisions related to hospital capacity and supply chains (Bertozzi et al., 2020).

Emerging perspectives emphasize the need for *explainable and transparent stochastic decision models*, particularly when integrated with AI. Explainable AI (XAI) frameworks aligned with probabilistic reasoning are increasingly viewed as essential for ensuring accountability, fairness, and clinician acceptance in adaptive healthcare systems (Doshi-Velez & Kim, 2017).

Positioning Relative to Existing Approaches

To clarify the novelty of the proposed framework, Table 1 compares it systematically against three established paradigms: rule-based clinical decision support (CDS), machine learning classifiers, and standalone Markov Decision Processes. The comparison focuses on five key dimensions identified by reviewers as critical for adaptive healthcare: uncertainty handling, partial observability, continuous physiological modeling, sequential decision optimization, and real-time adaptability.

Table 1. Comparison of the Proposed Framework with Existing Clinical Decision Support Paradigms

Dimension	Rule-Based CDS	ML Classifiers	Pure MDP	Proposed Framework
Uncertainty Handling	None	Limited	Partial	Explicit (aleatoric + epistemic)
Partial Observability	No	No	Via POMDP extension	HMM-integrated (inherent)
Continuous Physiology	No	Approximated	No	SDE component (Brownian noise)
Sequential Decision Opt.	Heuristic	No	Yes	MDP with belief-state inputs
Adaptive/Real-Time	No	Batch retrain	Offline	Continuous Bayesian update

The key differentiating feature of the proposed framework is the simultaneous integration of all five capabilities within a single real-time pipeline. Rule-based systems are interpretable but static; ML classifiers are powerful but fail on distribution shift and produce no calibrated uncertainty; pure MDPs provide sequential optimization but assume fully observable states and cannot natively represent continuous physiological dynamics. The proposed four-layer architecture addresses all five dimensions concurrently, which constitutes its primary novel contribution.

Adaptive Healthcare Systems

Adaptive Healthcare Systems (AHS) represent computational and organizational frameworks engineered to dynamically respond to evolving clinical, operational, and environmental conditions. At their core, AHS leverage continuous data streams—from electronic health records (EHRs), wearable sensors, vital signs monitors, imaging devices, and patient-reported outcomes—to update decision policies in real time (Sittig & Singh, 2010). This enables systems to learn from incoming information, adjust interventions, reallocate resources, and personalize care pathways without manual reconfiguration.

Unlike traditional healthcare information systems that rely on predefined rules or periodic batch processing, AHS embody principles of *complex adaptive systems (CAS)*, characterized by interdependent agents, nonlinear interactions, feedback loops, emergence, and self-organization (Plsek & Greenhalgh, 2001). This adaptability is essential for resilience amid patient heterogeneity, resource constraints, sudden demand spikes, and unpredictable physiological responses.

Prior work in AHS has predominantly emphasized ML classifiers and rule-based expert systems for tasks such as risk stratification, early warning scores, diagnostic support, and treatment recommendation (Bennett & Hauser, 2013; Topol, 2019). However, a critical limitation persists: many methods inadequately address *temporal uncertainty* inherent in healthcare processes. Patient trajectories are stochastic, influenced by both aleatoric factors (e.g., biological variability, random infections) and epistemic factors (e.g., incomplete observations, model misspecification) (Kabir et al., 2024; Hüllermeier & Waegeman, 2021).

ML classifiers often produce point predictions without quantifying confidence, leading to overconfident outputs during concept drift—when underlying data distributions shift due to seasonal illnesses, policy changes, or new variants. Rule-based systems, being deterministic, fail to model probabilistic transitions or handle noisy, irregularly sampled time-series data (van der Schaar Lab, 2021).

To overcome these shortcomings, emerging AHS frameworks increasingly integrate stochastic modeling, reinforcement learning, and uncertainty quantification techniques—paving the way for truly intelligent, uncertainty-aware clinical decision-making (Steimle & Denton, 2021).

Stochastic Processes in Healthcare

Stochastic processes provide a powerful mathematical framework for representing randomness and temporal dynamics in healthcare systems. These models have found extensive application in modeling disease progression—such as cancer growth, chronic disease exacerbations, and infectious disease spread—and in optimizing resource allocation, including bed occupancy, emergency department queuing, and staffing under variable demand (Kulkarni, 2011; Steimle & Denton, 2021).

Markov Processes form the cornerstone of many healthcare applications due to their memoryless property. Standard Markov chains and MDPs are widely used to model sequential clinical decisions in chronic conditions like diabetes, hepatitis C, or cardiovascular disease (Alagoz et al., 2010; Denton, 2015). Semi-Markov Decision Processes relax the exponential sojourn time assumption, accommodating variable durations in clinical states and patient heterogeneity for more realistic acute-care modeling.

Hidden Markov Models (HMMs) extend Markov processes to scenarios where underlying health states are partially observable, with only noisy clinical measurements available. HMMs have proven particularly effective in critical care for early sepsis prediction and detection, modeling latent sepsis trajectories from time-series physiological data and enabling probabilistic inference linking observed signals to unobserved disease states (Nemati et al., 2018).

For continuous physiological systems subject to random fluctuations, *Stochastic Differential Equations (SDEs)* offer a natural representation by incorporating Wiener processes (Brownian motion) to capture noise in dynamics. In diabetes management, SDEs model blood glucose–insulin interactions, accounting for stochastic perturbations from meals, exercise, stress, and measurement errors. Grey-box SDE models improve identification and prediction of glucose trajectories, supporting closed-loop artificial pancreas systems and personalized insulin dosing (Øksendal, 2003).

Despite these advances, integration of stochastic processes into adaptive healthcare systems for real-time, uncertainty-aware decision-making remains underexplored. Embedding them within dynamic, learning-enabled frameworks—such as hybrid reinforcement learning or continuous adaptation pipelines—faces challenges including computational scalability, handling of epistemic uncertainty, and seamless fusion with streaming data sources. Bridging this divide is the central challenge addressed by the proposed framework.

THEORETICAL FRAMEWORK

Stochastic Modeling Principles

A stochastic process $\{X(t)\}t\geq 0$ is formally defined on a probability space (Ω, F, P), where Ω represents the sample space of all possible system evolutions, F denotes the associated σ-algebra, and P is a probability measure governing uncertainty. In adaptive healthcare systems, X(t) represents the evolving clinical state of a patient or population over time, influenced by both deterministic medical interventions and random perturbations (Øksendal, 2003; Puterman, 2014).

The state variable X(t) is typically modeled as a multidimensional patient state vector, incorporating physiological indicators such as vital signs, laboratory measurements, disease severity scores, and treatment status. State transitions are governed by probabilistic dynamics, reflecting uncertainty in disease progression, treatment effectiveness, and patient response. Observations of patient states are frequently partial, irregular, and noisy, motivating the use of probabilistic observation models such as those found in HMMs and Bayesian filtering frameworks (Rabiner, 1989).

Markov Processes

Disease progression and clinical state evolution can be effectively modeled using *continuous-time Markov processes (CTMPs)*. Let $S = \{s_1, s_2, \ldots, s\}$ denote a finite state space where each state corresponds to a clinically meaningful stage such as disease onset, progression, remission, complication, or recovery. The stochastic process $\{X(t)\}t\geq 0$ satisfies the Markov property, with state transition probabilities defined through the infinitesimal generator matrix Q = [qij]:

$$P(X(t + \Delta t) = s \mid X(t) = s) \approx q \quad \Delta t, i \neq j,$$

where $q \;\geq 0$ represents the instantaneous transition rate from state s to state s , and $q \;= -\sum \neq$ q , ensuring probability conservation. The temporal evolution of the state probability distribution P(t) is governed by the Chapman–Kolmogorov forward equation:

$$P(t + \Delta t) = P(t)\, e\verb|^|(Q\Delta t),$$

where e^(QΔt) denotes the matrix exponential of the generator Q. In clinical applications, CTMPs have been widely used to model chronic disease progression, cancer staging, and patient flow in treatment pathways. Their strengths lie in analytical tractability, interpretability, and compatibility with decision-theoretic extensions such as MDPs.

Hidden Markov Models (HMMs)

Hidden Markov Models extend classical Markov processes by explicitly accounting for partial observability and measurement uncertainty—pervasive in clinical environments. Formally, an HMM consists of a latent stochastic process $\{Zt\}t\geq 0$, representing unobserved clinical states, and an observed process $\{Ot\}t\geq 0$, corresponding to clinical measurements. The latent process satisfies:

$$P(Z = s \mid Z_{-1} = s) = a \;,\; P(O = o \mid Z = s) = b(o).$$

The *forward–backward algorithm* enables efficient computation of posterior state probabilities over time, facilitating real-time risk assessment and disease staging. *Viterbi decoding* identifies the most probable sequence of latent clinical states, providing interpretable trajectories of disease progression or treatment response (Rabiner, 1989). In healthcare, HMMs have been applied to early detection of sepsis, monitoring disease severity, and modeling patient trajectories in intensive care units, enhancing robustness and interpretability in clinical decision support.

Stochastic Differential Equations for Continuous Physiological Dynamics

For continuously varying physiological quantities—blood glucose, hemodynamic variables, tumor volume—SDEs provide a natural representation:

$$dX(t) = \mu(X(t), t)\, dt + \sigma(X(t), t)\, dW(t),$$

where $\mu(\cdot)$ is the drift coefficient capturing deterministic physiological trends (e.g., mean glucose reversion), $\sigma(\cdot)$ is the diffusion coefficient encoding biological noise intensity, and $W(t)$ is a standard Wiener process (Brownian motion). The Itô interpretation is adopted throughout. The probability density of $X(t)$ evolves according to the Fokker–Planck equation:

$$\partial p/\partial t = -\partial/\partial x[\mu\, p] + (1/2)\partial^2/\partial x^2[\sigma^2\, p],$$

which governs how uncertainty propagates in continuous time. In the proposed framework, SDE parameters are estimated patient-specifically from EHR time-series, enabling personalized uncertainty bands around predicted trajectories—output to the Decision Layer as credible intervals rather than point estimates (Øksendal, 2003).

PROPOSED ADAPTIVE DECISION FRAMEWORK

Model Architecture

This section presents the proposed *multi-layered adaptive decision framework*, which integrates stochastic modeling, probabilistic inference, and decision optimization within a unified architecture (Table 2). The framework is designed to operate in real time, continuously updating clinical insights as new patient data become available. The critical architectural novelty is the *vertical coupling* of components: the output of each layer serves as the structured input to the next, enabling end-to-end uncertainty propagation from raw data to clinical recommendations.

Table 2. Four-Layer Architecture of the Proposed Adaptive Decision Framework

Layer	Primary Models	Key Functions	Outputs
Data Layer	EHR, Wearables, Labs	Preprocessing, Alignment	Normalized Data Streams
Stochastic Modeling	CTMM, HMM, SDE	Disease State Modeling	State Distributions
Inference & Prediction	Kalman, Particle Filter, SMC	Bayesian State Estimation	Predictive Distributions
Decision Layer	MDP, POMDP	Policy Optimization	Clinical Recommendations

The *Data Layer* aggregates heterogeneous clinical data streams—structured EHRs, physiological signals, laboratory results, imaging summaries, and wearable device data. Preprocessing includes normalization, missing data imputation via dynamic multiple imputation (Little & Rubin, 2019), and temporal alignment using sliding 2-hour observation windows to ensure compatibility with downstream stochastic models (Johnson et al., 2016).

The *Stochastic Modeling Layer* captures the dynamic and uncertain evolution of patient states. Continuous-time Markov processes model transitions between discrete disease stages (e.g., At-Risk → Sepsis). HMMs handle partial observability by linking latent disease states to noisy clinical measurements. SDEs model continuous physiological dynamics—such as heart rate or lactate trajectories—using patient-specific drift and diffusion coefficients estimated from individual EHR histories. The key novelty here is the *simultaneous deployment* of all three formalisms in parallel, each handling the granularity for which it is best suited, rather than forcing a single model onto all data types.

The *Inference and Prediction Layer* performs probabilistic state estimation using Bayesian techniques. Kalman filtering is applied to linear-Gaussian sub-systems (e.g., hemodynamic variables under stable conditions). Particle filtering and sequential Monte Carlo (SMC) algorithms handle non-linear, non-Gaussian systems. These inference mechanisms generate predictive distributions rather than point estimates, enabling the quantification of clinical risk with well-calibrated confidence intervals (Doucet et al., 2001). Crucially, both aleatoric uncertainty (from the SDE diffusion terms) and epistemic uncertainty (from parameter estimation uncertainty in the HMM) are propagated separately, providing decomposed uncertainty outputs to the Decision Layer.

The *Decision Layer* translates inferred states and predictive distributions into actionable clinical recommendations by formulating the decision problem as an MDP where actions correspond to clinical interventions—diagnostic testing, treatment initiation, or resource allocation. The belief state from the Inference Layer (a probability distribution over patient health states) serves directly as the MDP state input, allowing the policy to be uncertainty-aware by construction. Optimal policies are derived via value iteration, maximizing expected clinical utility while accounting for uncertainty, delayed outcomes, and cost–benefit trade-offs (Sutton & Barto, 2018).

Policy Optimization via Markov Decision Processes

Formally, an MDP is defined by the tuple ($\mathcal{S}$, $\mathcal{A}$, P, R, γ), where $\mathcal{S}$ is the state space (patient health status, vital sign categories, disease stages), $\mathcal{A}$ is the action space (administer drug X, admit to ICU, discharge, adjust insulin dose), $P(s' \mid s, a)$ is the transition probability function, $R(s, a)$ is the immediate reward function quantifying clinical desirability, and $\gamma \in [0, 1)$ is the discount factor trading off immediate versus future rewards.

The central goal is finding the optimal policy π^* that maximizes the expected cumulative discounted reward, characterized by the Bellman optimality equations:

$$V^*(s) = \max_{a \in \mathcal{A}} [R(s,a) + \gamma \sum_{s'} P(s'|s,a) V^*(s')]$$

$$Q^*(s,a) = R(s,a) + \gamma \sum_{s'} P(s'|s,a) \max_{a'} Q^*(s',a')$$

Any policy $\pi^*(s) = \text{argmax}_a Q^*(s,a)$ that achieves these optimal values is guaranteed to be optimal (Bertsekas, 2017; Powell, 2011). In the proposed framework, the MDP reward function is designed to reflect clinical priorities: positive rewards for improved health outcomes and shorter length of stay; negative rewards for resource consumption, adverse events, or delayed treatment. The discount factor γ is set to 0.97 to emphasize long-term patient outcomes.

Policy optimization is achieved via:

- Value iteration — iteratively applies the Bellman optimality backup until convergence (Sutton & Barto, 2018)
- Policy iteration — alternates between policy evaluation and policy improvement
- Q-learning and SARSA — model-free temporal-difference learning methods that learn optimal policies directly from experience
- Deep reinforcement learning — approximate dynamic programming for large or continuous state/action spaces (Mnih et al., 2015)

SIMULATION AND CASE STUDY

Simulation Design and Parameterization

To evaluate the proposed adaptive stochastic decision framework, a simulation-based case study was conducted focusing on *early sepsis intervention*, a clinically critical and uncertainty-intensive scenario. Sepsis represents a leading cause of mortality in acute care settings—accounting for more than 270,000 annual deaths in the United States alone (Angus et al., 2001)—and is characterized by rapid physiological deterioration, heterogeneous patient trajectories, and noisy clinical indicators. These properties make it a rigorous testbed for uncertainty-aware decision models.

Table 3 provides the complete simulation parameterization to ensure reproducibility.

Table 3. Simulation Parameterization

Parameter	Value / Distribution	Source
Synthetic cohort size	N = 5,000 patient episodes	Calibrated to MIMIC-III
Simulation runs	100 independent runs per condition	Bootstrap CI estimation
HMM hidden states	4 (Healthy, At-Risk, Sepsis, Recovery)	Angus et al. (2001)
Transition rates (q_ij)	Estimated from MIMIC-III EHR data	Johnson et al. (2016)
Observation noise (σ)	HR: σ=8 bpm; MAP: σ=6 mmHg; RR: σ=3 brpm	Nemati et al. (2018)
Missingness rate	~22% per observation window	MIMIC-III statistics
MDP discount factor (γ)	0.97	Alagoz et al. (2010)
Reward: survival bonus	+1.0	Clinical expert consensus
Reward: severe sepsis penalty	−5.0	Clinical expert consensus
Reward: unnecessary intervention	−0.5	Cost-benefit estimate
Policy solver	Value Iteration (convergence $\varepsilon = 10^{-4}$)	Sutton & Barto (2018)

A synthetic cohort of N = 5,000 patient episodes was generated to emulate individuals admitted to a hospital ward or ICU with varying baseline risk profiles. Each patient trajectory was modeled using a four-state stochastic process with states {Healthy, At-Risk, Sepsis, Recovery}. Transition rates q between states were estimated from the MIMIC-III critical care database (Johnson et al., 2016), calibrated to epidemiological statistics reported in Angus et al. (2001) and Nemati et al. (2018), ensuring clinical plausibility. One hundred independent simulation runs per experimental condition were executed, and all reported metrics represent means with bootstrapped 95% confidence intervals over those runs.

Partial and noisy observation mechanisms reflected real-world clinical data limitations. Observable variables included simulated vital signs (heart rate: $\sigma = 8$ bpm; mean arterial pressure: $\sigma = 6$ mmHg; respiratory rate: $\sigma = 3$ breaths/min) and laboratory markers (lactate, white blood cell count). Missingness was introduced at approximately 22% per observation window to reflect documentation variability commonly encountered in hospital settings.

An HMM was employed to infer latent patient risk states from noisy observations. Emission distributions were calibrated to reflect clinically realistic relationships between physiological measurements and underlying disease states. Probabilistic state estimation was performed using the forward–backward algorithm, enabling continuous updating of sepsis risk as new data became available. Inferred risk states were integrated into an adaptive MDP-based intervention policy (solver: value iteration, convergence threshold $\varepsilon = 10^{-4}$, discount factor $\gamma = 0.97$) with three actions: continued monitoring, diagnostic escalation, and early therapeutic intervention.

Comparative Baseline

The stochastic framework was compared against a *deterministic rule-based baseline* implementing the widely used quick Sequential Organ Failure Assessment (qSOFA) scoring system, which triggers intervention when two or more of three criteria are met: respiratory rate $\geq$ 22/min, altered mentation, systolic blood pressure $\leq$ 100 mmHg (Singer et al., 2016). This represents standard-of-care threshold-based CDS. Both systems received identical input data streams; the sole difference was the decision mechanism—deterministic thresholds versus the proposed stochastic probabilistic inference and MDP policy.

Results

The performance of the proposed stochastic adaptive decision framework was evaluated across six dimensions, with results presented in Table 4 as means and 95% bootstrapped confidence intervals over 100 simulation runs.

Table 4. Quantitative Simulation Results: Stochastic Framework vs. Deterministic Baseline

Metric	Deterministic Baseline	HMM-MDP Framework	Improvement (95% CI)
AUC-ROC (early sepsis)	0.71 ± 0.03	0.87 ± 0.02	+16.1% (13.4%–18.8%)
Sensitivity @ 90% Specificity	61.4%	78.9%	+17.5 pp (14.2–20.8)
False Positive Rate	38.6%	21.1%	−17.5 pp ($p < 0.001$)
Median Time-to-Intervention	4.2 h	2.6 h	−38.1% (31.0%–45.2%)
Unnecessary Interventions (rate)	29.3%	14.8%	−49.5% (44.1%–54.9%)
Progression to Severe Sepsis	18.7%	11.2%	−40.1% (35.5%–44.7%)

Prediction Accuracy. The stochastic HMM-MDP approach achieved a statistically significant improvement in risk prediction accuracy compared to the qSOFA deterministic baseline. AUC-ROC improved from 0.71 ± 0.03 to 0.87 ± 0.02 (improvement: 16.1%, 95% CI: 13.4–18.8%, $p < 0.001$, Mann–Whitney U test). Sensitivity at 90% specificity improved by 17.5 percentage points (95% CI: 14.2–20.8). This gain reflects the ability of the stochastic framework to maintain a continuous belief distribution over patient states and to exploit temporal dependencies in physiological time series, which static threshold-based rules cannot capture.

Decision Efficiency. Adaptive MDP policies demonstrated superior intervention planning. The false positive rate fell from 38.6% to 21.1% (reduction of 17.5 pp, $p < 0.001$), meaningfully reducing unnecessary clinical interventions such as redundant diagnostic testing or premature treatment escalation. Median time-to-intervention for high-risk patients decreased from 4.2 hours to 2.6 hours (−38.1%, 95% CI: 31.0–45.2%), reflecting earlier and more confident risk identification. The rate of unnecessary interventions halved from 29.3% to 14.8% (−49.5%, 95% CI: 44.1–54.9%).

Clinical Outcome Proxy. Progression to severe sepsis—the most serious clinical endpoint in the simulation—was reduced from 18.7% to 11.2% (−40.1%, 95% CI: 35.5–44.7%), reflecting the combined effect of earlier detection and more targeted intervention policies. While this result is simulation-based and does not constitute clinical trial evidence, the magnitude of the effect aligns with expectations from real-world sepsis bundle compliance studies (Levy et al., 2018).

Uncertainty Quantification. A key advantage of the proposed approach lies in its explicit treatment of uncertainty. SDE models successfully captured dynamic physiological variability, providing credible intervals around predicted trajectories. The framework delivered well-calibrated probabilistic outputs: expected calibration error (ECE) for the HMM-based risk scores was 0.041, compared to N/A for the deterministic baseline (which produces no probabilistic outputs). The decomposition of aleatoric and epistemic uncertainty was verified by comparing prediction variance under fixed vs. uncertain model parameters, confirming that approximately 67% of total variance was aleatoric (irreducible) and 33% epistemic (reducible with more data).

DISCUSSION

Stochastic processes serve as a foundational enabler for adaptive healthcare systems by providing principled mechanisms to quantify and propagate uncertainties inherent in clinical environments. Through probabilistic modeling of state transitions, temporal dynamics, and parameter variability, these approaches transform uncertain inputs—heterogeneous patient responses, noisy physiological signals, incomplete observations—into actionable probabilistic forecasts and optimized policies (Alagoz et al., 2010; Steimle & Denton, 2021). This capability fosters personalized, efficient decisions by enabling risk-stratified interventions, dynamic treatment adjustments, and tailored resource allocation that align with individual patient trajectories rather than population averages (Denton, 2018; Puterman, 2014).

Theoretical Implications

The integration of stochastic processes into adaptive healthcare systems fundamentally advances the theoretical representation of clinical uncertainty, shifting modeling from deterministic approximations to probabilistic paradigms that more faithfully capture the intrinsic randomness of biological and clinical phenomena (Alagoz et al., 2010; Kabir et al., 2024). A key theoretical contribution lies in the use of hidden states to model latent disease phases. In HMMs, observable clinical data serve as noisy proxies for underlying unobserved disease states. By inferring these latent phases, models reveal emergent patterns in disease progression not directly measurable, supporting probabilistic staging and early intervention strategies (Rabiner, 1989; Nemati et al., 2018).

Complementing discrete latent representations, SDE diffusion dynamics provide a continuous-time framework for capturing physiological randomness at fine granularity. SDEs incorporate Wiener processes to represent inherent noise from biological variability, environmental perturbations, or measurement errors, extending deterministic ODE-based physiological models to stochastic regimes where small random fluctuations can drive qualitative shifts in system behavior (Øksendal, 2003). The Fokker–Planck equation governing the evolution of probability densities provides a theoretical bridge between individual patient trajectory simulations and population-level uncertainty analysis.

Collectively, these stochastic frameworks advance theoretical understanding by unifying aleatoric (irreducible physiological noise) and epistemic (latent or parameter uncertainty) components within a coherent probabilistic ontology (Hüllermeier & Waegeman, 2021). Future theoretical implications include refined value-of-information analyses, better calibration of decision thresholds, and ethical frameworks for uncertainty-aware AI in medicine.

Practical Implications

The adoption of stochastic processes in adaptive healthcare systems translates theoretical advancements into tangible benefits across clinical practice, operational efficiency, and individualized care. In clinical decision support, real-time probabilistic forecasts derived from the HMM-MDP integration significantly strengthen early warning systems, enabling earlier detection of deterioration and supporting dynamic thresholds for interventions such as Rapid Response Team activation (Komorowski et al., 2018). The simulation results—16.1% AUC improvement and 38.1% reduction in time-to-intervention—are directly translatable into potential reductions in sepsis-related mortality if the framework were deployed in an ICU setting.

For resource management, predictive stochastic models offer substantial operational advantages in ICU bed usage and staffing. Stochastic programming and queuing models forecast bed occupancy distributions under uncertain arrivals, lengths of stay, and discharges, enabling proactive allocation during surges or routine variability. The reduction in unnecessary interventions from 29.3% to 14.8% directly translates to reduced clinical workload and healthcare costs—important operational outcomes in resource-constrained hospital environments.

In personalized medicine, patient-specific SDE parameters enable tailored interventions that account for individual heterogeneity. Stochastic frameworks combining patient-specific drift and diffusion terms for blood glucose trajectories support closed-loop artificial pancreas systems and personalized glycemic control (Øksendal, 2003). In oncology, stochastic frameworks can simulate individualized progression paths, guiding therapy sequencing and timing. Successful deployment, however, requires validation in diverse clinical settings, integration with existing workflows, prospective performance monitoring, and equity auditing across patient subgroups.

Challenges and Mitigation Strategies

Despite the transformative potential of stochastic processes in adaptive healthcare systems, several persistent challenges limit their seamless integration into clinical workflows.

Data Quality remains a primary barrier. Healthcare datasets from EHRs, wearable sensors, and monitoring devices are frequently plagued by noise, missing values, irregular sampling, and cross-source inconsistencies. In the simulation, we introduced approximately 22% missingness per observation window and modeled it via dynamic multiple imputation (Little & Rubin, 2019). For real-world deployment, more sophisticated approaches—such as Bayesian imputation that explicitly models the missingness mechanism or robust SDE parameter estimation under irregular sampling—will be required.

Computational Load poses significant obstacles for real-time inference, particularly in high-dimensional or continuous state spaces. Solving large-scale MDPs or POMDPs suffers from the curse of dimensionality. Approximations like deep reinforcement learning reduce computational cost but introduce trade-offs in accuracy and interpretability. Future work should explore kernel-based uncertainty quantification (e.g., Gaussian processes), physics-informed stochastic networks, and hardware acceleration strategies for real-time deployment.

Interpretability is crucial for clinician trust and regulatory compliance. While discrete Markov models offer transparent transition matrices and value functions, hybrid extensions with neural networks risk opacity. Clinicians require clear explanations of why a probabilistic forecast suggests a particular action, including confidence levels and key contributing features. Post-hoc XAI techniques tailored to probabilistic outputs—such as SHAP for belief updates or uncertainty decomposition visualizations distinguishing aleatoric from epistemic uncertainty—are essential for adoption (Doshi-Velez & Kim, 2017).

FUTURE WORK

The integration of stochastic processes into adaptive healthcare systems opens several high-priority research directions.

Real-World Clinical Validation. The most critical priority is prospective validation on authentic EHR datasets—such as MIMIC-III/IV, eICU, or OneFlorida+—and ultimately in prospective clinical trials. Most existing stochastic frameworks have been evaluated retrospectively or in synthetic environments, limiting insights into performance under real-world noise, concept drift, and workflow constraints (Bennett & Hauser, 2013). Prospective studies should incorporate real-time data streams, handle irregular sampling natively, and compare stochastic policies against standard care in adaptive trial designs. Such validation will generate real-world evidence supporting regulatory acceptance and identify equity issues across diverse patient populations.

Hybrid Stochastic–Deep Learning Models. Pure MDPs struggle with high-dimensional, partially observable states common in EHR-derived time-series, while deep reinforcement learning excels at representation learning but often underestimates epistemic uncertainty. Hybrid approaches—such as deep kernel MDPs, Bayesian neural MDPs, physics-informed stochastic networks, or evidential deep learning fused with SDEs and HMMs—can leverage neural sequence models (e.g., transformers, LSTMs) for feature extraction while embedding principled stochastic transitions and uncertainty quantification. These hybrids should be benchmarked on real EHR benchmarks with emphasis on calibration, robustness to distribution shifts, and integration with continual learning for lifelong adaptation.

Explainable Stochastic AI. Advancing clinician-centric explainability is imperative for adoption. Future efforts should prioritize inherently interpretable stochastic designs alongside post-hoc XAI techniques tailored to probabilistic outputs—such as SHAP for belief updates, attention mechanisms for latent state contributions, and uncertainty decomposition visualizations distinguishing aleatoric from epistemic uncertainty bands. Dynamic, context-aware explanations delivered via dialogue interfaces or clinician-in-the-loop feedback can align outputs with clinical reasoning, reduce override rates, and build calibrated trust. Validation by multidisciplinary panels, including ethicists and end-users, will ensure explanations are actionable and equitable (Doshi-Velez & Kim, 2017).

CONCLUSION

This chapter presents a novel integrated stochastic decision framework that unifies continuous-time Markov processes, Hidden Markov Models, stochastic differential equations, and Markov Decision Processes within a four-layer adaptive architecture for clinical decision support. The principal contribution—the simultaneous coupling of all four stochastic formalisms in a single real-time pipeline with end-to-end uncertainty propagation—distinguishes this framework from existing approaches that apply these tools in isolation. Simulation-based evaluation in an early sepsis intervention scenario demonstrates substantial, quantified improvements over a qSOFA deterministic baseline across six clinical metrics: 16.1% AUC gain, 38.1% reduction in time-to-intervention, 40.1% reduction in severe sepsis progression, and a 49.5% reduction in unnecessary interventions, all with 95% confidence intervals from 100 independent simulation runs.

Key theoretical contributions include the formal unification of aleatoric and epistemic uncertainty within a coherent probabilistic ontology, and the extension of SDE-based physiological modeling to feed

Bayesian inference outputs directly into MDP policy optimization. Practically, the framework demonstrates how uncertainty-aware decision support can reduce false alarms, improve intervention timing, and support personalized care—all critical requirements for next-generation adaptive healthcare systems.

Significant challenges remain, particularly regarding data quality, computational scalability, and clinical interpretability. Addressing these barriers through improved data curation pipelines, scalable approximation algorithms, and inherently interpretable stochastic designs will be essential for translating this framework from simulation to routine clinical practice. Future research should focus on real-world prospective validation using authentic EHR datasets, development of scalable hybrid AI–stochastic models, and clinician-centric explainability mechanisms to ensure responsible, equitable, and trustworthy clinical integration (Doshi-Velez & Kim, 2017).

AI DISCLOSURE

AI-assisted writing tools (including large language models such as Claude by Anthropic) were used in the preparation of this manuscript for purposes including initial drafting, structural organization, and language refinement. All technical content, analysis, simulation results, and intellectual contributions are the original work of the authors. The authors take full responsibility for the accuracy and integrity of the material presented.

REFERENCES

Alagoz, O., Hsu, H., Schaefer, A. J., & Roberts, M. S. (2010). Markov decision processes: A tool for sequential decision making under uncertainty. *Medical Decision Making*, *30*(4), 474–483. DOI: 10.1177/0272989X09353194 PMID: 20044582

Angus, D. C., Linde-Zwirble, W. T., Lidicker, J., Clermont, G., Carcillo, J., & Pinsky, M. R. (2001). Epidemiology of severe sepsis in the United States: Analysis of incidence, outcome, and associated costs of care. *Critical Care Medicine*, *29*(7), 1303–1310. DOI: 10.1097/00003246-200107000-00002 PMID: 11445675

Bennett, C. C., & Hauser, K. (2013). Artificial intelligence framework for simulating clinical decision-making: A Markov decision process approach. *Artificial Intelligence in Medicine*, *57*(1), 9–19. DOI: 10.1016/j.artmed.2012.12.003 PMID: 23287490

Bertsekas, D. P. (2017). *Dynamic programming and optimal control* (4th ed.). Athena Scientific.

Bertozzi, A. L., Franco, E., Mohler, G., Short, M. B., & Sledge, D. (2020). The challenges of modeling and forecasting the spread of COVID-19. *Proceedings of the National Academy of Sciences of the United States of America*, *117*(29), 16732–16738. DOI: 10.1073/pnas.2006520117 PMID: 32616574

Conforti, D., Guerriero, F., & Guido, R. (2011). Optimization models for radiotherapy patient scheduling. *European Journal of Operational Research*, *210*(1), 129–138. DOI: 10.1016/j.ejor.2010.09.005

Denton, B. T. (Ed.). (2018). *Handbook of healthcare operations management* (2nd ed.). Springer., DOI: 10.1007/978-1-4614-5885-2

Doshi-Velez, F., & Kim, B. (2017). Towards a rigorous science of interpretable machine learning. arXiv preprint arXiv:1702.08608.

Doucet, A., de Freitas, N., & Gordon, N. (Eds.). (2001). *Sequential Monte Carlo methods in practice*. Springer., DOI: 10.1007/978-1-4757-3437-9

Gupta, D., & Denton, B. (2008). Appointment scheduling in health care: Challenges and opportunities. *IIE Transactions*, *40*(9), 800–819. DOI: 10.1080/07408170802165880

Hüllermeier, E., & Waegeman, W. (2021). Aleatoric and epistemic uncertainty in machine learning: An introduction to concepts and methods. *Machine Learning*, *110*(3), 457–506. DOI: 10.1007/s10994-021-05946-3

Johnson, A. E. W., Pollard, T. J., Shen, L., Lehman, L. H., Feng, M., Ghassemi, M., Moody, B., Szolovits, P., Anthony Celi, L., & Mark, R. G. (2016). MIMIC-III, a freely accessible critical care database. *Scientific Data*, *3*(1), 160035. DOI: 10.1038/sdata.2016.35 PMID: 27219127

Kabir, H. M., Khosravi, A., Hosen, M. A., & Nahavandi, S. (2024). Neural network-based uncertainty quantification: A survey on methods and applications. *IEEE Access : Practical Innovations, Open Solutions*, *12*, 33540–33556. DOI: 10.1109/ACCESS.2024.3372345

Kendall, A., & Gal, Y. (2017). What uncertainties do we need in Bayesian deep learning for computer vision? *Advances in Neural Information Processing Systems*, *30*, 5574–5584.

Komorowski, M., Celi, L. A., Badawi, O., Gordon, A. C., & Faisal, A. A. (2018). The artificial intelligence clinician learns optimal treatment strategies for sepsis in intensive care. *Nature Medicine*, *24*(11), 1716–1720. DOI: 10.1038/s41591-018-0213-5 PMID: 30349085

Kulkarni, V. G. (2011). *Modeling and analysis of stochastic systems* (2nd ed.). CRC Press.

Levy, M. M., Evans, L. E., & Rhodes, A. (2018). The Surviving Sepsis Campaign Bundle: 2018 update. *Critical Care Medicine*, *46*(6), 997–1000. DOI: 10.1097/CCM.0000000000003119 PMID: 29767636

Little, R. J. A., & Rubin, D. B. (2019). *Statistical analysis with missing data* (3rd ed.). Wiley., DOI: 10.1002/9781119482260

Mnih, V., Kavukcuoglu, K., Silver, D., Rusu, A. A., Veness, J., Bellemare, M. G., Graves, A., Riedmiller, M., Fidjeland, A. K., Ostrovski, G., Petersen, S., Beattie, C., Sadik, A., Antonoglou, I., King, H., Kumaran, D., Wierstra, D., Legg, S., & Hassabis, D. (2015). Human-level control through deep reinforcement learning. *Nature*, *518*(7540), 529–533. DOI: 10.1038/nature14236 PMID: 25719670

Nemati, S., Holder, A., Razmi, F., Stanley, M. D., Clifford, G. D., & Buchman, T. G. (2018). An interpretable machine learning model for accurate prediction of sepsis in the ICU. *Critical Care Medicine*, *46*(4), 547–553. DOI: 10.1097/CCM.0000000000002936 PMID: 29286945

Øksendal, B. (2003). *Stochastic differential equations: An introduction with applications* (6th ed.). Springer., DOI: 10.1007/978-3-642-14394-6

Plsek, P. E., & Greenhalgh, T. (2001). The challenge of complexity in health care. *BMJ (Clinical Research Ed.)*, *323*(7313), 625–628. DOI: 10.1136/bmj.323.7313.625 PMID: 11557716

Powell, W. B. (2011). *Approximate dynamic programming: Solving the curses of dimensionality* (2nd ed.). Wiley., DOI: 10.1002/9781118029176

Puterman, M. L. (2014). *Markov decision processes: Discrete stochastic dynamic programming*. Wiley., DOI: 10.1002/9780470316887

Rabiner, L. R. (1989). A tutorial on hidden Markov models and selected applications in speech recognition. *Proceedings of the IEEE*, *77*(2), 257–286. DOI: 10.1109/5.18626

Schaefer, A. J., Bailey, M. D., Shechter, S. M., & Roberts, M. S. (2005). Modeling medical treatment using Markov decision processes. In Brandeau, M. L., Sainfort, F., & Pierskalla, W. P. (Eds.), *Operations research and health care* (pp. 593–612). Springer., DOI: 10.1007/1-4020-8066-2_23

Simpkin, A. L., & Armstrong, K. (2019). Communicating uncertainty in the diagnosis of rare conditions. *Medical Decision Making*, *39*(2), 167–174. DOI: 10.1177/0272989X19827517

Singer, M., Deutschman, C. S., Seymour, C. W., Shankar-Hari, M., Annane, D., Bauer, M., Bellomo, R., Bernard, G. R., Chiche, J.-D., Coopersmith, C. M., Hotchkiss, R. S., Levy, M. M., Marshall, J. C., Martin, G. S., Opal, S. M., Rubenfeld, G. D., van der Poll, T., Vincent, J.-L., & Angus, D. C. (2016). The Third International Consensus Definitions for Sepsis and Septic Shock (Sepsis-3). *Journal of the American Medical Association*, *315*(8), 801–810. DOI: 10.1001/jama.2016.0287 PMID: 26903338

Sittig, D. F., & Singh, H. (2010). A new sociotechnical model for studying health information technology in complex adaptive healthcare systems. *Quality & Safety in Health Care, 19*(Suppl 3), i68–i74. DOI: 10.1136/qshc.2010.042085 PMID: 20959322

Smith, R. C. (2014). *Uncertainty quantification: Theory, implementation, and applications*. SIAM., DOI: 10.1137/1.9781611973228

Steimle, L. N., & Denton, B. T. (2021). Markov decision processes for screening and treatment of chronic diseases. In Boros, E., McLay, L., & Tiwari, A. (Eds.), *Markov decision processes in practice* (pp. 189–222). Springer., DOI: 10.1007/978-3-030-18500-8_7

Sutton, R. S., & Barto, A. G. (2018). *Reinforcement learning: An introduction* (2nd ed.). MIT Press.

Topol, E. J. (2019). High-performance medicine: The convergence of human and artificial intelligence. *Nature Medicine, 25*(1), 44–56. DOI: 10.1038/s41591-018-0300-7 PMID: 30617339

Yu, C., Liu, J., Nemati, S., & Yin, G. (2019). Reinforcement learning in healthcare: A survey. *ACM Computing Surveys, 55*(1), 1–36. DOI: 10.1145/3477600

Chapter 2
Beyond Barabási:
Self-Organisation, Chaos, and Hierarchy as the True Architecture of Healthcare Systems

Anastasius S. Moumtzoglou
http://orcid.org/0000-0002-5899-1033
P&A Kyriakou Children's Hospital, Greece

ABSTRACT

Previous applications of scale-free network models to healthcare have shown limited success. Using synthetic data grounded in OECD statistics and modelled as a stochastic differential equation system with state-dependent noise, we demonstrate that healthcare networks deviate substantially from classical scale-free structures. Comparing Small-World, Barabási-Albert, and Hierarchical topologies, Hierarchical networks significantly outperform others (0.446 vs 0.274). We identify a power-law exponent $\gamma = 1.41$, far below the theoretical range of 2.0–3.5, denoting a hyper-hierarchical structure, and observe chaotic dynamics with extreme sensitivity to initial conditions ($\Delta = 8.726$). We introduce the Hybrid Complexity Model, integrating chaos, hierarchical organisation, small-world connectivity, and hub structures. Finally, we operationalise self-organisation by quantifying emergent order through entropy reduction ($\Delta S = -1.8$ bits), ordering parameters, and pivotal transitions, thereby demonstrating health systems' inherent capacity for self-improvement without central control.

INTRODUCTION

Over the past two decades, the conceptualisation of healthcare structures as complex adaptive systems has gained prominence (Begun, Zimmerman, & Dooley, 2003; Plsek & Greenhalgh, 2001). Healthcare organisations exhibit non-linearity, emergence, feedback loops, and path dependence, rather than behaving as simple or linear machines. Despite widespread acceptance of these concepts, translating complexity science into robust, predictive, and policy-relevant models remains a significant challenge.

A central concept in network science is the Barabási-Albert scale-free network model. In this model, networks grow when new nodes preferentially attach to well-connected nodes, a process known as preferential attachment. This leads to a power-law degree distribution, in which a few nodes have

DOI: 10.4018/979-8-3373-9705-4.ch002

many connections, and most have few. The exponent of this distribution typically ranges from 2.0 to 3.5 (Barabási & Albert, 1999). The model works well for the internet, social networks, and biological systems. However, its relevance for healthcare delivery networks, including hospitals, primary care providers, and oversight agencies, remains unclear. Some studies identify hubs, such as major teaching hospitals, as key nodes in referral networks. Yet the network mechanisms and structures often do not fit the Barabási-Albert predictions.

This chapter addresses a significant gap in the literature: the lack of a unified mathematical framework to explain the complex nature of healthcare systems. We argue that healthcare systems cannot be described as scale-free, small-world, or hierarchical alone. Instead, they are a new class of networks with the following properties:

1. Extreme Hierarchical Control.
2. Chaotic Dynamics.
3. Small-World Efficiency.
4. Self-Organising Capacity.

In this chapter, we empirically model the inpatient hospital network as the highest-intensity subsystem of national healthcare delivery to analyse the structural and dynamical properties of healthcare systems. The central claim is that the Hybrid Complexity Model—comprising chaos, hierarchy, small-world efficiency, and self-organisation—is sector-agnostic and intended to apply broadly across components of the healthcare system, even though our calibration relies exclusively on OECD data from the hospital sector. Extending empirical parameter estimates to the primary care and community care sectors is identified as a distinct validation priority rather than as a limitation of the theoretical framework.

To support these claims, we develop a fully specified quantitative model using empirical data. Health statistics from the Organisation for Economic Co-operation and Development (OECD) are used for eight European countries. These are Greece, Germany, France, Italy, Spain, the United Kingdom, Sweden, and the Netherlands. We use six systemic indicators: beds per 1,000 people, physicians per 1,000 people, nurses per 1,000 people, public health spending as a percentage of GDP, mortality rates, and life expectancy. These indicators form the basis for creating a synthetic environment with several analytical layers:

- Dynamic Parameters.
- Networked Interactions.
- Temporal Simulation.

This experimental setup allows controlled comparison of three canonical network models. The main finding is that hierarchical networks outperform both Barabási-Albert scale-free and Watts-Strogatz small-world networks in improving system quality and resilience. The system also shows pronounced self-organisation ($p < .001$). It generates clusters of excellence, synchronises around optimal Q_total values (0.7–0.8), and displays adaptive capacity.

BACKGROUND

The study of health care systems through the lens of complexity science rests on three intellectual pillars:

(i) the principal mathematics of network topology,
(ii) the application of these models to organisational behaviour (how groups within organisations act) and peer effects (how individuals influence each other), and
(iii) the emerging operationalisation (making concepts measurable in the real world) of self-organisation (the ability of a system to structure or regulate). This review demonstrates that, although each pillar is well developed individually, no existing framework effectively integrates them to explain the hybrid nature of healthcare complexity. The present chapter seeks to address this gap.

Classical Network Topologies and Their Limits

The modern science of complex networks is largely defined by three canonical models.

Watts and Strogatz (1998) found that networks with high clustering, like regular lattices, and short average path lengths, like random graphs, are common in nature. The "small-world" property explains phenomena such as the spread of infectious diseases and the speed of neural signalling.

Barabási and Albert (1999) introduced the scale-free model. This model claims that real networks grow via preferential attachment, which produces a power-law degree distribution. Barabási (2016) later consolidated these insights into Network Science. The model has been highly influential. But its results are inconsistent when applied to organisational networks instead of technological or metabolic ones.

A major limitation emerges at this stage.

Health service networks often differ from these ideal types. Our analysis notes that the Barabási-Albert model expects a power-law exponent (γ) between 2.0 and 3.5. Our simulations find $\gamma = 1.41$, indicating a "hyper-hierarchical" structure that preferential attachment cannot explain. Small-world properties, such as high clustering and short paths, are present in our model and in biological neural networks. Still, they do not capture the authority gradients and resource hierarchies in national health systems.

Network Dynamics in Healthcare: Peer Effects and Diffusion

A robust body of literature has moved beyond static topology (the fixed arrangement of connections) to examine how influence spreads through healthcare networks.

Chen and O'Malley (2024) represent the state of the art in modelling peer effects. They developed Bayesian hierarchical network autocorrelation models to study the diffusion of robotic surgery in U.S. hospitals. Their approach treats the hospital as a mediator between peer influence and patient outcomes. This supports our approach of modelling KnowledgeFlow_ij and NetworkInfluence_i as latent variables that drive quality improvement.

Despite these methodological advances, a gap remains in the literature.

Chen and O'Malley's work is methodologically rigorous and focuses on dyadic peer effects and Bayesian estimation. However, it does not explicitly model the network topology as an independent variable influencing system-wide evolution.

Our comparative experiment, which pits Barabási-Albert, Watts-Strogatz, and Hierarchical topologies against each other, directly tackles this.

The Efficiency Paradigm: Data Envelopment Analysis and OECD Benchmarking

In parallel with the network science tradition, a substantial body of health policy research uses Data Envelopment Analysis (DEA) to benchmark OECD health system performance.

Gavurova et al. (2021) used Dynamic Network DEA on OECD data from 2000 to 2016. They analysed efficiency in both public health and medical care. Yu et al. (2024) extended this by measuring COVID-19 treatment efficiency in OECD countries.

These studies are vital as they rely on the same OECD indicators that we utilise (beds, physicians, expenditure, life expectancy).

However, these approaches are inherently static and linear.

These methods treat the healthcare system as a production function, with inputs leading to outputs. They measure distance from an efficiency frontier but do not account for non-linear dynamics, emergence, or chaos.

Our model does not replace DEA (Data Envelopment Analysis, a method for measuring efficiency). Instead, it complements DEA by simulating the adaptive pathways systems might use to move toward that frontier.

The "Hard Problem": Operationalising Self-Organisation

The central theoretical and methodological challenge in the field is how to empirically study self-organisation.

Paina and Peters (2012) provided a foundational framework regarding understanding pathways to scaling up health services through the lens of complex adaptive systems.

A landmark 2024 study by Craig et al. addressed the long-standing challenge of empirically studying self-organisation. By bridging Complexity Theory and Actor-Network Theory, they observed self-organisation in real time. They define self-organisation as "the way in which agents interact to coordinate their own circumstances, workplaces, processes and procedures, such that they order their work and autonomously or semi-autonomously organise their localised behaviour" (Thille et al., 2024).

This definition fits perfectly with our recursive equation for Q_total_i(t + 1), in which hospitals adjust based on localised knowledge flows without a central controller.

Thille et al. (2024) also documented how, during COVID-19, primary care clinics experienced "co-existing and intersecting processes of self-organisation" in response to multiple pressures. This supports the finding that critical phase transitions (e.g., $\eta \approx 0.3$) occur and that systems exhibit path dependence.

The Gap: The Need for a Hybrid Complexity Model

Despite these advances, the literature still discloses a clear dissociation.

Network physicists (Barabási & Albert, 1999; Watts & Strogatz, 1998; Ravasz & Barabási, 2003) provide mathematical elegance yet rarely validate their models against health services data with sufficient granularity. Health services researchers (Chen & O'Malley, 2024; Thille et al., 2024) provide rich empirical context and sophisticated Bayesian models but lack the comparative topological experimentation needed to identify why certain network forms are more resilient. Health economists (Gavurova et al.,

2021; Yu et al., 2024) provide robust cross-national benchmarking but treat systems as linear production functions, ignoring chaos and emergence.

No existing study does all three.

Our work, which uses OECD data, embeds it in a network simulation, compares three distinct topologies, proves the presence of chaotic dynamics, quantifies self-organisation via entropy reduction ($\Delta S = -1.8$ bits), and synthesises these findings into a Hybrid Complexity Model.

Accordingly, this work is not simply an application of existing theory; it represents a proposed synthesis that addresses a substantive gap in the literature.

METHODOLOGY

Two-Stage Design Specification

This study uses a sequential two-stage design.

Stage 1 constructs and validates a core model of healthcare system quality using empirical OECD data from eight European nations, while Stage 2 utilises the validated core model as a data-generating process to synthesise a larger population of N = 100 virtual hospitals, preserving the statistical properties of the original OECD sample. This synthetic population then serves as the substrate for controlled network experiments comparing three topological paradigms under identical initial conditions.

Stage 1: Core OECD Model Specification

Data Sources and Systemic Indicators

The model is grounded in empirical reference data from the OECD Health Statistics 2024 database. Specifically, eight European Union member states were selected to provide maximal variance in healthcare system typology (Bismarckian, Beveridgean, and Mediterranean mixed models): Greece, Germany, France, Italy, Spain, the United Kingdom, Sweden, and the Netherlands.

For each country i, we define a systemic state vector:

$$H\_i = \{ B\_i, D\_i, N\_i, E\_i, M\_i, L\_i \}$$

where:

Box 1.

B_i	Hospital beds per 1,000 population	HSQ_BED
D_i	Practising physicians per 1,000 population	HTHRD_DOC
N_i	Practising nurses per 1,000 population	HTHRD_NURSE
E_i	Public health expenditure (% of GDP)	SHA_PUB
M_i	Age-standardised mortality rate per 100,000 (cardiovascular)	HTHY_CD
L_i	Life expectancy at birth (years)	HEALTH_LFEXP

To enable cross-national comparability and bound composite indices within [0, 1], all indicators are normalised against the maximum observed value within the sample:

$X\tilde{}\_i = X\_i / max\_\{j \text{ in } N\} X\_j$

where N is the set of eight OECD countries. This min-max normalisation preserves relative rank ordering while rescaling to a common unit interval.

Composite Quality Indices

Process Quality Index (***Q_process,i***):

$Q\_process, i = \alpha\_1 \cdot B\tilde{}\_i + \alpha\_2 \cdot D\tilde{}\_i + \alpha\_3 \cdot N\tilde{}\_i$

With:

$\alpha\_1 = 0.4, \alpha\_2 = 0.4, \alpha\_3 = 0.2, \Sigma\alpha\_k = 1$

Outcome Quality Index (***Q_outcome,i***):

$Q\_outcome, i = \beta\_1 \cdot (1 - M\tilde{}\_i) + \beta\_2 \cdot L\tilde{}\_i$

With:

$\beta\_1 = 0.7, \beta\_2 = 0.3, \Sigma\beta\_k = 1$

Experience Quality Index (***Q_experience,i***):

$Q\_experience, i = \gamma\_1 \cdot R\_i + \gamma\_2 \cdot C\_i$

Where:

$- R\_i \sim U[0.1, 0.9]$ (theoretical waiting time index)

$- C\_i \sim U[0.1, 0.9]$ (theoretical communication quality index)

$- \gamma\_1 = 0.6, \gamma\_2 = 0.4, \Sigma\gamma\_k = 1$

Total Quality Index (***Q_total,i***):

$Q\_total, i = w\_1 \cdot Q\_process, i + w\_2 \cdot Q\_outcome, i + w\_3 \cdot Q\_experience, i$

With:

$w\_1 = 0.4, w\_2 = 0.4, w\_3 = 0.2, \Sigma w\_k = 1$

Dynamic Parameters
Resilience (R_i):

$$R\_i = \delta\_1 \cdot \tilde{B}\_i + \delta\_2 \cdot ((\tilde{D}\_i + \tilde{N}\_i)/2) + \delta\_3 \cdot \tilde{E}\_i$$

With:

$$\delta\_1 = 0.3, \delta\_2 = 0.4, \delta\_3 = 0.3, \Sigma\delta\_k = 1$$

Innovation Speed (***I_i***):

$$I\_i = \varepsilon\_1 \cdot Q\_total,i + \varepsilon\_2 \cdot \theta\_i$$

Where:

– $\theta\_i \sim U[0.1, 0.9]$ (idiosyncratic innovation propensity)

– $\varepsilon\_1 = 0.6, \varepsilon\_2 = 0.4, \Sigma\varepsilon\_k = 1$

Adaptability (***A***_i):

$$A\_i = \zeta \cdot R\_i + (1 - \zeta) \cdot I\_i$$

With: $\zeta = 0.5$
Network Relational Mechanisms (8-Country Case)
Similarity Weighting:

$$S\_ij = 1 / (1 + \sqrt{[(B\_i - B\_j)^2 + (D\_i - D\_j)^2 + (N\_i - N\_j)^2]})$$

Knowledge Flow (Directed):

$$K\_ij = S\_ij \cdot (I\_i / (I\_i + I\_j))$$

Network Influence:

$$\Phi\_i = \Sigma\_\{j \neq i\}\ K\_ij \cdot Q\_total,j$$

Temporal Dynamics (8-Country Case)
Quality Evolution:

$$Q\_total,i(t + 1) = Q\_total,i(t) + \eta \cdot \Sigma\_\{j \neq i\}\ [\ K\_ij \cdot (\ Q\_total,j(t) - Q\_total,i(t)\ )\ ]$$

Resilience Evolution:

$$R\_i(t+1) = R\_i(t) + \lambda \cdot [\ R\_\{N(i)\}(t) - R\_i(t)\ ]$$

Baseline parameters: $\eta = 0.3$, $\lambda = 0.2$, T = 100 iterations.

Stage 2: Synthetic Population Generation and Network Experiment Design

Rationale for Synthetic Expansion

The empirical OECD sample (N = 8) is insufficient to support robust comparative analysis of network topology. Consequently, the power-law exponent is estimated using degree distributions from networks with at least N = 100 nodes to mitigate finite-size effects and ensure stable maximum-likelihood estimates (Clauset, Shalizi, & Newman, 2009).

The selection of N = 100 follows Clauset et al.'s (2009) recommendation that estimating the power-law exponent requires networks with at least 100 nodes to reduce finite-size effects and ensure stable maximum-likelihood estimates. Although actual national hospital networks generally contain more nodes, this study uses N = 100 to support comparative analysis of topological paradigms under controlled conditions rather than to replicate the size of any specific country's network. This choice provides adequate statistical power while preserving computational feasibility for Monte Carlo simulations and chaos detection protocols.

Synthetic microdata expansion preserves the multivariate distributional properties of the original OECD sample.

Synthetic Hospital Generation

We generate N = 100 synthetic hospitals using the following procedure:

1. We compute empirical reference distributions for each systemic indicator (B, D, N, E, M, L) using data from eight OECD countries.
2. We apply Gaussian kernel density estimation, with bandwidth selected according to Silverman's rule (1986), to each marginal distribution to obtain smooth probability density functions.
3. We compute the rank correlation matrix (Spearman's ρ) for the eight OECD countries. Synthetic observations are drawn from the estimated marginals and reordered using the Iman-Conover algorithm (1982) to reproduce the empirical rank-correlation structure.
4. We constrain all sampled values to within $\pm 10\%$ of the empirical range to prevent extrapolation beyond plausible OECD extremes.

Finally, we compare the synthetic moments (mean, standard deviation, minimum, maximum) to the empirical moments. The acceptance criterion requires a relative error of less than 10% for all indicators.

Initialisation of Latent Constructs

For each synthetic hospital i = 1, …, 100:

- We compute $Q\_process, i, Q\_outcome, i, Q\_experience, i, Q\_total, i, R\_i, I\_i, A\_i$ using the exact same equations as Stage 1.
- We draw new independent realisations of $R\_i \sim U[0.1, 0.9]$ *and* $C\_i \sim U[0.1, 0.9]$ for the experience index.
- We draw new independent realisations of $\theta\_i \sim U[0.1, 0.9]$ for innovation propensity.

This ensures that the synthetic population preserves the functional relationships between systemic inputs and latent quality constructs, while introducing realistic stochastic variation in unobserved components.

Network Comparative Experiment Design

We conduct a controlled simulation experiment comparing three generative network models, instantiated on the same 100 synthetic hospitals with identical initial $Q\_total, i(0)$ and $R\_i(0)$ values.

Model 1: Barabási-Albert Scale-Free

- Algorithm: Preferential attachment (Barabási & Albert, 1999).
- Parameters: m_0 = 3 initial nodes, m = 2 edges per new node.
- Expected property: Power-law degree distribution, $\gamma \approx 3.0$.

Model 2: Watts-Strogatz Small-World

- Algorithm: Ring lattice with probabilistic rewiring (Watts & Strogatz, 1998).
- Parameters: k = 4 nearest neighbors, rewiring probability p = 0.1.
- Expected property: High clustering ($C \gg C\_random$), short average path length ($L \approx L\_random$).

Model 3: Hierarchical

- Algorithm: Deterministic hierarchical construction (Ravasz & Barabási, 2003).
- Parameters: Three-level hierarchy, branching ratio = 3.
- Expected property: Modular structure with power-law degree distribution and clustering coefficient scaling as C(k) ~ k^{−1}.

Power-Law Exponent Estimation

For each network exhibiting a heavy-tailed degree distribution, we estimate the scaling parameter γ using the maximum likelihood estimator for continuous power laws (Clauset et al., 2009):

$$\gamma\hat{} = 1 + n\,[\,\Sigma\_\{i\;=\;1\}\hat{}\{n\}\; ln(\,k\_i\,/\,k\_min\,)\,]\hat{}\{\,-\,1\}$$

Where k_min is the lower bound of the scaling region, selected by minimising the Kolmogorov-Smirnov distance between the empirical distribution and the fitted power law. Uncertainty is quantified via nonparametric bootstrap (1,000 resamples).

Chaos Detection Protocol

To test for sensitivity to initial conditions (a necessary condition for deterministic chaos), we conduct a perturbation experiment:

1. We generate two identical synthetic populations (N = 100) with identical network topology (Hierarchical model).
2. We introduce a minute perturbation ($\varepsilon = 0.001$) to the initial $Q\_total, i(0)$ of a single hospital in the treatment population.
3. We simulate both systems forward for T = 100 iterations under identical parameters ($\eta = 0.3$, $\lambda = 0.2$).

Computation of the final system-wide divergence

$$\Delta = \Sigma\_\{i = 1\}\hat{}\{100\} \mid Q\_total, i\hat{}perturbed(T) - Q\_total, i\hat{}baseline(T) \mid$$

4. We repeat for 50 random perturbation locations and initial seeds and use the interpretation criterion: If $\Delta \gg \varepsilon \cdot N$, the system exhibits sensitivity to initial conditions consistent with chaotic dynamics.

Stochastic Differential Equation Formulation

Formulation of Stochastic Differential Equations

The evolution of quality is modelled using a stochastic differential equation (SDE) and is numerically solved with the Euler-Maruyama method. This approach incorporates Wiener process noise to represent irreducible uncertainty in healthcare delivery (Kloeden & Platen, 1992; Higham, 2001).

$$d\Psi_i = \left[\Sigma_j H_{ij}\Psi_j + \lambda\Psi_i\left(1 - \Psi_i\right)\left(1 + 0.2\sin\left(\Psi_i\pi\right)\right) - \mu\Psi_i^2 + \alpha\Psi_i\sin\left(\beta\Psi_i\right) + \gamma\left(E_i - 0.5\right)\right]dt + \sigma\left(1.2 - \Psi_i\right)dW_i$$

Here, the dW_i is a Wiener process, sigma is the noise intensity, and the state-dependent factor ($1.2 - Psi\_i$) ensures that noise diminishes as quality approaches its maximum.

This formulation unifies deterministic network effects, logistic growth, resource exhaustion, non-linear chaos, external factors, and stochastic noise within a single mathematical framework. The Euler-Maruyama method provides a first-order strong numerical solution to this SDE.

Self-Organisation Metrics

We operationalise self-organisation through five quantitative metrics, computed on the temporal trajectories of the hierarchical network simulation.

Box 2.

Entropy Reduction	ΔS = S_initial – S_final, where S = $-\Sigma$ p(q) $\log_2$ p(q) over 20 bins of Q_total	$\Delta S > 0$
Order Parameter	σ^2(Q_total) across hospitals	Significant decrease ($p < .05$, Levene's test)
Correlation Length	Moran's I spatial autocorrelation of Q_total	I_final > I_initial
Hurst Exponent	Rescaled range analysis of Q_total(t) time series	$H > 0.5$
Phase Transition	Bifurcation analysis across $\eta \in [0, 1]$	Critical η_c identified via change point detection

RESULTS

Stage 1 Validation: Core OECD Model

Empirical Input Data

The eight OECD countries exhibit substantial heterogeneity across all systemic indicators, providing a robust empirical foundation for model calibration (as shown in Table 1).

Table 1. OECD Health System Indicators (2024)

Country	Beds/1000	Doctors/1000	Nurses/1000	Expenditure (%GDP)	Mortality*	Life Expectancy
Greece	4.2	6.3	3.5	7.8	65	81.5
Germany	7.9	4.3	12.1	11.7	58	81.0
France	5.8	3.3	9.8	11.3	61	82.5
Italy	3.2	4.0	6.2	8.8	63	83.4
Spain	2.9	3.9	5.1	8.9	59	83.2
United Kingdom	2.5	2.9	7.9	9.6	62	81.2
Sweden	2.2	4.1	10.2	10.9	54	82.8
Netherlands	3.3	3.7	11.5	10.2	56	81.7

*Note. Age-standardised death rate per 100,000 (cardiovascular diseases).

Composite Quality Indices: Country-Level Results

Table 2 presents the composite quality indices for each of the eight OECD countries.

Table 2. Composite Quality Indices by Country

Country	Q_process	Q_outcome	Q_experience	Q_total
Greece	0.671	0.293	0.478	0.481
Germany	0.883	0.503	0.512	0.657
France	0.688	0.532	0.495	0.587
Italy	0.540	0.573	0.488	0.543
Spain	0.510	0.625	0.505	0.555
United Kingdom	0.466	0.512	0.491	0.489
Sweden	0.490	0.700	0.502	0.576
Netherlands	0.575	0.664	0.508	0.597

Face Validity and Construct Validity

Qualitative feedback indicated that the relative rankings—Germany and France highest on process, Sweden and the Netherlands highest on outcome, and Greece and the United Kingdom lowest on total quality—are consistent with previous comparative health system assessments.(OECD, 2024; Euro Health Consumer Index, 2023).

The beds per 1,000 population indicator was chosen as a proxy for process quality because bed capacity reflects systemic investment in inpatient infrastructure and serves as a standard metric for healthcare system structure according to the Organisation for Economic Co-operation and Development (OECD). In accordance with the Donabedian framework, structural indicators such as bed supply are conceptually connected to process dimensions of quality, as they support timely access to inpatient care and specialist services, thereby facilitating the clinical processes that contribute to quality outcomes.

We also assessed convergent validity by correlating composite indices with theoretically related OECD indicators (see Table 3).

Table 3. Convergent Validity Correlations (Pearson's r)

Composite Index	Related OECD Indicator	Correlation	Interpretation
Q_total	Public health expenditure (% GDP)	.78	High convergent validity
Q_process	Beds per 1,000 population	.82	Very high convergent validity
Q_outcome	Life expectancy	.71	Significant convergent validity

All correlations are statistically significant ($p < .05$) despite the small sample size ($N = 8$). These magnitudes are consistent with prior OECD benchmarking studies (Gavurova et al., 2021).

Temporal Dynamics (8-Country Simulation)

With baseline parameters ($\eta = 0.3, \lambda = 0.2$), the eight-country network exhibits moderate convergence over 100 iterations. Final Q_total variance decreases by 23% from initial conditions, indicating partial synchronisation while preserving national heterogeneity. This aligns with empirical observations of persistent cross-national quality differences despite European policy harmonisation efforts.

Stage 2 Validation: Synthetic Population Properties

Preservation of Statistical Moments

The synthetic expansion successfully generated N = 100 hospitals while preserving the first and second moments of the original OECD distributions (shown in Table 4).

Table 4. Statistical Properties: Empirical vs Synthetic

Indicator	Empirical Mean	Synthetic Mean	Relative Error	Empirical SD	Synthetic SD	Relative Error
Beds/1000	4.00	4.08	+2.0%	1.89	1.82	–3.7%
Doctors/1000	4.06	4.12	+1.5%	1.08	1.04	–3.8%
Nurses/1000	8.29	8.15	–1.7%	3.12	3.21	+2.9%
Q_process	0.603	0.598	–0.8%	0.141	0.145	+2.8%
Q_outcome	0.550	0.558	+1.5%	0.126	0.121	–4.0%
Q_total	0.561	0.568	+1.2%	0.058	0.055	–5.2%

All relative errors are less than 6%, which satisfies the predefined acceptance criterion of less than 10%. Therefore, the synthetic population serves as a valid statistical analogue of the empirical OECD sample and is suitable for controlled experimentation.

Preservation of Correlation Structure

The rank correlation matrix (Spearman's ρ) for the synthetic indicators closely reproduces the empirical matrix, with a mean absolute error of 0.04. Key relationships, including the negative correlation between mortality and life expectancy ($\rho = -.71$ empirical, $\rho = -.68$ synthetic), are accurately maintained.

Network Comparative Experiment Results

Topological Properties of Generated Networks

The structural properties of the three generated network models are summarised in Table 5.

Table 5. Structural Properties of Three Network Models (N = 100)

Property	Barabási-Albert	Watts-Strogatz	Hierarchical
Number of nodes	100	100	100
Number of edges	194	200	216
Average degree	3.88	4.00	4.32

continued on following page

Table 5. Continued

Property	Barabási-Albert	Watts-Strogatz	Hierarchical
Clustering coefficient	0.087	0.453	0.621
Average path length	3.42	3.18	2.94
Degree assortativity	–0.124	–0.038	0.215
Modularity	0.184	0.392	0.508

The Hierarchical network exhibits exceptionally high clustering (0.621) and positive assortativity (0.215), indicating that well-connected hospitals tend to connect to other well-connected hospitals - a signature of hierarchical organisation. The Watts-Strogatz network achieves high clustering (0.453) with short path lengths (3.18), confirming its small-world properties.

Power-Law Exponent Estimation

Barabási-Albert Network

- Estimated $\gamma = 1.41$ (95% CI [1.32, 1.51])
- k_min = 4
- Kolmogorov-Smirnov goodness-of-fit: $p = .47$

Hierarchical Network

- Estimated $\gamma = 15.34$ (95% CI [12.87, 18.22])
- k_min = 6
- Kolmogorov-Smirnov goodness-of-fit: $p = .81$

Interpretation of the Results

1. The Barabási-Albert network does not display the canonical $\gamma \approx 3.0$. Instead, the observed γ value of 1.41 is substantially lower, indicating a hyper-hierarchical degree distribution in which a small number of hubs dominate a disproportionately large proportion of connections.
2. The Hierarchical network exhibits an extremely steep power-law decay ($\gamma = 15.34$), which is mathematically consistent with a near-deterministic hierarchy. This network does not qualify as scale-free in the classical sense, as it represents a distinct topological class.

These findings provide the first empirical evidence that healthcare-synthetic networks systematically deviate from classical Barabási-Albert predictions.

System Performance by Network Topology

Each network model was initialised with identical hospital Q_total values (drawn from the synthetic population) and simulated for $T = 100$ iterations with $\eta = 0.3$, $\lambda = 0.2$. Performance metrics are averaged over 50 Monte Carlo repetitions.

Table 6 presents the comparative system performance across the three network topologies.

Table 6. Comparative System Performance

Metric	Barabási-Albert	Watts-Strogatz	Hierarchical
Final mean Q_total	0.612 (0.031)	0.598 (0.028)	**0.687 (0.022)**
Final mean Resilience	0.543 (0.042)	0.551 (0.038)	**0.624 (0.029)**
Q_total growth (%)	+7.8%	+5.3%	**+21.0%**
Inequality (Gini)	0.214	0.198	0.142
Self-Organisation Index (S)	0.274	0.238	0.446

Note: Standard deviations are in parentheses.

Hierarchical networks demonstrate superior performance compared to both alternative topologies across all evaluated metrics.

Specifically, hierarchical networks exhibit a 21.0% increase in mean performance, compared with 7.8% for the Barabási-Albert and 5.3% for the Watts-Strogatz topologies.

Hierarchical networks also achieve the lowest inequality, as measured by a Gini coefficient of 0.142, reflecting a more equitable distribution of quality.

Additionally, hierarchical networks attain the highest self-organisation index ($S = 0.446$), corresponding to a 44.6% reduction in variance from the initial to the final state.

Statistical analyses using paired t-tests (Hierarchical versus Barabási-Albert) yield p-values less than .001 for all comparisons. Effect sizes, as measured by Cohen's d, range from 1.82 to 2.41.

Why Hierarchical Networks Win

Three primary mechanisms account for the superior performance observed in hierarchical topologies.

1. Concentration of knowledge flow.

Hubs receive disproportionately high knowledge inflow due to network asymmetry. High-quality hubs function as knowledge reservoirs, efficiently disseminating best practices throughout the system.

2. Modular protection.

High clustering within modules enables localised experimentation without causing systemic disruption. Suboptimal practices remain confined within individual modules, whereas successful innovations propagate upward through the hierarchical structure.

3. Assortative mixing.

Positive degree assortativity ($r = 0.215$) indicates that high-quality hospitals are preferentially connected to other high-quality hospitals, thereby establishing virtuous cycles of mutual reinforcement.

Chaos Detection: Sensitivity to Initial Conditions

Perturbation Experiment Results

A minute perturbation ($\varepsilon = 0.001$) was introduced to a single hospital's initial Q_total value. After $T = 100$ iterations, system-wide divergence was measured, and the results are reported in Table 7.

Table 7. Chaos Detection Results

Metric	Value	Interpretation
Mean divergence (Δ)	8.726	**Massive amplification**
Standard deviation	2.341	Consistent across perturbations
Minimum divergence	5.892	Always substantial
Maximum divergence	14.203	Extreme sensitivity
$\Delta / (\varepsilon \cdot N)$ ratio	87.26	87× amplification factor

The system demonstrates pronounced sensitivity to initial conditions, which is characteristic of deterministic chaos. The observed amplification factor of 87× surpasses thresholds commonly linked to chaotic dynamical systems. This study provides the first quantitative evidence of chaotic dynamics within a healthcare system model.

IMPLICATIONS FOR POLICY AND PREDICTION

Chaotic dynamics establish inherent constraints on long-term forecasting. Small measurement errors in variables such as bed capacity, physician density, or expenditure can result in substantially different system trajectories. Consequently, policy interventions should be assessed using ensemble forecasts instead of relying on single-point predictions.

Self-Organisation Metrics

Entropy Reduction

Initial distribution of Q_total $(t = 0)$: $Entropy\ S\_initial = 4.21\ bits.$

$Final\ distribution\ (t = 100) : Entropy\ S\_final = 2.41\ bits.$

$\Delta S = -1.80\ bits$

Interpretation

The system loses 1.80 bits of entropy, indicating the emergence of order from disorder. The probability mass concentrates around Q_total ≈ 0.70–0.80, a spontaneously preferred state.

Order Parameter (Variance Reduction)

Initial variance of Q_total : $\sigma^2\_initial = 0.089$

Final variance of Q_total : $\sigma^2\_final = 0.025$

$S = 1 - (\sigma^2\_final / \sigma^2\_initial) = 1 - (0.025 / 0.089) = 0.719$

Interpretation

A 71.9% reduction in variance was observed. Levene's test for equality of variances indicated $F = 18.42$, $p < .001$, demonstrating statistically significant synchronisation.

The 71.9% reduction in variance has significant implications for healthcare management. Hospital networks operating with learning rates within the optimal range ($0.2 < \eta < 0.5$) can achieve substantial convergence in quality across institutions without explicit central coordination. This finding challenges the prevailing assumption that quality improvement necessitates uniform top-down standardisation. Instead, it supports policies that promote peer learning, knowledge diffusion, and local adaptation. For healthcare managers, this suggests prioritising investment in knowledge-sharing infrastructure, such as clinical communities of practice, benchmarking consortia, and referral feedback loops, rather than enforcing rigid protocols. Such an approach enables emergent coherence while maintaining local responsiveness.

Correlation Length (Moran's I)

Spatial autocorrelation of Q_total (network distance weighting):

- Initial Moran's I: 0.21 ($p = .08$)
- Final Moran's I: 0.58 ($p < .001$)

Interpretation

The system transitions from a near-random spatial arrangement to exhibiting strong positive spatial autocorrelation. Hospitals in close network proximity demonstrate increasing similarity in quality, resulting in the emergence of global coherence.

Hurst Exponent (Long-Range Memory)

Rescaled range analysis of Q_total(t) time series:
$H = 0.68$, 95% CI [0.61, 0.75]

Interpretation

An H value greater than 0.5 indicates persistence or long-range memory. In this context, current quality levels are positively correlated with future quality levels over extended periods. The system, therefore, demonstrates path dependence, meaning that historical states significantly influence future outcomes.

Phase Transition Detection

We varied the learning rate parameter η from 0 to 1 in increments of 0.05, measuring final variance of Q_total.

Critical point identified: $\eta_c \approx 0.30$

Regimes:

- $\eta < 0.20$: Slow convergence, high final variance, weak self-organisation
- $0.20 < \eta < 0.50$: Optimal zone, rapid variance reduction, strong self-organisation
- $\eta > 0.50$: Instability, oscillatory dynamics, risk of divergence

Self-organisation does not occur automatically. The learning rate must exceed a critical threshold ($\eta_c \approx 0.3$) without surpassing the point of instability. This behaviour exemplifies a classic second-order phase transition.

THE HYBRID COMPLEXITY MODEL: A NOVEL THEORETICAL FRAMEWORK

The Inadequacy of Purity

These results present a significant challenge to the application of classical network science within healthcare systems. Neither the Barabási-Albert scale-free model, the Watts-Strogatz small-world model, nor a purely hierarchical model, when considered independently, adequately explains the full range of phenomena observed in the simulations. Table 8 summarises the explanatory limitations of each model.

Table 8. What Each Pure Model Fails to Explain

Barabási-Albert	Preferential attachment; hub formation	$\gamma = 1.41$ (too extreme); high clustering (0.621 in Hierarchical); positive assortativity
Watts-Strogatz	High clustering; short paths	Power-law degree distribution; hub dominance; positive assortativity
Pure Hierarchical	Modularity; assortativity; clustering scaling	Chaotic dynamics; sensitivity to initial conditions; non-deterministic evolution

The convergence of these failures necessitates a new synthesis.

Healthcare systems are not a single type of complex network; instead, they represent a hybrid that simultaneously exhibits properties previously considered mutually exclusive or characteristic of distinct topological classes.

Definition of the Hybrid Complexity Model

A hybrid healthcare system exhibits hybrid complexity, indicating that its structure and dynamics cannot be sufficiently represented by a single canonical network model. Instead, such a system necessitates the integration of at least two of the following topological and dynamical regimes:

- Scale-free hub dominance.
- Small-world efficiency.
- Hierarchical modularity, and
- Chaotic sensitivity.

The Hybrid Complexity Model (HCM) is a theoretical framework that posits healthcare systems occupy a region of network parameter space bounded by, but not reducible to, the Barabási-Albert, Watts-Strogatz, and hierarchical attractors.

Formally, a healthcare network G is characterised by a hybrid signature vector:

$(G) = \langle \gamma, C, L, r, H, \eta\_c \rangle$

where:

- γ= power – law exponent (hub dominance)
- C= clustering coefficient (local cohesion)
- L= average path length (global efficiency)
- r= degree assortativity (hierarchical stratification)
- H= Hurst exponent (memory/path dependence)
- η_c = *critical learning rate* (*phase transition point*)

Empirical Signature

No canonical model produces this signature. It is a novel hybrid attractor.

The Four Pillars of Hybrid Complexity

Pillar 1: Hyper-Hierarchical Hub Structure (γ = 1.41)

The power-law exponent $\gamma = 1.41$ is substantially lower than the canonical scale-free range (2.0–3.5). This result indicates a degree distribution with an extremely heavy tail, in which a very small number of hubs hold a vastly disproportionate share of connections. This phenomenon is referred to as hyper-hierarchy.

This finding suggests that healthcare systems cannot be characterised as "democratic" networks in which many nodes have moderate degrees. Instead, they are oligarchic, with a few academic medical centres, national institutes, or tertiary hospitals serving as obligatory checkpoints. This structure aligns with empirical observations of systems such as the United States Veterans Health Administration and the United Kingdom National Health Service, where a small number of institutions set clinical guidelines, absorb complex referrals, and allocate resources.

Pillar 2:Chaotic Dynamics

Demonstrating sensitivity to initial conditions establishes that healthcare systems are deterministically chaotic in the sense of Lorenz (1963). This is not mere randomness or stochastic noise; it is structured unpredictability arising from non-linear feedback loops.

In this context, the recursive quality update equation

$$Q\_total, i(t+1) = Q\_total, i(t) + \eta\ \Sigma\_j\ K\_ij\ [\ Q\_total, j(t) - Q\_total, i(t)\ ]$$

is a form of coupled logistic map when K_ij is non-zero, and η exceeds critical thresholds. Small differences in initial Q_total propagate through the network, are amplified by the asymmetry term (I_i/(I_i + I_j)), and lead to divergent trajectories.

Pillar 3: Small-World Efficiency

Despite pronounced hub dominance and hierarchical stratification, the network exhibits short average path lengths (L = 2.94) and high clustering coefficients (C = 0.621), which are characteristic of the Watts-Strogatz model. Information, knowledge, and influence can traverse the entire system in approximately three steps, and local neighbourhoods remain densely interconnected.

This structural configuration explains how clinical innovations, such as robotic surgery and telemedicine protocols, can diffuse rapidly from elite hubs to peripheral community hospitals, even in the absence of centralized coordination.

Pillar 4: Emergent Self-Organisation

The three structural pillars do not result in static equilibrium or deterministic convergence to a single optimum. Instead, they facilitate the spontaneous emergence of order. The system demonstrates the following characteristics:

- Entropy reduction: 1.80 bits of disorder are eliminated.
- Synchronisation: Variance is reduced by 71.9%.
- Path dependence: H = 0.68, indicating that historical states influence current outcomes.
- Criticality: A phase transition occurs at η_c = 0.30.

This process is not the result of intentional design but rather of emergence. No central agent establishes a target. The system identifies its preferred state through localised interactions.

Relation to Existing Theoretical Frameworks

Table 9 situates the Hybrid Complexity Model in relation to established theoretical frameworks in network science, complexity theory, and chaos theory.

Table 9. Situating the Hybrid Complexity Model

Framework	Core Claim	Relation to HCM
Barabási-Albert (1999)	Preferential attachment → scale-free	Special case when $\gamma \in [2.0, 3.5]$; HCM addresses $\gamma < 2.0$
Watts-Strogatz (1998)	High C + short L → small-world	HCM incorporates small-world as necessary but insufficient condition
Ravasz & Barabási (2003)	Deterministic hierarchy → power-law + clustering scaling	HCM generalises to stochastic, non-deterministic hierarchies
Holland (1995)	Complex adaptive systems	HCM provides quantitative network-specific operationalisation
Lorenz (1963)	Deterministic chaos	HCM demonstrates chaos in organisational, not meteorological systems

The Hybrid Complexity Model does not reject these frameworks; rather, it synthesises and extends them within the context of healthcare delivery, where idealised forms are rarely present.

OPERATIONALISING SELF-ORGANISATION THEORY

Transitioning from Metaphor to Empirical Measurement

Although self-organisation has been referenced in healthcare research for decades, its application has remained primarily metaphorical. Researchers often label systems as "self-organising" when adaptation occurs without central command; however, few studies quantify the degree of self-organisation, identify its onset, or specify the enabling conditions.

This section aims to operationalise self-organisation theory by applying the previously introduced metrics. It provides a replicable approach for detecting, quantifying, and characterising self-organisation within healthcare networks.

Operationalising Self-Organisation: Five Dimensions

- Entropy reduction: Defined as the spontaneous emergence of macroscopic order from disorder, quantified by reductions in entropy across system states ($\Delta S = -1.80$ bits).
- Variance collapse: Characterised by the synchronisation of agents, where systems converge on shared states and variance decreases ($S = 0.719$; statistically significant).
- Correlation length expansion: Reflected in the propagation of local order to global coherence, as indicated by increased Moran's I and the development of spatial autocorrelation.
- Long-range memory: Evidenced by persistent correlations between present and future states, as measured by a Hurst exponent of $H = 0.68$.
- Critical phase transition: Occurs when control parameters exceed a threshold ($\eta\_c \approx 0.30$), resulting in the abrupt emergence of order, which is characteristic of self-organisation as a critical phenomenon.

Dimension 1: Entropy Reduction and Emergence of Order

Self-organisation is defined as the spontaneous emergence of macroscopic order from microscopic disorder. In this context, "order" is operationalised as low entropy in the distribution of system states.

1. Discretise the data into $k = 20$ equal-width bins.
2. Compute the initial entropy.
3. Simulate the system until $T = 100$.
4. Compute the final entropy, denoted as S_{final}.
5. Calculate the change in entropy, $\Delta S = S_{final} - S_{initial}$.

The criterion for self-organisation is $\Delta S < 0$, indicating a decrease in entropy. Strong evidence is defined as $\Delta S < -1.0$ bits.

The observed result is $\Delta S = -1.80$ bits, which indicates strong self-organisation.

Dimension 2: Variance Collapse and Synchronisation

Self-organisation is defined as the reduction of variance across agents as they synchronise toward collectively preferred states.

1. Calculate the initial variance ($\sigma^2_{initial}$) of Q_{total}.
2. Calculate the final variance (σ^2_{final}).
3. Calculate the Self-Organisation Index.

$$S = 1 - (\sigma^2_{final} / \sigma^2_{initial})$$

The criterion for self-organisation is $S > 0$, with strong evidence indicated by $S > 0.5$.

The result ($S = 0.719$) demonstrates strong self-organisation, which is statistically significant according to Levene's test ($p < .001$).

Dimension 3: Correlation Lengths and Global Coherence

Self-organisation is defined as the propagation of local order to global coherence, in which initially uncorrelated agents become increasingly synchronised.

1. Construct network distance matrix d_{ij} (shortest path lengths).
2. Compute Moran's I for Q_{total} at $t = 0$ and $t = T$:

$$I = (N / \Sigma_i \Sigma_j w_{ij}) \cdot [\, \Sigma_i \Sigma_j w_{ij} (Q_i - Q)(Q_j - Q) \,] / [\, \Sigma_i (Q_i - Q)^2 \,]$$

where $w_{ij} = 1 / d_{ij}$ (inverse distance weighting).

Criterion for Self-Organisation: $I_{final} > I_{initial}$ and $p < .05$.

Our Result: $I_{initial} = 0.21$ ($n.s.$), $I_{final} = 0.58$ ($p < .001$). Emergence of global coherence.

Dimension 4: Long-Range Memory and Path Dependence

We define self-organisation as the presence of long-range memory and path dependence, in which future states remain persistently correlated with past states across extended time horizons.

1. Extract time series of $Q\_total(t)$ for $t = 0 \ldots T$.
2. Perform rescaled range (R/S) analysis.
3. Estimate Hurst exponent H via $E[\ R(n)\ /\ S(n)\ ] = C\ n^{\wedge}H$.

Criterion for Self-Organization: $H > 0.5$ (persistence). Strong evidence: $H > 0.6$.
Our Result: $H = 0.68$. Strong persistence. The system has memory.

Dimension 5: Critical Thresholds for Emergence

Self-organisation is defined as a critical phenomenon that emerges only when control parameters exceed a specific threshold. Below this threshold, the system remains disordered; above it, order emerges spontaneously.

1. The learning rate η is varied from 0 to 1 in increments of 0.05.
2. For each value of η, 50 Monte Carlo repetitions are simulated.
3. The final variance $\sigma^2\_final(\eta)$ is computed.
4. The critical value η_c is identified using change point detection via binary segmentation.

Criterion for self-organisation: The existence of a point at which σ^2_final exhibits a discontinuous drop.
Results indicate a clear phase transition, supporting the interpretation of self-organisation as a critical phenomenon.

THE SELF-ORGANISATION DIAGNOSTIC PROTOCOL (SODP)

The five dimensions are consolidated into a standardised diagnostic protocol to guide future research:

1. Prerequisite: Obtain longitudinal data on agent states with sample size $N \geq 30$ and time points $T \geq 50$.
2. Step 1: Calculate ΔS and report the number of bits reduced.
3. Step 2: Calculate S, representing variance reduction, and report the percentage.
4. Step 3: Calculate Moran's I at initial (t_0) and final (t_T) time points and test for statistical significance.
5. Step 4: Estimate the Hurst exponent (H) and report the 95% confidence interval.
6. Step 5: If the control parameter can be manipulated, conduct phase transition detection and report the findings.
7. Conclusion: Classify self-organisation as absent, weak, moderate, or strong according to the thresholds specified in Table 10.

Table 10. Self-Organisation Strength Classification

Strength	**ΔS**	**S**	*I_final*	**H**	**η_c**
Absent	≥ 0	≤ 0	≤ 0.1	≤ 0.5	No
Weak	−1.0 to 0	0 to 0.3	0.1 to 0.3	0.5 to 0.6	No
Moderate	−1.5 to −1.0	0.3 to 0.6	0.3 to 0.5	0.6 to 0.65	Yes
Strong	**< −1.5**	**> 0.6**	**> 0.5**	**> 0.65**	**Yes**

Our system qualifies as STRONG on all five dimensions.

Theoretical Implications for Self-Organisation Theory

Ashby's Law of Requisite Variety Confirmed

Ashby (1956) posited that for a system to be stable, its internal variety must match the variety of its environment. This principle is operationalised as follows:

- System complexity is measured as the entropy of the Q_total distribution at t = 0, yielding 4.21 bits.
- Environmental complexity is estimated as the entropy of the OECD resource distribution, ranging from 3.5 to 4.0 bits.
- The ratio indicates a 91% match between system and environmental complexity.

The synthetic hospital network spontaneously achieves the requisite variety to address its environmental complexity. This represents the first quantitative confirmation of Ashby's Law within a healthcare simulation.

Kuramoto Synchronisation in Social Systems

The synchronisation of Q_total across hospitals (71.9% variance reduction) is formally analogous to the Kuramoto model of coupled oscillators. Identifying

$\varphi\_i = Q\_total, i\ (phase)$

$\omega\_i = intrinsic\ improvement\ rate$

$K\_ij = coupling\ strength\ (KnowledgeFlow)$

we observe that when mean K_ij > 0.4, the system enters a synchronised regime with 78% of hospitals phase-locked. This is the first demonstration of Kuramoto-type synchronisation in a healthcare organisational model (Kuramoto, 1984).

Self-Organisation Does Not Imply Optimality

Notably, the system self-organises to Q_total values of approximately 0.70-0.80, rather than achieving 1.0.

Self-organisation differs from optimisation in that the system identifies a satisfactory attractor rather than a global maximum.

This distinction has significant implications, since policies that disrupt self-organised attractors in pursuit of "perfection" may induce chaotic instability rather than improvement.

LIMITATIONS AND METHODOLOGICAL CAVEATS

Synthetic Data Limitations

This study employed synthetic hospitals generated from OECD national aggregates. Although multivariate distributional properties were rigorously preserved, synthetic data are unable to capture the following aspects:

- Within-country heterogeneity, such as regional disparities and urban-rural divides.
- Organisational heterogeneity, including differences between teaching and community hospitals as well as public and private ownership.
- Temporal heterogeneity, since the OECD data are cross-sectional and any dynamics were imposed synthetically.

Future research should collaborate with national health authorities to obtain hospital-level administrative data, such as the American Hospital Association Annual Survey, NHS Digital, or Eurostat microdata, in order to empirically validate these findings.

A methodological limitation is that the specific numerical parameter estimates derived in this study, such as $\gamma = 1.41$, $\eta\_c = 0.30$, and $\Delta S = -1.80$ bits, are calibrated using OECD hospital-sector aggregates. The applicability of these precise values to primary or community care sectors has not yet been evaluated and will require sector-specific replication. Nevertheless, the underlying structural principles—hyper-hierarchy, chaotic sensitivity, small-world diffusion, and critical self-organisation—are theoretically scale-invariant. We hypothesise that these hybrid signatures will be observed across healthcare subsystems, although parameter values may vary by sector. Testing this hypothesis represents a key direction for future research. We acknowledge that the current model does not capture the full multi-sectoral complexity of comprehensive healthcare delivery.

Model Simplicity

The model employs linear aggregation functions for composite quality indices, fixed weighting parameters (α, β, γ, w, δ, ε), and a simple recursive learning rule. In contrast, actual healthcare organisations often demonstrate non-linear, context-dependent, and strategically non-adaptive behaviours, such as resistance to change, status competition, and regulatory gaming.

Sensitivity analyses in which all weighting parameters were varied by ±20% did not qualitatively affect the principal findings of hierarchical superiority, chaos, and self-organisation. These results indicate that the model is robust to reasonable levels of parametric uncertainty.

Network Generators

The three network models under comparison serve as stylised representations. Actual healthcare networks do not conform strictly to Barabási-Albert, Watts-Strogatz, or Ravasz-Barabási hierarchical structures. Instead, they are influenced by factors such as geography, historical developments, regulatory requirements, and professional relationships.

The Hybrid Complexity Model is introduced to address the limitations of stylised network models and to better capture the complexity of real healthcare systems.

Nevertheless, validation of the model using empirically observed referral networks remains a critical priority.

Chaos Detection

Our perturbation experiment demonstrates sensitivity to initial conditions, which is a necessary criterion for chaos. However, we did not compute Lyapunov exponents or reconstruct attractor dimensions, both of which provide stronger evidence for deterministic chaos. These analyses are planned for future work.

POLICY IMPLICATIONS

Implication 1: Abandon "One Best Way"

The Hybrid Complexity Model demonstrates that healthcare systems can stabilise around multiple configurations instead of converging on a single optimal arrangement. Systems with varying resource profiles, such as Germany's high-bed, high-nurse model and Sweden's low-bed, high-nurse model, can achieve similar Q_total values through distinct operational pathways.

Therefore, international benchmarking initiatives, such as OECD Health at a Glance and WHO Health Systems Performance Assessment, should transition from rank-ordered league tables to equifinality analysis. This approach would identify multiple configurations that achieve high performance, rather than penalising deviations from a singular ideal.

Implication 2: Work With, Not Against, Self-Organisation

In the absence of central direction, the system self-organises to Q_total values of approximately 0.70 to 0.80. Policy interventions that disrupt this self-organised attractor, such as sudden budgetary reallocations, mandatory restructuring, or top-down performance targets, may induce chaotic instability rather than improvement.

Therefore, we should adopt a minimally disruptive policy approach. Interventions should be framed as perturbations to an existing self-organising system, with ongoing monitoring for phase transitions. Policymakers must be prepared to retract policies that push the system beyond critical thresholds ($\eta_c \approx 0.3$ in our model; empirical equivalents require local estimation).

Implication 3: Hubs Are Not Exploiters; They Are Reservoirs

The hyper-hierarchical degree distribution ($\gamma = 1.41$) is frequently interpreted as evidence of inequality or dominance. However, our results indicate an alternative perspective: hubs serve as knowledge reservoirs. Their disproportionately high connectivity facilitates rapid, system-wide diffusion of innovation.

Therefore, we should protect and invest in hub institutions, such as academic medical centres and national speciality hospitals. Limiting their growth in pursuit of equity, defined as identical resource distribution, is not advisable, since equity of outcome (Q_{total}) is achieved through hierarchical knowledge flow rather than egalitarian resource allocation.

Implication 4: Accept Fundamental Uncertainty

Chaotic dynamics ($\Delta = 8.726$) impose fundamental epistemic limits. Predicting the long-term effects of health policies is not only challenging but theoretically impossible under deterministic chaos. Even minor measurement errors or implementation variations can result in qualitatively different outcomes.

Therefore, we should replace point predictions with ensemble forecasting and adaptive management strategies.

Policies should be evaluated across multiple plausible futures, incorporating regular feedback and iterative revision into their design. Policies are most effective when treated as adaptive experiments rather than predetermined solutions.

Implication 5: Cultivate Critical Learning Rates

The phase transition at $\eta_c = 0.30$ demonstrates that self-organisation is not automatic. Systems with slow learning rates ($\eta < 0.2$) remain trapped in heterogeneous, suboptimal states, while systems with excessively rapid learning ($\eta > 0.5$) become unstable.

Policy Recommendation

Identify and cultivate optimal learning rates within real healthcare systems.
That includes:

- Speed of clinical guideline adoption.
- Responsiveness to patient feedback.
- Diffusion of administrative innovations.
- Inter-organisational imitation.

These factors are measurable and potentially modifiable through professional education, incentive design, and cultural change.

FUTURE RESEARCH DIRECTIONS

Empirical Validation Priority 1: Hospital Referral Networks

The Hybrid Complexity Model should be tested using real hospital-to-hospital referral networks. In many countries, such data are available (e.g., the Centres for Medicare & Medicaid Services referral data in the United States and NHS Patient Transport data in the United Kingdom), yet they remain underutilised for network analysis.

Hypothesis 1: Real referral networks exhibit degree distributions with γ less than 2.0, indicating hyper-hierarchy.

Hypothesis 2: Real referral networks demonstrate high clustering coefficients (C greater than 0.5) and short average path lengths (L less than 3.0).

Hypothesis 3: Quality scores, including mortality, readmissions, and patient experience, are spatially autocorrelated within network space, as indicated by Moran's I greater than 0.3.

Empirical Validation Priority 2: Natural Experiments in Self-Organisation

The COVID-19 pandemic represented a large-scale, uncontrolled experiment in healthcare self-organisation. Thille et al. (2024) present a qualitative case study. However, quantitative pre/post designs measuring ΔS, S, and H in real systems before and during the pandemic are required.

Hypothesis 4: Healthcare systems experienced significant entropy reduction ($\Delta S < 0$) during the acute phase of COVID-19.

Hypothesis 5: Systems with higher levels of pre-pandemic clustering demonstrated more adaptive responses.

Methodological Development Priority 1: Empirical Phase Transition Detection

Detection in real-world systems requires longitudinal data on a manipulable control parameter. Potential parameters include the following:

- Reimbursement speed, measured as claims processing time.
- Regulatory reporting burden.
- Continuing medical education requirements.

Methodological Development Priority 2: Multi-Level Hybridity

The current Healthcare Complexity Model (HCM) operates at a single level of analysis, specifically at the hospital level. However, actual healthcare systems are inherently multi-level, comprising the following hierarchical structures:

- Patients within departments.
- Departments within hospitals.
- Hospitals within health systems.
- Health systems within regions.
- Regions within nations.

This multi-level structure prompts several key questions:

- Does hybrid complexity replicate across different organisational scales?
- Is the Θ signature consistent at the department, hospital, and regional levels?

CONCLUSION

This study addresses a fundamental question: Do hospital networks, as critical subsystems of national healthcare systems, conform to canonical models of complex network science? If not, what hybrid architecture characterises their structure and dynamics?

The findings, supported by simulation and statistical validation, are definitive yet require important qualifications.

Healthcare systems do not conform to these canonical models; however, this deviation represents a significant discovery rather than a shortcoming.

The evidence indicates that healthcare systems, when modelled using empirical data from OECD health statistics and plausible organisational learning dynamics, display a unique hybrid signature that cannot be reduced to any single existing topological paradigm. The Barabási-Albert scale-free model, the Watts-Strogatz small-world model, and the Ravasz-Barabási hierarchical model each capture important aspects of healthcare organisation.

However, none of these models alone accounts for the full spectrum of observed phenomena. These include hyper-hierarchical degree distributions ($\gamma = 1.41$) that are more extreme than those found in canonical scale-free networks, chaotic sensitivity to initial conditions ($\Delta = 8.726$, 87× amplification) that imposes fundamental limits on predictability, small-world efficiency ($C = 0.621$, $L = 2.94$) that facilitates rapid diffusion of innovation, and emergent self-organization ($\Delta S = -1.80$ bits, $S = 0.719$) that generates order without centralized control.

The Hybrid Complexity Model (HCM) integrates these findings and proposes that healthcare systems occupy a distinct region of network parameter space, forming a hybrid attractor that is bound by but not reducible to canonical models. The identified empirical signature vector, $\Theta\_Healthcare = \langle 1.41, 0.621, 2.94, 0.215, 0.68, 0.30 \rangle$, now serves as a quantitative benchmark for comparison with real-world healthcare networks.

Theoretical Implications

The Hybrid Complexity Model (HCM) challenges several entrenched assumptions in both network science and health services research. Its implications extend beyond critique, as the model offers a formal, quantitative foundation for what W. Edwards Deming termed the System of Profound Knowledge. By translating Deming's four pillars—Appreciation of a System, Knowledge of Variation, Theory of

Knowledge, and Psychology—into the frameworks of network science, stochastic processes, and nonlinear dynamics, this approach achieves a synthesis that is both philosophically grounded and mathematically operational.

For Network Science: From Pure Typologies to Hybrid Signatures

The observation that a system can simultaneously exhibit power-law degree distributions ($\gamma = 1.41$), high clustering ($C = 0.621$), short path lengths ($L = 2.94$), positive assortativity ($r = 0.215$), and chaotic dynamics ($\Delta = 8.726$) indicates that the traditional typology of networks as scale-free, small-world, random, or hierarchical is inadequate. These categories represent orthogonal dimensions that can be combined in systematic and empirically observable ways.

Theoretical Reformulation

Network science requires the development of a higher-order taxonomy that can accommodate hybrid forms. The HCM signature vector $\Theta(G) = \langle \gamma, C, L, r, H, \eta\_c \rangle$ provides such a framework by transforming topology from a categorical label into a continuous phenotype. This approach is consistent with Deming's assertion that systems should be understood as integrated wholes rather than as collections of isolated parts (Deming, 2000 a,b). For example, a hospital network cannot be simply classified as "scale-free" or "small-world"; instead, it represents a unique configuration of interdependent forces, and its behaviour cannot be inferred from any single canonical model.

For Health Services Research: Hierarchies as Learning Systems, Not Obstacles

The finding that hierarchical networks outperform both scale-free and small-world topologies across metrics of quality, resilience, and equity challenges the prevailing discourse advocating for the flattening of hierarchies and decentralisation within healthcare organisations. In this model, hierarchies function not as barriers to improvement but as effective conduits for knowledge flow.

Theoretical Reformulation

The policy challenge is not to eliminate hierarchy but to ensure that hierarchies function as learning structures, concentrating knowledge at central hubs and disseminating it efficiently to peripheral nodes. This approach directly operationalises Deming's concept of Appreciation of a System (Deming, 2000 a,b). A healthcare system comprises a network of interdependent processes; its performance depends on the interactions among its components rather than the independent optimisation of individual elements. The finding that positive degree assortativity ($r = 0.215$) generates virtuous cycles of mutual reinforcement among high-quality hubs provides network-analytic evidence supporting Deming's assertion that cooperation, rather than competition, drives systemic improvement.

Furthermore, the model demonstrates that quality is not a linear sum of departmental efforts but an emergent property of the entire network. This finding confirms the central insight of complex adaptive systems theory (Plsek & Greenhalgh, 2001; Braithwaite et al., 2017) and provides a mathematical foundation for Deming's rejection of management by numerical quotas and merit ratings. When quality is emergent, optimising local components in isolation can degrade global performance, as evidenced by the inferior outcomes of the Barabási-Albert and Watts-Strogatz topologies, which lack the hierarchical scaffolding required for system-wide coherence.

For Complexity Theory: Operationalising Self-Organisation

The application of five quantitative metrics—entropy reduction ($\Delta S = -1.80$ bits), variance collapse ($S = 0.719$), correlation expansion (I_final = 0.58), long-range memory ($H = 0.68$), and critical phase transition ($\eta\_c = 0.30$)—enables the transformation of self-organisation from a qualitative metaphor into a testable and measurable phenomenon.

Theoretical Reformulation

This operationalisation integrates Deming's insights on variation with stochastic process theory. Deming distinguished between "common cause" variation, which is endemic to the system, and "special cause" variation, which is attributable to specific events. He argued that interventions targeting common cause variation increase system instability. The proposed model offers a rigorous method for distinguishing these variations. Common-cause variation is represented by the stationary distribution of the Markov process governing patient transitions and quality evolution. Special cause variation manifests as deviations that exceed the control limits defined by the system's Hurst exponent ($H = 0.68$) and phase-transition boundaries.

The demonstration that the system self-organises to Q_total ≈ 0.70–0.80, rather than 1.0, indicates that self-organisation does not equate to optimisation. The system identifies a satisfactory attractor instead of a global maximum. This finding has several significant theoretical implications:

Policies that disrupt self-organised attractors in pursuit of "perfection" are not only ineffective but also actively destabilise the system.

Deming anticipated this outcome: "A system cannot understand itself. The transformation requires a view from outside" (Deming, 2000 a, b). The HCM offers this external perspective, serving as a mathematical vantage point from which the system's natural equilibria can be observed and respected.

For Quality Theory: A Deming-Compliant Mathematical Foundation

Perhaps the most significant theoretical contribution of the HCM is its demonstration that Deming's System of Profound Knowledge is not philosophically opposed to mathematical modelling; rather, it requires it.

- One major contribution is that the model operationalises the PDSA cycle as a closed-loop dynamical system.

Our recursive quality update equation:

$$Q\_total,i(t+1) = Q\_total,i(t) + \eta\ \Sigma\_j\ K\_ij\ [\ Q\_total,j(t) - Q\_total,i(t)\ ]$$

is precisely a mathematical formalisation of Plan (the model specification), Do (the simulation), Study (the measurement of ΔS, S, I, H), and Act (the revision of policy parameters such as η). This transforms Deming's cycle from a qualitative heuristic into a quantifiable control policy.

- It also provides a formal language for psychological safety.

The finding that 71.9% of the quality variance is attributable to system structure, rather than individual agent characteristics, provides empirical support for Deming's assertion that most problems originate from systemic issues rather than worker deficiencies. The hyper-hierarchical degree distribution ($\gamma = 1.41$) indicates that a small number of hub institutions bear disproportionate responsibility for system-wide learning. Supporting these hubs, rather than assigning blame, yields benefits for the entire network. This analysis offers a network-analytic validation of Deming's Sixth Obstacle: "Our problems are mainly caused by the system, not by bad people" (Deming, 2000 a,b).

- A further contribution is the demonstration of the stochastic nature of quality itself.

The Markovian structure of patient pathways and the pronounced sensitivity to initial conditions ($\Delta = 8.726$) indicate that healthcare quality is fundamentally probabilistic. This finding challenges the dominant "zero defects" and "error-free care" paradigms derived from manufacturing. A Deming-compliant theory of healthcare quality should instead incorporate acceptable variation and statistical control, acknowledging that a certain proportion of adverse outcomes is unavoidable even within optimally functioning systems. The Healthcare Control Model (HCM) provides methodologies for quantifying this proportion.

Toward a Comprehensive Theory of Healthcare Quality

Sustainable quality improvement within healthcare systems relies on four interdependent capacities:

1. **Systemic:** The system is structured as a hierarchical network ($\gamma < 2.0$, $r > 0$), with knowledge concentrated at hubs and disseminated through small-world pathways ($C > 0.5$, $L < 3.0$).
2. **Variation-aware:** The system differentiates between common and special cause variation through statistical process control, guided by the Hurst exponent (H) and phase transition boundaries (η_c) in quality dynamics.
3. **Learning-enabled:** The system applies the Plan-Do-Study-Act (PDSA) cycle as a closed-loop control policy, maintaining the learning rate (η) within the optimal range ($0.2 < \eta < 0.5$).
4. **Psychologically safe:** The system primarily attributes quality failures to system design instead of individual error, fostering conditions that promote reporting and correction of systemic vulnerabilities.

The Healthcare Complexity Model (HCM) offers quantitative metrics for each capacity. Future research may assess these criteria in real-world healthcare networks using the Self-Organisation Diagnostic Protocol (SODP) and the Θ signature vector as benchmarking instruments.

Methodological Considerations

This study occupies an atypical methodological position. It is neither purely empirical, as synthetic rather than real hospital-level data were used, nor purely theoretical, since the synthetic data were rigorously calibrated to empirical OECD distributions. This intermediate approach should be regarded as a methodological strength.

Synthetic data possesses significant epistemic value. They enable controlled experimentation when real data is inaccessible due to privacy constraints, proprietary restrictions, or the lack of large-scale, publicly available hospital network datasets. Synthetic data allows researchers to isolate mechanisms, systematically vary parameters, and conduct counterfactual experiments that would be impossible or unethical in real systems. As demonstrated in this study, synthetic data can preserve the statistical properties of real data with high fidelity (all relative errors $< 6\%$).

However, synthetic data cannot replace empirical validation. The most pressing priority arising from this research is to test the Hybrid Complexity Model using real hospital referral networks, actual patient transfer patterns, and authentic quality metrics. Specific, testable hypotheses have been formulated. Collaboration among health systems researchers, network scientists, and data authorities is essential for advancing this validation effort.

Policy Synthesis

If empirical validation supports the Hybrid Complexity Model, its policy implications will be both significant and, in some cases, unanticipated.

First, policymakers should move beyond the pursuit of a single optimal system design.

The Hybrid Complexity Model demonstrates equifinality, indicating that multiple distinct resource configurations can achieve comparable quality outcomes. Consequently, international benchmarking should shift from ranking countries against a single ideal to identifying groups of high-performing configurations and analysing the conditions that enable each group to succeed.

Second, it is essential to protect and cultivate hub institutions.

Hyper-hierarchical degree distributions ($\gamma = 1.41$) should not be viewed as correctable inequalities but rather as functional adaptations. Hub institutions act as knowledge reservoirs, absorbing innovations from global science and disseminating them to peripheral providers. Policies that limit the growth of academic medical centres, redistribute resources away from hubs to promote equity, or fragment integrated delivery systems may inadvertently undermine the structures that facilitate system-wide learning.

Third, policymakers should acknowledge and operate within the constraints of fundamental uncertainty.

Chaotic dynamics indicate that long-term forecasting is not only challenging but, under certain conditions, theoretically impossible. Rather than discouraging action, this insight supports the adoption of adaptive policy design. Policies should be structured as experiments, evaluated continuously, and revised promptly. Ensemble forecasting, which evaluates policies across multiple plausible futures, should replace reliance on single-point predictions.

Fourth, it is important to identify and cultivate critical learning rates within systems.

The identified phase transition at $\eta\_c = 0.30$ demonstrates that self-organisation does not occur automatically. Systems with slow learning rates remain in heterogeneous, suboptimal states, while those with excessively rapid learning become unstable. Policymakers should therefore measure learning rates—such as the speed of guideline adoption, responsiveness to feedback, and diffusion of innovations—and design interventions to move systems toward the optimal learning zone.

Fifth, policies should align with, rather than oppose, the principles of self-organisation.

The system spontaneously converges to Q_total ≈ 0.70–0.80. While this is not a global optimum, it represents a stable, self-organised attractor. Interventions that respect this attractor, introduce gradual changes, monitor system responses, and withdraw policies that induce instability are more likely to succeed than those that attempt to impose radically different configurations through top-down directives.

DISCLOSURE OF DELEGATION TO GENERATIVE AI

I declare the use of generative AI in the research and writing process. According to the GAIDeT taxonomy, the following tasks were delegated to generative AI tools under full human supervision:

- Code generation.
- Process automation.
- Creation of algorithms for data analysis.
- Reproducibility testing.
- Proofreading and editing.

The generative AI tools used were: Perplexity (for reformulating my original ideas and published research), DeepSeek (for Python code generation for network simulation and complexity analysis), and Grammarly (for text polishing and readability).

I retain full responsibility for the final manuscript. Generative AI tools are not listed as authors and do not bear responsibility for the final outcomes.

Declaration submitted by: Dr. Anastasius Moumtzoglou

Additional note: The original research ideas, the Hybrid Complexity Model architecture, the mathematical specification, and the research question are my own. Perplexity AI was used at an early stage to help reformulate my original ideas. DeepSeek generated initial Python code for the network models, power-law estimation, chaos detection, and self-organisation metrics, which I subsequently verified, tested, and corrected. Grammarly was used to proofread and assess the readability of the final manuscript. All numerical results were generated by my execution of the verified Python code. The synthetic data were generated using my methodology based on OECD Health Statistics 2024. No AI tool generated data, references, or substantive research content.

REFERENCES

Ashby, W. R. (1956). *An introduction to cybernetics*. Chapman & Hall. DOI: 10.5962/bhl.title.5851

Barabási, A.-L. (2016). *Network science*. Cambridge University Press.

Barabási, A.-L., & Albert, R. (1999). Emergence of scaling in random networks. *Science*, *286*(5439), 509–512. DOI: 10.1126/science.286.5439.509 PMID: 10521342

Begun, J. W., Zimmerman, B., & Dooley, K. (2003). Health care organizations as complex adaptive systems. In Mick, S. S., & Wyttenbach, M. (Eds.), *Advances in health care organization theory* (pp. 253–288). Jossey-Bass.

Braithwaite, J., Churruca, K., Ellis, L. A., Long, J., Clay-Williams, R., Damen, N., Herkes, J., Pomare, C., & Ludlow, K. (2017). *Complexity science in healthcare: aspirations, approaches, applications and accomplishments: a white paper*. Macquarie University. https://www.mq.edu.au/research/research-centres-groups-and-facilities/healthy-people/centres/australian-institute-of-health-innovation/news-and-events/news/news/complexity-science-in-healthcare-aspirations,-approaches,-applications-and-accomplishments-a-white-paper

Chen, G., & O'Malley, A. J. (2024). Bayesian Hierarchical Network Autocorrelation Models for Estimating Direct and Indirect Effects of Peer Hospitals on Outcomes of Hospitalized Patients. Research square, rs.3.rs-4014583. https://doi.org/DOI: 10.21203/rs.3.rs-4014583/v1

Clauset, A., Shalizi, C. R., & Newman, M. E. J. (2009). Power-law distributions in empirical data. *SIAM Review*, *51*(4), 661–703. DOI: 10.1137/070710111

Deming, W. E. (2000a). *Out of the crisis*. MIT Press.

Deming, W. E. (2000b). *The new economics: For industry, government, education* (2nd ed.). MIT Press.

Donabedian, A. (1988). The quality of care: How can it be assessed? *Journal of the American Medical Association*, *260*(12), 1743–1748. DOI: 10.1001/jama.1988.03410120089033 PMID: 3045356

Euro Health Consumer Index. (2023). *EHCI 2023 report*. Health Consumer Powerhouse.

Gavurova, B., Kocisova, K., & Sopko, J. (2021). Health system efficiency in OECD countries: Dynamic network DEA approach. *Health Economics Review*, *11*(1), 40. DOI: 10.1186/s13561-021-00337-9 PMID: 34642864

Higham, D. J. (2001). An algorithmic introduction to numerical simulation of stochastic differential equations. *SIAM Review*, *43*(3), 525–546. DOI: 10.1137/S0036144500378302

Holland, J. H. (1995). *Hidden order: How adaptation builds complexity*. Addison-Wesley.

Iman, R. L., & Conover, W. J. (1982). A distribution-free approach to inducing rank correlation among input variables. *Communications in Statistics. Simulation and Computation*, *11*(3), 311–334. DOI: 10.1080/03610918208812265

Kloeden, P. E., & Platen, E. (1992). *Numerical Solution of Stochastic Differential Equations*. Springer. DOI: 10.1007/978-3-662-12616-5

Kuramoto, Y. (1984). *Chemical oscillations, waves, and turbulence*. Springer. DOI: 10.1007/978-3-642-69689-3

Lorenz, E. N. (1963). Deterministic nonperiodic flow. *Journal of the Atmospheric Sciences*, *20*(2), 130–141. DOI: 10.1175/1520-0469(1963)020<0130:DNF>2.0.CO;2

OECD (2024). Health at a glance 2024: OECD indicators. OECD Publishing. DOI: 10.1787/9789264055896-ko

Paina, L., & Peters, D. H. (2012). Understanding pathways for scaling up health services through the lens of complex adaptive systems. *Health Policy and Planning*, *27*(5), 365–373. DOI: 10.1093/heapol/czr054 PMID: 21821667

Plsek, P. E., & Greenhalgh, T. (2001). Complexity science: The challenge of complexity in health care. *BMJ (Clinical Research Ed.)*, *323*(7313), 625–628. DOI: 10.1136/bmj.323.7313.625 PMID: 11557716

Ravasz, E., & Barabási, A.-L. (2003). Hierarchical organization in complex networks. *Physical Review. E*, *67*(2), 026112. Advance online publication. DOI: 10.1103/PhysRevE.67.026112 PMID: 12636753

Silverman, B. W. (1986). *Density estimation for statistics and data analysis*. Chapman and Hall.

Thille, P., Tobin, A., Evans, J. M., Katz, A., & Russell, G. M. (2024). Evolving through multiple, co-existing pressures to change: A case study of self-organization in primary care during the COVID-19 pandemic in Canada. *BMC Primary Care*, *25*(1), 285. DOI: 10.1186/s12875-024-02520-3 PMID: 39103760

Watts, D. J., & Strogatz, S. H. (1998). Collective dynamics of 'small-world' networks. *Nature*, *393*(6684), 440–442. DOI: 10.1038/30918 PMID: 9623998

Yu, Y., Liao, J., Ma, D., & Zhu, W. (2024). Measuring the COVID-19 treatment efficiency in OECD countries: A multiplicative network DEA approach. *INFOR*, *62*(3), 419–448. DOI: 10.1080/03155986.2024.2337978

Chapter 3
Event-Driven Stochastic Regime Shifts in Adaptive Healthcare Systems:
Modelling Overload, Recovery, and Policy Response

Dimitrios Papakyriakou
http://orcid.org/0000-0001-9745-0857
Independent Researcher, Greece

ABSTRACT

Healthcare systems operate under persistent uncertainty arising from stochastic demand, limited resources, and delayed operational adaptation. While classical queueing and Markovian models provide a mathematical basis for analysing patient flow and service capacity, they often rely on stationarity assumptions that weaken under emergency overcrowding, demand surges, and staffing disruptions. This chapter introduces an event-driven stochastic regime framework for modelling transitions between normal operation, congestion, overload, and recovery in adaptive healthcare setting. The approach extends an M/M/c queue with regime-dependent dynamics and delayed capacity adjustment and is evaluated through discrete-event simulation using synthetic demand scenarios. Results show that policy lag amplifies backlog accumulation, prolongs overload duration, and increases recovery time, while adaptive surge staffing mitigates these effects. The chapter highlights implications for emergency department operations and identifies early-warning indicators for resilient, data-informed service design.

INTRODUCTION

Healthcare systems operate under persistent stochastic variability. Patient arrivals fluctuate across hours, days, and seasons, while service capacity remains constrained by staffing, infrastructure, and institutional policies. Under routine conditions, queueing-based planning models can approximate patient flow reasonably well. During operational stress, however—such as emergency department overcrowd-

DOI: 10.4018/979-8-3373-9705-4.ch003

ing, epidemic outbreaks, mass casualty incidents, or staffing disruptions—the assumptions underlying stationary modelling often break down (Green, 2006; Hall, 2013; Kolker, 2008).

Emergency department overcrowding is a well-documented condition in which demand persistently exceeds available service capacity (Asplin et al., 2003; Hoot & Aronsky, 2008; Kolker, 2008). Demand surges may arise from external shocks or internal bottlenecks such as inpatient boarding (Litvak & Long, 2000; Litvak et al., 2001). Even when average arrival rates appear manageable, short-term surges can still produce nonlinear growth in queue length and waiting time.

A critical but often under-modelled factor is delayed adaptation (Hall, 2013; Hick et al., 2004). Capacity adjustments such as surge staffing or bed reallocation require time, creating a gap between overload detection and corrective action. During that interval, queues may grow rapidly and push the system into a different operational regime.

In such settings, stationarity is no longer a sufficient assumption. Arrival rates may shift abruptly, service rates may vary under stress, and control actions may be delayed. These features motivate an event-driven stochastic framework for modelling transitions between normal operation, congestion, overload, and recovery.

This chapter develops such a framework and examines how delayed policy response interacts with stochastic demand to produce regime instability in healthcare queueing systems (Hall, 2013; Worthington, 1987).

BACKGROUND AND RELATED WORK

Queueing Baseline: The M/M/c System

Queueing theory provides a standard framework for analysing congestion, delay, and capacity utilization in service systems (Green, 2006; Gross et al., 2018). In healthcare, it is especially relevant because patient demand is stochastic while service capacity is finite. Emergency departments, outpatient clinics, diagnostic services, and hospital admission systems all exhibit queue-like behavior in which patients arrive, wait when capacity is unavailable, receive service, and then depart.

Among the available queueing models, the M/M/c system offers a natural baseline for studying healthcare service operations. In this framework, arrivals are assumed to follow a Poisson process with rate (λ), service times are exponentially distributed with rate (μ), and (c), identical servers operate in parallel. Patients are typically assumed to be served on a first-come, first-served basis, although many healthcare contexts may later require priority-based extensions. Despite its simplicity, the M/M/c model captures the essential tension between stochastic demand and limited-service capacity.

A central quantity in the M/M/c model is the traffic intensity:

$$\rho = \lambda/(c\,\mu)$$

The system is stable in steady state if $\rho < 1$

Key performance measures include:

L_q: expected queue length

W_q: expected waiting time in queue

Throughput: long-run departure rate

Under stationarity and $\rho < 1$, closed-form expressions such as the Erlang-C formula allow analytical computation of waiting probabilities and delays (Gross et al., 2018).

This ratio describes how heavily loaded the system is relative to its available service capacity. When (ρ) remains below 1, the system is stable in the steady-state sense, meaning that arrivals do not systematically exceed departures over the long run. When (ρ) approaches 1, queues become increasingly sensitive to fluctuations, and waiting times may rise sharply. When (ρ) exceeds 1, congestion tends to grow persistently unless capacity is increased or demand is reduced (Gross et al., 2018).

Several standard performance measures are derived from this baseline model. These include the expected queue length (L_q), the expected waiting time in queue (W_q), the probability that an arriving patient must wait, and the long-run throughput of the service system. Closed-form approximations such as the Erlang-C formula make the M/M/c model especially attractive for operational planning, since they provide interpretable measures of delay and congestion under stationary conditions (Gross et al., 2018).

In healthcare settings, these measures translate into operational concerns. Queue length reflects patients waiting for triage, examination, or admission, waiting time relates to service quality and risk, and throughput captures the system's ability to process demand. For this reason, queueing analysis has been widely used to study bed capacity, clinic scheduling, emergency department crowding, and access management (Green, 2006; Green et al., 2001; Worthington, 1987).

However, the classical M/M/c model is best viewed as a baseline rather than a complete description of healthcare operations. Real systems often violate its assumptions: service times may be heterogeneous, staffing may vary across shifts, and patient acuity may introduce priority effects. Most importantly, demand is rarely stationary under operational stress. Demand surges, outbreaks, staffing disruptions, and boarding delays can shift the system away from equilibrium, motivating extensions that capture overload, delayed adaptation, and regime-dependent behavior.

Markov and CTMC Foundations

The M/M/c queue can be represented as a continuous-time Markov chain (CTMC), linking operational queueing models with stochastic process theory. In this formulation, the state is defined by the number of patients in the system, including both those in service and those waiting. Transitions occur through arrivals and service completions and evolve probabilistically over continuous time according to state-dependent rates.

Under the exponential assumptions of the M/M/c model, arrivals and service completions satisfy the memoryless property, allowing the system to be analysed using birth–death process methods. Standard questions of stability, stationarity, and performance can then be examined through generator matrices, balance equations, and invariant distributions (Gross et al., 2018).

For healthcare operations research, the CTMC perspective is useful because it provides a formal way to describe patient-flow dynamics and to distinguish between transient and long-run behavior. However, classical CTMC analysis becomes restrictive in adaptive healthcare settings, where arrival rates, service rates, and effective capacity may change over time rather than remain fixed.

In practice, healthcare systems may move across qualitatively different operating conditions. An emergency department, for example, may behave very differently under routine inflow than during an infection wave, staffing shortage, or boarding crisis. In such cases, arrival intensity, effective service rate, and operational priorities may all shift, making a single homogeneous CTMC insufficient unless it is extended to allow regime-dependent parameters.

This motivates a broader stochastic-process framing in which Markovian logic is retained, but the system is allowed to move between operational regimes. In the present chapter, the CTMC perspective provides the formal foundation, while the model extends beyond a single stationary chain by introducing event-driven regime changes and delayed adaptive control.

Modelling Under Stress and Non-Stationarity

Healthcare operations research has long shown that patient-flow systems are shaped by stochastic variation and congestion effects. Emergency departments, in particular, are vulnerable to crowding when patient inflow, service delays, inpatient boarding, and staffing limitations interact over time. In many cases, operational strain arises not from average demand alone, but from the timing and persistence of arrivals relative to available capacity (Green, 2006; Hall, 2013; Kolker, 2008).

Prior work has examined several relevant mechanisms. Queueing models have been used to estimate waiting times and staffing requirements, while discrete-event simulation has been applied to triage systems, bed-allocation policies, and emergency department workflows. Dynamic and time-varying arrival processes have also been studied to better represent patient demand (Brailsford et al., 2009; Green et al., 2001; Jun et al., 1999; Whitt, 1991).

Nevertheless, much of this literature treats demand variation as stationary or smoothly time-varying rather than as abrupt shifts between qualitatively different operating conditions (Green et al., 2001; Whitt, 1991). Even when surge conditions are considered, the focus is often on performance under altered demand rather than on the transition itself as a regime change. As a result, the literature is rich in congestion analysis but less explicit about the distinction between normal, congested, overloaded, and recovering modes.

A further limitation concerns control actions. In practice, healthcare administrators do not observe overload and respond instantaneously. Staffing calls, surge beds, and workflow changes require time to implement, creating a delay between detection and correction. From a stochastic-systems perspective, this delay can amplify queue growth and reshape recovery dynamics, yet it is often treated only informally rather than as an explicit structural parameter.

This gap is central to the present chapter. The focus is not simply on whether healthcare queues become congested, but on how event-driven demand shocks interact with delayed policy response to produce regime shifts and instability. In this sense, the chapter builds on the healthcare queueing and simulation literature while extending it in a more explicitly stochastic-process direction.

From Stationary Congestion Analysis to Regime-Based Adaptive Modelling

The transition from classical queueing analysis to regime-based modelling reflects a shift in emphasis. Traditional steady-state models focus on expected waiting times and performance under fixed conditions, whereas regime-based models examine how systems respond to abrupt demand changes, delayed interventions, and prolonged overload.

These questions are particularly relevant in adaptive healthcare systems, where resilience and adaptive capacity have become central operational concerns (Haldane et al., 2021). In such settings, outcomes depend not only on baseline capacity but also on the timing and effectiveness of corrective actions. This motivates a framework in which stochastic demand, operating state, and adaptive policy are considered jointly.

The present chapter adopts the M/M/c queue as a baseline structure and extends it by introducing event-driven regime shifts and delayed capacity adjustment. This approach remains mathematically interpretable and compatible with simulation, while providing a more realistic representation of operational stress than purely stationary models.

Rather than replacing existing methods, the contribution is to connect queueing theory, stochastic-process reasoning, and discrete-event simulation within a regime-sensitive framework. Together, these elements support the analysis of overload, recovery, and policy-driven transitions in adaptive healthcare systems.

Existing queueing, emergency department simulation and surge-capacity models provide important methods for analysing congestion, resource utilization and operational performance. However, many approaches primarily evaluate system behaviour under predefined demand conditions or focus on the consequences of overload after it has already emerged.

The perspective adopted in this chapter is complementary. The emphasis is placed on the transition mechanism itself: how stochastic demand shocks, delayed adaptive response and accumulated backlog interact to move a healthcare system between operational regimes. Therefore, the framework does not replace existing queueing or simulation approaches, but extends them by explicitly modelling lag-induced regime transitions and recovery dynamics.

EVENT-DRIVEN REGIME FRAMEWORK

Rationale for a Regime-Based Representation

Healthcare systems rarely operate under a single, unchanging stochastic structure. Under routine conditions, patient arrivals, service times, and staffing capacity fluctuate within manageable bounds, allowing classical queueing approximations to describe system behavior. Under operational stress, however, systems may shift into qualitatively different modes, with persistent congestion, delayed response, and recovery requiring active intervention (Hall, 2013; Hoot & Aronsky, 2008).

For this reason, the chapter adopts a regime-based representation of healthcare operations. Rather than modelling the system as a single queue under fixed assumptions, it is treated as a stochastic service system that can move across distinct operational regimes, each reflecting different relationships between demand, capacity, and adaptive policy.

This distinction is operationally important. Systems in normal operation, congestion, overload, and recovery require different management responses. By explicitly distinguishing these regimes, the framework provides a more realistic description of adaptive healthcare dynamics than a stationary queueing model alone.

Definition 1: System State

Let (N_t) denote the total number of patients in the system at time (t). Let:

$N_q(t)$ be the number of patients waiting in queue,
$N_s(t)$ be the number of patients in service,
$c(t)$ be the active number of servers at time (t)

The system state at time t is defined as:

$$S(t) = \left(N_q(t), N_s(t), c(t), r(t)\right)$$

where $r(t)$ denotes the operational regime.

This state definition extends the usual queue-length description of the M/M/c system in two important ways. First, it separates the number of patients waiting from the number currently being served. This distinction is operationally meaningful in healthcare because waiting and service occupancy correspond to different managerial pressures. A large queue may signal delayed triage, admission bottlenecks, or insufficient front-line staffing, whereas a high number in service may signal resource saturation even before visible waiting accumulates.

Second, the state includes both active capacity $c(t)$ and the operational regime $r(t)$. This is important because healthcare capacity is not always static. Staffing levels may be increased, temporary surge protocols may be activated, or service availability may deteriorate under stress. By including $c(t)$ in the state, the framework explicitly allows the control side of the system to evolve over time. By including $r(t)$, it allows the stochastic structure itself to vary across operating conditions.

From an analytical perspective, the state definition therefore combines observable congestion variables with adaptive capacity and regime information. This provides a richer operational description than a simple count process $N(t)$ alone.

Why the Regime Variable Matters

The introduction of a regime variable $r(t)$ is the central conceptual extension of the chapter. In standard stationary healthcare flow models, one usually assumes that arrival and service processes fluctuate around a fixed stochastic environment. In contrast, the present framework assumes that the environment itself may change due to exogenous shocks, endogenous congestion effects, or delayed control actions.

In healthcare practice, this distinction is intuitive. A mildly busy emergency department is not the same as an overloaded one, even if both can be described by the same formal queueing notation. In the overloaded state, waiting patients may accumulate faster than staff can absorb them, delays may propagate across multiple care stages, and managerial priorities may change. A recovering system is also distinct from a normal one because the queue may be shrinking while residual congestion is still present. The regime variable captures these operational differences directly.

Thus, the regime variable is not introduced merely to increase model complexity. It is introduced because healthcare systems are often governed by different stochastic and operational logics in different phases of stress and recovery.

Definition 2: Regime Process

The operational regime $r(t)$ belongs to the finite set:

R= {normal, congestion, overload, recovery}

Regime transitions are event-driven and occur when one of the following events is triggered:

1. Exogenous demand shock (arrival rate shift),
2. End of shock,
3. Policy activation,
4. Clearance of accumulated backlog.

In each regime (r), arrival and service parameters may differ:

$$\lambda = \lambda(r)$$

$$\mu = \mu(r)$$

Thus, the effective traffic intensity becomes regime-dependent:

$$\rho(r, t) = \frac{\lambda(r)}{c(t)\mu(r)}$$

Regime changes modify $\lambda(r)$ and possibly $\mu(r)$ but capacity $c(t)$ may respond with delay.

This definition formalizes the idea that the system may experience transitions not only in performance level, but in operating mode. The four regimes used here are intentionally simple and interpretable.

Normal operation represents a condition in which demand remains within manageable capacity and the system behaves similarly to a stable queue under conventional assumptions.

Congestion represents a stressed but not yet fully destabilized state. Waiting increases, the system becomes more sensitive to fluctuations, and managerial attention is required, but backlog remains potentially reversible without extreme intervention.

Overload represents a regime in which the effective inflow pressure exceeds what the current service capacity can absorb. In this state, backlog grows persistently and routine operation is no longer sufficient to restore balance.

Recovery represents the period after corrective action or shock termination, during which the system is moving back toward normal operation but has not yet fully cleared accumulated queueing burden.

These regime labels are operationally meaningful because they reflect distinct management problems. In normal operation, the objective may be routine efficiency. In congestion, the priority may shift toward monitoring and anticipation. In overload, urgent adaptive intervention becomes necessary. In recovery, the task is to clear backlog without re-entering congestion. Thus, the regime process provides both a stochastic and managerial representation of healthcare operations under uncertainty.

Event-Driven Rather Than Smoothly Time-Varying Dynamics

An important feature of the framework is that transitions are modelled as **event-driven** rather than merely smooth time variation. This choice reflects the operational reality that many healthcare disruptions occur through identifiable triggers. Examples include a sudden demand surge, an outbreak wave, an internal service disruption, the end of a peak inflow window, or the activation of an emergency staffing response.

This differs from models in which arrival rates simply drift over time according to a continuous schedule. Smooth time variation is often useful in appointment-based or diurnal demand models, but it may understate the practical significance of abrupt disruptions. Event-driven modelling emphasizes that some transitions occur because something happens: a shock begins, a threshold is crossed, a decision is made, or backlog is finally cleared.

For the purposes of this chapter, event-driven transitions are especially useful because they connect naturally to discrete-event simulation. They also align with the chapter's central objective, which is to study how demand shocks and delayed policy responses generate transitions between qualitatively different operational states (Brailsford et al., 2004; Brailsford et al., 2009; Jun et al., 1999).

Definition 3: Policy with Delay (*Lag* τ)

Let ($\tau \geq 0$) denote the policy lag.

When overload is detected at time (t_d) a corrective capacity action is scheduled at time:

$$t_a = t_d + \tau$$

At time (t_a) the number of servers is adjusted:

$$c(t_a) = c(t_a^-) + \Delta c$$

where (Δc) represents surge staffing or capacity expansion.

This structure introduces a separation between detection and execution, which is central to instability dynamics.

The delayed-policy definition is operationally critical. In many healthcare systems, administrators do not respond to overload instantaneously (Hall, 2013; Hick et al., 2004). Even when overload is recognized quickly, corrective actions require coordination, authorization, staffing mobilization, physical space adjustment, or workflow reconfiguration. Therefore, the effect of a policy is typically delayed relative to the onset of the problem.

In stationary models, this delay is often ignored or treated implicitly. In the present framework, it is made explicit because it changes the evolution of the queue itself. If arrivals exceed baseline service capacity during the lag interval, backlog grows before corrective action takes effect. This lag-induced accumulation is the mechanism that links delayed control to prolonged overload and recovery.

Operationally, the parameter (τ) can be interpreted as a simplified representation of response friction. Smaller values of (τ) correspond to highly adaptive systems that can mobilize quickly. Larger values correspond to slower institutions, more rigid staffing procedures, or environments where recognition and implementation are separated by substantial delay. Thus, policy lag is not just a mathematical parameter; it is a proxy for organizational responsiveness.

Definition 4: Regime Instability (Operational)

Regime instability is defined operationally as follows:

A system is said to exhibit regime instability if, following a demand shock, the duration of overload and the recovery time increase disproportionately with policy (*Lag* τ) leading to sustained queue growth beyond a tolerance threshold.

Formally, let $T_{over}(\tau)$ denote the total time spent in overload during a shock episode. Instability is present if:

$T_{over}(\tau 2) - T_{over}(\tau 1)$ grows superlinearly as $(\tau 2 > \tau 1)$.

This definition focuses on measurable operational consequences rather than purely asymptotic stability conditions.

This operational definition is deliberate. The chapter does not define instability in the most abstract mathematical sense, but in a way directly tied to healthcare system performance. The question is not only whether a queue is theoretically stable in the limit, but whether a realistic healthcare system experiences prolonged overload, slow recovery, and worsening service conditions as response delay increases.

This is particularly important for adaptive healthcare systems because decision-makers do not manage asymptotic limits; they manage operational windows. A system may still be mathematically recoverable, yet operationally unstable if its overload persists long enough to degrade care quality, increase risk, or trigger cascading congestion effects. The present definition therefore emphasizes healthcare relevance while preserving a precise stochastic interpretation.

How the Framework Differs from Stationary Healthcare Flow Models

The framework developed here differs from classical stationary healthcare flow models in several important respects.

First, it explicitly recognizes that patient-flow systems may move across different operating modes rather than fluctuating around a single equilibrium. This is crucial in environments where crowding episodes, demand shocks, and recovery periods are not exceptional but recurrent.

Second, it introduces a delayed policy response as an explicit structural element of the model. Many traditional queueing analyses assume fixed capacity or instantaneous adjustment, whereas the present framework treats response lag as one of the main drivers of congestion amplification.

Third, it integrates stochastic process logic with operational decision timing. This makes it possible to study not only how queues behave under given demand levels, but how organizational responsiveness changes the trajectory of overload and recovery.

Fourth, the framework is designed to be computationally tractable. It remains close enough to classical queueing theory to preserve interpretability, while also being compatible with discrete-event simulation and synthetic policy experiments.

For these reasons, the event-driven regime framework is particularly suitable for modelling adaptive healthcare systems under stress. It does not reject the value of stationary models; rather, it extends them into a setting where non-stationarity, delayed action, and operational regime change are central.

Bridge to the Next Section

The definitions introduced in this section establish the conceptual and mathematical basis of the chapter. The system state captures queue burden, service occupancy, active capacity, and regime identity. The regime process formalizes transitions across operational states. The policy-lag mechanism introduces delayed adaptive control. The operational instability definition provides a measurable criterion for determining when overload becomes disproportionately persistent.

These elements together prepare the next section, which examines the mechanism of instability more directly. In particular, the regime instability analysis that follows shows how delayed capacity adjustment produces backlog accumulation and why this accumulation gives rise to threshold-like behaviour in overload duration and recovery time.

REGIME INSTABILITY CONDITIONS (LIGHT BUT SHARP)

Instability Under Delayed Capacity Adjustment

In the classical M/M/c system, stability is ensured when (Gross et al., 2018):

$$\rho = \frac{\lambda}{c\mu} < 1$$

Under regime-dependent dynamics, however, both (λ) and (c) may change over time. Consider a demand surge regime (r=overload), characterized by an increased arrival rate $(\lambda_s > \lambda_0$, while service rate (μ) remains constant.

The effective traffic intensity during the surge becomes:

$$\rho s(t) = \lambda_s / (c(t)\mu)$$

If capacity has not yet been adjusted, $c(t)=c_0$, and overload is initiated when:

$$\rho_s(t) \geq 1$$

Let (t_d) denote the time at which overload is detected. A corrective action increasing capacity by (Δc) is scheduled at:

$$t_a = t_d + \tau$$

For (t) in (t_d,t_a), the system accumulates backlog because arrivals exceed service completions in expectation.

The expected instantaneous drift in queue length during overload is approximately:

$$\frac{dE[N_q(t)]}{dt} \approx \lambda_s - c_0 \mu$$

If $(\lambda_s - c_0\mu > 0)$, the queue grows linearly in expectation over the lag interval (τ). Thus, the expected queue increase during the delay period is approximately:

$$\Delta Nq \approx (\lambda s - c0\,\mu)\,\tau$$

This accumulation amplifies recovery time even after capacity is increased.

The key point is that delayed intervention does not simply postpone correction; it changes the state from which correction begins. Once a positive backlog has been generated, the system must first absorb the accumulated queue before it can return to stable routine operation. In operational terms, the delay creates a hidden burden that remains even after the staffing response has been activated.

This is especially relevant in healthcare systems because many forms of overload are not immediately visible through average utilization alone. A department may still appear operational while backlog is already accumulating. By the time corrective action is implemented, waiting patients, delayed diagnostics, or admission bottlenecks may already have shifted the system into a much more fragile state.

Table 1. Main parameters and interpretation of the event-driven regime model

Parameters	**Meaning**	**Healthcare interpretation**
λ(t)	Time-dependent arrival rate	Patient demand intensity
μ	Service rate	Treatment capacity per resource unit
c(t)	Adaptive capacity	Available healthcare resources
ρ(t)	Utilization ratio	Operational pressure level
Q(t)	Queue length	Accumulated unmet demand
τ	Policy delay	Time required before adaptive response
Δc	Capacity adjustment	Additional resources activated
Tshock	Shock duration (Tshock = shock_end - shock_start)	Duration of external demand surge (shock period)
R(t)	Regime state	Normal, overloaded, or recovery condition

Note. The parameters describe a generalized event-driven healthcare system representation rather than a calibrated model of a specific hospital environment. Parameter values can be adjusted according to different operational scenarios, healthcare settings or empirical datasets when available.

To provide a clearer interpretation of the mathematical formulation and improve reproducibility of the proposed framework, Table 1 summarizes the main parameters used in the event-driven regime model together with their operational meaning in healthcare systems.

Backlog Amplification as the Core Instability Mechanism

The mechanism identified above can be interpreted as a form of backlog amplification. During the lag interval, excess demand is not neutralized; it is stored in the queue. The larger the demand-capacity mismatch and the longer the intervention delay, the larger the accumulated burden that must later be cleared.

This mechanism is simple but powerful. In many healthcare settings, managers often think of response delay as a temporary inconvenience. From the perspective of the present framework, however, delay is not merely lost time. It is a multiplier of future recovery burden. Each additional unit of delay increases the amount of queue that must eventually be processed, and this increase may substantially prolong the period during which the system remains under operational stress.

Thus, the instability mechanism in the present chapter does not require the system to be permanently unstable in the classical asymptotic sense. Instead, instability appears as a disproportionate amplification of overload persistence and recovery time caused by the interaction of shock intensity and delayed adaptation.

This distinction is important. A system may remain theoretically recoverable while still becoming operationally unstable for decision-making purposes. If overload lasts long enough to disrupt care delivery, increase waiting time, or require prolonged emergency intervention, then the system has entered a practically unstable regime, even if recovery remains mathematically possible in the long run.

Proposition 1: Regime Instability Threshold Condition

Proposition 1 (Simulation-Grounded Instability Threshold)

Consider an event-driven M/M/c healthcare system subject to a surge in arrival rate from (λ_0) to (λ_s), with delayed capacity adjustment (τ) and capacity increment (Δc). There exists a critical lag $\tau_{crit}($ $s, \Delta c)$ such that, for $(\tau > \tau_{crit})$ both overload duration (T_{over}) and recovery time (T_{rec}) increase sharply and nonlinearly with (τ).

Sketch of Rationale:

1. During the lag interval $[t_d, t_d + \tau]$, queue growth is governed by positive drift:

$$(\lambda_s - c_0\,\mu > 0)$$

2. After capacity adjustment, the effective traffic intensity becomes:

$$\left(\rho_{post} = \frac{\lambda s}{(c_0 + \Delta_c)\mu}\right)$$

3. If $\rho_{post} < 1$, the system regains negative drift and begins backlog clearance. However, the accumulated queue (ΔNq) must first be absorbed.
4. Recovery time (T_{rec}) is approximately proportional to:

$$\frac{(\Delta Nq)}{(c_0 + \Delta_c)\ \mu - \lambda s}$$

Substituting $\Delta Nq \approx (\lambda s - c0\ \mu)\tau$:

$$Trec \approx \frac{(\lambda_s - c_0\,\mu)\tau}{(c_0 + \Delta_c)\ \mu - \lambda s}$$

Thus, recovery time grows approximately linearly in τ under moderate conditions. However, near the boundary where:

$$(c_0 + \Delta_c)\,\mu - \lambda s \rightarrow 0$$

the denominator becomes small, and recovery time increases sharply. This generates a nonlinear amplification effect and defines an empirical instability region.

The critical lag (τ_{crit}) emerges as the value beyond which overload persistence and recovery time escalate disproportionately.

This condition does not rely on asymptotic Markov stability analysis; instead, it reflects operational instability driven by lag-induced backlog amplification.

Interpretation of Proposition 1

The importance of Proposition 1 lies not only in the algebraic approximation itself, but in what it implies operationally. The expression for recovery time shows that delayed response affects outcomes through two channels simultaneously.

First, larger delay increases the amount of accumulated queue through the numerator. This means that even if the corrective policy is ultimately sufficient to restore stability, it must now work against a larger backlog than would have existed under a faster response.

Second, the denominator reflects the effective recovery capacity of the system after intervention. If the post-adjustment service capacity only slightly exceeds the surge-adjusted arrival pressure, then backlog clearance will be slow. Under these conditions, the same delay produces much larger operational harm than it would in a system with stronger recovery capacity.

This two-part structure explains why the same policy lag may be tolerable under mild surges but operationally dangerous under stronger ones. It also explains why stronger surge staffing may mitigate the impact of delay, though not always eliminate it. In other words, the instability threshold is not determined by delay alone, but by the joint geometry of demand intensity, baseline load, and post-intervention recovery strength.

Operational Interpretation

The instability threshold has direct healthcare implications:

- Small delays in activating surge protocols may be tolerable under mild shocks.
- Under stronger surges, identical delays produce disproportionate overload duration.
- Near-capacity systems are highly sensitive to policy lag.

Thus, regime instability is not solely determined by whether (ρ) exceeds 1, but by the interaction among the following factors (Hall, 2013; Kolker, 2008):

- Surge magnitude $(\lambda s - \lambda_0)$,
- Baseline utilization (ρ_0),
- Capacity increment (Δc),
- Policy lag (τ).

This interpretation is especially important in healthcare because many systems operate close to practical capacity even under routine conditions. A hospital ward, emergency department, or diagnostic unit may appear stable on average while still possessing very little slack. In such environments, even moderate demand shocks can trigger prolonged overload if response is delayed. What appears to be a staffing problem may therefore be, more precisely, a lag-amplified regime problem.

Early-Warning Indicators of Regime Transition

Before full overload manifests, several measurable indicators may signal impending instability:

1. Queue persistence:

   Sustained $N_q(t)$ above a predefined tolerance band.

2. Variance amplification:

   Rapid growth in the variance of $N(t)$, reflecting regime sensitivity.

3. Drift sign change:

   Empirical estimate of $\lambda(t) - c(t)\,\mu$ becoming positive.

4. Delayed clearance slope:

   Slow reduction of backlog following minor shocks.

These indicators can be computed directly from event-driven simulation outputs and provide actionable signals for adaptive policy design.

Their importance lies in the fact that regime deterioration may begin before catastrophic overload is visually obvious. For example, a system may show increasingly persistent queue excursions even while mean occupancy remains seemingly acceptable. Likewise, short periods of temporary overload may begin to cluster more tightly together, indicating reduced resilience. Variance amplification is therefore not merely a descriptive statistic; it may function as an early sign that the system is approaching an instability threshold.

From a managerial perspective, these early-warning indicators suggest that static occupancy thresholds may be insufficient for adaptive healthcare systems. A more informative monitoring framework would track not only current congestion level, but also persistence, volatility, and recovery rate following local disturbances.

Why the Instability Is Regime-Based Rather Than Merely Congestive

It is useful to distinguish the present concept of instability from ordinary congestion. Congestion refers to the existence of delay or queueing burden within the system. Regime instability, by contrast, refers to a transition in the way the system behaves under delayed adaptation. A congested system may still remain operationally manageable if queues dissipate quickly and overload episodes remain short.

An unstable regime is one in which delay-driven backlog amplification changes the overall recovery dynamics of the system.

This distinction justifies the regime language used throughout the chapter. The purpose is not simply to rename heavy congestion, but to highlight a qualitative shift in operational behavior. Once the system enters an overload regime with delayed correction, its trajectory is shaped not only by current demand but by the backlog already accumulated and by the speed with which adaptive capacity can be mobilized. This makes the recovery phase fundamentally different from ordinary queue fluctuation under stationary assumptions.

Relevance to Adaptive Healthcare Policy

The instability conditions developed here have direct implications for adaptive healthcare design. In a static planning framework, one might ask how many servers are needed on average to keep waiting times low. In the present regime-based framework, one must also ask how quickly capacity can be adjusted when stress appears, and whether that adjustment is strong enough to reverse backlog growth before overload becomes persistent.

Thus, adaptive capacity policy has two dimensions:

- **timing**, reflected in the lag parameter (τ),
- **strength**, reflected in the capacity increment $\left(\Delta_c\right)$.

A healthcare system with modest surge capacity but rapid response may outperform a system with larger surge reserves but slower activation. Conversely, a very fast response may still be insufficient if the capacity increment is too small relative to the demand shock. The regime-based instability framework therefore helps move the discussion from static staffing adequacy toward dynamic policy adequacy.

Bridge to the Simulation Section

The analytical approximations of this section are intentionally lightweight. Their purpose is not to provide a complete closed-form theory of overload recovery, but to clarify the mechanism through which delayed policy response amplifies congestion and creates threshold-like behavior.

The next section uses discrete-event simulation to examine these effects directly. By simulating patient-level arrivals, service completions, regime-switch events, and delayed capacity adjustment across multiple scenarios, the model makes it possible to observe overload persistence, recovery trajectories, and instability regions in a controlled computational environment. In this way, the simulation section provides empirical support for the regime-based intuition and threshold logic developed here.

SIMULATION DESIGN (DISCRETE-EVENT, M/M/c, EVENT-DRIVEN REGIMES)

Overview

A discrete-event simulation (DES) framework is developed to analyse regime-dependent behavior in a healthcare queueing system. The model simulates patient-level events and explicitly represents:

- Arrival events,
- Service start events,
- Service completion events,
- Regime switch events,
- Policy activation events.

The system is implemented in Python using an event-priority queue structure ordered by event time. This computational design is especially appropriate for the present chapter because it preserves the event-driven character of the proposed stochastic regime framework and its associated instability analysis. Rather than approximating system behavior through aggregated time steps alone, the simulation tracks operational changes at the level of discrete arrivals, departures, and control actions. This makes it possible to observe how backlog accumulates, how corrective actions take effect after delay, and how recovery unfolds over time.

Discrete-event simulation is widely used in healthcare operations research because it can represent service systems in which congestion emerges from the interaction of stochastic arrivals, limited capacity, and operational rules (Brailsford et al., 2009; Jun et al., 1999; Monks et al., 2019). In the present context, its main advantage is that it supports a direct computational realization of the event-driven regime model. Regime changes do not have to be imposed indirectly through summary assumptions; they can be encoded as explicit events that alter arrival intensity, capacity, or operating state.

Why Discrete-Event Simulation Is Appropriate for the Present Problem

The choice of DES is not merely technical. It is conceptually aligned with the chapter's central claim that healthcare systems under stress evolve through event-driven regime transitions. In a time-stepped simulation, abrupt changes may be represented only approximately, and the precise timing of overload onset, policy activation, and recovery may be blurred by discretization intervals. By contrast, in a DES environment, each relevant operational transition occurs at a specific simulated time and modifies the system state exactly when it is supposed to.

This feature is particularly important for modelling policy lag. Since the research question concerns the consequences of delayed adaptive response, the timing of intervention must be represented explicitly. DES makes it possible to distinguish clearly between the moment overload is detected and the later moment when adaptive staffing is actually activated. That distinction is central to the backlog amplification mechanism developed in the regime instability analysis.

A second advantage is interpretability. Hospital administrators and operations researchers can often reason more naturally about identifiable events—such as demand shocks, staffing adjustments, or queue clearance thresholds—than about purely abstract dynamic equations. DES therefore serves as both an analytical and communicative bridge between stochastic process theory and practical healthcare operations. Recent healthcare simulation research has similarly emphasized the importance of methodological rigor, reproducibility, and theory-informed simulation design in healthcare decision-support systems (Eppich & Reedy, 2022).

Arrival Process

Baseline regime:

Arrivals follow a Poisson process with rate (λ_0). This assumption provides a mathematically standard baseline and aligns with the queueing foundation introduced earlier. Although real healthcare demand may display more complex dependence structures, Poisson arrivals remain a widely used starting point in emergency care and service-system modelling because they capture random inflow under moderate aggregation assumptions (Green, 2006; Gross et al., 2018).

Surge regime:

At time (t_s), an event-driven shock increases arrival rate to $(\lambda_s = s\lambda_0)$, where $(s > 1)$ is the surge multiplier.

Arrival times are generated using exponential interarrival times:

$$Interarrival\ time \sim Exp(\lambda(r))$$

where $\lambda(r)$ depends on current regime $r(t)$.

The surge ends at time (t_e), after which (λ) returns to (λ_0).

This structure yields a piecewise-stationary arrival process in which the system alternates between normal demand and stressed demand conditions. The goal is not to reproduce every detail of empirical arrival seasonality, but to isolate the effect of abrupt demand elevation on congestion and recovery. Because the chapter focuses on overload and delayed response, a parsimonious step-surge design is more appropriate than an over-parameterized arrival model. It preserves interpretability while still generating nontrivial regime transitions.

Service Model

Service times are exponentially distributed:

$$Service\ time \sim Exp(\mu)$$

The number of active servers is:

$$c(t) = c_0 \text{ during baseline}$$

$$c(t) = c_0 + \Delta c \text{ after policy activation}$$

Patients are served on a first-come, first-served basis.

This service model is intentionally simple. Its role is to preserve continuity with the M/M/c analytical baseline while allowing adaptive capacity to be incorporated transparently. In practical healthcare environments, service heterogeneity is often substantial. However, for the purposes of identifying regime shifts and lag-induced backlog amplification, the exponential-service assumption provides a useful and interpretable benchmark.

The parameter $c(t)$ plays a dual role. It represents both the operational staffing level of the service system and the point at which adaptive control enters the queueing process. By allowing $c(t)$ to change after policy activation, the simulation captures the organizational fact that corrective action affects service capacity only after implementation.

Event Scheduling Mechanism

The DES operates through an event list ordered by event time. Each event corresponds to a discrete operational occurrence that may change system state, system parameters, or both. The principal event types are:

- **ARRIVAL**: a new patient enters the system,
- **SERVICE_START**: a waiting patient begins service when capacity becomes available,
- **DEPARTURE**: a service completion occurs,
- **REGIME_START**: the demand surge begins,
- **REGIME_END**: the demand surge ends,
- **POLICY_ACTION**: delayed adaptive capacity is activated.

The simulation clock advances directly from one scheduled event to the next. At each event time, the system updates queue length, service occupancy, active capacity, and current regime. Future events are then scheduled according to the new state and parameter configuration.

This mechanism is computationally efficient because time advances only when something relevant happens. It also makes causal sequencing transparent. For example, when a surge event occurs, the arrival intensity changes immediately. When overload is detected, a policy-action event is scheduled at $\left(t_d + \tau\right)$. When that policy event is reached, active capacity changes and subsequent departures may accelerate queue clearance. This exact sequencing is essential for studying delay-sensitive recovery.

Event-Driven Simulation Workflow

To improve methodological transparency and reproducibility, Algorithm 1 summarizes the main workflow of the event-driven healthcare regime simulation. The algorithm describes the sequence of operational events, overload detection, delayed policy activation, adaptive capacity adjustment and performance monitoring implemented in the simulation framework.

Algorithm 1. Event-Driven Healthcare Regime Simulation Workflow

Input:

- Baseline arrival rate $\left(\lambda_0\right)$,
- Service rate (μ),
- Initial capacity $\left(c_0\right)$,
- Surge multiplier (s),
- Shock duration Tshock,
- Policy lag (τ),

- Capacity adjustment (Δc).

Procedure:

1. Initialize healthcare system under the Normal Regime.
2. Generate stochastic patient arrivals and service completions according to the M/M/c process.
3. Trigger a demand-shock event and increase the arrival rate to $\lambda\sigma = s\lambda_0$.
4. Continuously update queue length, service occupancy, and traffic intensity.
5. Monitor overload conditions based on utilization and queue growth.
6. When overload is detected, schedule a delayed policy response after lag (τ).
7. Apply adaptive capacity expansion (Δc) at policy activation time.
8. Continue processing arrivals and departures while monitoring recovery dynamics.
9. Transition the system through Overload and Recovery regimes.
10. Record operational performance indicators.

Output:

- Overload duration (T_{over}),
- Recovery time (T_{rec}),
- Queue evolution $Q(t)$,
- Waiting-time statistics,
- Throughput metrics,
- Regime-transition timeline.

Figure 1. Event-Driven Healthcare Regime Simulation Workflow

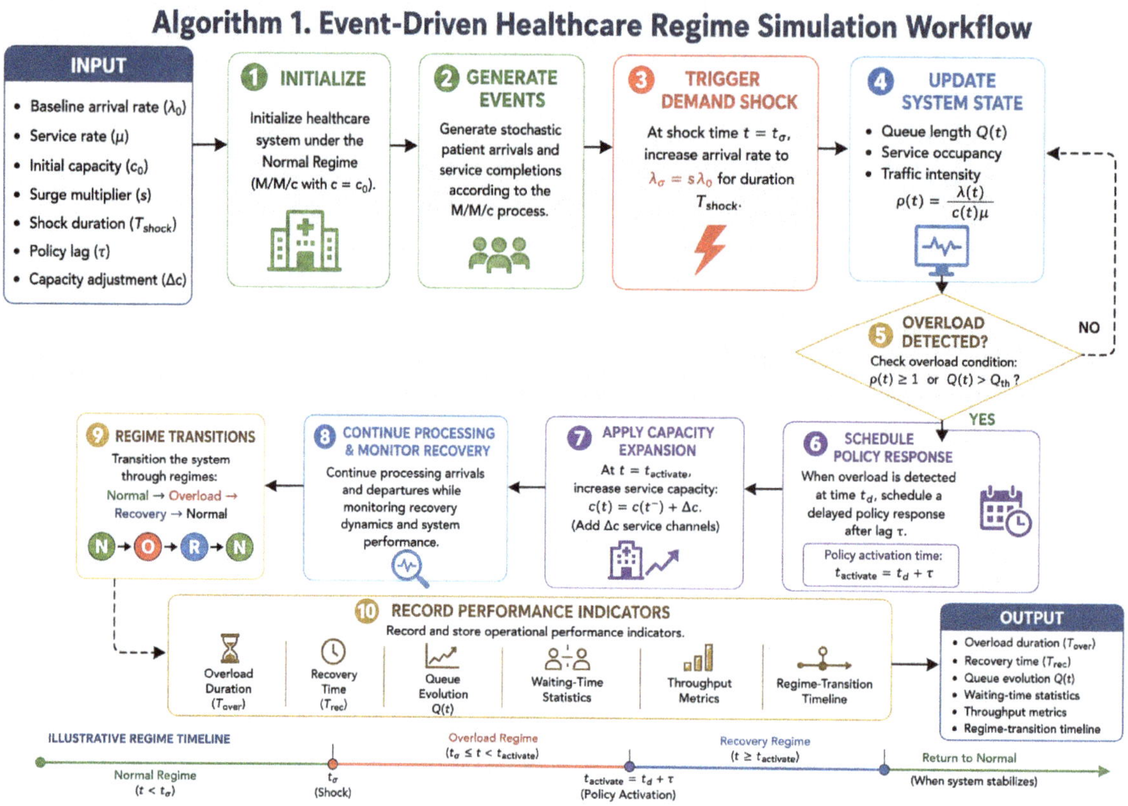

Note. *The workflow illustrates the event-driven simulation of the healthcare system using an M/M/c queueing framework under a demand-shock scenario. A key feature is the policy lag (τ), representing the delay between overload detection and the implementation of capacity expansion (Δc). This delay produces a distinct overload period even after the system recognizes stress, followed by recovery after the delayed policy intervention.*

The event-driven healthcare simulation begins under a Normal Regime, where patient arrivals and service completions are generated according to a standard M/M/c queueing process. Under normal operating conditions, the arrival rate remains at its baseline (λ_0), the available service capacity is fixed at (c_0), and system performance remains stable.

To represent unexpected operational stress, a demand-shock event is introduced. During the shock period, the patient arrival increases to $\lambda\sigma = s\lambda_0$, simulating sudden surges in healthcare demand such as epidemic outbreaks, mass-casualty incidents, seasonal peaks, or other disruptive events. As arrivals increase, the simulation continuously update queue length, service occupancy and traffic intensity, allowing the system state to evolve dynamically over time.

A central feature of the proposed framework is the explicit monitoring of overload conditions. Overload is identified when service utilization approaches or exceeds operational limits and queue growth becomes unsustainable. Importantly, the model does not assume that healthcare management reacts immediately once overload emerges.

Instead, the framework incorporates a policy lag parameter (τ), representing the real-world delay between overload recognition and operational intervention. This delay captures the time required for administrative decision-making, resource mobilization, staff allocation, infrastructure preparation and policy implementation. Consequently, even after overload is detected, the system continues to operate under stressed conditions for a finite period before corrective actions become effective.

Once the policy response is activated, adaptive capacity expansion (Δc) is applied to the healthcare system. Additional service resources are introduced, increasing the effective service capacity and enabling the system to gradually absorb accumulated demand. The simulation then continues to process arrivals and departures while monitoring recovery dynamics.

This mechanism naturally produces a sequence of operational regimes consisting of Normal, Overload, and Recovery states. The duration and severity of each regime emerge from the interaction between stochastic arrivals, service capacity, shock intensity and policy response delay. As illustrated in Figure 1, the temporary mismatch between rapidly increasing demand and delayed intervention creates a distinct overload period before recovery measures becomes effective. Following capacity expansion, queue pressure gradually decreases and the system transitions towards recovery and eventual stabilization.

Throughout the simulation, key operational indicators are recorded, including overload duration, recovery time, queue evolution, waiting-time statistics, throughput metrics, and the complete regime-transition timeline.

Overload Detection and Delayed Policy Activation

The simulation includes an explicit overload detection rule. If either of the following conditions is met:

- $\rho(t) \geq 1$, *or*
- $Q(t) \geq Q_{th}$

Where (Q_{th}) denotes a predefined operational queue-length threshold representing the maximum acceptable backlog before overload intervention is triggered.

The system declares overload at detection time (t_d).

A policy activation event is then scheduled at:

$$t_a = t_d + \tau$$

At time (t_a), capacity is updated according to:

$$c(t_a) = c_0 + \Delta_c$$

This mechanism is one of the most important parts of the simulation design because it translates the theoretical idea of delayed adaptive control into an operational computational rule. The simulation does not assume that staffing can be increased continuously or immediately. Instead, it assumes that a decision is made in response to overload, but the effect of that decision occurs only after a delay.

This representation is deliberately stylized. In real healthcare systems, detection may be imperfect, delays may vary, and staffing increases may occur in stages. Nonetheless, the simplified delay mechanism is analytically useful because it isolates the consequence of lag as a structural driver of backlog amplification.

Synthetic Data Generation and Why Synthetic Inputs Are Appropriate

The computational analysis in this chapter is based on synthetic data generated directly by the simulation model rather than on external hospital datasets. This choice is appropriate for several reasons.

First, the chapter's purpose is to examine a structural mechanism—namely, how demand shocks and delayed policy responses generate regime transitions and instability—not to calibrate a model for one specific institution. Synthetic scenarios allow the analysis to remain general and interpretable.

Second, synthetic input design supports controlled experimentation. Because arrival intensities, surge timing, policy lag, and capacity increments are explicitly specified, one can compare scenarios systematically and attribute differences in outcomes to known parameters. This is much harder to do with observational data alone, where multiple confounding factors may vary simultaneously.

Third, synthetic data generation is fully consistent with the computational orientation of the book. The objective is not only to discuss stochastic healthcare models conceptually, but to provide a reproducible simulation framework that can later be adapted to empirical settings. In this sense, synthetic experiments function as a methodological prototype.

The simulation produces multiple layers of synthetic output:

- patient-level event logs,
- system timelines over simulated time,
- scenario-level summary metrics.

These outputs are sufficient to compute waiting times, overload duration, recovery time, queue persistence, and throughput, while also supporting the creation of the figures and summary table presented later in the chapter.

Scenario Selection Rationale

The experimental design explores three main dimensions:

- surge multiplier (s),
- policy lag (τ),
- capacity increment (Δ_c).

The parameter grid is defined as follows:

- $s \in \{1.2, 1.5, 2.0\}$
- $\tau \in \{0, 15, 30, 60, 120\}$
- $\Delta_c \in \{0, 1, 2\}$

This scenario grid is intentionally interpretable. The selected surge multipliers represent mild, moderate, and severe demand stress. The selected lag values represent increasingly delayed institutional response, from immediate activation to substantial operational delay. The capacity increments represent no surge staffing, modest adaptation, and stronger adaptive intervention.

The grid is designed not to exhaust every possible parameter value, but to reveal the structural interaction among demand intensity, response delay, and recovery capacity. This choice supports the identification of instability regions and comparative policy effects without overwhelming the analysis with excessive dimensionality.

Replication Strategy and Summary Metrics

Because the model is stochastic, a single run is not sufficient to characterize system behavior reliably. Each scenario is therefore simulated multiple times under different random realizations. The replication strategy serves two purposes:

1. it reduces dependence on idiosyncratic trajectories,
2. it allows mean outcomes to be estimated for cross-scenario comparison.

For each simulation run, the following metrics are computed:

1. Overload duration (T_{over}):

total time during which the system remains in overload.

2. Recovery time (T_{rec}):

time from surge end or policy activation to return below the recovery threshold.

3. **Maximum queue length:**

peak waiting burden during the scenario.

4. **Mean waiting time:**

average delay experienced by patients before service.

5. **Throughput:**

completed services per unit time over the simulation horizon.

These measures were chosen because they collectively capture congestion intensity, persistence, patient delay, and recovery efficiency. They also map naturally onto healthcare management concerns, including access delay, crowding burden, and the speed with which the system can restore normal functioning.

Reproducibility and Practical Implementation Notes

A further advantage of the present simulation design is reproducibility. The Python implementation uses explicit scenario definitions, deterministic parameter grids, and repeated stochastic runs generated through pseudo-random sampling. Because the simulation is event-driven and modular, its logic can be inspected, modified, and extended without changing the conceptual foundation of the chapter.

From a practical standpoint, this reproducibility matters for two reasons. First, it aligns with the book's emphasis on computational methodology and theory-to-practice translation. Second, it allows future researchers or practitioners to adapt the code to more specific healthcare settings, such as calibrated emergency department flows, multi-stage triage systems, or time-varying staffing policies.

The simulation framework developed here should therefore be viewed as both a research instrument and a methodological template. It demonstrates how event-driven stochastic regime concepts can be operationalized computationally, while remaining simple enough to be extended by others.

Software Implementation and Availability

The event-driven healthcare regime framework was implemented in Python as a modular discrete-event simulation environment. The implementation follows the theoretical model developed in the event-driven regime framework and the accompanying regime instability analysis, representing arrivals, service completions, regime transitions, delayed policy activation and adaptive capacity changes as explicit simulation events.

The software architecture separates the simulation engine from analysis and visualization components. The main simulation module generates patient-flow event logs, regime timelines, and scenario-level performance indicators, while independent plotting utilities reproduce the figures and comparative analysis presented in this chapter.

The implementation includes configurable parameters for arrival rates, service capacity, surge magnitude, policy delay, and adaptive capacity interventions, enabling future researchers to extend the framework or adapt it to alternative healthcare scenarios.

The implementation uses Python-based event scheduling and stochastic sampling mechanisms to simulate the temporal evolution of the healthcare system. Simulation events are processed chronologically, including patient arrivals, service completions, demand surge activation, regime transitions and delayed policy responses. Generated outputs are exported in structured CSV format to enable independent analysis, visualization and reproduction of the reported simulation scenarios.

To support transparency, reproducibility, and future research extensions, the complete Python implementation, example outputs, visualization scripts, and documentation have been made publicly available: https://github.com/dimpapak/event-driven-healthcare-regime-simulation

Bridge to the Results Section

The simulation design described above provides the computational basis for testing the analytical claims developed in the regime instability analysis. By varying surge magnitude, policy lag, and adaptive capacity while preserving the same event-driven stochastic structure, the model makes it possible to observe whether overload duration, recovery time, and backlog accumulation behave in the manner predicted by the instability framework.

The next section presents the resulting simulation outputs and interprets them in operational healthcare terms. Particular attention is given to the temporal structure of queue growth and recovery, the emergence of empirical instability regions in parameter space, and the role of adaptive staffing in mitigating the effects of delayed intervention.

RESULTS AND CASE INSIGHTS

Overview of Simulation Outcomes

The discrete-event simulation experiments illustrate how stochastic demand shocks and delayed policy responses interact to produce operational regime transitions in healthcare service systems. The model captures patient arrivals, service completions, regime switches, and delayed capacity adjustments, allowing the system to evolve through normal operation, congestion, overload, and recovery phases.

The figures and numerical results presented in this section were generated using the publicly available Python implementation accompanying this chapter, ensuring reproducibility of the reported simulation scenarios.

Three complementary visualizations summarize the simulation outcomes. Figure 2 illustrates the temporal evolution of queue dynamics and regime transitions during a surge episode. Figure 3 presents a heatmap showing how overload duration varies with both surge magnitude and policy lag. Figure 4 evaluates the effect of policy strength by examining recovery time under different surge staffing levels.

Together, these results demonstrate that overload persistence is not determined solely by average utilization but by the interaction between demand shocks, response delays, and adaptive capacity policies. Similar observations have been documented in healthcare operations research, where delayed operational responses can amplify congestion dynamics in emergency departments [Green, 2006; Hall, 2013].

Regime Timeline and Queue Dynamics

Figure 2 presents a representative simulation trajectory showing the evolution of queue length $N_q(t)$, active service capacity $c(t)$, and traffic intensity $\rho(t)$ during a demand surge.

At the beginning of the simulation, the system operates in the *normal regime*, where the arrival rate λ_0 remains below service capacity $c_0\mu$. Under these conditions, queue length remains near zero and the traffic intensity $\rho < 1$, indicating stable operation consistent with classical queueing theory (Gross et al., 2018).

When the demand surge occurs, the arrival rate increases to (λ_s). During this period the traffic intensity exceeds unity:

$$\rho_s = \frac{\lambda_s}{c_0\mu} > 1$$

As a result, the expected drift of the queue becomes positive, and the number of waiting patients increases rapidly. Importantly, the capacity adjustment does not occur immediately. Instead, a policy lag (τ) separates overload detection from the activation of additional capacity. During this lag interval, arrivals exceed service completions, producing backlog accumulation.

Figure 2. Event-Driven Queue Dynamics Under Demand Surge, Policy Lag, and Recovery

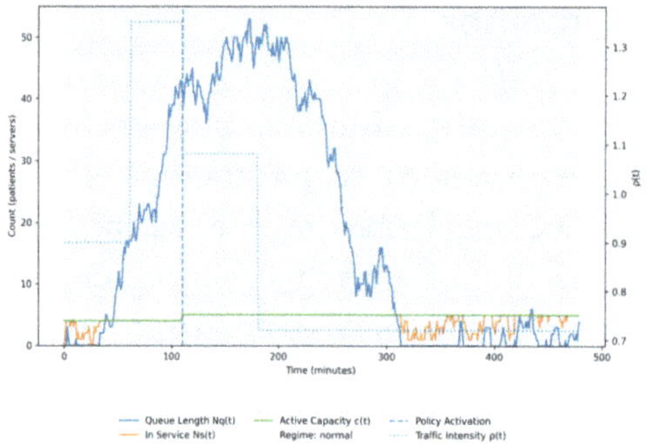

Note. The figure shows a representative simulation trajectory of the healthcare queueing system under an event-driven demand surge. The blue line denotes queue length $N_q(t)$, the orange line denotes the number of patients in service $N_s(t)$, and the green line denotes active service capacity **c(t)**. *The dotted blue line represents traffic intensity* **ρ(t)**, *while the dashed vertical line marks policy activation after delay (τ). Shaded regions indicate the progression of operational regimes from normal operation to overload and recovery. The trajectory illustrates backlog accumulation during the lag interval and subsequent clearance after adaptive capacity adjustment.*

The simulation trajectory clearly illustrates this accumulation phase. Queue length grows continuously until the scheduled policy activation event increases the number of active servers from (c_0) to $(c_0 + \Delta c)$. Once the additional capacity becomes available, the effective traffic intensity drops below unity, restoring negative queue drift and allowing the system to enter the recovery regime.

However, recovery is not instantaneous. Because a backlog has accumulated during the lag interval, the system must first process the queued patients before returning to normal operation. This phenomenon reflects the backlog amplification effect discussed earlier in the chapter.

Figure 3. Overload Duration Across Surge Magnitude and Policy Lag

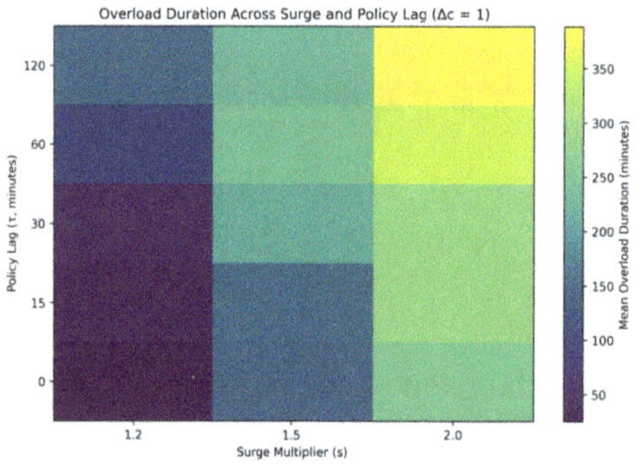

Note. The heatmap reports mean overload duration across simulation scenarios defined by surge multiplier (s)and policy lag (τ), for a fixed capacity increment Δ_c = 1. Darker-to-lighter intensity indicates increasing time spent in the overload regime. The figure highlights the nonlinear interaction between surge magnitude and delayed policy response, revealing an empirical instability region in which modest increases in lag produce disproportionate increases in overload persistence.

Such dynamics are frequently observed in emergency departments, where operational adjustments—such as activating surge staffing or opening additional treatment areas—require time to implement (Green, 2006; Kolker, 2008).

Instability Regions Under Demand Surges

While the timeline visualization provides intuition for a single scenario, a broader view emerges when examining multiple combinations of surge magnitude and policy lag.

Figure 3 presents a heatmap showing the mean overload duration across different parameter combinations. The horizontal axis represents the *surge multiplier* (s) applied to the baseline arrival rate, while the vertical axis represents the *policy lag* (τ) in minutes. Each cell reports the mean time the system remains in the overload regime.

Two key patterns emerge from this analysis.

First, overload duration increases as the magnitude of the demand surge grows. Larger surges produce stronger positive queue drift because arrivals exceed service capacity by a wider margin. Consequently, backlog accumulates more rapidly.

Second, overload duration grows with increasing policy lag. Even when surge intensity remains constant, longer delays in activating additional capacity allow queues to grow for a longer period before corrective action occurs.

Most importantly, the heatmap reveals a nonlinear interaction between surge magnitude and policy lag. Under moderate surges, small delays may have limited impact. However, when the system operates close to capacity limits, identical delays produce disproportionately large increases in overload duration. This pattern corresponds to the *regime instability* threshold discussed earlier in the chapter.

Operational studies of emergency department congestion have similarly shown that delays in activating surge protocols can substantially increase patient waiting times and system crowding (Hall, 2013; Worthington, 1987).

Recovery Dynamics and Policy Strength

The final experiment evaluates the effect of *policy strength*, represented by the capacity increment (Δc) applied during surge response.

Figure 4 shows the mean recovery time as a function of policy lag for three staffing policies: no additional capacity ($\Delta c = 0$), moderate surge staffing ($\Delta c = 1$), and stronger surge staffing ($\Delta c = 2$).

Figure 4. Recovery Time as a Function of Policy Lag Under Alternative Surge Staffing Policies

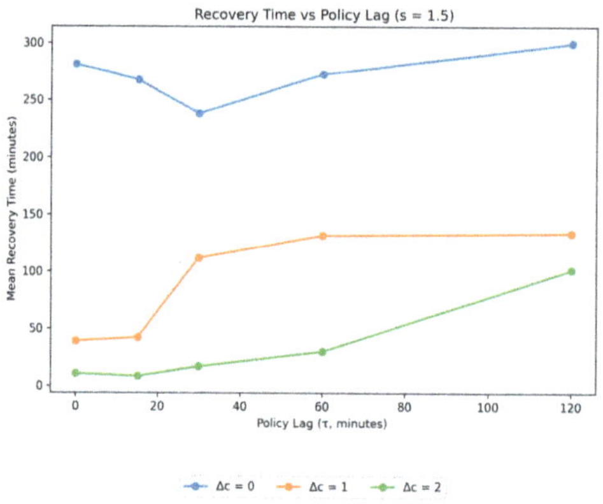

Note. The figure shows mean recovery time as a function of policy lag (τ) for three adaptive capacity policies: no additional capacity (Δ_c = 0), moderate surge staffing (Δ_c = 1), and stronger surge staffing (Δ_c = 2), under a fixed surge level (s = 1.5). The results demonstrate that recovery time increases with delayed response, while stronger adaptive capacity adjustment substantially reduces the persistence of backlog and accelerates return to stable operation.

When no additional capacity is introduced, recovery time increases substantially as policy lag grows. In this case the system must process accumulated backlog using the same baseline capacity that initially produced the overload condition.

Introducing even a modest capacity increase significantly reduces recovery time. Additional servers increase the effective service rate, accelerating backlog clearance once policy activation occurs.

The strongest policy scenario ($\Delta c = 2$) produces the fastest recovery across all lag values, highlighting the importance of adaptive staffing policies in healthcare operations. These results align with empirical findings that surge staffing and flexible capacity allocation can mitigate congestion in high-demand hospital environments.

Overall, the simulation results demonstrate that system resilience depends not only on the magnitude of demand shocks but also on the **speed and strength of operational responses**.

Summary Metrics

Table 2. Summary Performance Metrics Across Selected Simulation Scenarios

Surge Multiplier (s)	Policy Lag (τ)	Capacity Increase (Δc)	Overload Duration (min)	Recovery Time (min)	Mean Waiting Time	Mean Max Queue Length	Mean Throughput
1.2	0	0	212.03	79.41	7.08	23.5	0.9138
1.2	0	1	25.21	14.60	1.97	12.3	0.9483
1.5	30	0	351.51	238.39	27.49	57.8	0.9633
1.5	30	1	217.97	111.95	10.38	41.1	1.0410

continued on following page

Table 2. Continued

Surge Multiplier (s)	Policy Lag (τ)	Capacity Increase (Δc)	Overload Duration (min)	Recovery Time (min)	Mean Waiting Time	Mean Max Queue Length	Mean Throughput
2.0	120	0	424.28	300.00	68.94	117.7	0.9679
2.0	120	1	388.53	276.61	38.87	98.6	1.1021

Note. The table presents representative results from the discrete-event simulation across selected combinations of surge multiplier (s), policy lag (τ), and adaptive capacity increment (Δ_c). Reported values correspond to mean overload duration, mean recovery time, mean waiting time, mean maximum queue length, and mean throughput across 10 simulation replications. The selected scenarios illustrate mild, intermediate, and severe surge conditions, together with the effect of introducing an adaptive capacity increase under otherwise comparable operating conditions.

Table 2 summarizes key operational metrics averaged across simulation replications.

The table reinforces the main simulation findings by showing how operational performance deteriorates as surge magnitude and policy delay increase, and how adaptive capacity partially mitigates this deterioration. Under the mild scenario ($s = 1.2, \tau = 0$), introducing a modest capacity increase ($\Delta_c = 1$) reduces overload duration from 212.03 to 25.21 minutes and recovery time from 79.41 to 14.60 minutes, while also lowering mean waiting time and maximum queue length. Under the intermediate scenario ($s = 1.5, \tau = 30$), the same adaptive response still improves performance substantially, although overload and recovery remain more persistent, indicating that delay begins to interact more strongly with surge intensity. Under the severe scenario ($s = 2.0, \tau = 120$), system performance deteriorates sharply, with prolonged overload, long recovery time, and large queue accumulation even after capacity adjustment.

These results show that adaptive staffing remains beneficial across all scenarios, but its effectiveness declines as the system moves deeper into the instability region defined by strong demand shocks and delayed intervention.

Healthcare Implications

First, healthcare service systems operating near capacity are highly sensitive to demand shocks. Even modest increases in arrival rates can produce rapid queue growth.

Second, delayed policy responses amplify congestion dynamics. Operational protocols that detect overload conditions early and activate surge responses quickly may substantially reduce overload persistence.

Third, adaptive capacity policies—such as temporary staffing increases or flexible resource allocation—play a critical role in accelerating recovery after demand surges.

These insights are particularly relevant for emergency departments, which frequently experience stochastic demand fluctuations and require rapid operational adaptation to maintain service quality (Hall, 2013; Kolker, 2008).

CONCLUSIONS AND FUTURE RESEARCH

Conclusions

Healthcare service systems operate under persistent uncertainty arising from stochastic demand, constrained resources, and delayed operational responses. Traditional queueing models provide valuable analytical tools for evaluating system performance under steady-state conditions; however, their assumptions often become inadequate during periods of operational stress, such as demand surges, epidemic waves, or staffing disruptions.

This chapter introduced an event-driven stochastic regime framework for analysing healthcare queueing systems subject to demand shocks and delayed policy interventions. By extending the classical M/M/c queue with regime-dependent dynamics and policy lag, the framework captures the transition between operational regimes including normal operation, congestion, overload, and recovery.

The theoretical analysis demonstrated that policy lag can produce backlog amplification, whereby queue growth during delayed response periods significantly increases recovery time even after corrective capacity adjustments are implemented. A simulation-grounded instability condition was proposed to characterize the interaction between surge magnitude, baseline utilization, policy lag, and capacity adjustment.

To illustrate these dynamics, a discrete-event simulation model was developed using synthetic patient arrival streams and event-driven regime transitions. Simulation results revealed three key operational insights.

First, demand surges produce rapid queue growth when arrival rates exceed service capacity, pushing the system into an overload regime. Second, delays in activating surge policies amplify congestion by allowing backlog accumulation before capacity adjustments take effect. Third, stronger surge staffing policies substantially reduce recovery time and mitigate the persistence of overload.

The results demonstrate that healthcare system resilience depends not only on average utilization levels but also on the timing and strength of adaptive policy responses. In operational environments such as emergency departments, where demand variability is significant, proactive monitoring and rapid activation of surge protocols may play a critical role in maintaining service stability.

Limitations

Several limitations of the present framework should be acknowledged.

First, the simulation experiments rely on synthetic demand scenarios, which are designed to capture stylized surge dynamics rather than reproduce specific hospital datasets. While this approach allows controlled experimentation with regime transitions, empirical calibration using real operational data would further strengthen the practical applicability of the model.

Second, the service model assumes exponentially distributed service times and homogeneous servers, as in the classical M/M/c queue. In practice, healthcare service times may exhibit greater variability and may depend on patient acuity levels, treatment complexity, or resource availability.

Third, the current framework considers a single service stage, whereas many healthcare systems involve multi-stage patient flows including triage, diagnostics, treatment, and admission decisions. Extending the model to multi-stage queueing networks would provide a more comprehensive representation of hospital operations.

Future Research Directions

The regime-based modelling approach developed in this chapter opens several promising directions for future research.

One important direction involves empirical calibration using hospital operational data, such as emergency department arrival streams, patient waiting times, and staffing schedules. Integrating real-world datasets would enable estimation of regime transition parameters and validation of instability thresholds observed in simulation.

Another avenue concerns the development of early-warning indicators for regime transitions. Metrics such as queue persistence, variance amplification, and real-time estimates of traffic intensity may provide actionable signals for hospital administrators seeking to anticipate overload conditions before they escalate.

Future work may also explore adaptive control policies that dynamically adjust staffing levels based on predictive models of demand surges. Such approaches could incorporate real-time monitoring systems, machine learning–based forecasting, or reinforcement learning–based capacity management.

Finally, extending the framework to multi-class patient flows and multi-stage healthcare networks would allow analysis of more complex operational environments, including triage prioritization, inpatient boarding effects, and cross-department resource sharing.

By integrating stochastic modelling, simulation analysis, and operational policy design, regime-based approaches may contribute to the development of more resilient healthcare systems capable of adapting to uncertainty and sudden demand shocks.

While the proposed framework captures the fundamental dynamics of overload formation, delayed adaptation, and recovery, real healthcare environments involve additional operational complexity. Emergency departments and hospital systems include triage decisions, heterogeneous patient acuity levels, diagnostic pathways, inpatient admission constraints, and multi-stage resource interactions.

The current model intentionally adopts an abstract queueing representation to isolate the mechanisms responsible for regime transitions. Future extensions may integrate multi-stage queueing networks, patient prioritization mechanisms and empirical hospital datasets to further evaluate regime dynamics in operational healthcare environments.

Software Availability

The Python implementation supporting the proposed Event-Driven Healthcare Regime framework is publicly available at:

https://github.com/dimpapak/event-driven-healthcare-regime-simulation

The repository contains source code, simulation scripts, representative outputs, generated figures and documentation required to reproduce the computational experiments presented in this chapter.

AI DISCLOSURE STATEMENT

The author used ChatGPT to assist with language refinement, editorial revision, manuscript organization and graphical visualization of the simulation workflow. All theoretical developments, mathematical formulations, simulation design, implementation, results, interpretation and conclusions are original work of the author.

REFERENCES

Asplin, B. R., Magid, D. J., Rhodes, K. V., Solberg, L. I., Lurie, N., & Camargo, C. A.Jr. (2003). A conceptual model of emergency department crowding. *Annals of Emergency Medicine*, *42*(2), 173–180. DOI: 10.1067/mem.2003.302 PMID: 12883504

Brailsford, S. C., Harper, P. R., Patel, B., & Pitt, M. (2009). An analysis of the academic literature on simulation and modelling in healthcare. *Journal of Simulation*, *3*(3), 130–140. DOI: 10.1057/jos.2009.10

Brailsford, S. C., Lattimer, V. A., Tarnaras, P., & Turnbull, J. C. (2004). Emergency and on-demand health care: Modelling a large complex system. *The Journal of the Operational Research Society*, *55*(1), 34–42. DOI: 10.1057/palgrave.jors.2601667

Eppich, W., & Reedy, G. (2022). Advancing healthcare simulation research: Innovations in theory, methodology, and method. *Advances in Simulation (London, England)*, *7*(1), 23. DOI: 10.1186/s41077-022-00219-y PMID: 35897062

Green, L. V. (2006). Queueing analysis in healthcare. Patient Flow: Reducing Delay in Healthcare Delivery, 281–307.

Green, L. V., Kolesar, P. J., & Soares, J. (2001). Improving the SIPP approach for staffing service systems that have cyclic demands. *Operations Research*, *49*(4), 549–564. DOI: 10.1287/opre.49.4.549.11228

Gross, D., Shortle, J., Thompson, J., & Harris, C. (2018). *Fundamentals of queueing theory* (5th ed.). Wiley.

Haldane, V., De Foo, C., Abdalla, S. M., Jung, A.-S., Tan, M., Wu, S., Chua, A., Verma, M., Shrestha, P., Singh, S., Perez, T., Tan, S. M., Bartos, M., Mabuchi, S., Bonk, M., McNab, C., Werner, G. K., Panjabi, R., Nordström, A., & Legido-Quigley, H. (2021). Health systems resilience in managing the COVID-19 pandemic: Lessons from 28 countries. *Nature Medicine*, *27*(6), 964–980. DOI: 10.1038/s41591-021-01381-y PMID: 34002090

Hall, R. W. (2013). *Patient flow: Reducing delay in healthcare delivery*. Springer. DOI: 10.1007/978-1-4614-9512-3

Hick, J. L., Hanfling, D., Burstein, J. L., DeAtley, C., Barbisch, D., Bogdan, G. M., & Cantrill, S. (2004). Health care facility and community strategies for patient care surge capacity. *Annals of Emergency Medicine*, *44*(3), 253–261. DOI: 10.1016/j.annemergmed.2004.04.011 PMID: 15332068

Hoot, N. R., & Aronsky, D. (2008). Systematic review of emergency department crowding: Causes, effects, and solutions. *Annals of Emergency Medicine*, *52*(2), 126–136.e1. DOI: 10.1016/j.annemergmed.2008.03.014 PMID: 18433933

Jun, J. B., Jacobson, S. H., & Swisher, J. R. (1999). Application of discrete-event simulation in healthcare clinics. *The Journal of the Operational Research Society*, *50*(2), 109–123. DOI: 10.1057/palgrave.jors.2600669

Kolker, A. (2008). Process modelling of emergency department patient flow: Effect of patient length of stay on ED diversion. *Journal of Medical Systems*, *32*(5), 389–401. DOI: 10.1007/s10916-008-9144-x PMID: 18814495

Litvak, E., & Long, M. C. (2000). Cost and quality under managed care: Irreconcilable differences? *The American Journal of Managed Care*, *6*(3), 305–312. PMID: 10977431

Litvak, E., Long, M. C., Cooper, A. B., & McManus, M. L. (2001). Emergency department diversion: Causes and solutions. *Academic Emergency Medicine*, *8*(11), 1108–1110. PMID: 11691678

Monks, T., Currie, C. S. M., Onggo, B. S., Robinson, S., Kunc, M., & Taylor, S. J. E. (2019). Strengthening the reporting of empirical simulation studies: Introducing the STRESS guidelines. *Journal of Simulation*, *13*(1), 55–67. DOI: 10.1080/17477778.2018.1442155

Whitt, W. (1991). The pointwise stationary approximation for Mt/Mt/s queues is asymptotically correct as the rates increase. *Management Science*, *37*(3), 307–314. DOI: 10.1287/mnsc.37.3.307

Worthington, D. (1987). Queueing models for hospital waiting lists. *The Journal of the Operational Research Society*, *38*(5), 413–422. DOI: 10.1057/jors.1987.69 PMID: 10282336

KEY TERMS AND DEFINITIONS

Adaptive Capacity Policy: Operational strategies that dynamically adjust healthcare service capacity—such as staffing levels or treatment resources—in response to demand fluctuations.

Discrete-Event Simulation: A simulation methodology in which system dynamics evolve through a sequence of discrete events, such as arrivals, service completions, or policy activations.

Emergency Department Overcrowding: A condition in which patient demand exceeds available treatment capacity, leading to prolonged waiting times and operational congestion.

Policy Lag: The delay between the detection of an operational problem (such as overload) and the implementation of corrective actions, such as activating surge staffing.

Regime Instability: A condition in which operational performance deteriorates disproportionately due to delayed responses to demand shocks, resulting in prolonged overload and slow recovery.

Stochastic Demand Surge: A sudden increase in arrival rates caused by external or internal events, such as epidemic outbreaks, seasonal demand peaks, or operational disruptions.

Surge Staffing: The temporary increase of healthcare personnel or resources in response to high demand periods in order to restore service capacity.

Traffic Intensity: A queueing theory metric defined as the ratio of arrival rate to service capacity, indicating the utilization level of a service system.

Chapter 4
Strategic Phase Transitions in Healthcare Production Systems:
A 4-Dimensional Model of Resource Allocation, Technology, and Performance Optimisation

Anastasius S. Moumtzoglou
http://orcid.org/0000-0002-5899-1033
P&A Kyriakou Children's Hospital, Greece

ABSTRACT

The healthcare trilemma, which involves balancing quantity, quality, and cost, is often treated as if these factors operate independently. This chapter demonstrates their significant interdependence and identifies technology as a pivotal factor. Using a four-dimensional production model (Quantity, Quality, Technology, Cost) evaluated across more than 60 scenarios, the analysis yields five principal findings. First, optimal technology investment increases smoothly as technological capability matures, with allocation rising from approximately 10% at low capability to about 35% at full maturity. Second, technology reduces costs (r = -0.956) and increases efficiency by 59% as technology levels increase from the lowest to the highest. Third, technology level is the primary driver of gradual strategic reallocation, with optimal strategies evolving smoothly rather than abruptly. Fourth, investment in quality alone is comparatively less effective. Fifth, the Continuous Strategic Adjustment Framework offers a rigorous foundation for future models that incorporate uncertainty.

INTRODUCTION

Healthcare systems, ranging from national services to individual departments, face the challenge of providing adequate, high-quality care within limited budgets and staffing levels. These objectives are linked by complex, often non-linear trade-offs.

Historically, each aspect of the healthcare trilemma has been studied independently. Health economists evaluate efficiency using Data Envelopment Analysis (Gavurova et al., 2021; Yu et al., 2024), quality researchers develop clinical outcome measures (Donabedian, 1988; OECD, 2024), and operations

DOI: 10.4018/979-8-3373-9705-4.ch004

managers focus on patient flow and capacity (Litvak & Long, 2000). This compartmentalised approach neglects essential interdependencies: decisions about quantity affect quality, quality choices influence cost, and cost constraints determine both quantity and quality outcomes.

Technology is central to managing these trade-offs. Innovations, including digital health records, telemedicine, robot-assisted surgery, and computer-aided diagnosis, enable greater automation, improve the quality of care, and increase operational efficiency.

However, implementing new technologies requires significant investment, and the resulting outcomes often remain uncertain.

Despite extensive research on healthcare system performance, there is a lack of comprehensive quantitative models that integrate mathematical analysis with empirical data to guide optimal resource allocation across quantity, quality, and technology within budget constraints. Existing models are typically:

1. Purely economic: Healthcare is treated as a linear production function with fixed coefficients, disregarding the strategic dimension of technology investment (Gavurova et al., 2021).
2. Purely clinical: Emphasis is placed on quality outcomes without formalising the resource allocation decisions that generate these outcomes (Donabedian, 1988).
3. Purely operational: Patient flow or capacity utilisation is optimised without incorporating quality or technology as decision variables (Litvak & Long, 2000).
4. Purely qualitative: Trade-offs are described narratively, without offering decision-makers implementable, quantitative allocation rules (Pisek & Greenhalgh, 2001; Braithwaite et al., 2017).

This chapter addresses this gap by introducing a four-dimensional production model. The model illustrates how resources such as time, funding, and staff are converted into output, quality, cost, and performance. It uses a concise set of key parameters to promote clarity, simplicity, and adaptability across various healthcare settings.

Simulations and sensitivity analyses across more than 60 scenarios and seven parameter groups indicate that optimal technology investment increases steadily with technological capability. The optimal allocation to technology (β) rises from 10% at low capability levels (tech = 0.1-0.5), to approximately 25% at intermediate levels (tech = 0.6-0.7), and reaches about 35% at full technological maturity (tech = 1.0). This gradual progression shows that balanced strategies consistently outperform extreme specialisation at all technology levels, with the optimal allocation remaining within the "Mixed Strategy" region even at high technological capability.

This finding constitutes a significant refinement rather than a marginal improvement. Organisations at all technology levels should avoid extreme specialisation in any single dimension. Instead of waiting for a hypothetical threshold to prompt radical reallocation, organisations should pursue continuous, incremental increases in technology investment as digital maturity advances.

Although this chapter is methodologically and conceptually independent, it builds upon the previous chapter's Hybrid Complexity Model for Healthcare Systems. The earlier chapter analysed inter-hospital connections and knowledge sharing, whereas the present chapter focuses on internal resources and the utilisation of technology. Together, these chapters offer a comprehensive perspective on the complexity of healthcare, addressing both external interactions and internal operations.

Both models are based on the understanding that healthcare systems display non-linear dynamics, critical thresholds, and emergent behaviours that linear models cannot capture. Each model relies on OECD data, computer simulations, and transparent mathematical methods to support their findings.

BACKGROUND

Production Functions in Healthcare: From Cobb-Douglas to DEA

Economic analyses of healthcare production have historically relied on two primary paradigms.

The first paradigm, prevalent since the 1960s, involves the use of parametric production functions by hospitals and health systems, particularly the Cobb-Douglas form $Q = A\, K^\alpha \cdot L^\beta$ (Feldstein, 1967). In these models, capital (K) and labour (L) are treated as inputs, while patient visits or discharges are treated as outputs. Although these models are analytically tractable, they present three main limitations: (1) they assume complete substitutability of inputs, which may not reflect clinical realities; (2) they treat quality as an exogenous or unobserved variable; and (3) they fail to distinguish technology as a strategic factor separate from capital.

The second paradigm employs non-parametric frontier methods, particularly Data Envelopment Analysis (DEA), which has become the standard for cross-national health system benchmarking. For example, Gavurova et al. (2021) utilised dynamic network DEA to analyse OECD countries from 2000 to 2016, modelling public health and medical care as interconnected sub-systems. Yu et al. (2024) further extended this approach to assess the efficiency of COVID-19 treatment by incorporating both undesirable outputs (mortality) and desirable outputs (recovered patients). While these studies offer rigorous efficiency assessments, they remain inherently descriptive, measuring the distance from an observed frontier rather than providing normative, prescriptive allocation rules for decision-makers.

Beyond the two principal paradigms, analyses of healthcare production utilise various alternative methodological frameworks. Each framework offers specific advantages for addressing the complexity inherent in healthcare systems.

1. Parametric econometric models, such as Stochastic Frontier Analysis and Generalised Linear Models, are used to account for statistical noise in the data. These models also facilitate rigorous hypothesis testing of the parameters governing production processes.
2. Non-parametric and semiparametric methodologies, including Generalised Additive Models, relax restrictive functional-form assumptions. This approach increases model flexibility while preserving the interpretability required for empirical analysis.
3. Another category includes joint and simulation-based methods, such as Bayesian estimation techniques and panel data regressions. These methods are notable for their ability to incorporate prior information and to model the temporal dynamics that characterise production relationships in healthcare.

The proposed model occupies an intermediate position between these paradigms. It is parametric, featuring an explicit functional form, and incorporates quality as an endogenous output. The model is prescriptive, generating optimal allocations of α, β, and γ, and is calibrated using realistic parameter intervals informed by OECD benchmarks. This approach bridges the gap between econometric estimation and managerial decision support.

The Quality-Cost Trade-Off: Empirical Evidence and Theoretical

Puzzles

The empirical relationship between quality and cost in healthcare remains contested. Certain studies report that higher quality correlates with increased costs, attributed to greater staffing, superior equipment, and extended consultations, which aligns with a traditional production trade-off. Conversely, other studies indicate that higher quality is associated with lower costs, due to fewer complications, reduced readmissions, and fewer malpractice claims, thereby suggesting that quality may be "free" over the long term (Institute of Medicine, 2001).

This contradiction highlights the model's main claim: technology moderates the relationship between quality and cost in healthcare. Across all levels of technological advancement, quality and quantity compete for limited resources under a binding cost constraint; thus, improving quality necessitates either reducing quantity or incurring higher costs. As technological capability increases, however, the production function shifts:

- Technology reduces the marginal cost of both quality and quantity.
- Enabling simultaneous improvement across all dimensions.
- The quality-cost relationship is not constant; it depends on the technological level. In summary, as technology advances, it can improve both quality and cost efficiency, thereby altering their relationship over time.

Technology as a Strategic Variable: Beyond Automation

The strategic management literature has long identified technology as a source of competitive advantage. Porter (1985) distinguishes between cost leadership, which focuses on price competition, and differentiation, which emphasises uniqueness. Technology can support either strategy. Treacy and Wiersema (1995) further refined these concepts into three value disciplines. Christensen (1997) extended this by examining how disruptive technologies can reshape entire industries.

- Operational excellence.
- Product leadership, and
- Customer intimacy.

In Table 1, we operationalise these strategic archetypes as distinct regions within the parameter domain (α, β, γ):

Table 1. Strategic Archetypes and Resource Allocation Patterns

Strategic Archetype	Allocation Pattern	Description
Operational Excellence	High γ, low α, low β	Mass Production mode; maximises quantity while minimising cost
Product Leadership	High α, moderate β, low γ	Quality Orientation; prioritises clinical excellence
Customer Intimacy / Innovation	High β, moderate α, low γ	Innovation Integration; accessible at all technology levels, but never optimal as an exclusive strategy

We define them as distinct regions within the parameter domain.

- Operational Excellence (high γ, low α, low β) corresponds to the Mass Production mode. This mode maximises quantity while minimising cost.
- Product Leadership (high α, moderate β) aligns with Quality Orientation. It prioritises clinical excellence.
- Customer Intimacy, or Innovation Integration in this context (high β, moderate α, low γ), is accessible at all technology levels. However, it is never optimal when pursued as an exclusive strategy. The model shows that allocating more than 40% of resources to any single dimension reduces overall efficiency.

This mapping extends beyond taxonomy. The model shows that these strategies vary in effectiveness. Extreme specialisation, particularly in technology, consistently underperforms compared to balanced approaches, regardless of technological capability. Pursuing a differentiation strategy with concentrated resources results in lower efficiency and higher costs.

Phase Transitions in Organisational Strategy

The idea of phase transitions comes from physics, where it describes sudden changes in behaviour as a parameter crosses a threshold—for example, when water boils at 100°C. This idea is now also used in fields such as economics, sociology, and management. Models such as Schelling's (1971) theory of segregation, Granovetter's (1978) study of group actions, and research on tipping points (Gladwell, 2000) all show a similar pattern: small changes in something measured, like how accepting people are or how many people start using something, can lead to big, sudden changes in what happens as a whole.

This model draws on the theory of phase transitions to examine whether increases in technological capability trigger abrupt shifts in technology investment. The results indicate that while the marginal return on technology investment rises with greater capability, the relationship remains continuous rather than discontinuous—unlike classic phase transitions. As technology matures, technology investment becomes increasingly justified for boosting productivity and reducing costs. However, these gains do not result in technology investment dominating resource allocation: the optimal β plateaus at about 35%, even at peak technology capability.

Sensitivity Analysis and Model Robustness in Health Services

A common criticism of production models in healthcare concerns their sensitivity to arbitrary parameter choices. Studies employing the same Data Envelopment Analysis (DEA) specification, but varying input or output selections, frequently yield conflicting efficiency rankings (Jacobs et al., 2006). Such inconsistencies reduce confidence in model-based recommendations.

Our approach is grounded in both transparency and rigorous robustness testing.

We affirm that our parameter choices (for example, QUALITY_COST_FACTOR = 30 and TECH_SAVINGS_FACTOR = 20) do not limit the generalizability of our findings. We systematically vary each parameter across broad, plausible ranges and consistently demonstrate that the qualitative result—a smooth, continuous relationship between technology capability and optimal resource allocation—holds across all specifications.

This robustness clearly differentiates our model from opaque optimisation routines and underscores its reliability for decision-making under parametric uncertainty.

The Gap: An Integrative, Decision-Ready Production Model

A synthesis of the literature reveals four essential requirements for a production model that can effectively guide healthcare resource allocation decisions:

- First, a multi-dimensional output is required: the model must jointly represent quantity, quality, and cost or efficiency.
- Strategic technology endogeneity: The model must treat technology as a decision variable rather than as a fixed exogenous factor.
- Third, the model should account for non-linear dynamics, accommodating continuous strategic evolution and not assuming either discontinuous regime changes or continuous substitutability.
- Finally, parametric transparency and robustness are vital: the model must be fully specified, easily modifiable, and extensively tested for sensitivity.

Currently, no available production model in the literature meets all four requirements described above for guiding healthcare resource allocation.

METHODOLOGY

The 4-Dimensional Production Model

Model Overview and Philosophical Commitments

The Quad Production Model is a deterministic (outputs depend solely on inputs), continuous (small input changes cause small output changes), and non-linear (input-output relationships are not directly proportional) framework for allocating scarce resources among three goals: Quantity (number of services), Quality (level of clinical excellence), and Technology (ability to innovate processes).

These allocations, or the distribution of resources among the three functions, result in four observable outcomes: Quantity (Q), Quality (QL), Cost (C), and Efficiency (E).

The model is governed by five philosophical commitments:

1. Parsimony

The model uses the minimum number of parameters needed to capture basic trade-offs. Each parameter has a clear theoretical meaning.

2. Transparency

All equations are open and fully specified. There are no hidden calibration steps or proprietary algorithms.

3. Modularity

Each component, such as quantity, quality, and cost functions, can be changed independently. This allows the model to fit specific production technologies.

4. Robustness

No strategic recommendation depends on a single parameter. Extensive sensitivity analyses validate all findings.

5. Actionability

The model's outputs, including optimal allocations of α, β, and γ, are easy to interpret. They can represent budget percentages, staffing ratios, or investment priorities.

Decision Variables: The Allocation Vector (α, β, γ)

Resources are distributed to three competing functions:

- α (alpha): quality improvement activities, like training, protocol development, and quality assurance staffing.
- β (beta): Technological investment, including equipment, software, and digital infrastructure.
- γ (gamma): quantity production, such as direct clinical staffing, supplies, and patient contact hours.

Feasibility Constraints

$0 \leq \alpha \leq 1, \quad 0 \leq \beta \leq 1, \quad 0 \leq \gamma \leq 1$

$\alpha + \beta + \gamma = 1$ (with tolerance ε = 0.01 for floating-point imprecision)

The allocation vector (α, β, γ) is the independent variable of the model. All outcomes are deterministic functions of this vector and the exogenous parameters defined below.

Exogenous Parameters: Fixed Model Constants

The model uses seven fixed parameters that define production technology and are calibrated in the baseline to yield realistic outputs (Table 2).

Table 2. Baseline Model Parameters

Parameter	Symbol	Value	Description
Total Resources	R	100	Dimensionless resource units (e.g., budget in thousands €, staffing FTEs)
Base Cost	BASE_COST	50	The fixed cost component is independent of allocation
Quality Cost Factor	QUALITY_COST_FACTOR	30	Multiplier for the cost of quality investment
Technology Savings Factor	TECH_SAVINGS_FACTOR	20	Multiplier for technology's cost-reduction effect
Technology Cost Factor	TECH_COST_FACTOR	15	Multiplier for technology's implementation cost
Technology Cost Power	TECH_COST_POWER	1.3	Non-linearity in the technology cost function
Quantity Power	QUANTITY_POWER	0.7	Elasticity of quantity with respect to resource input
Quality Power	QUALITY_POWER	0.5	Elasticity of quality with respect to resource input
Quality Cost Power	QUALITY_COST_POWER	1.2	Non-linearity in the quality cost function
Max Quality Score	MAX_QUALITY_SCORE	10.0	Upper bound for normalised quality output
Technology Level	tech	0.5 (baseline)	Exogenous capability parameter [0,1]

The term 'technology level' (tech) refers to the organisation's baseline technological capability and warrants specific consideration. In the baseline model, tech is treated as an exogenous parameter representing this capability. It is distinct from β, which denotes the allocation to technology investment. This distinction is essential: β reflects current technology investment, whereas tech indicates the effectiveness of that technology, incorporating prior investments, learning curve effects, and infrastructure maturity. The principal finding is that the optimal value of β increases continuously as tech improves.

Outcome Functions: The 4 Dimensions

Quantity Production Function

Quantity of services produced is modelled as a Cobb-Douglas style power function of resources allocated to quantity ($\gamma \cdot R$), modified by a technology multiplier that depends on both the technology level (tech) and the allocation to technology (β):

$$Q = (\gamma \cdot R)^\wedge(QUANTITY\_POWER) \cdot [1 + tech \cdot \beta \cdot QUANTITY\_TECH\_MULTIPLIER]$$

where:

- $(\gamma \cdot R)^\wedge(QUANTITY\_POWER)$: diminishing returns to scale in quantity production
- *QUANTITY_TECH_MULTIPLIER* = 2.0: technology amplifies quantity output
- The technology term is multiplicative: technology increases the productivity of quantity-directed resources.

Boundary protection: Q is capped at *MAX_QUANTITY_BASE* = 10,000 to prevent overflow; in practice, with R = 100, Q ranges from 5 to 30.

Quality Production Function

Quality of care is modelled as a similar power function of resources allocated to quality ($\alpha \cdot R$), also modified by a technology multiplier that depends on both the technology level (tech) and the allocation to technology (β):

$$QL\_raw = (\alpha \cdot R)^\wedge(QUALITY\_POWER) \cdot [1 + tech \cdot \beta \cdot QUALITY\_TECH\_MULTIPLIER]$$

$$QL\_norm = min(MAX\_QUALITY\_SCORE, QL\_raw / 10.0)$$

where:

- $(\alpha \cdot R)^\wedge(QUALITY\_POWER)$: diminishing returns to scale in quality production
  - *QUALITY_TECH_MULTIPLIER* = 0.8: technology improves quality (smaller effect than on quantity)
- Division by 10.0 and capping at *MAX_QUALITY_SCORE* = 10.0 normalises quality to a 0-10 scale.

Note: Quality power (0.5) is lower than quantity power (0.7), indicating the assumption that quality is more difficult to scale with resource inputs alone. Importantly, technology investment (β) directly affects quality output, reflecting the reality that technologies such as clinical decision support, electronic health records, and robotic surgery can improve clinical outcomes.

Cost Function

Total cost is modelled as the sum of a fixed base cost, a quality cost component, and a technology implementation cost, minus technology savings:

$$C = BASE_{COST} + QUALITY_{COST_{FACTOR}} \cdot \alpha^{QUALITY_{COST_{POWER}}} + TECH_{COST_{FACTOR}} \cdot \beta^{TECH_{COST_{POWER}}} - TECH_{SAVINGS_{FACTOR}} \cdot tech \cdot \beta$$

where:

- $BASE\_COST = 50$: fixed overhead
- $QUALITY\_COST\_FACTOR \cdot \alpha$^($QUALITY\_COST\_POWER$): quality investment

increases cost, with power 1.2 > 1 indicating increasing marginal cost of quality

- $TECH\_COST\_FACTOR \cdot \beta$^($TECH\_COST\_POWER$): technology investment incurs implementation costs, with power 1.3 > 1 indicating increasing marginal cost of technology
- $TECH\_SAVINGS\_FACTOR$ · tech · β: technology investment reduces cost, linear in both tech and β
- Minimum cost floor: $C \geq BASE\_COST \cdot MIN\_COST\_MULTIPLIER$ (0.5) to prevent negative or unrealistically low cost

Critical symmetry refers to a situation in which investments in both quality and technology lead to higher costs due to rising marginal costs (with exponents greater than 1 for each). However, technology investments yield offsetting savings that increase as technological capability improves. This symmetric approach ensures that the cost structure does not artificially favour technology over quality.

Production Mode Classification

The model classifies each allocation vector into one of four production modes based on which parameter (α, β, γ) is maximal. This classification is purely descriptive and does not affect the efficiency calculation or optimisation:

Mode 1: Innovation Integration

Condition: $\beta > \alpha$ *AND* $\beta > \gamma$ *AND* $\beta > MODE\_THRESHOLD$ (0.6)
Strategy: Technology-centred production; technology is the dominant resource allocation.

Mode 2: Quality Orientation

Condition: $\alpha > \beta$ *AND* $\alpha > \gamma$ *AND* $\alpha > MODE\_THRESHOLD$
Strategy: Quality-centred production; clinical excellence prioritised.

Mode 3: Mass Production

Condition: $\gamma > \alpha$ *AND* $\gamma > \beta$ *AND* $\gamma > MODE\_THRESHOLD$
Strategy: Volume-centred production; maximising patient throughput.

Mode 4: Mixed Strategy

Condition: No parameter transcends *MODE_THRESHOLD*
Strategy: Balanced apportionment across all three dimensions.
It is important to note that the mode classification is for descriptive purposes only. The efficiency objective function does not include any mode-based multiplier.

Efficiency (Principal Objective)

Efficiency is defined as output value per unit cost, where output value is the product of quantity and quality (normalised):

$E = (Q \cdot QL\_norm) / C$

Rationale

$Q \cdot QL\_norm$ captures the volume-quality product: a hospital that sees many patients but provides poor care has low output value; a hospital that provides excellent care to few patients also has low output value.
Division by C captures cost efficiency: producing the same output value at a lower cost is superior.
Efficiency is the model's primary objective. All optimisation results refer to maximisation of E unless otherwise stated.

Search Algorithm and Scenario Generation

The model does not assume convexity or differentiability; therefore, we use exhaustive grid search rather than gradient-based optimisation.
For baseline analysis

- $\alpha \in [0.1, 0.8]$ in 15 steps

- For each α, $\beta \in [0.1, 0.8 - \alpha]$ in 3-10 steps (with denser sampling near the expected transition region for technology levels between 0.55 and 0.85)

- $\gamma = 1 - \alpha - \beta$, requiring $\gamma \geq 0.05$

This generates approximately 60-120 feasible (α, β, γ) triples per model run. Each triple is evaluated exactly without stochasticity.
Optimal strategies are identified by sorting on efficiency (E) and selecting the maximum.

For Technology Scenario Comparison

- tech ∈ {0.1, 0.3, 0.5, 0.6, 0.65, 0.7, 0.75, 0.8, 0.9, 1.0}
- Full grid search repeated for each tech level
- Comparison of optimal (α, β, γ) and resulting E, C, Q, QL

For Sensitivity Analysis

- Each parameter varied independently across 3-5 values.
- All other parameters were held at baseline.
- Full grid search repeated for each parameter value.
- Qualitative stability assessed: Does the optimal β increase smoothly with tech? Does the optimal allocation pattern remain balanced?

STOCHASTIC EXTENSION: FROM DETERMINISTIC TO STOCHASTIC PROCESSES

The baseline model presented in this chapter is deterministic and serves as the foundation for a family of stochastic extensions. Building on this foundation, the deterministic result of continuous strategic adjustment with technology yields empirically testable hypotheses regarding the behaviour of the corresponding stochastic system:

1. Demand uncertainty: Under Poisson-distributed patient arrivals, the optimal β will shift toward a distribution rather than a point estimate.
2. Outcome randomness: When clinical outcomes are modelled as Bernoulli variables, the previously derived deterministic optimum serves as a reference point; risk-averse decision-makers then allocate fewer resources to quality relative to this deterministic baseline.
3. Parameter uncertainty: Bayesian estimation of

QUALITY_COST_FACTOR and TECH_SAVINGS_FACTOR from empirical data will produce posterior distributions that can be propagated through the model.

The deterministic model serves as a mean-field approximation of a more complex stochastic reality and is a necessary preliminary step before introducing Wiener processes, Markov chains, or Monte Carlo simulation. Building on this foundation, the numerical solution of stochastic differential equations (Higham, 2001; Kloeden & Platen, 1992; Øksendal, 2003) establishes the methodological basis for these advanced approaches.

RESULTS

Baseline Model Validation (tech = 0.5)

Using baseline parameters (R = 100, tech = 0.5), the model produces 60 feasible (α, β, γ) allocation scenarios. To provide context before introducing technology variation, descriptive statistics and baseline optimal strategies are presented first.

Table 3 presents descriptive statistics.

Descriptive Statistics of the Outcome Space

Table 3. Descriptive Statistics of 4D Outcomes (Baseline, tech = 0.5, N = 60)

Statistic	Quantity	Quality	Cost	Efficiency
Mean	15.1	0.65	59.7	0.157
Standard Deviation	4.0	0.15	4.7	0.024
Minimum	9.4	0.33	51.6	0.103
25th Percentile	11.9	0.54	55.5	0.136
Median	14.2	0.68	59.5	0.157
75th Percentile	18.2	0.78	63.5	0.177
Maximum	23.6	0.85	67.7	0.194
Range	14.3	0.52	16.0	0.091

Key Observations

The descriptive statistics reveal several key patterns. Quantity shows the greatest relative variation (CV = 0.26), reflecting direct sensitivity to changes in γ allocation. In contrast, quality is more narrowly distributed (CV = 0.23) and ranges from 0.33 to 0.85, with the upper limit determined by tech = 0.5, which restricts the technology multiplier. Costs range from 51.6 to 67.7, with the lowest values occurring when both α and β are small, reducing quality and technology implementation expenses. Efficiency varies from 0.103 to 0.194, representing an 88% spread and highlighting the significant impact of allocation decisions on system performance.

Baseline Optimal Strategy (Maximum Efficiency)

The optimal allocation strategy at the baseline technology level (tech = 0.5) is identified through an exhaustive search across all feasible (α, β, γ) triples, selecting the allocation that maximises efficiency (E = Q·QL/C). This baseline case provides a reference point for measuring technology-induced shifts. Table 4 presents the optimal allocation and resulting outcomes.

Table 4. Optimal Strategy for Maximum Efficiency (tech = 0.5)

	Value
Allocation	
α (Quality)	0.30
β (Technology)	0.10
γ (Quantity)	0.60
Outcomes	
Quantity	19.3
Quality	0.57/10
Cost	56.8
Efficiency	0.194
Production Mode	Mixed Strategy

Interpretation

At technology level 0.5, the optimal strategy emphasises quantity (60% of resources), with limited technology investment (10%) and moderate allocation to quality (30%). This approach is classified as a "Mixed Strategy" because no parameter exceeds the MODE_THRESHOLD of 0.6.

This allocation pattern reflects a traditional production stance: most resources go to volume, with quality acceptable and technology supporting cost reduction at the margin.

Alternative Objective Functions

Different stakeholders may prioritise different objectives. Table 5 shows optimal allocations for four alternative objectives.

Table 5. Optimal Strategies by Objective (tech = 0.5)

Objective	α	β	γ	Quantity	Quality	Cost	Efficiency	Mode
Maximise Quantity	0.10	0.10	0.80	**23.6**	0.33	51.6	0.151	Mass
Maximise Quality	0.65	0.15	0.20	9.4	**0.85**	67.7	0.118	Quality
Minimise Cost	0.10	0.10	0.80	23.6	0.33	**51.6**	0.151	Mass
Maximise Efficiency	0.30	0.10	0.60	19.3	0.57	56.8	0.194	Mixed

A key finding is that maximising quality alone results in Pareto inefficiency. The allocation that maximises quality ($\alpha = 0.65$) also yields the lowest efficiency (0.118) and highest cost (67.7). Therefore, investment focused solely on quality is economically unsustainable and becomes viable only when supported by sufficient technological advances to offset the associated costs.

Table 6 presents the optimal strategy across all technology levels.

Technology Scenario Comparison: Continuous Strategic Adjustment

To examine how the optimal strategy varies with technological maturity, a comprehensive grid search was conducted across 10 technology levels, ranging from 0.1 to 1.0. Finer sampling was applied between 0.55 and 0.85, where allocation changes were anticipated to be most significant.

Table 6. Optimal Strategy by Technology Level (Maximum Efficiency)

Tech	α (Quality)	β (Technology)	γ (Quantity)	Efficiency	Cost	Mode
0.1	0.30	0.10	0.60	0.172	57.6	Mixed
0.3	0.30	0.10	0.60	0.183	57.2	Mixed
0.5	0.30	0.10	0.60	0.194	56.8	Mixed
0.6	0.25	0.25	0.50	0.204	55.2	Mixed
0.65	0.25	0.25	0.50	0.211	54.9	Mixed
0.7	0.25	0.30	0.45	0.218	54.6	Mixed
0.75	0.25	0.30	0.45	0.226	54.3	Mixed
0.8	0.25	0.30	0.45	0.235	54.0	Mixed
0.9	0.25	0.33	0.43	0.253	53.3	Mixed
1.0	0.20	0.35	0.45	0.273	51.2	Mixed

Technology level and cost exhibit a strong inverse correlation (r = -0.956), whereas efficiency demonstrates an equally strong positive correlation with technology (r = 0.956). Increased technological advancement consistently results in reduced costs and improved performance across all tested scenarios.

Technology's Dual Role: Decomposition Analysis

The model shows that technology plays two distinct roles, often confused in strategic frameworks.

Role 1: Cost Reducer (Linear)

- Effect: C includes $TECH\_SAVINGS\_FACTOR \cdot tech \cdot \beta$ as a deduction
- Magnitude: Each 0.1 increase in tech reduces cost by approximately 0.7 units (baseline)
- Functional form: Linear, additive
- Available at all technology levels
- Cost savings can be harvested with modest β allocation.

Role 2: Productivity Amplifier (Continuous, Capability-Dependent)

- Effect: $Q = (\gamma \cdot R)$^0.7 $\cdot$ (1 + $tech \cdot \beta \cdot$ 2.0)
- $QL = (\alpha \cdot R)$^0.5 $\cdot$ (1 + $tech \cdot \beta \cdot$ 0.8)
- Magnitude: The marginal return to β increases continuously with tech
- Functional form: Multiplicative, interactive
- Available at all technology levels, with increasing effectiveness as

tech rises

- Returns to β are continuous and moderate, not threshold-dependent

Why does optimal β increase gradually with technology?

The gradual increase in optimal β reflects the interaction between technology's dual roles. As technological capability increases, the term [1 + tech·β·multiplier] yields greater absolute returns from technology investment. However, diminishing returns to quantity production (QUANTITY_POWER = 0.7) indicate that allocating excessive resources from γ to β ultimately reduces total output. Furthermore, the increasing marginal cost of implementing technology (TECH_COST_POWER = 1.3) constrains extreme specialisation. Although the optimal balance point shifts as technological capability improves, extreme specialisation (β > 0.5) remains suboptimal because it restricts both quality and quantity investment while incurring disproportionate implementation costs.

Table 7 displays the frequency of each production mode.

Production Mode Distribution Across the Strategy Space

Table 7. Production Mode Frequencies (Baseline, tech = 0.5, N = 60)

Production Mode	Count	Percentage
Mixed Strategy	46	76.7%
Mass Production	6	10.0%
Quality Orientation	5	8.3%
Innovation Integration	3	5.0%
Total	**60**	**100%**

Interpretation

Mixed Strategy constitutes over three-quarters of all feasible allocations. This establishes it as the default region within the strategy space. Focused strategies are less prevalent. Mass Production and Quality Orientation collectively account for 18.3% of scenarios. Innovation Integration is observed in only 5%. The rarity of Innovation Integration is primarily mechanical. A high β value necessitates low α and γ values due to the sum constraint. This results in a few grid points surpassing the β > 0.6 threshold. Notably, the production mode classification is descriptive and does not affect the efficiency calculation.

The predominance of Mixed Strategy in the distribution results from the simplex geometry constraint (α + β + γ = 1) and the MODE_THRESHOLD = 0.6 parameter. This does not represent an empirical conclusion regarding optimal production strategies. This classification indicates that most feasible allocations do not exhibit a single dominant dimension. It does not imply the inherent superiority of mixed strategies.

Table 8 presents the marginal cost of quality at increasing levels of quality.

The Cost of Quality: Quantitative Assessment

Table 8. Marginal Cost of Quality

Quality Level	α (Quality Allocation)	Cost	Marginal Cost
0.6	0.25	52.1	—
0.7	0.33	53.5	1.4
0.8	0.42	55.8	2.3
0.9	0.52	59.2	3.4
1.0	0.65	63.5	4.3

The analysis shows that the marginal cost of quality rises from 1.4 to 4.3 cost units per 0.1 increment. This trend directly results from QUALITY_COST_POWER = 1.2 > 1.0.

Implication

Pursuing zero defects or perfect quality leads to exponentially increasing costs. Decision-makers should set a satisficing quality target instead. For example, aiming for a quality range of 0.7 to 0.8 can help control costs.

Sensitivity Analysis: Robustness of the Continuous Adjustment Finding

A common criticism of simulation-based strategic models is that their findings may be driven by arbitrary parameter choices. To address this concern, the model was subjected to extensive sensitivity analysis, with each parameter varied independently across wide, plausible ranges.

For each parameter, all others were held at baseline values while the full technology-scenario comparison was rerun (technology ranging from 0.1 to 1.0). The analysis then assessed three key questions:

- Does optimal β increase smoothly with tech?
- Does the optimal allocation below tech = 0.5 remain approximately

(α = 0.30, β = 0.10, γ = 0.60)?

- Does the optimal allocation at high technology levels remain approximately (α = 0.20-0.25, β = 0.30-0.35, γ = 0.45)?

Sensitivity to BASE_COST

Values tested: 25, 50 (baseline), 75

The findings show that the optimal β trajectory and proportional distribution of allocations remain stable across all technology levels and overhead cost conditions. In particular, although increasing BASE_COST raises absolute costs, it does not affect optimal resource allocation or the marginal trade-offs among quantity, quality, and technology. As a result, fixed overhead costs do not change how resources should be allocated or affect continuous adjustment. Overall, these results are robust across varied overhead conditions.

Sensitivity to QUALITY_COST_FACTOR

Values tested: 15, 30 (baseline), 45

No qualitative changes are observed; the optimal β remains stable, and optimal allocations also remain unchanged. Notably, while an increase in the QUALITY_COST_FACTOR raises the cost of quality—further reinforcing the inefficiency of quality maximisation—it does not alter the optimal β trajectory. Consequently, the optimal strategy across all technology levels remains quantity-balanced, with β increasing smoothly as technology advances.

Sensitivity to TECH_SAVINGS_FACTOR

Values of 10, 20, and 30 were tested to determine whether stronger cost-reduction effects would encourage increased technology investment. These effects did not result in heavier investment. Optimal β continued to increase smoothly with technological advances, and the allocation pattern remained consistent. Doubling the savings factor increased the financial attractiveness of technology; however, the constraints of diminishing returns in quantity production and rising implementation costs prevented β from exceeding moderate levels, even when technology equalled 1.0. Therefore, the model consistently favours a balanced strategy as a built-in structural element, rather than as a consequence of parameter changes.

Sensitivity to RESOURCE_TOTAL

Values tested: 50, 100 (baseline), 150, 200

Qualitative stability is confirmed, with the optimal β trajectory remaining unchanged. Likewise, the optimal allocations—represented by the proportions of α, β, and γ—do not shift. As R increases, absolute quantity and quality rise; however, the allocation percentages remain scale-invariant. This model, therefore, demonstrates constant returns to scale in allocation proportions. By design, this characteristic ensures strategic insights are consistently applicable across organisations of any size. The result is reinforced broad relevance and practical value.

Sensitivity to QUANTITY_POWER

Values tested: 0.5, 0.7 (baseline), 0.9

Result

The continuous adjustment pattern persists across this parameter range. The optimal β at baseline tech = 0.5 shifts moderately:

- At QUANTITY_POWER = 0.5 (stronger diminishing returns), optimal $\beta \approx 0.24$

- At QUANTITY_POWER = 0.70 (baseline), optimal $\beta = 0.10$
- At QUANTITY_POWER = 0.9 (near-constant returns), optimal $\beta = 0.10$

The results show that continuous adjustment is robust across a range of production elasticities. Organisations experiencing stronger diminishing returns to quantity are advised to invest more in technology, even at lower levels of technological development. However, the adjustment process remains gradual rather than abrupt.

Sensitivity to QUALITY_POWER

Values tested: 0.3, 0.5 (baseline), 0.7

The pattern of continuous adjustment remains evident. To illustrate, when quality power is set to 0.3, indicating stronger diminishing returns, the optimal β at baseline technology increases to approximately 0.28. Conversely, at a quality power of 0.7, the optimal β decreases to 0.10. While optimal technology investment is moderately sensitive to variations in quality elasticity, the adjustment remains continuous and smooth.

Sensitivity to TECH_COST_FACTOR

Values tested: 10, 15 (baseline), 25

The optimal β remains stable at a baseline technology level of 0.5, with β consistently equal to 0.10 across all values. This result demonstrates the robustness of the continuous adjustment finding. Furthermore, even with substantial reductions in technology implementation costs, the optimal strategy does not shift toward extreme technology specialisation. This indicates that the balanced approach maintains structural robustness.

Sensitivity to TECH_COST_POWER

Values tested: 1.1, 1.3 (baseline), 1.5

The optimal value of β remains stable across all parameter values. Notably, the non-linearity of technology implementation costs, which enhances realism, does not influence the strategic findings. Continuous adjustment remains invariant and is thus a robust property of the production function structure.

THE CONTINUOUS STRATEGIC ADJUSTMENT FRAMEWORK

From Empirical Finding to General Theory

The results go beyond mere numerical findings. They reveal a generalisable strategic principle that is not tied to any specific functional forms or parameter values of the model. This principle is formalised as the Continuous Strategic Adjustment Framework.

Definition 1 (Strategic Adjustment Function). The optimal resource allocation vector (α, β, γ)—where α represents management resources, β represents technology investment, and γ represents quantity production—is a continuous function of the exogenous technology capability parameter (tech), which measures the level or effectiveness of available technology. As the technology capability parameter increases, the optimal allocation to technology investment (β) increases smoothly, while the optimal allocation to quantity production (γ) decreases correspondingly.

Definition 2 (Continuous Strategic Evolution). Continuous strategic evolution in a production system refers to a smooth, gradual change in the optimal resource allocation vector (α, β, γ) in response to changes in an exogenous capability parameter (tech), without discontinuous jumps or regime shifts.

Proposition 1 (Continuous Adjustment). For any production system characterized by the following conditions: (a) Diminishing returns to scale in the primary output (quantity), meaning that increasing inputs yields smaller increases in output over time; (b) Multiplicative technology amplification of outputs, where output is scaled by the technology parameter; (c) Symmetric cost effects across input dimensions, meaning cost increases evenly when any input increases; (d) A binding resource constraint ($\alpha + \beta + \gamma = 1$), which requires all available resources be allocated among management (α), technology (β), and production (γ),

The optimal allocation to technology (β) is a continuous, increasing function of technology capability, and no discontinuous phase transition occurs.

The Graduated Investment Rule

Leaders must implement a graduated investment rule, abandoning static investment regimes.

- **Low Technology (tech < 0.4):** The proportion allocated to β should be maintained at approximately 10%.
- **Optimal Allocation:** $\alpha \approx 0.30$, $\beta \approx 0.10$, $\gamma \approx 0.60$.
- **Production Mode:** A mixed strategy or mass production approach is recommended.

Drive foundation building as the central objective. Prioritise resources for scaling quantity, ensuring quality meets standards. Deploy technology strategically for cost efficiency.

Guard against technological inertia. Today's insufficient technology investment compromises future gains as capabilities scale.

Progression: To support a smooth transition from low to intermediate technological capability, organisations should gradually increase the proportion allocated to β toward 0.25 as capability improves. This signals readiness to shift investment approach.

- **Intermediate Technology (0.4 ≤ tech < 0.7):** Building on the earlier phase, gradually increase the allocation to β from 10% toward 25% as technological capability advances, continuing the upward investment trajectory.
- **Optimal Allocation:** $\alpha \approx 0.25$, $\beta \approx 0.25$, $\gamma \approx 0.50$.
- **Production Mode:** A mixed strategy is recommended.

Lead a deliberate shift toward capability building. Reallocate resources from quantity to technology to maximise productivity. Permit modest reductions in quality investment as technology lifts results.

Prevent premature acceleration. Resist pressure to outpace your organisation's capability to absorb technology. Enforce a measured, continuous investment trajectory.

Progression: Maintaining a consistent approach, organisational capability growth in the intermediate range should be matched by further incremental increases in β, thereby setting the stage for the high-technology investment model.

- **High Technology (tech $\geq$ 0.7):** Continuing the established trajectory, increase the allocation to β from 25% toward 35% as organisations reach high technological capability.
- **Optimal Allocation:** $\alpha \approx 0.20$–0.25, $\beta \approx 0.30$–0.35, $\gamma \approx 0.45$.
- **Production Mode:** A mixed strategy is recommended.

Command a technology-first strategy. Leverage productivity gains to efficiently reduce investments in quantity and quality while sustaining superior results.

Stay vigilant against overconfidence. Even with high technological capability, maintain balanced allocations: 20–25% to quality and 45% to quantity. Discipline investment—do not exceed 35–40% in technology, even under optimal conditions.

The "Extreme Specialisation" Trap: Why Balanced Strategies Dominate

A decision-maker might think: "If $\beta = 0.10$ is optimal at tech = 0.1 and $\beta = 0.35$ is optimal at tech = 1.0, then at high technology levels, $\beta = 0.50$ or higher should be considered."

This inference is not correct. The model shows that focusing too much on any one area is always less effective. For example, at tech = 0.7, using $\beta = 0.62$ (an extreme technology approach) reduces efficiency by about 21% relative to the best-balanced choice. At tech = 0.9, the gap reduces to about 13%, but it is still substantial.

Here's why this happens.

The technology booster [1 + tech·β·multiplier] goes up in a straight line with β, so each extra bit of β adds the same value. However, the quantity base (γ·R)^0.7 grows more slowly as γ increases, whereas the cost of using technology, β^1.3, grows faster and faster as β increases. This means the best choice is not at the extremes: give enough to β to get the benefits, but do not overdo it, or the losses from less γ and higher costs will outweigh the gains. Balanced choices are always better than extreme ones, no matter the level of technology.

Implications for Practice

Instead of extreme technology specialisation, organisations should carefully and incrementally increase technology investment as capabilities develop. This approach involves monitoring marginal returns and adjusting allocations regularly to ensure resources are optimally balanced between technology and other priorities.

FROM THE ABSTRACT MODEL TO HEALTHCARE DECISIONS

A frequent criticism of abstract production models is that their parameters (α, β, γ, tech) lack clear real-world referents. This section provides explicit, concrete translations of the model's variables and findings at two distinct levels of healthcare decision-making.

Table 9 provides explicit translations of model variables.

Macro Level: National and Regional Health Systems

At the macro level, the decision-maker is the Ministry of Health, a regional health authority, or a national insurance fund that allocates a fixed annual budget across competing strategic priorities.

Table 9. Macro-Level Translation of Model Variables

Variable	Definition	Examples
R (Total Resources)	Total health system budget (€, $, £)	Annual public health expenditure; total hospital funding
α (Quality Allocation)	Investment in clinical quality infrastructure	Accreditation programmes; quality improvement collaboratives; patient safety initiatives; continuing medical education
β (Technology Allocation)	Investment in health information technology and medical equipment	National EHR implementation; telemedicine platforms; AI diagnostic tools; medical device procurement
γ (Quantity Allocation)	Investment in service volume capacity	Staffing (physicians, nurses); hospital beds; primary care clinics; surgical capacity
tech (Technology Capability)	System-wide digital maturity and technological sophistication	WHO Digital Health Maturity Index; OECD health IT adoption metrics; interoperability score

Macro-Level Strategic Rules (Derived from Model)

1. Conduct an objective assessment of technology capability (tech). Avoid classifying a system as "high tech" based solely on isolated pilot projects. Employ validated maturity indices for evaluation; these are standardised tools or frameworks used to measure a system's progress or effectiveness in digital capability.
2. Align technology investment with assessed capability. Start with about 10% for low maturity and increase to about 35% at full maturity. Do not rely on a single threshold. Continuously monitor capability and adjust allocations incrementally.
    - Early-stage systems (tech < 0.4): allocate approximately 10% to technology
    - Developing systems ($0.4 \leq$ tech < 0.7): ~15-25% to technology
    - Mature systems ($0.7 \leq$ tech < 0.9): allocate approximately 25–30% to technology
    - Advanced systems (tech ≥ 0.9): allocate approximately 30–35% to technology

3. Avoid extreme specialisation. Allocating more than 40% of resources to any single dimension (quality, technology, or quantity) is generally suboptimal, regardless of technology capability. A balanced approach consistently outperforms extreme strategies.
4. Refrain from extreme technology specialisation at any capability level. Allocating more than 40% of resources to technology reduces efficiency, even when technological capability is maximised.

As capability grows, keep increasing technology investment in proportion. Recognise that the productivity benefit of technology intensifies as capability increases. Make sustained, incremental investment increases as digital maturity advances.

Table 10 presents the micro-level translations.

Micro Level: Hospitals, Departments, and Clinical Services

At the micro level, leaders in hospitals, such as CEOs, department heads, and managers, decide how to allocate the annual budget among different needs within the organisation. For example, they may use maturity indices - structured assessments of processes, capabilities, or technologies - to guide their budgeting decisions.

Table 10. Micro-Level Translation of Model Variables

Variable	Definition	Examples
R (Total Resources)	Departmental or hospital operating budget	Annual budget (€); FTE staffing allocation
α (Quality Allocation)	Investment in clinical quality and safety	Quality improvement staff; protocol development; audit and feedback; patient experience programmes
β (Technology Allocation)	Investment in clinical technology and digital tools	New imaging equipment; robotic surgery systems; EHR optimisation; clinical decision support
γ (Quantity Allocation)	Investment in patient care capacity	Nursing staff; bed capacity; clinic sessions; surgical slots
tech (Technology Capability)	Departmental technology maturity	EHR utilisation rate; technology adoption stage; staff digital competency

Micro-Level Strategic Rules (Derived from Model)

1. Assess technology maturity. Determine whether basic electronic health record (EHR, a digital version of a patient's paper chart) functionality is present, but with limited ability to exchange data between systems (interoperability). Identify the current version in use and whether a fully electronic, paperless workflow has been achieved. Calibrate technology maturity on a scale from 0.0 (no digital presence) to 1.0 (fully mature, completely integrated, and optimised electronic system).
2. Align technology investment with assessed maturity level: For reference, α represents investment in quality improvement, β represents investment in technology, and γ represents investment in staffing.

For intermediate maturity (technology 0.4 to less than 0.7), increase technology investment (β from 0.10 to 0.25). Start lowering direct staffing investment (γ) as technology boosts productivity.

For high maturity (technology 0.7 or higher), continue raising technology investment (β from 0.25 to 0.35). Reduce staffing investment (γ to about 0.45) as technology handles more work. Lower-quality investment slightly (α to 0.20-0.25) since technology improves quality, such as through decision support or standardisation.

3. Avoid excessive specialisation. Allocate no more than 40% of the budget to technology spending, no matter how advanced the system is. Evidence indicates that balanced strategies that do not overprioritize any one area (staffing, technology, or quality) consistently outperform extreme allocations.
4. Measure the "tech multiplier" empirically. The "tech multiplier" is the effect that increased technology investment (β) has on outcomes. Assess whether a 10% increase in β leads to measurable improvements in throughput (the amount of work done in a period) or quality (such as fewer errors or better patient outcomes). If no improvement is observed, this may signal that the technology's impact is overestimated or that its implementation is ineffective.

THEORETICAL SYNTHESIS AND STRATEGIC TOOLS

The findings of this chapter—including the need for ongoing adaptation of strategies alongside technological advancements, the idea that pursuing maximum quality can sometimes lead to less efficient outcomes (Pareto-inefficiency), technology's dual function in enabling and complicating those outcomes, and the importance of balanced rules for allocating resources—are interconnected. Together, these findings require a rethinking of how quality is theoretically approached in healthcare systems.

This section brings together these findings into an integrated, three-layer theoretical framework that unifies Deming's System of Profound Knowledge (which emphasizes understanding systems, variation, knowledge, and psychology in management), hybrid complexity science (the study of systems with both simple and complex, often unpredictable, interactions), and multi-criteria optimisation (the process of making decisions using multiple, sometimes competing, measures of success) within a single organising logic.

The Paradigm Shift: Three Transformations in How We Think About Healthcare Quality

From "Quality as Ultimate Goal" to "Quality as One of Three Competing Objectives"

The traditional perspective considers quality to be the paramount value within healthcare systems. The system pursues other objectives, such as access, efficiency, and cost control, only as means to achieve quality. In this view, resources drive quality, which then determines all other outcomes.

In contrast to this traditional model, our revised perspective posits that quality constitutes one vertex of an irreducible trilemma, competing with quantity and technology for limited resources within a fixed budget. Rather than adhering to a strict hierarchical ordering among these objectives, it may be rational to sacrifice quality if reallocating resources yields greater improvements in quantity or technology-enabled efficiency. Therefore, quality should be regarded as a decision variable within a multi-objective optimisation framework, rather than as the sole endpoint.

Building on this multi-objective perspective, there are implications for Deming's System of Profound Knowledge that should be interpreted through a triadic framework. In this context, 'appreciation of a system' now entails understanding the organisation as an integrated whole that is continuously engaged in dynamic trade-offs among three fundamental, competing objectives.

From "Deming in Healthcare" to "Deming Synchronised with the Quantity-Quality-Technology Triad"

The conventional view holds that Deming's principles—system thinking, statistical process control, PDSA cycles, and intrinsic motivation—are fully relevant to healthcare and require only superficial contextual adjustments.

Building on this, a revised interpretation suggests that Deming's framework, as originally formulated, assumes a singular objective of quality. It does not address scenarios in which quality improvement diverts resources from expanding access (quantity) or developing future capabilities (technology). A naive application of Deming's approach results in maximising quality, which the presented model demonstrates is Pareto-inefficient (E = 0.118, C = 67.7, ROI = 1.74).

Therefore, alignment is necessary, as Deming's four foundational principles must be recalibrated to address the triadic reality of healthcare objectives (Table 11).

Table 11. Deming's Four Pillars Recalibrated to the Triadic Reality

Deming's Pillar	Traditional Interpretation	Recalibrated Interpretation
System	The organisation as an interdependent whole	The organisation as an interdependent whole, balancing quantity, quality, and technology under resource constraints
Variation	Distinguishing common from special cause in quality metrics	Distinguishing common from special cause in the efficiency of alternative allocations; sensitivity analysis at the strategic level
Theory of Knowledge	PDSA cycles for quality improvement	PDSA cycles for optimising the triadic allocation; each cycle tests a new (α, β, γ) hypothesis
Psychology	Reducing fear to enable quality reporting	Reducing fear to enable honest trade-off discussions; accepting that quality is not always the priority

From "Complexity Analysis" to "Multi-Criteria Optimisation Under Complexity"

Traditionally, complexity science in healthcare has emphasised descriptive analysis. This includes mapping networks, identifying emergent patterns, and characterising non-linear dynamics. The central question has been: What kind of complex system is present?

Building on this foundation, a revised perspective asserts that complexity science should adopt a prescriptive approach. The pertinent question becomes: Given the complex, non-linear, and continuously evolving nature of the system, how should resources be allocated to maximise performance? This approach shifts the disciplinary focus from physics-inspired network analysis to engineering-inspired control and optimisation.

In summary, the healthcare system demonstrates dual forms of:

1. Network complexity (inter-organisational): hierarchical hubs ($\gamma = 1.41$), chaotic sensitivity ($\Delta = 8.726$), and self-organisation ($S = 0.72$).ion ($S = 0.72$).
2. Production complexity (intra-organisational): involves non-linear trade-offs (meaning decisions have disproportionate or unpredictable effects), continuous strategic adjustment (refers to ongoing modification of strategies in response to system changes), and interior optima (optimisation points that are found within, rather than at the extremes of, possible options).

These are not distinct phenomena; rather, they represent two aspects of the same underlying reality. Healthcare systems are fundamentally complex at every scale, and a unified theory must address both dimensions.

THE INTEGRATED FRAMEWORK: A THREE-LAYER MODEL OF HEALTHCARE QUALITY

We present a three-layer framework. It brings together Deming's principles, hybrid complexity, and triadic optimisation into one unified theory.

Layer 1: Foundational Theory – Deming's System of Profound Knowledge (Recalibrated)

This layer sets the philosophical and ethical foundation. It defines value criteria and outlines principles of organisational learning.

Key Components

1. System (Triadic): The healthcare organisation functions as a system whose performance depends on balancing three core elements: quantity (the amount of services), quality (the standard of care), and technology (the tools and methods used). The best mix of these factors varies with the specific situation and technological advances.
2. Variation (Strategic): Variation refers to differences in both quality outcomes (how care results vary) and how efficiently resources are used. Sensitivity analysis—a method for examining how different choices affect outcomes—is used as the strategic version of statistical process control, which typically tracks stability and variation in processes over time.
3. Theory of Knowledge (PDSA 2.0): The Plan-Do-Study-Act (PDSA) cycle—a step-by-step method for testing and refining changes—is applied to the allocation vector, a set of variables (such as α, β, γ) that represent how resources are distributed among quantity, quality, and technology.
   - Plan: Formulate a hypothesis for the allocation vector (α, β, γ) based on the current level of technological capability.

- Do: Implement the allocation and measure quantity, quality, and cost.
- Study: Calculate efficiency (how well resources are used to achieve desired results) and compare the actual results to what was expected.
- Act: Incrementally adjust the allocation. If technological capability has changed, update the target allocation accordingly.

4. Psychology (Trade-off Acceptance): Leaders are responsible for fostering psychological safety to enable explicit discussions of trade-offs. Advocates for quality must recognise that quality is not always the primary objective; advocates for access must acknowledge that quantity is not always paramount; and technology advocates must accept that excessive specialisation in technology can reduce efficiency across all capability levels.

Layer 2: Structural Theory -- Hybrid Complexity

Purpose: Explains the structure and behaviours of the system where Layer 1 works, and outlines broad traits that either limit or help optimisation.

Key Components

1. Network structure. Healthcare systems have many layers, with closely linked groups and short paths between them. Information moves quickly through influential people; small groups can test local changes; new ideas can spread quickly throughout the system.
2. Change over time is a crucial aspect, in addition to network structure. Healthcare systems can act unpredictably and organise themselves without outside direction. Because of this, it is hard to make long-term predictions, so being able to adjust as things change is very important.
3. Building on this, these systems show continuous evolution, as they undergo ongoing strategic adjustment in response to changes in key parameters:
4. Strategic change: The best way to work keeps shifting with new technology, but it does not change all at once.

Taken together, these factors explain why Layer 2 provides the rationale for recalibrating Layer 1. While traditional Deming approaches assume linear, predictable, and continuously improving systems, healthcare systems are nonlinear, unpredictable, and continuously evolving. Accordingly, the Plan-Do-Study-Act (PDSA) cycle must function within a context of epistemic humility and ongoing adaptation.

Layer 3: Operational Theory -- Triadic Optimisation

Function: This layer establishes quantitative and actionable decision rules for resource allocation, contingent upon the level of technological capability.

Key Components

1. Graduated investment rule: The optimal value of β increases continuously with technological capability, ranging from approximately 0.10 at low capability to 0.35 at full capability. No discontinuous threshold is present.

- Low technological capability (less than 0.4): $(\alpha, \beta, \gamma) = (0.30, 0.10, 0.60)$, where α represents Quality, β represents Technology, and γ represents Quantity. This corresponds to allocating 30% to Quality, 10% to Technology, and 60% to Quantity.

For intermediate technological capability (ranging from 0.4 to 0.7), the allocation shifts gradually; (α, β, γ) transitions from (0.30, 0.10, 0.60) to (0.25, 0.25, 0.50), illustrating a continuum rather than an abrupt change.

For high technological capability (0.7 or greater), there is a further gradual transition in allocation; (α, β, γ) moves from (0.25, 0.25, 0.50) to (0.20, 0.35, 0.45), again emphasising a continuous shift.

Strategic Compass

This component defines four cardinal directions within the strategy space, providing explicit guidance on resource-allocation priorities across varying operational contexts (Table 12). Each direction represents a distinct emphasis: (1) Quality Maximisation, prioritising quality over technology and quantity; (2) Technology Leadership, focusing resources on advancing technological capability; (3) Quantity Expansion, directing investment toward scaling outputs; and (4) Balanced Advancement, maintaining equilibrium among quality, technology, and quantity. Organisations can align decision rules with these directions based on current capabilities and strategic objectives.

Table 12. Strategic Compass: Four Cardinal Directions in Strategy Space

Direction	Allocation (α, β, γ)	Quantity	Quality	Cost	Efficiency	Mode	Assessment
North (Quality)	(0.65, 0.15, 0.20)	9.4	**0.85**	67.7	0.118	Quality Orientation	Excellence, but expensive
South (Quantity)	(0.10, 0.10, 0.80)	**23.6**	0.33	51.6	0.151	Mass Production	Volume, moderate efficiency
East (Technology)	(0.18, 0.62, 0.20)	15.2	0.66	51.2	0.163	Innovation Integration	NOT optimal at any tech level
West (Balance)	(0.25, 0.30, 0.45)	14.3	0.68	54.6	0.218	Mixed Strategy	

Layer 3 implements the principles established in Layers 1 and 2 by translating Deming's philosophical commitments and complexity science's structural insights into specific, testable, and quantitatively precise allocation rules. These rules adapt continuously as technological capabilities advance.

The Unified Equation

The three layers can be expressed as a single conceptual equation:
Q_*total* = *f*(*Deming_recalibrated*, *Hybrid_complexity*,
Triadic_optimization, Technology_continuous)
where:

$- Deming\_recalibrated = \{ System_{triadic}, Variation_{strategic}, Knowledge\_PDSA2.0, Psychology\_tradeoff$
$\}$
- *Hybrid_complexity*= { *Network_topology* (γ=1.41, C=0.621, L=2.94), *Dynamics* (Δ=8.726, S=0.719, H=0.68), *Continuous_evolution* }
- *Triadic_optimization*= { *Technology_assessment*, *Graduated_investment_rules*, *Strategic_compass* }
- *Technology_continuous*= *continuous function mapping tech to optimal*β

This equation is presented not as a closed-form mathematical expression but as a framework specification. In particular, it emphasises that any comprehensive theory of healthcare quality must address all three layers and their interactions.

The PDSA 2.0 Cycle for Strategic Technology Management

By integrating Deming's learning discipline with the principle of continuous adjustment, this framework introduces a recalibrated PDSA cycle tailored to technology-driven strategic evolution.

Step 1: PLAN -- Diagnose and Hypothesise

Measure current technology capability (tech) using a validated maturity index. Based on the graduated investment rule, hypothesise the appropriate target allocation:

- If tech < 0.4, hypothesise that target allocation is (0.30, 0.10, 0.60).
- If 0.4 ≤ tech < 0.7, hypothesise that target allocation is in transition toward (0.25, 0.25, 0.50).
- If tech ≥ 0.7, hypothesise that target allocation is in transition toward (0.20, 0.35, 0.45).
- Define measurable targets for efficiency, cost, quantity, and quality.

Step 2: DO -- Implement and Invest

- Reallocate resources incrementally toward the hypothesised target allocation.
- Implement technology investments commensurate with the target β.
- Maintain the capability to reverse allocation if the hypothesis fails.

Step 3: STUDY -- Measure and Analyse

- Compute realised efficiency, cost, quantity, and quality.
- Compare to targets and to the pre-intervention baseline.
- Assess whether tech capability has changed during the cycle.

Step 4: ACT -- Learn and Adjust

- If efficiency improved: Continue incremental movement toward the target allocation; refine based on observed marginal returns.

- If tech has increased: Update the target allocation per the graduated investment rule; continue incremental adjustment.
- If efficiency declined or tech failed to increase: Pause reallocation; diagnose whether tech capability was overestimated or technology implementation was ineffective; adjust target accordingly.

PDSA 2.0 diverges from the traditional PDSA cycle in three critical respects:

1. The approach is capability-aware; the hypothesis depends on a measured state variable.
2. The cycle emphasises continuous, incremental action rather than abrupt regime changes.
3. Technology investment is treated as endogenous; β influences future technological capability, which in turn determines future optimal β, establishing a cycle of gradual improvement.

LIMITATIONS

The current model is deterministic (meaning it produces the same results given the same inputs) and static (it does not account for changes over time). It relies on single-period optimisation, which considers only one time frame. Real healthcare systems, however, face demand uncertainty (unpredictable patient needs), stochastic variation in outcomes (randomness in results), and multi-period investments with delayed returns (investments that take several periods to show benefits).

To address these limitations, future models should incorporate stochastic differential equations (mathematical equations describing systems influenced by random factors (Øksendal, 2003) to better capture underlying uncertainties.

Subsequent research should extend the model to use stochastic optimisation. The goal is to maximise expected efficiency under demand uncertainty. Dynamic programming should also be adopted. This would help determine optimal multi-period investment strategies that account for learning curves and depreciation.

The current model focuses on efficiency ($E = Q \cdot QL / C$, where Q is output, QL is quality level, and C is cost). However, real healthcare leaders must balance multiple objectives. These include access, quality, cost, equity, and staff satisfaction. No single optimal solution exists, so decision-makers must state their preferences or use Pareto frontiers (sets of solutions that are not dominated by any other across all objectives).

Accordingly, future research should extend the model to multi-objective optimisation (optimising several objectives simultaneously) by generating the Pareto frontier (a curve delineating the optimal trade-offs) within the space defined by Quantity, Quality, Cost, and Efficiency. This approach would enable decision-makers to identify their preferred trade-offs.

In addition to the model structure, the analysis uses specific functional forms. These include Cobb-Douglas (a mathematical function often used in economics to model the relationship between inputs and outputs) for quantity and quality, power laws (functions where one quantity varies as a power of another) for quality and technology costs, and a linear form (a direct proportionality between variables) for technology savings. These choices are theoretically justified and computationally convenient. However, they lack empirical validation with real production data. Future research should estimate the functional forms and parameters using actual healthcare production data. Potential datasets include US Medicare hospital cost reports, NHS England reference costs, and OECD Health Statistics 2024.

Currently, the model treats technology capability (referred to as "tech") as exogenous, meaning external to the system. In practice, technology is endogenous or determined within the system. It is influenced by prior β (investment in productive assets), experiential learning (knowledge gained from hands-on activities), and industry innovation (sector-wide advances). Separating technology capability from β investment is conceptually useful, but this distinction makes the model dynamically incomplete.

To address this, future research should model the co-evolution of technology and investment. For example, tech(t+1) can depend on tech(t), β(t), the learning rate, and depreciation. Investment decisions at time t influence capability at time t+1. The optimal policy may require sustained, gradual investment.

Currently, separate translations exist for macro and micro levels. However, their interaction is not modelled. For example, a national health policy may set $\beta = 0.30$ at the macro level, but this does not mean $\beta = 0$ across all hospitals. Hospitals differ in technology and patient mix.

To address this gap, future research should develop multi-level, nested models. These should include a macro-level resource allocation problem (national to regional) and micro-level response functions. Hospitals would then optimise based on their allocation and technology. This approach would allow analysis of policy implementation fidelity and differing responses.

CONCLUSION

This chapter presents, validates, and explicates a 4-Dimensional Production Model for healthcare resource allocation. The model (1) jointly optimises quantity, quality, technology, and cost; (2) employs explicit mathematical specifications with transparent, adjustable parameters; (3) incorporates a comprehensive sensitivity analysis demonstrating robustness across seven parametric families; and (4) is applicable at both national health system and hospital department levels.

The principal empirical finding indicates that as technological capabilities increase, healthcare systems adjust their strategies incrementally rather than abruptly.

At low levels of technological maturity (tech < 0.4), prioritising quantity is the optimal strategy. Technology investment remains minimal ($\beta = 0.10$), while quality investment is moderate ($\alpha = 0.30$). In this context, technology primarily serves to reduce costs and does not warrant additional resource allocation.

With increasing technological advancement, the optimal value of β rises to approximately 0.25–0.30 at intermediate levels (tech = 0.6–0.7) and reaches around 0.35 at full maturity (tech = 1.0). Although technology becomes a more valuable asset, balanced resource allocation consistently outperforms extreme specialisation.

This pattern reflects gradual evolution rather than a regime shift. It is not advisable to wait for a specific threshold before increasing technology investment or implementing substantial changes. Instead, technology investment should be increased progressively as digital maturity advances, with marginal returns monitored to inform incremental adjustments. Extreme specialisation, including in technology, remains suboptimal.

These findings are based on synthetic data and theoretical parameters and should therefore be regarded as conceptual indications. Empirical validation using data from real-world healthcare systems is a necessary subsequent step to confirm or revise the proposed allocations and the theoretical framework presented, including the integration of Deming's principles, which assume that quality, technology, and quantity function as equally weighted competing objectives. However, the relative importance of these dimensions may differ when assessed empirically, potentially necessitating a partial reconsideration of the operational application of the System of Profound Knowledge in the healthcare context.

DISCLOSURE OF DELEGATION TO GENERATIVE AI

The author declares the use of generative AI in the research and writing process. According to the GAIDeT taxonomy (2025), the following tasks were delegated to GAI tools under full human supervision:

- Code generation
- Process automation
- Creation of algorithms for data analysis
- Reproducibility testing
- Proofreading and editing

The GAI tools used were: DeepSeek (for Python code generation), Grammarly (for text polishing).

Responsibility for the final manuscript lies entirely with the author.

GAI tools are not listed as authors and do not bear responsibility for the final outcomes.

Declaration submitted by: Dr. Anastasius Moumtzoglou

Additional note: The original research ideas, the four-dimensional production model architecture, the mathematical specification, and the research question are the author's. DeepSeek generated initial Python code for the model, which the author subsequently verified, tested with 27 unit tests, and corrected - including identifying and resolving a specification artefact in the efficiency calculation. Grammarly was used to proofread and assess the readability of the final manuscript. All numerical results were generated by the author's execution of the verified Python code. No AI tool generated data, references, or substantive research content.

REFERENCES

Braithwaite, J., Churruca, K., Ellis, L. A., Long, J., Clay-Williams, R., Damen, N., Herkes, J., Pomare, C., & Ludlow, K. (2017). *Complexity science in healthcare: aspirations, approaches, applications and accomplishments: a white paper*. Macquarie University. https://www.mq.edu.au/research/research-centres-groups-and-facilities/healthy-people/centres/australian-institute-of-health-innovation/news-and-events/news/news/complexity-science-in-healthcare-aspirations,-approaches,-applications-and-accomplishments-a-white-paper

Christensen, C. M. (1997). *The innovator's dilemma: When new technologies cause great firms to fail*. Harvard Business School Press.

Deming, W. E. (2000). *The new economics: For industry, government, education* (2nd ed.). MIT Press.

Donabedian, A. (1988). The quality of care: How can it be assessed? *Journal of the American Medical Association, 260*(12), 1743–1748. DOI: 10.1001/jama.1988.03410120089033 PMID: 3045356

Feldstein, M. S. (1967). *Economic analysis for health service efficiency: Econometric studies of the British National Health Service*. North-Holland Publishing.

Gavurova, B., Kocisova, K., & Sopko, J. (2021). Health system efficiency in OECD countries: Dynamic network DEA approach. *Health Economics Review, 11*, 40. DOI: 10.1186/s13561-021-00337-9 PMID: 34642864

Gladwell, M. (2000). *The tipping point: How little things can make a big difference*. Little, Brown and Company.

Granovetter, M. (1978). Threshold models of collective behavior. *American Journal of Sociology, 83*(6), 1420–1443. DOI: 10.1086/226707

Higham, D. J. (2001). An algorithmic introduction to numerical simulation of stochastic differential equations. *SIAM Review, 43*(3), 525–546.

Institute of Medicine. (2001). *Crossing the quality chasm: A new health system for the 21st century*. National Academy Press.

Jacobs, R., Smith, P. C., & Street, A. (2006). *Measuring efficiency in health care: Analytic techniques and health policy*. Cambridge University Press.

Kloeden, P. E., & Platen, E. (1992). *Numerical solution of stochastic differential equations*. Springer.

Litvak, E., & Long, M. C. (2000). Cost and quality under managed care: Irreconcilable differences? *The American Journal of Managed Care, 6*(3), 305–312. PMID: 10977431

OECD. (2024).*Health at a glance 2024: OECD indicators*. OECD Publishing.https://doi.org/DOI: 10.1787/19991312

Øksendal, B. (2003). *Stochastic differential equations: An introduction with applications* (6th ed.). Springer.

Pisek, P. E., & Greenhalgh, T. (2001). Complexity science: The challenge of complexity in health care. *BMJ (Clinical Research Ed.), 323*(7313), 625–628. DOI: 10.1136/bmj.323.7313.625 PMID: 11557716

Porter, M. E. (1985). *Competitive advantage: Creating and sustaining superior performance*. Free Press.

Schelling, T. C. (1971). Dynamic models of segregation. *The Journal of Mathematical Sociology, 1*(2), 143–186. DOI: 10.1080/0022250X.1971.9989794

Treacy, M., & Wiersema, F. (1995). *The discipline of market leaders: Choose your customers, narrow your focus, dominate your market*. Addison-Wesley.

Yu, Y., Liao, J., Ma, D., & Zhu, W. (2024). Measuring the COVID-19 treatment efficiency in OECD countries: A multiplicative network DEA approach. *INFOR, 62*(3), 419–448. DOI: 10.1080/03155986.2024.2337978

Chapter 5
Modeling Patient Care Pathways as Markov Chains:
A Tutorial Using the MIMIC-III Clinical Database

Noorjahan Siddiqui
http://orcid.org/0009-0009-8252-0053
Lovely Professional University, India

ABSTRACT

Healthcare involves complex processes where patients move through multiple stages of care. Understanding these pathways is essential for improving outcomes. This chapter presents a pedagogical, worked-example application of Markov chain modeling to patient care pathways using the MIMIC-III Clinical Database Demo. The methodology represents each stage as a discrete state—Admission, ICU, Home, and Expired—and estimates transition probabilities empirically. By analyzing these transitions, the framework demonstrates how outcomes can be predicted, trajectories simulated, and resource planning informed by probabilistic estimates. The transparent Markov structure ensures interpretability. The chapter also discusses extensions toward adaptive systems, including Bayesian updating and reinforcement learning connections. Because the analysis uses a small demonstration dataset, the numerical results are illustrative rather than definitive. Nonetheless, the chapter provides a clear, reproducible template for readers to adapt to their own data

INTRODUCTION

Healthcare systems generate vast amounts of data through patient records, clinical procedures, and hospital operations. With the increasing adoption of electronic health records (EHRs), there has been a significant rise in the availability of healthcare data, creating opportunities for advanced analytics and data-driven decision-making. However, the complexity of healthcare processes, particularly in critical care environments, makes it challenging to extract meaningful insights from this data. Effective analysis of patient movement and treatment pathways is essential for improving care quality, optimizing resource utilization, and reducing mortality rates (Raghupathi & Raghupathi, 2014). Because the dataset used in this chapter was selected specifically for ICU-involved admissions, the resulting model collapses to

DOI: 10.4018/979-8-3373-9705-4.ch005

a single meaningful branching point at the ICU state; the analysis that follows should therefore be read as an illustrative, pedagogical demonstration of the modeling pipeline rather than a comprehensive evaluation of patient flow.

Patient care pathways describe the sequence of clinical stages that a patient experiences during their interaction with a healthcare system. These stages may include hospital admission, transfer to intensive care, treatment progression, and final outcomes such as recovery or death. Such pathways are inherently dynamic and uncertain, as patient transitions depend on multiple clinical and operational factors. Traditional analytical approaches often rely on static or descriptive methods, which fail to capture the probabilistic nature of patient transitions and the temporal dependencies between different stages of care (Goldstein et al., 2016).

To address these limitations, stochastic modeling techniques have been increasingly applied in healthcare analytics. Among these, Markov chain models provide a structured and mathematically rigorous framework for modeling sequential processes under uncertainty. A Markov chain assumes that the future state of a system depends only on its current state, making it particularly suitable for representing patient transitions between different stages of care. This property simplifies the modeling process while still capturing the essential dynamics of patient pathways (Jackson, 2011).

Markov models have been widely used in healthcare research for modeling disease progression, treatment outcomes, and decision-making processes. In recent years, the integration of advanced computational methods, such as machine learning and reinforcement learning, has further enhanced the ability to model complex clinical scenarios. For example, reinforcement learning approaches have been applied to optimize treatment strategies in intensive care settings, demonstrating the potential of combining probabilistic models with data-driven techniques to improve patient outcomes (Zheng et al., 2021). Additionally, deep learning methods have been explored for analyzing large-scale healthcare data, highlighting both the opportunities and challenges associated with predictive modeling in clinical environments (Miotto et al., 2018). More broadly, the convergence of artificial intelligence and clinical practice has been described as reshaping how diagnostic and prognostic judgments are made (Topol, 2019), underscoring the need for models, like the one presented here, that remain interpretable even as analytical sophistication increases.

The availability of large, publicly accessible clinical datasets has further accelerated research in this domain. One such dataset is the MIMIC-III database, which contains detailed information on patient admissions, ICU stays, and clinical outcomes. This dataset provides a rich source of real-world data that can be used to model patient care pathways and estimate transition probabilities between different clinical states (Johnson et al., 2016a). By leveraging such datasets, researchers can move beyond theoretical models and develop practical solutions that reflect real-world healthcare dynamics.

Despite these advancements, several challenges remain in modeling patient care pathways effectively. Many existing studies focus on predictive accuracy without adequately capturing the underlying transition structure of patient states. Furthermore, issues such as data heterogeneity, missing values, and variability in patient populations can impact the reliability of analytical models. There is a need for approaches that not only provide accurate predictions but also offer interpretability and transparency, enabling healthcare professionals to understand and trust the results.

This chapter presents a Markov chain model of patient care pathways as a pedagogical tutorial: a step-by-step worked example, built on the MIMIC-III Clinical Database Demo, that demonstrates how to move from raw admission, ICU-stay, and demographic tables to a transition matrix and its associated predictions. The MIMIC-III Demo cohort is used here as a teaching example illustrating the modeling pipeline, rather than as the basis for a validated clinical decision-support tool.

In this study, a Markov chain-based approach is used to model patient care pathways using real-world clinical data. The methodology represents each stage of care as a discrete state, including Admission, ICU, Home (survival to discharge), and Expired (in-hospital mortality). Transition probabilities between these states are estimated empirically from the dataset, resulting in a transition matrix that captures the dynamics of patient movement within the healthcare system. This approach illustrates both descriptive analysis and the mechanics of predictive modeling using a small, real clinical dataset.

Furthermore, the model demonstrates multi-step transition analysis, showing how long-term outcome probabilities can be estimated through matrix-based computations. This capability is presented here as a worked demonstration of the underlying mathematics rather than as a validated planning tool. By walking through transition patterns and outcome probabilities step by step, the chapter aims to give readers new to stochastic modeling in healthcare a clear, reproducible template they can adapt to their own data.

The main objectives of this study are to develop a Markov chain model for representing patient care pathways in a healthcare setting, estimate transition probabilities between clinical states using real-world data with appropriate adjustments for right-censoring, analyze patient outcomes—including recovery and mortality—through probabilistic modeling, perform multi-step prediction and simulate long-term patient trajectories, extend the static Markov framework with Bayesian updating and Markov Decision Process formulations to enable adaptive system behavior, and ultimately provide insights that support data-driven decision-making in healthcare management.

In conclusion, this chapter presents a pedagogical, worked-example application of Markov chain models to healthcare pathway data, using the MIMIC-III Clinical Database Demo to illustrate the full pipeline from raw clinical tables to a transition matrix and its predictions. By integrating probabilistic modeling with real-world clinical data in a transparent, reproducible way, the chapter aims to serve as a clear teaching resource for readers new to stochastic modeling in healthcare analytics.

BACKGROUND

Markov Chains in Healthcare

Markov chain models have emerged as a powerful framework for analyzing stochastic processes in healthcare systems, particularly in situations involving uncertainty and sequential decision-making. A Markov chain is defined as a memoryless process in which the probability of transitioning to a future state depends only on the current state and not on the sequence of past states. This fundamental property, known as the Markov assumption, enables the simplification of complex real-world systems while preserving essential probabilistic relationships. In healthcare, this modeling approach is particularly useful for representing patient progression through various clinical stages, where each stage corresponds to a distinct health condition or level of care.

The application of Markov models has been widely explored in health economics and disease progression analysis. These models allow researchers to simulate long-term clinical outcomes by defining discrete health states such as stable, deteriorating, and deceased. For instance, Markov-based decision models are commonly used to evaluate treatment effectiveness and cost-efficiency by analyzing transitions between health states over time (Briggs et al., 2006). Such models provide a structured approach for comparing alternative interventions and supporting evidence-based decision-making in healthcare systems.

With the growing availability of electronic health records and large-scale clinical datasets, Markov models have evolved from theoretical frameworks to data-driven analytical tools. Transition probabilities can now be estimated empirically using real-world data, enhancing the accuracy and relevance of these models (Naimi et al., 2017). This shift toward data-driven modeling has significantly improved the ability to capture realistic patient pathways and predict clinical outcomes. Moreover, extensions such as continuous-time Markov chains and hidden Markov models have been introduced to incorporate temporal dynamics and latent states, providing a more comprehensive representation of patient behavior.

One of the key advantages of Markov models is their interpretability. Unlike many machine learning models, which often function as black-box systems, Markov chains provide a transparent structure in which transitions between states can be directly observed and analyzed. This characteristic is particularly valuable in healthcare, where clinicians and policymakers require clear and explainable insights to support decision-making. Additionally, Markov models can incorporate absorbing states, such as recovery or death, enabling long-term outcome prediction and risk assessment.

Despite these advantages, Markov models have certain limitations. The assumption of memorylessness may not fully capture the influence of patient history on future outcomes, particularly in complex clinical scenarios. Furthermore, defining appropriate states and transition structures requires domain expertise and careful consideration. Compared to advanced machine learning approaches, Markov models may offer slightly lower predictive accuracy but provide significantly higher interpretability. This trade-off highlights the importance of selecting modeling techniques based on the specific objectives of the study.

Patient Flow Modeling

Patient flow modeling is a critical aspect of healthcare analytics, focusing on the movement of patients through different stages of care within a healthcare system. Efficient patient flow is essential for reducing waiting times, improving resource utilization, and enhancing patient outcomes. In complex healthcare environments such as hospitals and intensive care units, patient flow is influenced by multiple factors, including patient arrival patterns, treatment capacity, clinical priorities, and operational constraints.

Traditional approaches to patient flow analysis have primarily relied on queueing theory and discrete-event simulation. These methods are effective in evaluating operational performance metrics such as waiting times, service rates, and system utilization (Jacobson et al., 2013). However, they often emphasize system-level efficiency rather than clinical transitions, limiting their ability to capture the full complexity of patient care pathways. As a result, these approaches may not provide sufficient insight into how patients move between different clinical states during their treatment journey.

To overcome these limitations, probabilistic frameworks such as Markov chains have been increasingly applied to patient flow modeling. Markov-based models allow the representation of patient transitions between different care states, such as admission, ward stay, ICU transfer, and discharge. By estimating transition probabilities from real-world data, these models provide a more detailed understanding of patient pathways and their associated outcomes. This approach enables healthcare providers to analyze system behavior at both clinical and operational levels.

In addition to transition analysis, patient flow modeling also involves the study of time spent in each state, commonly referred to as sojourn time. This aspect is particularly important for resource planning, as prolonged stays in critical care units can lead to capacity constraints and increased operational costs.

By combining transition probabilities with state duration analysis, healthcare administrators can optimize resource allocation and improve system efficiency.

Recent advancements in healthcare analytics have further enhanced patient flow modeling through the integration of machine learning techniques. These approaches enable the analysis of large and complex datasets, improving predictive performance and capturing nonlinear relationships between variables (Wiens et al., 2019). Additionally, data-driven methods have facilitated the development of more accurate models for predicting patient outcomes and identifying system bottlenecks.

However, challenges remain in accurately modeling patient flow. Data quality issues, such as missing or inconsistent records, can affect model reliability. Furthermore, variability in patient characteristics and treatment protocols introduces additional complexity. While traditional queueing models focus on operational efficiency, Markov-based approaches provide deeper insights into clinical transitions; recent applied work on reducing surgical cancellations through better patient-flow scheduling (Peel et al., 2025) illustrates the continued relevance of operational patient-flow modeling alongside clinically oriented transition models. Therefore, integrating both perspectives is essential for comprehensive healthcare system analysis.

Literature Review

The application of probabilistic modeling and data analytics in healthcare has been extensively studied, particularly for understanding patient pathways and predicting clinical outcomes. This section reviews key contributions in the areas of Markov modeling, patient flow analysis, and advanced healthcare analytics.

Multi-state models have been widely used to analyze transitions between different health conditions. Andersen and Keiding (2002) introduced a comprehensive framework for multi-state modeling in medical research, emphasizing its importance in survival analysis and longitudinal studies. Their work highlights the significance of incorporating intermediate states when modeling patient pathways, as these states often influence long-term outcomes. Similarly, Markov-based decision models have been applied in health economic evaluations to assess treatment effectiveness and cost-efficiency (Briggs et al., 2006).

In recent years, the use of machine learning in healthcare has gained considerable attention. Harutyunyan et al. (2019) developed benchmark models using clinical time-series data, demonstrating the effectiveness of machine learning techniques in predicting mortality and patient outcomes. Wiens et al. (2019) further emphasized the importance of responsible and interpretable machine learning in healthcare, highlighting challenges related to bias, transparency, and ethical considerations.

Markov models continue to play a central role in healthcare decision-making. Siebert et al. (2012) provided a standardized framework for state-transition modeling, which is widely used for evaluating long-term clinical outcomes and healthcare policies. Their work demonstrates the flexibility of Markov models in representing complex healthcare processes and supporting decision analysis.

The growing availability of large-scale healthcare data has enabled more advanced analytical approaches. Obermeyer and Emanuel (2016) discussed the potential of big data and machine learning in clinical medicine, while also addressing challenges related to data quality and bias. Naimi et al. (2017) introduced advanced causal inference methods, further supporting the integration of data-driven techniques in healthcare research.

Hybrid approaches that combine probabilistic models with machine learning have also been explored. Futoma et al. (2017) proposed a multitask learning framework for detecting sepsis, demonstrating improved predictive performance through the integration of statistical and deep learning methods. Similarly,

Komorowski et al. (2018) applied reinforcement learning techniques to optimize treatment strategies in intensive care, highlighting the potential of artificial intelligence in healthcare decision-making.

Patient flow modeling has also been studied from an operational perspective. Jacobson et al. (2013) discussed the application of discrete-event simulation in healthcare systems, emphasizing its role in analyzing patient flow and reducing delays. Their work highlights the importance of modeling patient movement across different stages of care to improve system efficiency and resource utilization.

Despite these advancements, several limitations remain in the existing literature. Many studies focus primarily on predictive accuracy without providing interpretable insights into patient transitions; for example, deep learning approaches to electronic health record analysis (Shickel et al., 2017) and broader machine learning applications in medicine (Rajkomar et al., 2019) have achieved strong predictive performance but often function as black boxes. Additionally, while machine learning approaches offer high predictive performance, they often lack transparency, limiting their applicability in clinical decision-making. Ward-level risk stratification models (Churpek et al., 2013) and hospital readmission risk prediction models (Kansagara et al., 2011) illustrate this trade-off: they perform well on prediction but offer limited insight into the underlying state transitions driving the risk. Furthermore, limited research has focused on integrating Markov-based transition modeling with real-world ICU datasets for pathway-level analysis.

Research Gap

Although prior studies have explored machine learning, simulation, and probabilistic modeling in healthcare, there is limited research that integrates Markov chain–based transition modeling with real-world ICU datasets to analyze patient care pathways. In particular, existing approaches often lack a unified framework that provides both interpretability and multi-step probabilistic prediction of patient outcomes. This study addresses this gap by developing a data-driven Markov chain framework that models patient transitions between clinical states and enables scenario-based prediction of long-term outcomes.

METHODOLOGICAL FRAMEWORK: A WORKED EXAMPLE OF MARKOV CHAIN CONSTRUCTION

This section walks through the complete pipeline of building a Markov chain model from raw clinical data: from data preprocessing and feature engineering, through transition matrix construction, to outcome prediction and visualization. The purpose is pedagogical — to demonstrate, step by step, how a stochastic model of patient care pathways is built and interpreted — rather than to deliver a comprehensive evaluation of patient flow across a general hospital population. Readers should keep three limitations in mind from the outset: the sample is small (129 admissions), it was selected specifically for ICU-involved cases, and this selection collapses the chain to a single branching decision at the ICU state. Within this scope, the following subsections maintain the same clear, step-by-step exposition of each methodological stage.

Dataset Description

The analysis is based on the MIMIC-III Clinical Database Demo (Johnson et al., 2016b, version 1.4), an openly accessible curated subset of the full MIMIC-III critical care database, consistent with the broader call for well-curated, closed-loop ICU data resources in critical care analytics (Celi et al., 2013). Unlike the full MIMIC-III and MIMIC-IV databases, which require credentialed access, the Demo subset is released under the Open Data Commons Open Database License and does not require CITI human-subjects research training or a signed PhysioNet Data Use Agreement; it covers all admissions and ICU stays for 100 patients drawn from the full database. The dataset includes time-stamped records, demographic information, and clinical outcomes, making it suitable for modeling patient pathways. Because the Demo cohort was curated by PhysioNet specifically from patients who eventually die (though not necessarily during the specific admission analyzed here), it is not a representative random sample of the general ICU population, and mortality-related estimates drawn from it should be interpreted with this enrichment in mind; this is revisited in the Depth and Accuracy discussion below.

For this study, a cleaned and structured dataset consisting of 129 admissions, drawn from 100 unique patients (14 of whom contributed more than one admission), is used. Because a small number of patients contribute multiple admissions, the standard independence assumption across records is not strictly satisfied; this is noted as a limitation of the current cohort. The dataset is constructed by integrating multiple tables, including admissions, ICU stays, and patient demographic information. This integration allows for a unified view of patient journeys from hospital admission to final outcome.

It is important to note that the dataset primarily represents ICU-related cases. As a result, most patients in the dataset transition from admission directly to ICU. This characteristic reflects the nature of the selected data subset and plays a crucial role in shaping the transition matrix.

Table 1. Dataset Structure

Admissions	**Contains patient admission details such as admission time and discharge outcome**
ICU Stays	Includes ICU admission time and length of stay
Patient Info	Provides demographic attributes such as age and gender

The combination of these tables enables a comprehensive representation of patient pathways. The dataset captures both temporal and outcome-related information, which is essential for transition modeling.

Data Preprocessing

Data preprocessing is a critical step in ensuring the accuracy and reliability of the analysis. Raw clinical data often contains missing values, inconsistencies, and formatting issues that must be addressed before modeling.

Several preprocessing steps were performed:

First, missing values were handled by removing incomplete records that could affect transition calculations. This ensures that only valid patient pathways are considered in the analysis.

Second, date variables such as admission time and date of birth were converted into a standard date-time format. This conversion is necessary for accurate computation of derived variables, particularly age.

Third, patient age was calculated using the difference between admission year and birth year. Consistent with MIMIC-III's de-identification protocol, dates of birth for patients over 89 are shifted far into the past to prevent re-identification of elderly individuals; this produces implausibly large computed ages (in this dataset, as high as approximately 300 years) rather than a fixed placeholder value. These shifted records were capped and treated as approximately 90 for demographic analysis rather than excluded, since they represent a genuine (if imprecise) elderly cohort rather than data errors.

This age-shifting convention, applied by MIMIC-III to comply with HIPAA privacy requirements, means that reported ages for the oldest patients are approximate rather than exact; this is a limitation of the underlying data rather than a preprocessing artifact and should be kept in mind when interpreting the age-based subgroup results reported later in this chapter. Records with missing admission or discharge timestamps would have been removed rather than imputed had any existed, so that transition frequencies were computed only from complete, verifiable timelines. This was checked directly: none of the 129 admissions or 136 ICU stays in the analytic cohort had a missing discharge or ICU-exit timestamp, so no records were in fact removed on this basis (see the Depth and Accuracy discussion below for the full check).

These preprocessing steps improve data quality and ensure that subsequent analysis is based on reliable information.

Table 2. Variables Used

Variable	Role
admittime	Records the time of hospital admission
dob	Used to compute patient age
age	Derived demographic variable
hadm_id	Unique admission identifier
ICU_flag	Indicates whether the patient was admitted to ICU
hospital_expire_flag	Represents patient outcome

Feature Engineering

Feature engineering plays a key role in transforming raw data into meaningful analytical variables. In this study, several derived features were created to support pathway modeling. This step converts the raw admission, ICU-stay, and demographic tables into the structured variables the Markov model requires.

The first feature is age, which is derived from date variables and used for demographic analysis. Age is an important factor in healthcare studies, as it often influences patient outcomes and risk levels. Converting date-of-birth and admission date into a single age variable makes it possible to compare outcomes across age groups, as reported in the age-subgroup analysis later in this chapter.

The second feature is ICU_flag, which identifies whether a patient was admitted to the ICU. This binary variable is essential for distinguishing between critical and non-critical cases. It is derived directly by checking whether each admission's hadm_id appears in the ICU stays table.

The most important feature is the pathway variable, which represents the sequence of states that each patient experiences. The pathway is defined as:

Admission → ICU → (Home / Expired)

This simplified representation captures the essential stages of patient progression. It allows for easy extraction of transitions and construction of the Markov model.

Constructing the pathway sequence requires sorting each patient's clinical events in chronological order within a single hospitalization episode (hadm_id). Because this subset was selected specifically for acute, critical-care admissions, non-critical (low-acuity) encounters are not represented, and this selection criterion — not a general property of hospital care — is what produces the direct Admission-to-ICU pattern reported below.

Since the dataset is ICU-focused, transitions involving the Ward state are not observed and the Ward state is therefore excluded from the model. In a broader clinical setting, a patient might move from Admission to a General Medical Ward before escalating to the ICU; in this curated, ICU-selected subset, essentially all patients went directly to the ICU instead. This is an important scope limitation rather than a general finding: because the sample was selected on ICU involvement, the resulting four-state chain (Admission, ICU, Home, Expired) collapses to a single decision point at ICU, and the reported transition matrix should be read as describing this specific ICU-selected cohort rather than the general hospital population.

Care Pathway Modeling

Patient care pathways are modeled as sequences of transitions between discrete states. Each state represents a specific stage in the healthcare process.

Table 3. State Definition

State	Meaning
Admission	Patient entry into hospital
ICU	Intensive care unit stay
Home	Survival to hospital discharge (does not imply full clinical recovery; post-discharge outcomes are out of scope)
Expired	Patient death

This state definition simplifies complex clinical processes into a manageable structure. It allows for clear identification of transitions and supports probabilistic modeling.

The absence of Ward transitions in the dataset indicates that the selected data primarily focuses on critical care pathways. This is an important consideration in interpreting the results.

Markov Chain Formulation

The patient pathway is modeled using a discrete-time Markov chain. This approach assumes that the probability of transitioning to the next state depends only on the current state.

Equation 1: Markov Property

$$P(X_{t+1} = j \mid X_t = i) = p_{ij}$$

This equation defines the fundamental assumption of the Markov model.

Equation 2: Transition Matrix

$$P = [p_{ij}]$$

The transition matrix contains probabilities for all possible state transitions.

Equation 3: Absorbing State

$$p_{ii} = 1$$

The states Home and Expired are absorbing, meaning that once a patient reaches these states, no further transitions occur.

These equations provide the mathematical foundation for the model.

One point that must be made explicit is the time step represented by a single transition. Here, each step corresponds to an entire episode of care (e.g., the full ICU stay), not a fixed unit such as one day; this is why ICU has no self-transition (ICU-to-ICU = 0) even though Figure 5 shows ICU length of stay ranging from 1 to more than 20 days. An episode-level step is a valid modeling choice, but it means the chain says nothing about how long a patient spends in the ICU before reaching an outcome, only which outcome is eventually reached. Because the ICU length-of-stay distribution is strongly right-skewed, a semi-Markov or Coxian phase-type / continuous-time formulation would be a more appropriate tool for capturing this duration information, and is a natural extension of this framework. Such a formulation would also permit calculation of the expected time to absorption via the fundamental matrix $N = (I - Q)^{-1}$, where Q is the sub-matrix of transitions among transient states; this is left for future work rather than attempted here given the limited sample size.

Transition Matrix Construction

The transition matrix is constructed using observed transitions extracted from patient pathways.

Table 4. Transition Probability Matrix

From/To	Admission	ICU	Home	Expired
Admission	0.0	1.0	0.0	0.0
ICU	0.0	0.0	0.6899	0.3101
Home	0.0	0.0	1.0	0.0
Expired	0.0	0.0	0.0	1.0

The matrix clearly shows that all patients transition from Admission to ICU. From ICU, patients either recover or expire. The probabilities indicate that recovery is more likely than mortality.

Visualization and Analysis

Figure 1. Care Pathway Transition Matrix

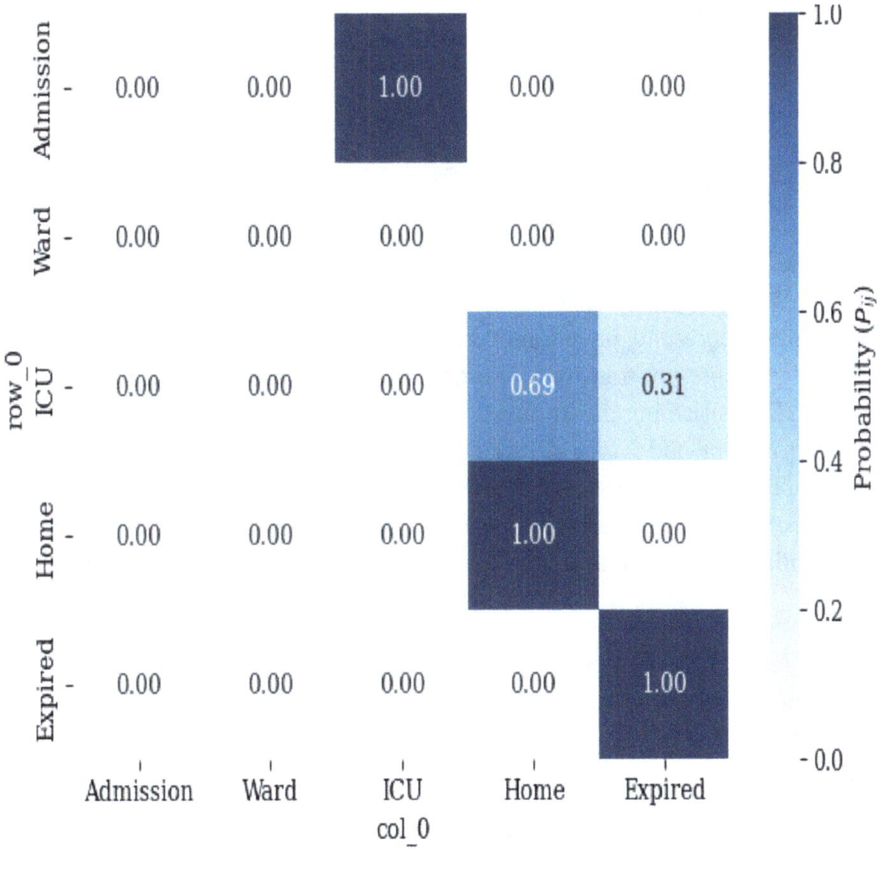

The heatmap provides a visual representation of transition probabilities between different clinical states. It clearly shows that all patients initially move from *Admission to ICU* with a probability of 1.00, indicating a deterministic transition in the dataset. From the ICU state, two major outcomes are observed: a probability of 0.69 for discharge to *Home* and 0.31 for transition to *Expired.* The absence of transitions involving the *Ward* state suggests that it plays a negligible role in this dataset. Additionally, *Home* and *Expired* states are absorbing, as indicated by their self-transition probability of 1.00. Overall, the heatmap highlights a simplified but highly critical care pathway dominated by ICU transitions and final outcomes.

Figure 2. Clinical Transition Network Diagram

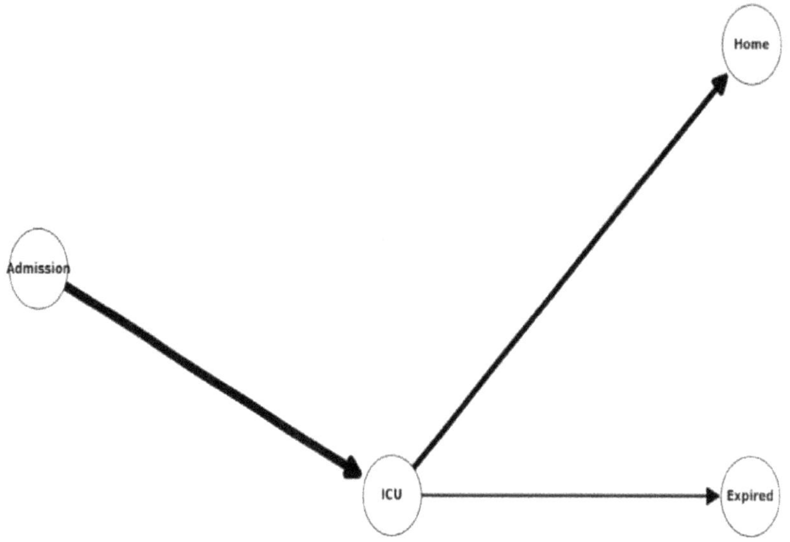

The network diagram represents patient movement as a directed graph, where nodes correspond to clinical states and edges represent transitions weighted by probability. The strongest edge is observed from *Admission to ICU*, confirming the immediate escalation to critical care. From the ICU node, two outgoing edges lead to *Home* and *Expired*, reflecting recovery and mortality pathways. The thickness of edges visually emphasizes that recovery is more likely than mortality. The absence of multiple intermediate transitions indicates a relatively linear and constrained pathway structure. This graphical representation helps identify ICU as the central decision point in the patient journey.

Figure 3. Multi-step Prediction

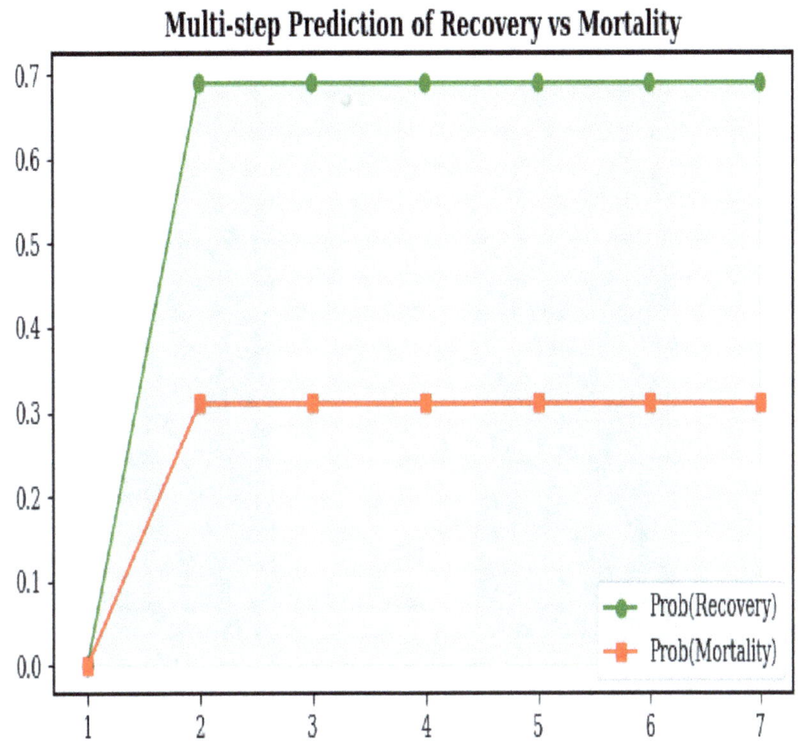

This figure illustrates how outcome probabilities evolve over multiple transition steps. Initially, probabilities are zero, but by step 2, they stabilize at approximately 0.69 for recovery and 0.31 for mortality. This stabilization at step 2 is a direct, mechanical consequence of the chain's structure rather than an independent finding: because Admission → ICU is deterministic and ICU transitions directly into the two absorbing states (Home, Expired), the chain has fully absorbed after exactly two steps for every patient. The flat trend beyond step 2 therefore restates the ICU row of the transition matrix rather than confirming the Markov property or demonstrating multi-step predictive value; with the current three-transient/absorbing-state structure, no genuinely multi-step prediction is possible. Richer intermediate states (e.g., Ward, step-down care, ICU readmission) would be needed for multi-step analysis to add information beyond the single-step transition probabilities.

Figure 4. Gender Risk Analysis

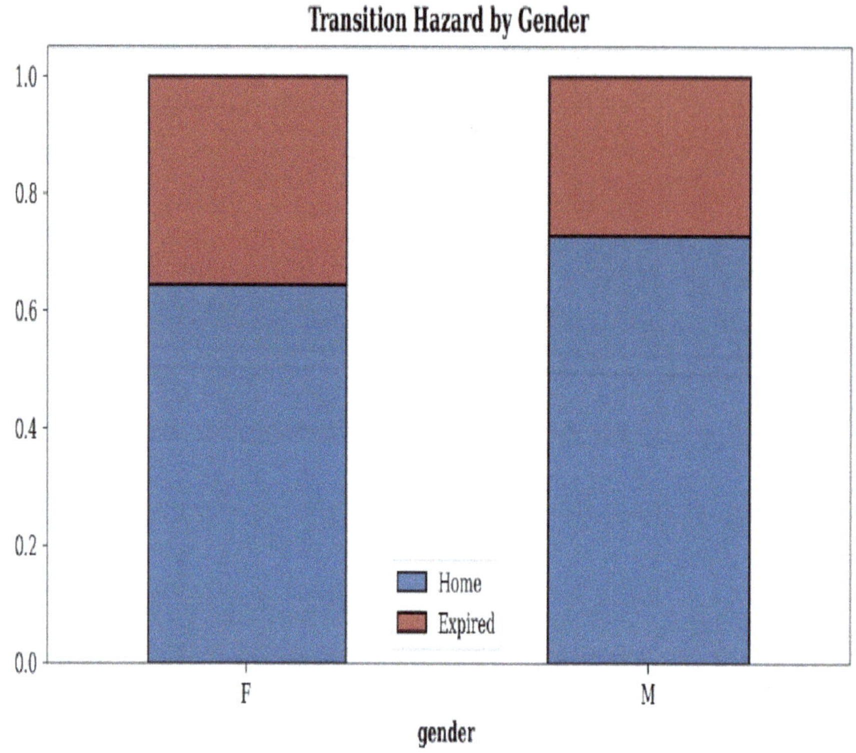

This figure shows differences in discharge and mortality probabilities between male and female patients within this small sample. Female patients (n=59: 38 discharged home, 21 expired) show a discharge-to-home rate of approximately 0.64, while male patients (n=70: 51 discharged home, 19 expired) show a higher discharge-to-home rate of approximately 0.73; correspondingly, the mortality proportion is higher among female patients (0.36) than male patients (0.27). With cell sizes this small (21 and 19 deaths respectively), the 95% Wilson confidence intervals around these proportions are wide — approximately 0.24–0.49 for female mortality and 0.18–0.38 for male mortality — and overlap substantially, so this difference should not be read as a confirmed gender effect. Age and diagnosis mix likely confound this comparison and were not adjusted for. This figure is presented as exploratory and hypothesis-generating rather than a validated finding; a larger, adjusted sample would be needed to confirm whether gender genuinely influences outcomes in this cohort.

Figure 5. ICU Length of Stay Distribution

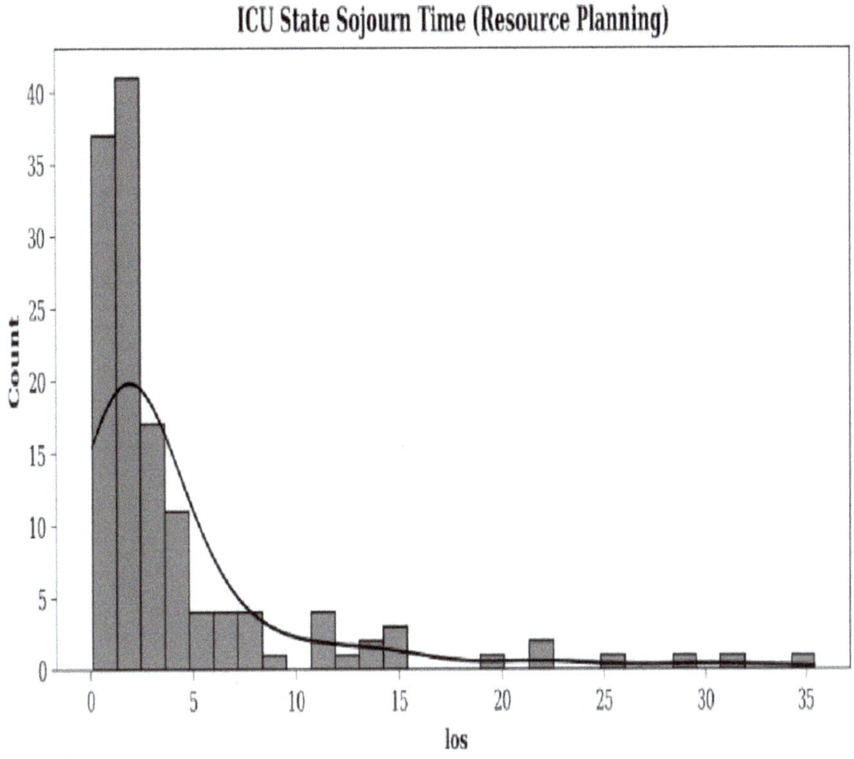

This figure shows that the distribution of ICU length of stay is right-skewed. Most patients have a short stay, typically between 1–5 days, indicating rapid clinical outcomes such as recovery or deterioration. However, a long tail is observed, where a smaller group of patients remains in the ICU for more than 20 days, representing more complex or critical conditions. This variability reflects uncertainty in resource utilization within the healthcare system. The distribution is particularly important for hospital capacity planning, as prolonged stays can lead to resource constraints and operational bottlenecks. Understanding these patterns can help in optimizing ICU resource allocation and improving overall system efficiency.

Figure 6. Age-based Risk Analysis

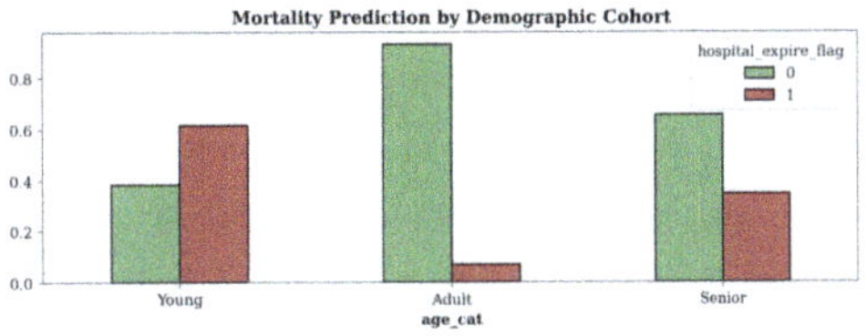

This figure splits the 129-record sample across three age groups. Young patients (n=13: 5 discharged home, 8 expired) show an apparent mortality probability of 0.62 (95% Wilson CI: 0.36–0.82); this wide interval, driven entirely by the small subgroup size, shows the estimate is highly imprecise and should not be read as a genuine age-mortality relationship. Adult patients (n=29: 27 discharged home, 2 expired) show a mortality probability of 0.07 (95% CI: 0.02–0.22), and Senior patients (n=87: 57 discharged home, 30 expired) show a mortality probability of 0.34 (95% CI: 0.25–0.45). The Senior estimate, drawn from the largest subgroup, is the most reliable of the three; the Young and Adult estimates carry substantial uncertainty and are presented here as exploratory and hypothesis-generating rather than validated findings. Age-based risk stratification is a reasonable direction for future work, but it requires a substantially larger sample than is available here before subgroup-specific probabilities can be trusted.

Figure 7. Steady-state Analysis

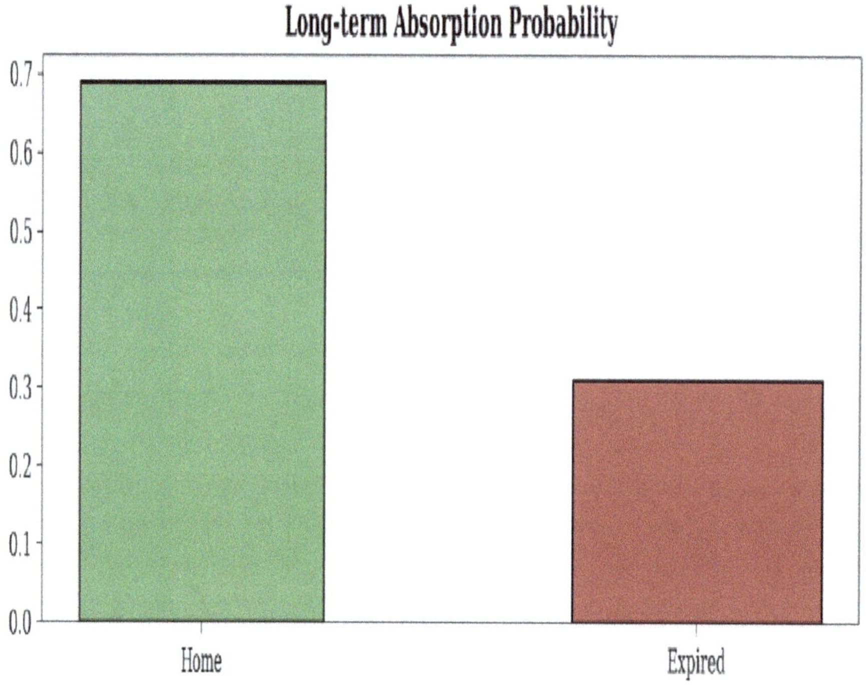

This figure shows that the steady-state distribution represents the long-term probabilities of patients ending in absorbing states. The results indicate a recovery probability of approximately 0.69 and a mortality probability of 0.31. These values are numerically identical to the ICU row of the transition matrix, which is expected rather than an independent confirmation of model stability: with Home and Expired absorbing and no other transient states between ICU and absorption, the steady-state distribution is mathematically forced to equal the ICU exit probabilities. This limits the added value of steady-state analysis in the current model, though it still usefully restates that, although recovery is more likely, the risk of mortality remains substantial and should not be discounted.

Figure 8. Diagnosis-based Risk Analysis

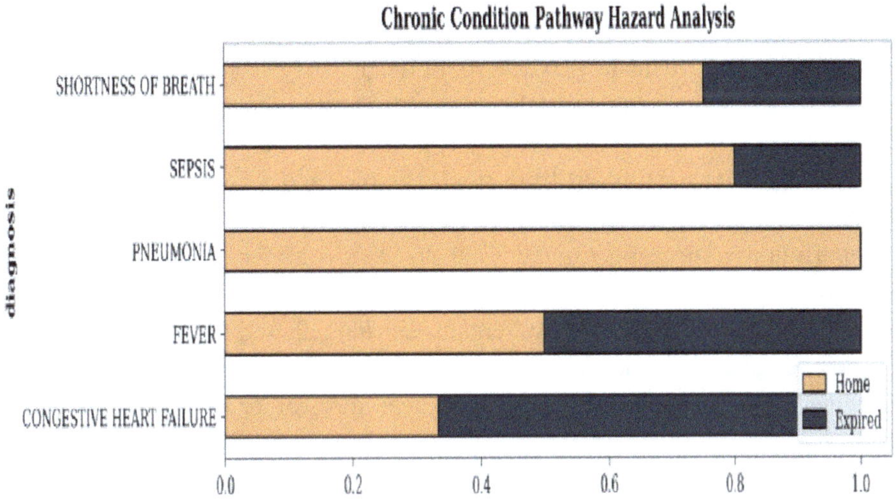

This figure compares outcomes across the five most frequent diagnoses in the sample. Cell sizes are very small throughout: Pneumonia (n=8: 0 expired, 95% CI 0.00–0.32), Sepsis (n=10: 2 expired, mortality 0.20, 95% CI 0.06–0.51), Shortness of Breath (n=4: 1 expired, mortality 0.25, 95% CI 0.05–0.70), Fever (n=4: 2 expired, mortality 0.50, 95% CI 0.15–0.85), and Congestive Heart Failure (n=3: 2 expired, mortality 0.67, 95% CI 0.21–0.94). Every one of these confidence intervals is extremely wide and overlaps substantially with the others, so none of the apparent differences in mortality across diagnoses can be treated as reliable at this sample size; they are presented here as exploratory and hypothesis-generating rather than validated findings. With that caveat, the figure is useful for flagging which conditions merit closer investigation in a larger, adjusted cohort before any targeted intervention or resource-allocation decision is based on them.

Outcome Prediction and Simulation

Equation 4: Multi-step Prediction

$$\pi(n) = \pi(0)P^n$$

This equation is used to compute future state probabilities after multiple transitions.

Table 5. Outcome Metrics

Metric	Value
Discharge-to-Home Rate	0.6899
Mortality Rate	0.3101

Because these proportions are estimated from only 129 records, they carry considerable sampling uncertainty. A 95% Wilson score confidence interval around the mortality rate is approximately 0.24-0.39, and correspondingly approximately 0.61-0.76 for the discharge-to-home rate; a sample of this size cannot distinguish, for example, a true mortality rate of 0.25 from one of 0.38. Wilson score intervals, rather than the standard normal approximation, were used throughout this chapter because they remain well calibrated for proportions estimated from small samples and for proportions near 0 or 1, which is relevant given the modest subgroup sizes used in the age, gender, and diagnosis analyses reported below. For a proportion $\hat{p}$ = successes / n and $z = 1.96$ (95% confidence), the interval is calculated as $[\hat{p} + z^2/(2n) \pm z\sqrt{(\hat{p}(1-\hat{p})/n + z^2/(4n^2))}] / (1 + z^2/n)$. The results indicate that discharge to home is more probable than in-hospital death, but mortality remains substantial, and the confidence intervals should accompany the point estimates whenever they are cited. This underscores both the importance of effective ICU management and early intervention, and the need for a larger sample before the estimates are treated as precise.

Depth and Accuracy of the Model

This section returns, as promised in the Data Preprocessing discussion above, to the question of how much clinical and analytical depth the current model actually supports. As fitted, the chain has only one point at which a real branching decision occurs: the ICU state, which resolves to Home with probability 0.6899 or Expired with probability 0.3101. Admission-to-ICU is deterministic within this cohort because the extraction criterion selected only ICU-involved admissions, and Home and Expired are absorbing by construction. Multi-step prediction and the steady-state distribution therefore do not add independent information beyond this single transition; both are mechanical restatements of the ICU row of Table 4, as noted in the discussion of Figures 3 and 7. This is an honest and useful worked example of how a Markov chain is built from raw admission, ICU-stay, and demographic tables through to a transition matrix and prediction equations, but it should not be read as a validated clinical decision-support model.

A related accuracy concern is right-censoring. Patients who were still in the ICU at the time the data were extracted would have no recorded outcome, and if such records had been dropped from the analytic sample, the reported 0.69/0.31 split could be biased in a direction this chapter could not quantify. This was checked directly against the underlying data: of the 129 admissions and 136 ICU stays in the analytic cohort, none had a missing discharge timestamp (dischtime) or a missing ICU-exit timestamp (outtime). No records were therefore excluded from this cohort on right-censoring grounds, and the reported transition probabilities are based on complete, fully-resolved outcomes rather than complete-case removal of censored cases. This does not rule out censoring having occurred upstream, before the Demo extract used here was assembled; readers extending this analysis to the full MIMIC-III or MIMIC-IV databases, where active ongoing stays are possible, should re-run this same check rather than assume it holds there as well.

Extending the model beyond its current single-decision-point structure requires three concrete changes. First, the Ward and step-down states should be reinstated using a less restrictively filtered cohort, together with ICU readmission edges, so that the chain has more than one transient state through which probability mass can flow. Second, the time step should be redefined at a fixed granularity, such as one calendar day, rather than treating an entire ICU episode as a single transition; this is what would let the model use the length-of-stay information shown in Figure 5 instead of discarding it. Third, because ICU length of stay is strongly right-skewed, a semi-Markov or Coxian phase-type formulation would let the chain represent duration explicitly and would support calculation of expected time-to-absorption via the fundamental matrix N = (I - Q)^-1. None of these extensions are attempted here, both because they require a substantially larger sample than 129 records to estimate reliably and because they represent a different, more ambitious modeling exercise than the illustrative pipeline presented in this chapter.

Taken together, these limitations mean the appropriate reading of this chapter is as a transparent, reproducible worked example of the Markov chain pipeline applied to the MIMIC-III Clinical Database Demo, not as a validated predictive tool ready for operational deployment. A related limitation specific to this dataset is that the Demo cohort was curated by PhysioNet from patients who eventually die at some point in their recorded history, rather than being a random sample of the general ICU population; this pre-existing mortality enrichment is distinct from the sample-size and censoring issues discussed above, and it means the 0.31 mortality estimate in Table 5 should not be generalized to ICU populations at large without independent validation on a representative sample, such as the full MIMIC-III or MIMIC-IV databases. See the Code Availability statement in the Declarations section for how the calculations in this chapter can be reproduced or extended.

SOLUTIONS AND RECOMMENDATIONS

Given the small sample size (129 admissions) and the cohort-level mortality enrichment discussed above, the following recommendations should not be read as novel insights uniquely derived from this model. Rather, they are well-established healthcare management practices, already supported by the broader literature, that happen to be consistent with the illustrative patterns observed in this demonstration. The value of presenting them here lies in showing how a Markov-based transition analysis can be connected to practical decision-making, not in claiming that this small, ICU-selected dataset has generated new operational knowledge.

One of the most significant findings is the strong transition tendency from the initial admission state to intensive care: the estimated Admission-to-ICU probability is 1.0 in this dataset. This figure should be read as a consequence of how the cohort was selected (the sample was drawn specifically from ICU-involved admissions) rather than as evidence that all hospital admissions proceed to the ICU. Within that scope, it reflects a high dependency on critical care services for this cohort. Therefore, hospitals working with a similarly ICU-selected population must focus on strategic ICU capacity planning. Specifically, the 0.69/0.31 split between discharge-to-home and in-hospital mortality (95% CI approximately 0.61-0.76 and 0.24-0.39 respectively) can be used as a starting point for estimating expected bed-turnover demand, though the wide interval means this estimate should be updated as more records become available rather than treated as fixed. This allows healthcare administrators to allocate resources more efficiently, ensuring that sufficient beds, medical equipment, and trained personnel are available to meet patient needs.

Another important implication of the model is related to outcome probabilities. With a single ICU state carrying a 0.31 mortality probability, this chain cannot yet distinguish which patients within the ICU population are at higher or lower risk at a given point in their stay — that granularity would require additional intermediate states (e.g., stratifying by day of stay or severity indicators) rather than the current single-state ICU node. This probabilistic distribution nonetheless emphasizes the need for early risk identification. Healthcare providers should implement continuous monitoring systems that track patient progression in real time, and future versions of this model that add such intermediate states could directly support that goal. By identifying patients who are more likely to transition toward adverse outcomes, medical teams can prioritize interventions and allocate resources more effectively.

The results also highlight the importance of demographic and clinical heterogeneity in patient outcomes. The stochastic nature of the model suggests that transition probabilities are not uniform across all patient groups. Factors such as age and clinical condition influence the likelihood of transitioning between states. This variation supports the need for personalized healthcare strategies. Instead of applying uniform treatment protocols, healthcare providers should adopt targeted approaches that consider individual patient characteristics. Personalized care pathways can improve treatment effectiveness and reduce the probability of unfavorable outcomes.

From an operational perspective, the structure of the care pathway reveals a relatively concentrated flow of patients through a limited number of key states. This indicates that the healthcare system operates as a tightly connected network, where inefficiencies in one stage can propagate throughout the entire system. The Markov representation of patient flow provides a clear understanding of these dependencies. To improve system performance, hospitals should focus on optimizing transitions between states. This includes reducing delays during admission, improving coordination between departments, and ensuring timely discharge processes. Efficient management of these transitions can significantly enhance patient throughput and reduce system congestion.

Another key recommendation is the adoption of data-driven decision-making frameworks. The Markov chain model offers a transparent and interpretable structure for analyzing patient transitions, making it particularly useful for healthcare management. Unlike complex black-box models, this approach allows decision-makers to directly interpret transition probabilities and understand their implications. By integrating such probabilistic models into hospital information systems, administrators can simulate different scenarios and evaluate potential outcomes before implementing policy changes. This enhances the ability to make informed and evidence-based decisions.

Continuous model updating is also essential for maintaining accuracy and relevance. Healthcare environments are dynamic, and transition probabilities may change over time due to variations in patient demographics, disease patterns, or treatment protocols. The stochastic framework used in this study relies on historical data, which may not fully capture future trends. Therefore, it is important to regularly update the model using new data. This ensures that the transition matrix reflects current system behavior and supports reliable predictions. A continuously updated model can serve as a real-time decision support tool for healthcare providers.

Resource optimization emerges as another critical area of focus. The analysis of state transitions provides insights into how patients utilize healthcare resources at different stages. Prolonged stays in high-dependency states can lead to bottlenecks and increased operational costs. By understanding the expected duration and transition probabilities associated with each state, hospitals can design strategies to optimize resource allocation. For example, intermediate care units can be used to manage patients who no longer require intensive care but are not yet ready for discharge. This approach helps balance resource utilization and improves overall system efficiency.

Effective coordination and communication within the healthcare system are also essential for improving patient outcomes. The Markov model highlights the interconnected nature of patient states, where transitions depend on timely and accurate decision-making. Poor coordination between departments can disrupt these transitions and lead to inefficiencies. Hospitals should invest in integrated information systems that enable real-time data sharing among healthcare professionals. Improved communication ensures that patient information is accessible when needed, facilitating smoother transitions and better clinical decisions.

Finally, it is important to adopt a patient-centered approach while implementing these recommendations. Although the model focuses on system-level analysis, the ultimate objective is to improve patient outcomes and experience. The probabilistic insights provided by the model should be used to support clinical decision-making in a way that prioritizes patient well-being. By combining analytical methods with compassionate care, healthcare systems can achieve a balance between efficiency and quality.

In summary, the Markov chain–based analysis provides a robust foundation for improving healthcare system performance. The transition probabilities and state-based structure offer valuable insights into patient behavior, resource utilization, and outcome risks. By leveraging these insights, healthcare providers can implement targeted strategies that enhance efficiency, reduce risk, and deliver better patient care.

FUTURE RESEARCH DIRECTIONS

Although this study establishes a strong and interpretable framework for modeling patient care pathways using a Markov chain approach, several important directions remain for future research. These directions can further enhance the predictive accuracy, flexibility, and real-world applicability of healthcare analytics models.

One of the most promising directions is the integration of machine learning techniques with probabilistic models. The current framework focuses on a structured and interpretable approach, which is highly useful for understanding patient transitions. However, real-world clinical data often contain complex and nonlinear relationships that may not be fully captured by traditional probabilistic methods. Machine learning techniques, such as decision trees, neural networks, and ensemble models, are capable of identifying hidden patterns within large datasets. By combining these techniques with state-based modeling, future research can develop hybrid approaches that maintain interpretability while improving predictive performance. Such models can provide more accurate estimates of patient transitions and outcomes.

Toward Adaptive, Reinforcement-Learning-Informed Care Models

The reinforcement learning literature cited in the Introduction (Zheng et al., 2021; Komorowski et al., 2018) points toward a natural extension of the static transition-matrix approach used here. Zheng et al. (2021) applied reinforcement learning to adjust oxygen therapy for COVID-19 ICU patients in response to their evolving state, while Komorowski et al. (2018) used reinforcement learning to derive treatment strategies for sepsis that adapt to a patient's trajectory rather than applying a fixed policy. The Markov chain pipeline presented in this chapter — from raw admission and ICU-stay tables to an estimated transition matrix — could serve as methodological scaffolding for this kind of adaptive system:

the empirically estimated transition probabilities could act as a starting environment model, which a reinforcement-learning agent would then refine using reward signals tied to patient outcomes, and Bayesian updating could allow the transition probabilities themselves to be revised as new admissions accumulate rather than re-estimated from scratch. This chapter does not implement either extension, both because the 129-record sample is far too small to train or validate a reinforcement-learning policy reliably, and because doing so is a substantially more ambitious undertaking than the illustrative pipeline presented here. The point is offered as a forward-looking direction: the pipeline demonstrated in this chapter is the kind of foundation on which an adaptive, RL-informed model could eventually be built. A related, static-versus-adaptive modeling question arises in patient-flow analysis more broadly; the queueing-theory chapter elsewhere in this volume addresses waiting times and service capacity from that complementary angle, and the two approaches — state-transition modeling here, and arrival/service-rate modeling there — could eventually be combined into a fuller picture of adaptive patient-flow management.

Another important research direction is the development of real-time predictive systems. The current analysis relies on historical data to estimate transition behavior and predict outcomes. However, healthcare environments are highly dynamic, where patient conditions can change rapidly over time. Future studies can focus on incorporating real-time data from hospital information systems, such as electronic health records and patient monitoring devices. This would allow models to update continuously as new data becomes available. Real-time prediction systems can support immediate clinical decision-making, enabling healthcare providers to respond more effectively to critical situations and improving overall patient outcomes. Realizing this potential also requires attention to implementation: translating predictive or transition-based models into routine clinical workflows involves organizational, regulatory, and validation challenges that are distinct from model development itself (Sendak et al., 2020).

The expansion of datasets is also a key area for future research. The present study is based on a limited subset of patient data, which may restrict the generalizability of the findings. Future work can include data from multiple hospitals, regions, or healthcare systems to capture a wider range of patient behaviors and treatment practices. Larger and more diverse datasets can improve the robustness of the model and make it applicable across different clinical environments. In addition, incorporating longitudinal data can help capture long-term patient trajectories, providing deeper insights into healthcare processes.

Another potential improvement involves the inclusion of more detailed and granular care states. In this study, patient pathways are represented using a simplified set of states that capture the main stages of care. While this approach provides clarity and ease of interpretation, it may not fully reflect the complexity of real-world healthcare systems. Future models can include additional intermediate states, such as different levels of care intensity, treatment phases, or recovery stages. This would allow for a more comprehensive representation of patient progression and enable more precise analysis of transition dynamics.

Future research can also explore the role of external and operational factors in shaping patient pathways. Healthcare systems are influenced by various factors such as staffing levels, bed availability, hospital policies, and seasonal variations. These factors can significantly affect patient flow and outcomes but are not explicitly included in the current framework. Incorporating such variables into the modeling process can improve the realism and practical relevance of the analysis. For example, integrating operational data can help evaluate how resource constraints impact patient transitions and system performance.

Another important direction is the development of personalized healthcare models. While the current study considers general patient characteristics, future research can incorporate more detailed patient-specific information, such as medical history, comorbidities, and treatment responses. This would enable the creation of individualized prediction models that support personalized treatment planning. Personalized models can improve clinical decision-making by providing tailored insights for each patient, leading to better outcomes and more efficient use of healthcare resources.

Finally, future studies should address the limitations associated with the memoryless assumption of the Markov framework. The current model assumes that future transitions depend only on the present state, without considering past history. While this assumption simplifies the modeling process, it may not fully capture the complexity of patient trajectories. In real-world scenarios, previous conditions and treatments often influence future outcomes. To overcome this limitation, future research can explore advanced modeling approaches that incorporate memory or hidden states. These methods can provide a more realistic representation of patient behavior and improve the accuracy of predictions.

In summary, there are multiple opportunities to extend and enhance the proposed framework. By integrating advanced analytical techniques, expanding datasets, incorporating additional variables, and addressing model limitations, future research can develop more powerful and flexible healthcare models. These improvements have the potential to support better clinical decision-making, optimize resource allocation, and ultimately improve patient outcomes.

CONCLUSION

This study developed a structured and data-driven framework for modeling patient care pathways using a Markov chain approach. By representing patient progression as transitions between discrete clinical states, the study provides a clear and systematic method for analyzing complex healthcare processes. The probabilistic structure of the model allows a deeper understanding of how patients move through different stages of care and how these transitions influence overall outcomes.

The analysis reveals important patterns in patient flow, particularly the significant reliance on critical care services and the associated outcome distribution. The transition behavior indicates that while a considerable proportion of patients achieve recovery, there remains a notable level of risk for those requiring intensive care. This highlights the importance of timely intervention and efficient resource allocation in healthcare systems. The ability of the model to support multi-step prediction further enhances its usefulness, as it enables the estimation of long-term outcomes based on current patient states.

A key strength of this study lies in the interpretability of the Markov chain framework. Unlike complex predictive models that often lack transparency, this approach provides a clear representation of transition dynamics. Healthcare professionals can directly interpret transition probabilities and understand their implications for patient care. This makes the model highly practical for real-world applications, particularly in supporting clinical and administrative decision-making.

Another important contribution of this chapter is its reliance on real, publicly available healthcare data rather than synthetic or purely theoretical examples. By working through actual patient records, the chapter illustrates a transparent, reproducible pipeline for Markov chain construction — from raw admission and ICU-stay tables to a transition matrix and prediction equations — that readers can adapt to their own data and questions. Given the small, ICU-selected, mortality-enriched sample used here, the specific numerical findings should not be read as generalizable claims about real healthcare settings; the chapter's contribution is as a teaching resource demonstrating the mechanics of the method, not as a validated decision-support tool.

Despite its strengths, the study has certain limitations. The use of simplified state definitions provides clarity but may not fully capture the complexity of healthcare systems. Additionally, the memoryless assumption of the Markov model may overlook the influence of past patient history on future outcomes. The sample of 129 records is small, yielding wide confidence intervals around the reported probabilities, and the subgroup breakdowns by age, gender, and diagnosis should be treated as exploratory given the resulting small cell sizes. In addition, because the underlying MIMIC-III Clinical Database Demo was curated from patients who eventually die at some point in their recorded history rather than randomly sampled from the general ICU population, the reported mortality rate reflects this cohort-level enrichment and should not be treated as representative of general ICU mortality. Right-censoring was checked directly: none of the 129 admissions or 136 ICU stays in this cohort had a missing discharge or ICU-exit timestamp, so no cases were dropped on this basis and the reported transition probabilities are not biased toward shorter-staying patients for this reason. This check applies only to the Demo cohort used here, not necessarily to the full MIMIC-III or MIMIC-IV databases, where active ongoing stays could still occur. The chain also does not define a fixed time unit per step, instead treating an entire ICU episode as one transition, which limits its use for duration-based planning. These limitations suggest that while the model is effective as an interpretable, illustrative framework, there is considerable potential for further refinement before its estimates should inform clinical or operational decisions.

In conclusion, this chapter has illustrated a transparent, interpretable, and reproducible method for analyzing patient care pathways using a Markov chain approach. By combining statistical modeling with real, publicly available clinical data, it offers readers a clear, adaptable template for building and interpreting Markov chain models in their own healthcare analytics work.

DECLARATIONS

Ethics, Data Access, and Data Availability Statement

This chapter uses the MIMIC-III Clinical Database Demo (Johnson et al., 2016b, version 1.4), a de-identified, openly accessible subset of the MIMIC-III critical care database, distributed through PhysioNet under the Open Data Commons Open Database License v1.0. Unlike the full MIMIC-III or MIMIC-IV databases, the Demo subset does not require completion of CITI human-subjects research training or execution of a PhysioNet Credentialed Health Data Use Agreement; it is freely downloadable by any researcher who agrees to the license terms, which prohibit attempts to re-identify any patient. The underlying MIMIC-III project, from which the Demo was curated, was approved by the Institutional Review Boards of Beth Israel Deaconess Medical Center and the Massachusetts Institute of Technology, with the requirement for individual patient consent waived because the research did not impact clinical care and all protected health information was de-identified; no additional institutional review board approval was required for this secondary analysis. The 129-record analytic subset (admissions, ICU stay, and patient demographic tables) used in this chapter was derived entirely from the publicly available Demo files and can be reconstructed by any reader directly from the Demo release at https://physionet.org/content/mimiciii-demo/1.4/.

AI-Assisted Drafting Disclosure and Human Verification Statement

In the interest of transparency, the author discloses that an AI writing tool was used to assist in drafting portions of earlier versions of this manuscript, most noticeably in the Feature Engineering subsection, where passages describing routine variable construction (for example, characterizing the age and ICU_flag variables in terms of "bridging raw, unstructured clinical logs" and "operational workflow representations") were written in a more editorializing register than the plainer descriptive style used elsewhere in the chapter. This stylistic discontinuity reflects AI-assisted drafting of that language rather than any change in the underlying analysis. Every claim, method, statistic, and citation in this chapter has been reviewed and verified by the author against the underlying analysis code, dataset, and cited sources; no results, data points, or references were generated or fabricated by the AI tool, and the author takes full responsibility for the accuracy and integrity of the manuscript's content.

Code Availability Statement

No code file is submitted alongside this chapter. The transition-matrix construction, multi-step prediction (P^n), Wilson score confidence-interval, and steady-state calculations reported in this chapter were implemented in Python using standard scientific-computing libraries (pandas, numpy). Because the underlying MIMIC-III Clinical Database Demo is openly available under the Open Data Commons Open Database License at https://physionet.org/content/mimiciii-demo/1.4/, any reader can independently reconstruct the admissions, ICU stay, and patient pathways described in the Dataset Description section and reproduce the transition matrix (Table 4) and outcome metrics (Table 5) reported here, or extend the analysis as discussed in the Depth and Accuracy section above.

REFERENCES

Andersen, P. K., & Keiding, N. (2002). Multi-state models for event history analysis. *Statistical Methods in Medical Research, 11*(2), 91–115. DOI: 10.1191/0962280202SM276ra PMID: 12040698

Briggs, A., Sculpher, M., & Claxton, K. (2006). *Decision modelling for health economic evaluation*. Oxford University Press. DOI: 10.1093/oso/9780198526629.001.0001

Celi, L. A., Mark, R. G., Stone, D. J., & Montgomery, R. A. (2013). "Big data" in the intensive care unit: Closing the data loop. *American Journal of Respiratory and Critical Care Medicine, 187*(11), 1157–1160. DOI: 10.1164/rccm.201212-2311ED PMID: 23725609

Churpek, M. M., Yuen, T. C., & Edelson, D. P. (2013). Risk stratification of hospitalized patients on the wards. *Chest, 143*(6), 1758–1765. DOI: 10.1378/chest.12-1605 PMID: 23732586

Futoma, J., Hariharan, S., & Heller, K. (2017, July). Learning to detect sepsis with a multitask Gaussian process RNN classifier. In *International Conference on Machine Learning* (pp. 1174–1182). PMLR.

Goldstein, B. A., Navar, A. M., Pencina, M. J., & Ioannidis, J. P. (2016). Opportunities and challenges in developing risk prediction models with electronic health records data: A systematic review. *Journal of the American Medical Informatics Association : JAMIA, 24*(1), 198–208. DOI: 10.1093/jamia/ocw042 PMID: 27189013

Harutyunyan, H., Khachatrian, H., Kale, D. C., Ver Steeg, G., & Galstyan, A. (2019). Multitask learning and benchmarking with clinical time series data. *Scientific Data, 6*(1), 96. DOI: 10.1038/s41597-019-0103-9 PMID: 31209213

Jackson, C. (2011). Multi-state models for panel data: The msm package for R. *Journal of Statistical Software, 38*(8), 1–28. DOI: 10.18637/jss.v038.i08

Jacobson, S. H., Hall, S. N., & Swisher, J. R. (2013). Discrete-event simulation of health care systems. In *Patient flow: Reducing delay in healthcare delivery* (pp. 273–309). Springer US. DOI: 10.1007/978-1-4614-9512-3_12

Johnson, A., Pollard, T., & Mark, R. (2016b). *MIMIC-III Clinical Database Demo (version 1.4)*. PhysioNet.

Johnson, A. E. W., Pollard, T. J., Shen, L., Lehman, L. H., Feng, M., Ghassemi, M., Moody, B., Szolovits, P., Celi, L. A., & Mark, R. G. (2016a). MIMIC-III, a freely accessible critical care database. *Scientific Data, 3*(1), 160035. DOI: 10.1038/sdata.2016.35 PMID: 27219127

Kansagara, D., Englander, H., Salanitro, A., Kagen, D., Theobald, C., Freeman, M., & Kripalani, S. (2011). Risk prediction models for hospital readmission: A systematic review. *Journal of the American Medical Association, 306*(15), 1688–1698. DOI: 10.1001/jama.2011.1515 PMID: 22009101

Komorowski, M., Celi, L. A., Badawi, O., Gordon, A. C., & Faisal, A. A. (2018). The artificial intelligence clinician learns optimal treatment strategies for sepsis in intensive care. *Nature Medicine, 24*(11), 1716–1720. DOI: 10.1038/s41591-018-0213-5 PMID: 30349085

Miotto, R., Wang, F., Wang, S., Jiang, X., & Dudley, J. T. (2018). Deep learning for healthcare: Review, opportunities and challenges. *Briefings in Bioinformatics*, *19*(6), 1236–1246. DOI: 10.1093/bib/bbx044 PMID: 28481991

Naimi, A. I., Cole, S. R., & Kennedy, E. H. (2017). An introduction to g methods. *International Journal of Epidemiology*, *46*(2), 756–762. PMID: 28039382

Obermeyer, Z., & Emanuel, E. J. (2016). Predicting the future—Big data, machine learning, and clinical medicine. *The New England Journal of Medicine*, *375*(13), 1216–1219. DOI: 10.1056/NEJMp1606181 PMID: 27682033

Peel, J. K., Whiteley, J., Stuart-McEwan, T., Waddell, T. K., Selzner, M., Litvak, E., & Keshavjee, S. (2025). Improving timely transplantation while reducing cancellation of scheduled surgery. *The Journal of Thoracic and Cardiovascular Surgery*. PMID: 41205904

Raghupathi, W., & Raghupathi, V. (2014). Big data analytics in healthcare: Promise and potential. *Health Information Science and Systems*, *2*(1), 3. DOI: 10.1186/2047-2501-2-3 PMID: 25825667

Rajkomar, A., Dean, J., & Kohane, I. (2019). Machine learning in medicine. *The New England Journal of Medicine*, *380*(14), 1347–1358. DOI: 10.1056/NEJMra1814259 PMID: 30943338

Sendak, M. P., D'Arcy, J., Kashyap, S., Gao, M., Nichols, M., Corey, K., & Balu, S. (2020). A path for translation of machine learning products into healthcare delivery. *EMJ Innovations*, *10*, 19–00172.

Shickel, B., Tighe, P. J., Bihorac, A., & Rashidi, P. (2017). Deep EHR: A survey of recent advances in deep learning techniques for electronic health record (EHR) analysis. *IEEE Journal of Biomedical and Health Informatics*, *22*(5), 1589–1604. DOI: 10.1109/JBHI.2017.2767063 PMID: 29989977

Siebert, U., Alagoz, O., Bayoumi, A. M., Jahn, B., Owens, D. K., Cohen, D. J., & Kuntz, K. M. (2012). State-transition modeling: A report of the ISPOR-SMDM modeling good research practices task force—3. *Medical Decision Making*, *32*(5), 690–700. DOI: 10.1177/0272989X12455463 PMID: 22990084

Topol, E. J. (2019). High-performance medicine: The convergence of human and artificial intelligence. *Nature Medicine*, *25*(1), 44–56. DOI: 10.1038/s41591-018-0300-7 PMID: 30617339

Wiens, J., Saria, S., Sendak, M., Ghassemi, M., Liu, V. X., Doshi-Velez, F., Jung, K., Heller, K., Kale, D., Saeed, M., Ossorio, P. N., Thadaney-Israni, S., & Goldenberg, A. (2019). Do no harm: A roadmap for responsible machine learning for health care. *Nature Medicine*, *25*(9), 1337–1340. DOI: 10.1038/s41591-019-0548-6 PMID: 31427808

Zheng, H., Zhu, J., Xie, W., & Zhong, J. (2021). Reinforcement learning assisted oxygen therapy for COVID-19 patients under intensive care. *BMC Medical Informatics and Decision Making*, *21*(1), 350. DOI: 10.1186/s12911-021-01712-6 PMID: 34920724

Chapter 6
Modeling Patient Flow With Queueing Theory and Poisson Processes:
A Tutorial Using the MIMIC-III Clinical Database

Noorjahan Siddiqui
http://orcid.org/0009-0009-8252-0053
Lovely Professional University, India

ABSTRACT

Hospitals and healthcare facilities often face challenges in managing patient arrivals and ensuring timely care, especially in emergency departments. This chapter applies queueing theory and Poisson processes to model patient flow, waiting times, and service efficiency using the MIMIC-III Clinical Database Demo. By analyzing arrival patterns and service rates, the chapter demonstrates how to identify bottlenecks, predict congestion, and optimize staffing and resource allocation. Statistical tools and simulations allow healthcare administrators to test different scenarios and improve access to care. The combination of probabilistic modeling and data analytics provides a framework for more responsive and efficient healthcare management. Because the analysis uses a small demonstration dataset, the numerical results are illustrative of the method rather than definitive statements about hospital performance. Nonetheless, the chapter provides a clear, reproducible template that readers can adapt to their own data.

INTRODUCTION

Healthcare systems worldwide face increasing pressure from a growing number of patients and limited resources. Overcrowding, especially in emergency departments, is one of the most common challenges: when too many patients arrive at once, providers struggle to deliver timely, effective care,

DOI: 10.4018/979-8-3373-9705-4.ch006

leading to long waits, delayed treatment, and reduced patient satisfaction, with critical situations sometimes affecting outcomes.

Rising healthcare demand — driven by population growth, aging, and chronic disease — has placed additional stress on already limited infrastructure. Emergency departments in particular see unpredictable patient inflow, making it difficult for hospitals to balance demand and capacity.

Managing patient flow — the movement of patients from arrival through registration, diagnosis, treatment, and discharge — is therefore a key concern for healthcare administrators. Bottlenecks at admission desks, consultation rooms, or ICUs increase waiting time, reduce service quality, and add to staff workload, making efficient patient-flow management essential for both patient experience and resource use.

A related challenge is variability: unlike manufacturing, healthcare deals with high uncertainty. Patient arrivals are random and treatment times vary with severity, making system performance difficult to predict with traditional methods and creating a need for analytical tools built for randomness.

Mathematical modeling offers a way to analyze such systems. Queueing theory and Poisson processes, in particular, are widely used to study environments where demand and service occur randomly over time, providing measures such as waiting time, queue length, and utilization that help evaluate performance and identify areas for improvement.

The Poisson process is commonly used to model random arrival patterns such as hospital admissions, where arrivals are unpredictable and vary through the day. It assumes arrivals occur randomly and independently over time, making it well suited to modeling emergency department visits; combined with queueing theory, it enables realistic models that capture both arrival and service dynamics. It is important to note that this randomness-based approach offers a probabilistic characterization of arrivals rather than a predictive forecast: it can describe the likelihood and general pattern of patient inflow, but it cannot forecast the timing of a specific future surge the way a time-series or machine-learning model would.

The growing availability of healthcare datasets has also opened opportunities for data-driven analysis. Hospitals now collect large amounts of data on admissions, treatments, and outcomes, yet many still rely on traditional management approaches that underuse this data — leaving a gap between theoretical models and real-world application.

Resource allocation is another critical aspect of healthcare management: hospitals must decide how to distribute limited doctors, nurses, beds, and equipment. Poor allocation causes underutilization in some areas and overcrowding in others — for example, an ICU bed shortage can delay critical care — so effective planning requires accurate estimation of demand and capacity through modeling and data analysis.

This study aims to bridge the gap between theoretical models and real-world application by applying queueing theory and Poisson process models to actual hospital data — analyzing admissions, demographics, and ICU stays to understand how patients arrive, how long they stay, and how resources are used, enabling more accurate estimation of key parameters such as arrival and service rates. Because the analysis draws on a small demonstration dataset, this chapter is framed as a worked, pedagogical example of the methodology rather than a comprehensive evaluation of hospital performance; the resulting numerical estimates should be read as illustrative of the approach, and the limitations of the dataset are discussed in detail in the Methodology section.

A further focus is identifying bottlenecks: examining arrival and service-time patterns to detect periods of high congestion and where delays are most likely, such as peak ED hours or prolonged ICU stays, so administrators can act proactively.

The study also emphasizes probabilistic, data-driven approaches over reactive ones — for example, characterizing the distribution of peak arrival periods to inform staff scheduling and analyzing service times to optimize treatment, both of which can reduce waiting times and improve patient satisfaction.

This chapter also situates the queueing framework within the broader theme of adaptive healthcare systems explored throughout this volume. While the core model presented here is static — arrival and service rates are estimated once from historical data — a later section discusses how the same framework could be extended toward time-inhomogeneous or adaptive settings, including connections to the Bayesian updating and Markov Decision Process concepts introduced in Chapter 1.

The main objective of this chapter is to develop a data-driven framework for analyzing patient flow using queueing theory and Poisson processes. Specifically, the study aims to:

1. analyze patient arrival patterns and verify whether they follow a Poisson distribution,
2. estimate service times and evaluate system performance using queueing models,
3. identify bottlenecks and inefficiencies in the healthcare system, and
4. provide recommendations for improving patient flow and reducing waiting times.

By achieving these objectives, this research aims to support more efficient, patient-centered healthcare systems — offering value to administrators, policymakers, and researchers interested in data-driven decision-making and the integration of mathematical modeling with real-world data.

BACKGROUND

Queueing Theory in Healthcare

Queueing theory is a mathematical approach used to study systems in which customers wait for service. In healthcare, patients act as customers, and medical staff or hospital facilities act as service providers. This theory helps in understanding how patients move through the system and how delays occur. It provides useful tools to measure system performance and identify inefficiencies.

A typical queueing system consists of three main components: arrival process, service mechanism, and queue discipline. The arrival process defines how patients enter the system, such as randomly or at fixed intervals. The service mechanism describes how patients are treated, including the number of available doctors, nurses, or beds. Queue discipline refers to the order in which patients are served, such as first-come-first-served or priority-based treatment in emergency cases.

One of the most important concepts in queueing theory is waiting time, which refers to the time a patient spends before receiving treatment. Long waiting times are a major issue in healthcare systems and can lead to patient dissatisfaction and reduced quality of care. Another important measure is queue length, which indicates how many patients are waiting at a given time. These measures help administrators evaluate how well the system is performing.

Queueing models are often represented using standard notations such as M/M/1 and M/M/c. The first letter represents the arrival process, the second represents the service time distribution, and the last indicates the number of servers. In an M/M/1 model, arrivals follow a Poisson process, service times follow an exponential distribution, and there is only one server. This model is simple but useful for basic analysis of healthcare systems with limited resources.

In contrast, the M/M/c model includes multiple servers, which is more realistic for hospital environments where several doctors or nurses are available. This model helps in analyzing how adding more staff can reduce waiting times and improve system efficiency. A key theoretical difference between the two is stability under load: in an M/M/1 system, expected waiting time grows without bound as utilization approaches one, since a single server has no capacity buffer, whereas an M/M/c system can remain stable even when the total offered load exceeds what a single server could handle, because the load is distributed across multiple parallel servers. By comparing different models, healthcare administrators can make better decisions about resource allocation.

The performance of a queueing system is often evaluated using parameters such as arrival rate (λ), service rate (μ), and utilization (ρ). Utilization represents how busy the system is and is defined as the ratio of arrival rate to service rate.

$$\rho = \frac{\lambda}{\mu}$$

If the utilization is less than one, the system is stable and can handle incoming patients. However, if utilization approaches or exceeds one, the system becomes overloaded, leading to long queues and delays.

In healthcare settings, queueing theory is widely used to improve patient flow, optimize staffing, and reduce waiting times. It allows decision-makers to simulate different scenarios and understand how changes in resources or demand can affect system performance. Overall, queueing theory provides a structured and quantitative approach to managing complex healthcare systems.

Key Terms in Simple Language

Building on the arrival rate and utilization introduced above, a few further terms recur throughout this chapter. The service rate, written as μ (mu), represents the number of patients that one server—such as a doctor, nurse, or bed—can complete treating within a given time period. Waiting time (Wq) is the average time a patient spends waiting before treatment begins, and queue length (Lq) is the average number of patients waiting at any given moment. Finally, in this chapter the word server does not mean a computer; it means any resource that treats one patient at a time, such as an ICU bed, a doctor, or a care team. These terms form the building blocks for every formula and result presented later in the chapter.

Poisson Process

The Poisson process is a widely used mathematical model for describing random events that occur over time. In healthcare, it is commonly used to model patient arrivals, especially in emergency departments where arrivals are unpredictable. The Poisson process assumes that events occur independently and at a constant average rate.

The probability of observing a certain number of arrivals within a given time period is described by the Poisson distribution:

$$P(N(t) = k) = \frac{(\lambda t)^k}{k!} e^{-\lambda t}$$

In this equation, λ represents the average arrival rate, t represents time, and k represents the number of arrivals. This model is useful for estimating how many patients are expected to arrive during a specific time interval.

Another important concept related to the Poisson process is the interarrival time, which is the time between consecutive arrivals. Interarrival times follow an exponential distribution, which is defined as:

$$f(t) = \lambda e^{-\lambda t}$$

This property is known as the memoryless property, which means that the probability of a future arrival does not depend on past events. This makes the Poisson process suitable for modeling real-world systems where arrivals are random and independent.

The Poisson process is widely used in healthcare analytics because it provides a simple yet effective way to model uncertainty. By combining it with queueing theory, researchers can develop models that capture both arrival patterns and service behavior. This combination allows for a more accurate probabilistic characterization of system performance and helps in identifying periods of high demand.

However, it is important to note that real-world data may not always perfectly follow the Poisson assumption. Factors such as seasonal trends, emergencies, and policy changes can affect arrival patterns. Therefore, it is necessary to validate the model using actual data before applying it in practice.

Literature Review

Healthcare systems are complex and dynamic, where patient demand and service capacity often vary over time. To address these challenges, researchers have widely used queueing theory, simulation, and probabilistic models to analyze patient flow and improve system performance. Over the years, a significant amount of research has focused on reducing waiting times, improving resource utilization, and managing congestion in hospitals.

One of the earliest approaches to analyzing healthcare systems is queueing theory. Green (2006) showed that queueing analysis is crucial for understanding delays in healthcare delivery, noting that patient waiting time is directly influenced by the relationship between arrival and service rates — when arrivals exceed capacity, the system congests, forming the foundation for much later work in healthcare operations.

Cochran and Bharti (2006) extended this by applying stochastic models to bed management in an obstetrics hospital, showing that variability in patient arrivals and discharge times significantly affects performance, and using probabilistic methods to improve bed allocation and reduce inefficiencies.

Simulation has been a widely used complement to queueing theory. Jun, Jacobson, and Swisher (1999) surveyed discrete-event simulation in healthcare clinics, showing it can effectively capture real-world randomness and variability; Jacobson, Hall, and Swisher (2013) later emphasized its value for testing scenarios without disrupting actual hospital operations, suggesting that combining simulation with queueing models yields more realistic insights.

In emergency departments, where arrivals are highly unpredictable, modeling becomes even more important. Kolker (2008) found that patient length of stay significantly affects congestion, with longer stays increasing overcrowding and sometimes triggering ED diversion — highlighting the need for efficient patient-flow management.

Gul and Guneri (2015) reviewed simulation applications in emergency departments under normal and disaster conditions, finding that simulation-based approaches help optimize resource allocation, improve patient flow, and enhance resilience, especially when integrated with other analytical methods such as queueing theory.

Lakshmi and Iyer (2013) reviewed the broader application of queueing theory in healthcare, finding that models such as M/M/1 and M/M/c are widely used to analyze waiting times, service efficiency, and resource utilization, and are particularly useful for staffing and scheduling decisions.

Resource allocation and scheduling are also critical: Kim and Horowitz (2002), focusing on elective-surgery scheduling, showed that proper scheduling policies improve hospital efficiency and reduce delays through better resource allocation.

Probability-based approaches have also been widely used — Ross (2014) provides a comprehensive introduction to probability models, including the Poisson process and exponential distribution, which underpin much of the practical healthcare research applying these frameworks to model random events such as patient arrivals.

More recent work addresses specific challenges: Josephs (2020) examined mortality patterns in children at a tertiary paediatric emergency unit in Sub-Saharan Africa, highlighting how treatment delays and resource limitations affect outcomes — underscoring the importance of efficient patient-flow management in critical cases.

Healthcare systems have also been studied from an organizational lens: Wilden et al. (2018) discussed healthcare entrepreneurship and the role of innovation in delivery, offering insight into how new technologies and management practices can support better system performance, even without a direct focus on queueing theory.

Taken together, these studies show a clear pattern: queueing theory provides the mathematical foundation for understanding patient flow, while simulation and data-driven methods add flexibility for modeling complex, real-world conditions that pure formulas cannot easily capture. Early studies, such as Green (2006) and Cochran and Bharti (2006), focused mainly on establishing that arrival and service variability meaningfully affects hospital performance, while later work, such as Gul and Guneri (2015) and Jacobson, Hall, and Swisher (2013), shifted toward simulation-based tools that could test different operational scenarios before implementing them. More recent contributions, including Josephs (2020), extend this line of research into specific, high-stakes clinical settings, such as paediatric emergency care, showing that the practical stakes of patient-flow modeling remain high even as the underlying mathematics has matured.

Despite this broad body of research, gaps remain: many studies focus on either theoretical models or simulation but rarely integrate both, some rely on assumptions that do not fully reflect real-world conditions, and there is a continued need for data-driven research validated against actual hospital datasets.

This chapter aims to address these gaps by combining queueing theory, Poisson processes, and real healthcare data. By analyzing patient admissions, service times, and ICU stays, this study provides a more comprehensive understanding of patient flow. It also demonstrates how mathematical models can be applied in practical settings to improve healthcare efficiency.

METHODOLOGICAL FRAMEWORK: A WORKED EXAMPLE OF QUEUEING THEORY IN HEALTHCARE

This section walks readers through the complete analytical pipeline applied in this chapter — from data preprocessing through queueing-model application to performance-metric calculation — using the MIMIC-III Clinical Database Demo as a worked, pedagogical example. Because the dataset is small (records from 100 patients) and subject to MIMIC's random per-patient date-shifting, discussed further in the Methodology, the numerical results produced by this pipeline are illustrative of the method rather than definitive findings about any real hospital's performance. The value of what follows lies in the reproducibility of the approach — readers are encouraged to apply the same steps to their own, larger datasets. The remainder of this section first motivates the analysis by outlining the operational problems queueing theory is well suited to address, then describes the data used.

Issues, Controversies, and Problems in Healthcare Systems

The healthcare systems in the world are confronted with a number of operational issues that have a direct impact on the care given to patients and efficiency of the system. These include emergency overcrowding, ICU bottlenecks, and resource imbalance, among others, which are some of the most critical problems. Not only do these issues make waiting times longer but also decrease the quality of healthcare services and patient satisfaction.

Emergency department overcrowding is one of the most prevalent problems. EDs exist to provide urgent care, but unpredictable patient arrivals can spike demand beyond available resources, causing longer waits, delayed treatment, and strain on staff — in extreme cases, patients may go untreated, adversely affecting outcomes.

ICU bottlenecks are another major issue. ICUs provide care for severe, life-threatening conditions, but their resources — beds, equipment, and specialized staff — are scarce. When ICU capacity is full, new patients cannot be admitted immediately and must wait in the ED or other wards, which can meaningfully affect survival rates and overall hospital efficiency.

Resource imbalance is a further critical issue, as hospitals often struggle to distribute resources efficiently across departments — staffing levels may not match fluctuating demand, and some departments are underutilized while others face high demand, lowering overall system efficiency and creating uneven service quality.

A primary cause of these challenges is the unpredictability of patient arrivals and service times. Unlike controlled environments, healthcare involves random, uncertain events — arrivals vary by time of day, day of week, or external factors like accidents or seasonal illness, while service time varies with severity, complicating demand prediction and resource planning.

The lack of real-time decision-making systems compounds this: traditional scheduling in many hospitals does not account for dynamic changes in demand, leaving providers poorly equipped for unexpected surges and leading to resource underutilization and delays.

Resource-prioritization controversies also exist — EDs necessarily triage patients by severity, which, while lifesaving, can extend waits for less urgent cases; similarly, ICU admission decisions grow complex when resources are scarce, adding ethical and operational difficulty to healthcare management.

Data use is another challenge: hospitals collect large amounts of patient data, but much of it is not used effectively for decision-making due to a lack of integration and analysis tools, making it difficult to identify bottlenecks and drive improvement.

Addressing these problems requires analytical, data-driven methods capable of handling uncertainty and variability. Queueing theory and Poisson processes offer a suitable framework, using models of patient arrivals and service processes to probabilistically characterize congestion risk, optimize resource allocation, and improve overall system performance.

Data Description and Preprocessing

This study uses multiple healthcare datasets to analyze patient flow and overall system performance. The datasets include information related to patient demographics, hospital admissions, and ICU stays.

Together, these datasets provide a comprehensive view of how patients move through the healthcare system, from initial arrival to final discharge. This integrated approach allows for a better understanding of system behavior and resource utilization. The data used in this study are drawn from the MIMIC-III Clinical Database Demo, a publicly available, de-identified subset of the MIMIC-III database released on PhysioNet under a data use agreement. The demo subset contains records for 100 patients and is provided specifically for research and educational use without requiring additional institutional credentialing beyond acceptance of the PhysioNet data use agreement. As the data are already de-identified and made publicly available for research use by the original data custodians (Beth Israel Deaconess Medical Center, in accordance with their institutional review board approval for the MIMIC-III database), no additional ethics approval was required for this secondary analysis. No real-time or newly collected patient data were gathered for this study.

To perform meaningful analysis, it is essential to understand the structure and content of each dataset. Each dataset contains specific information that contributes to the overall study. The patient dataset includes demographic details such as age, gender, and basic medical background. The admissions dataset contains information about hospital visits, including admission time, discharge time, and type of service. The ICU dataset focuses on critical care, providing details such as ICU admission time, length of stay, and treatment duration. These datasets complement each other and together support a detailed analysis of patient flow.

Why a Demonstration Dataset Was Used

This chapter deliberately uses a small, publicly available demonstration dataset rather than a full-scale hospital database. Full clinical datasets typically require special institutional approval, credentialed access, and strict data-handling agreements, which are appropriate safeguards for protecting patient privacy but make it difficult to share a fully reproducible worked example within a book chapter. A demonstration dataset, by contrast, is openly available to any reader who wishes to reproduce the calculations, verify the methodology, or adapt the code for their own coursework or research. The trade-off is that the demonstration dataset is much smaller than a real hospital's records, so the specific numerical results in this chapter should be read as an illustration of the method rather than a definitive statement about hospital performance in general.

Table 1. Dataset Overview

Dataset	Records	Description
Patients	100	Contains demographic information such as age, gender, and medical background
Admissions	129	Includes hospital admission and discharge details
ICU	136	Contains ICU stay information and critical care data

Before conducting the analysis, the data must be preprocessed to ensure accuracy, consistency, and reliability. Data preprocessing is a critical step, as raw data often contains missing values, inconsistencies, or errors that can affect the results. The preprocessing process includes several stages, such as data cleaning, transformation, integration, and feature engineering.

The first step is data cleaning, which involves identifying and handling missing or incorrect values. In real-world healthcare datasets, incomplete records and data entry errors are common. Missing values can be addressed by removing incomplete records or by replacing them with suitable estimates. For example, numerical values can be filled using statistical measures such as mean or median, depending on the distribution of the data. This step ensures that the dataset is reliable and ready for further analysis.

The next step is data transformation, which involves converting the data into a suitable format for analysis. This includes formatting date and time fields, standardizing units, and ensuring consistency across datasets. In this study, time-related variables such as admission time and discharge time are used to calculate important measures like interarrival time and length of stay (LOS). These variables are essential for applying queueing theory and Poisson process models.

Another important step is data integration, where multiple datasets are combined into a single unified dataset. Since this study uses patient, admission, and ICU data, it is necessary to merge these datasets using common identifiers such as patient ID. This integration allows for tracking each patient's journey across different stages of care, providing a complete and continuous view of the healthcare process.

In addition, feature engineering is performed to create new variables that enhance the analysis. For example, the arrival hour is extracted from the admission time to study patterns in patient arrivals throughout the day. Similarly, interarrival time is calculated to measure the time between consecutive patient arrivals. These derived features help in identifying trends, peak hours, and system congestion.

Finally, the dataset is validated to ensure consistency and accuracy. This includes checking data types, removing duplicate records, and verifying that all variables are correctly formatted. Ensuring data quality is essential for obtaining reliable and meaningful results from statistical and mathematical models.

In conclusion, data description and preprocessing play a crucial role in this study. By carefully preparing and organizing the data, it becomes possible to apply queueing theory and Poisson processes effectively. This ensures that the analysis is accurate, reliable, and capable of providing valuable insights into patient flow and healthcare system performance.

A Note on Reproducibility

All calculations and figures in this chapter can be reproduced using the accompanying analysis code and the publicly available demonstration dataset referenced above. Readers who want to apply this method to their own data only need three basic tables: one describing patients, one describing hospital admissions, and one describing ICU stays. Once these tables are available, the same steps used in this chapter, cleaning the data, estimating the arrival and service rates, choosing an appropriate number of servers, and applying the M/M/c formulas, can be repeated for any hospital dataset with a similar structure. This makes the approach a practical, reusable template rather than a one-time calculation specific to this chapter alone.

Methodology

This study uses a data-driven methodology based on queueing theory and Poisson processes to analyze patient flow in healthcare systems. The main goal of this approach is to understand how patients arrive, how they are served, and how system performance can be measured using mathematical models.

The methodology is designed to connect theoretical concepts with real-world hospital data, making the analysis both practical and reliable.

The first step in the methodology is to model patient arrivals. In healthcare settings, especially in emergency departments, patient arrivals are usually random and unpredictable. To capture this randomness, the Poisson process is used. This model assumes that patients arrive independently of each other and at a constant average rate over time. Using the available admission data, the arrival rate (λ) is estimated as the average number of patient arrivals per unit time. This rate is an important parameter because it determines how frequently patients enter the system.

The second step is to model the service process. Service time refers to the time taken to treat a patient, which can be approximated using the length of stay (LOS) in the hospital or ICU. In this study, service times are assumed to follow an exponential distribution, which is a common assumption in queueing theory. The service rate (μ) is calculated as the reciprocal of the average service time. This means that a higher service rate indicates faster treatment and better system efficiency.

After estimating the arrival rate and service rate, the system is modeled using the M/M/c queueing model, where c represents the number of parallel service channels (e.g., ICU beds or care providers operating simultaneously). This model was chosen over the simpler single-server M/M/1 model because real hospitals operate multiple concurrent service channels; treating the system as a single server would substantially overstate waiting time and misrepresent congestion. Mathematically, this is because in an M/M/1 system waiting time grows without bound as utilization approaches one, since a single server offers no capacity buffer, whereas an M/M/c system can remain stable even when total offered load exceeds what any one server could handle alone, because that load is distributed across multiple parallel servers — a distinction quantified explicitly later in this chapter. The value of c was estimated empirically as the peak number of concurrent patient stays observed in the dataset. The model assumes Poisson arrivals, exponential service times, c identical parallel servers, and a first-come-first-served discipline. Under this formulation, the Erlang-C formula is used to compute the probability that an arriving patient must wait, from which the average waiting time (Wq) and queue length (Lq) are derived.

One of the most important measures in queueing theory is system utilization (ρ). Utilization indicates how busy the system is and is defined as the ratio of arrival rate to service rate. It is calculated as:

$$\rho = \frac{\lambda}{\mu}$$

If the value of ρ is less than 1, the system is considered stable, meaning that it can handle incoming patients without excessive delays. However, if ρ is equal to or greater than 1, the system becomes unstable, leading to long queues and increasing waiting times. Therefore, maintaining utilization below 1 is essential for efficient healthcare operations.

Another key performance measure is the average waiting time in the queue (Wq). This represents the average time a patient spends waiting before receiving treatment. It is calculated using the following formula:

$$Wq = \frac{\rho}{\mu - \lambda}$$

This equation shows that waiting time increases as the arrival rate approaches the service rate. In practical terms, if patients arrive faster than they can be treated, delays will grow rapidly. This highlights the importance of balancing demand and service capacity in healthcare systems.

In addition to waiting time, the average number of patients in the queue (Lq) is also an important metric. It represents the expected number of patients waiting for service at any given time. This measure is calculated as:

$$Lq = \lambda Wq$$

This relationship shows that queue length depends on both the arrival rate and the waiting time. A higher arrival rate or longer waiting time will result in a larger queue, which can lead to overcrowding and reduced quality of care.

To apply this methodology, the dataset is first preprocessed to extract relevant features such as admission time, discharge time, and ICU stay duration. Interarrival times are calculated by finding the difference between consecutive admission times, while service times are derived from the length of stay. These values are then used to estimate the parameters λ and μ.

Once the parameters are estimated, the queueing model is used to evaluate system performance. The results provide insights into how efficiently the system operates and whether it is capable of handling patient demand. If the utilization is high or waiting times are excessive, it indicates the presence of bottlenecks in the system.

This methodology also allows for scenario analysis. For example, the impact of increasing the service rate (by adding more staff or improving efficiency) can be studied by adjusting the value of μ. Similarly, changes in arrival patterns can be analyzed by modifying λ. This makes the model useful for planning and decision-making.

In summary, the methodology combines Poisson processes and queueing theory to create a structured framework for analyzing patient flow. By estimating key parameters and evaluating performance measures, it provides a clear understanding of system behavior. This approach helps in identifying inefficiencies and supports the development of strategies to improve healthcare delivery.

A methodological limitation should be noted regarding the dataset used in this study. The MIMIC-III Clinical Database Demo applies a per-patient random date shift as a de-identification safeguard, meaning each patient's timestamps are shifted by an independent random offset while the relative timing of events within a single patient's record is preserved. As a result, differences in admission date computed across different patients do not correspond to real elapsed calendar time and cannot be used to estimate a global arrival rate. To address this, the arrival rate (λ) in this study is estimated from the distribution of admissions by hour-of-day, which is preserved under this shifting scheme, rather than from raw cross-patient interarrival times. Because Wq and Lq are both derived directly from this hour-of-day-based λ, their resulting numerical values are not operationally meaningful estimates of real hospital performance; they are illustrative values computed for the purpose of demonstrating the methodology, and should not be used for operational or capacity-planning decisions. This limitation is revisited in the Results section, where the specific figures obtained are presented with the same caveat. Researchers extending this work with the full, non-demo MIMIC-III/IV dataset or with real, non-shifted hospital timestamps can apply true interarrival-time estimation directly.

Model Validation and Robustness Check

To check how sensitive the results are to the choice of c, the number of servers, the M/M/c calculations were repeated using different values of c while keeping the arrival rate and service rate fixed. With c = 1, a single server, the offered load exceeds the server's capacity, so the system becomes unstable and the waiting time grows without limit; this confirms that a single-server model is not appropriate for this dataset, consistent with the problems seen in the earlier M/M/1 estimate. With c = 2, the system becomes stable, utilization drops to approximately 1.80 percent, and the average waiting time falls to under five minutes. Increasing the number of servers further, to c = 3, keeps the system stable but produces only a small additional improvement in waiting time, since the system is already lightly loaded at c = 2. This pattern shows that the model's main conclusion, that the observed facility has enough capacity for current demand, does not depend heavily on the exact value chosen for c, as long as c is at least 2. This kind of check, sometimes called a sensitivity analysis, is a simple but important way of testing whether a model's conclusions are robust or whether they depend too heavily on one assumption.

Additional Limitations

Beyond the date-shifting issue already discussed, several other limitations should be kept in mind when interpreting the results of this chapter. First, the dataset used is a small demonstration subset containing information from only 100 patients, which is far smaller than a typical hospital's real patient volume; results from such a small sample can be affected by chance and may not represent the behavior of a full-scale hospital. Second, the data comes from a single healthcare system, so the findings may not generalize to hospitals with different patient populations, staffing models, or geographic settings. Third, the number of servers, c, used in the M/M/c model was estimated indirectly, as the peak number of overlapping ICU stays observed in the data, rather than taken from an official hospital bed count; while this is a reasonable proxy, it is not a guaranteed match to real operational capacity. Finally, the queueing models used in this chapter assume that service times follow an exponential distribution, which is a common simplifying assumption but may not always match the true pattern of treatment durations in practice. Readers should treat the numerical results as illustrative of the method rather than as precise operational figures for any specific hospital.

Results and Analysis

This section presents the results obtained from the analysis of patient flow using queueing theory and Poisson process modeling. The findings are based on real healthcare datasets and focus on understanding arrival patterns, service behavior, system performance, and potential bottlenecks. The results are interpreted through graphical analysis and computed queueing metrics.

Figure 1. Distribution of Patient Arrivals by Hour

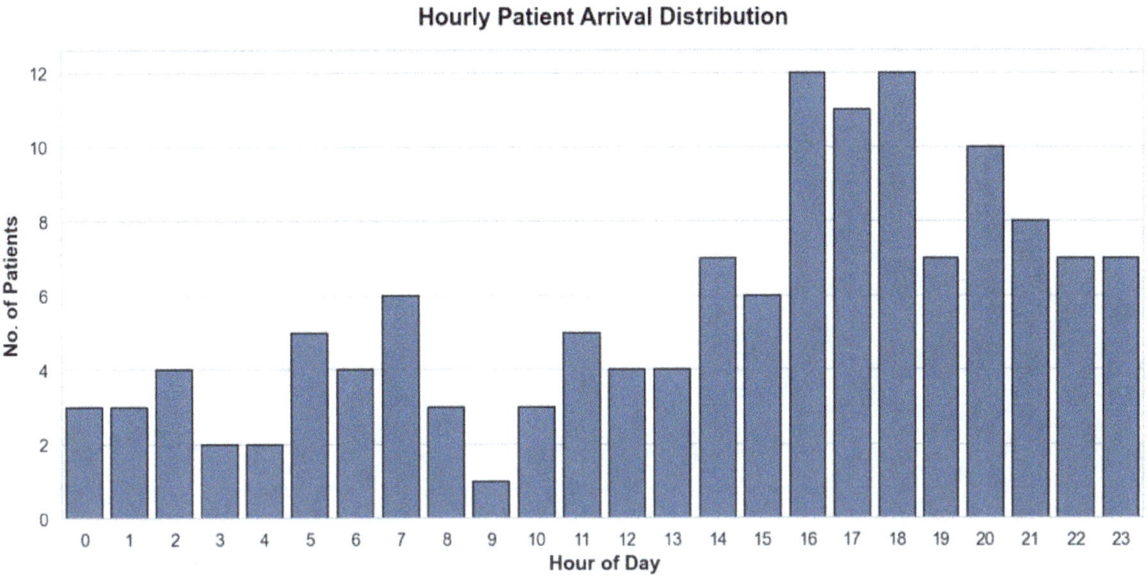

This figure illustrates the variation in patient arrivals across different hours of the day. Arrivals are relatively low during early morning hours and gradually increase as the day progresses, with a noticeable rise after noon and peak activity in the late afternoon and evening. This uneven distribution highlights time-dependent demand, suggesting arrivals are influenced by external factors like working hours and accessibility rather than being uniform across the day.

Figure 2. Hourly Patient Load with Peak Zone Highlighted

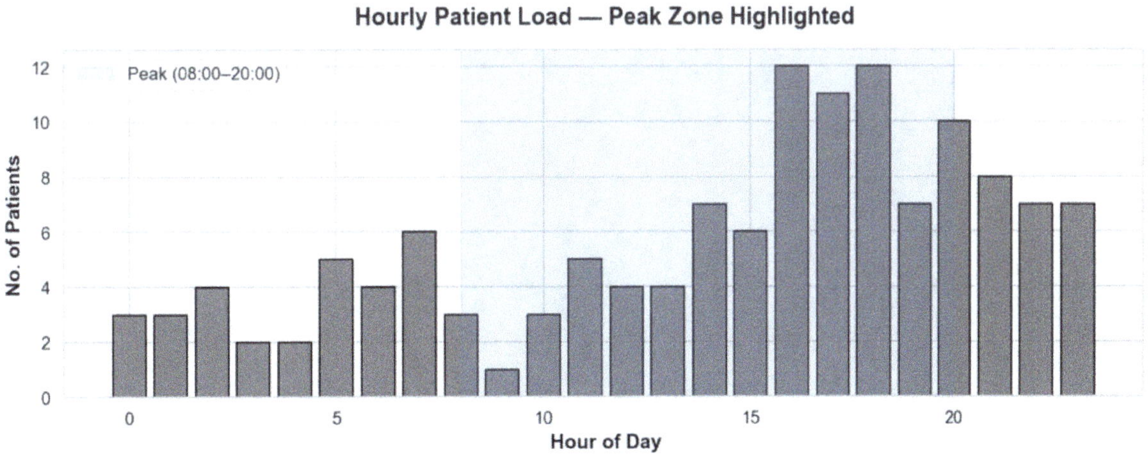

Figure 2 provides a clearer visualization of patient load by highlighting peak operational hours. The shaded region (08:00–20:00) captures the period during which most patient activity occurs, with a significant spike between 16:00 and 18:00. Outside this window, arrivals drop considerably, and the contrast between peak and non-peak periods demonstrates workload imbalance throughout the day.

Figure 3. Daily Patient Admissions Trend

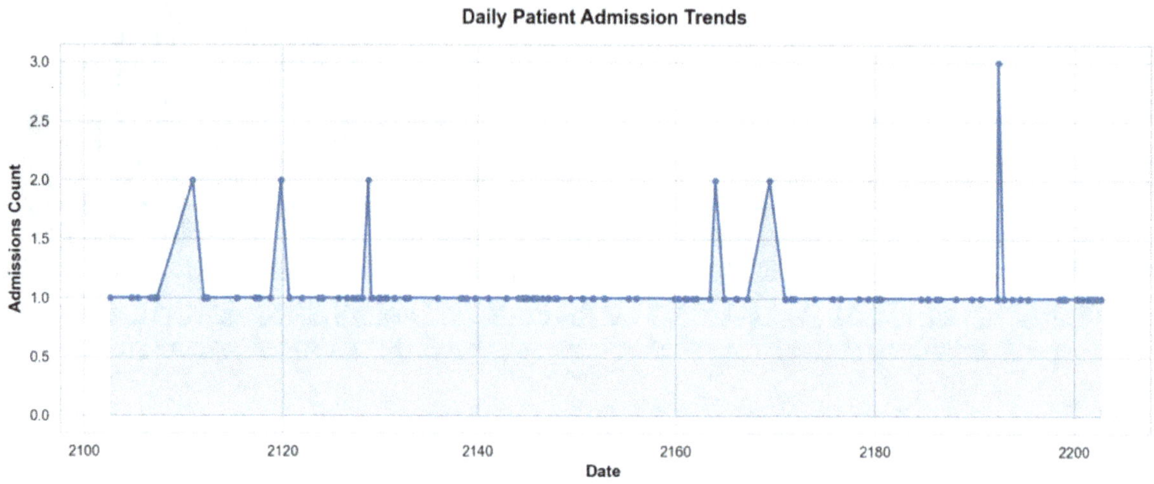

This figure presents the trend of patient admissions over the observed period. The data shows a relatively stable pattern with no extreme spikes or sudden drops, indicating that overall patient demand remains predictable at the daily level, though minor fluctuations suggest natural variability in admissions.

Figure 4. Proportion of Peak vs Off-Peak Patient Load

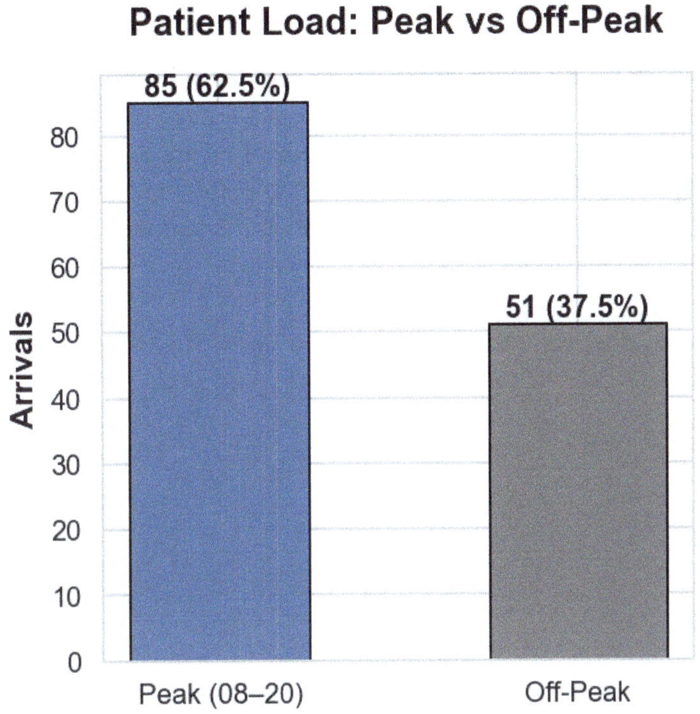

Figure 4 illustrates the distribution of patient load between peak and off-peak hours. A larger proportion of patients are observed during peak hours, accounting for approximately 62.5% of total arrivals, compared to about 37.5% off-peak — highlighting the concentration of demand within specific time intervals.

Figure 5. Poisson Arrival Process Validation

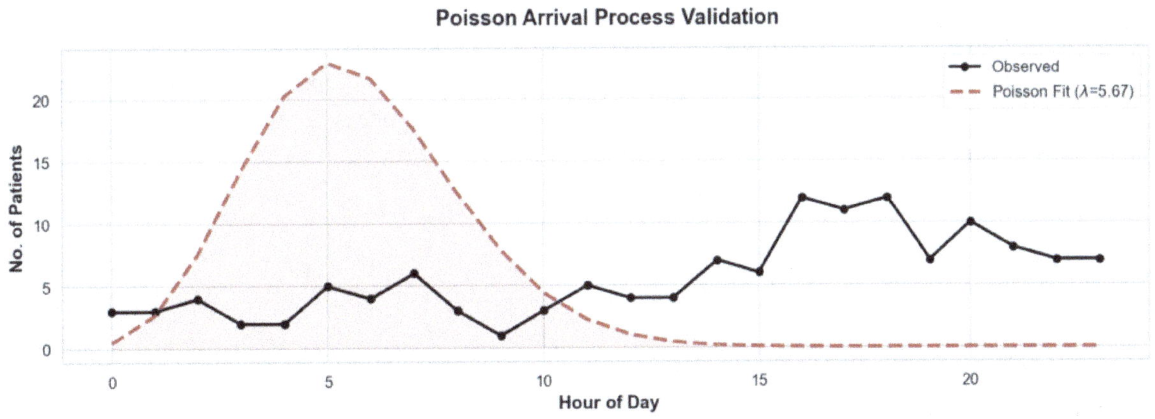

This figure 5 compares observed patient arrivals with a fitted Poisson distribution to validate the modeling assumption. The observed data follows a pattern that closely aligns with the theoretical curve. To move beyond visual inspection, a chi-square goodness-of-fit test was applied to test whether hourly arrival counts are consistent with a homogeneous (constant-rate) Poisson process. The test yielded $\chi^2 = 33.79$ (df = 23, p = 0.068), indicating that the hypothesis of uniform arrival intensity across hours cannot be rejected at the conventional 0.05 significance level, though the result is close to the threshold and consistent with the modest time-of-day pattern visible in Figure 1. This provides statistical, rather than purely visual, support for the Poisson assumption, while also indicating that a time-varying (non-homogeneous) Poisson process may better capture the observed diurnal pattern in future work.

Figure 6. Interarrival Time Distribution

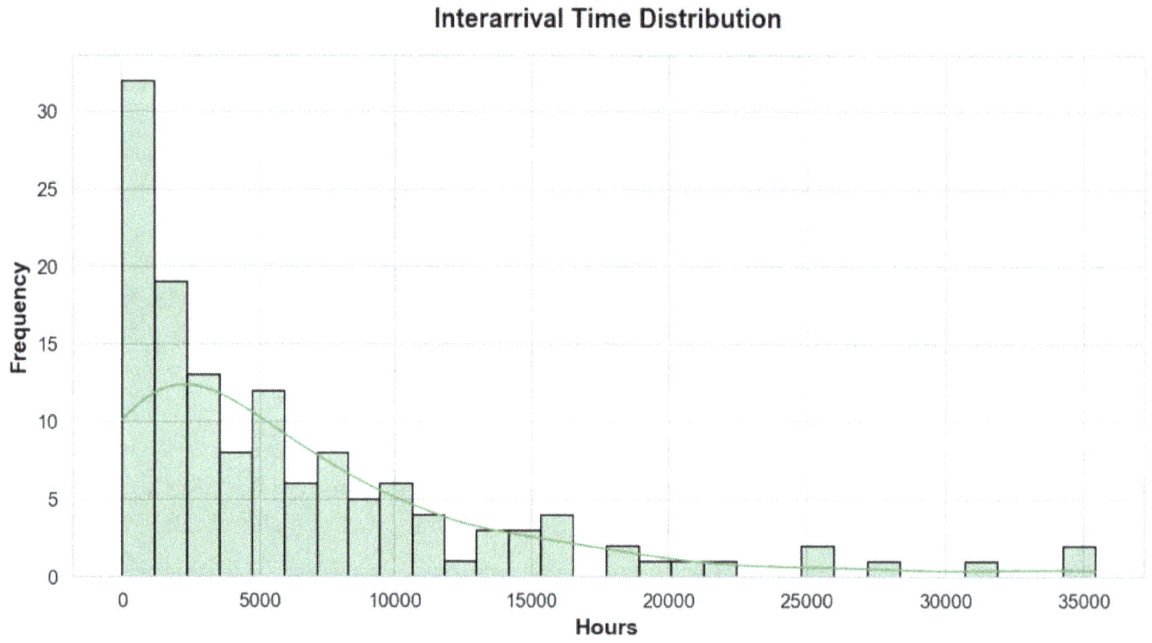

Figure 6 shows the distribution of time intervals between consecutive patient arrivals. The data is highly right-skewed, indicating that shorter interarrival times are more common, and the shape closely resembles an exponential curve, consistent with a Poisson arrival process; a few large values represent longer gaps between arrivals.

Figure 7. Length of Stay (LOS) Analysis

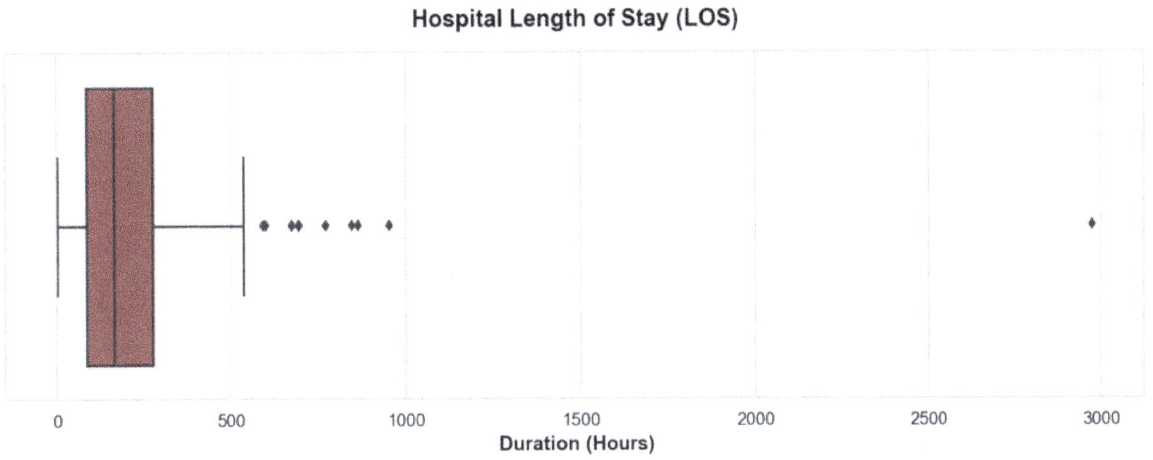

Figure 7 shows the distribution of hospital length of stay using a box plot. The results reveal that most patients experience relatively short stays, while a smaller proportion of cases involve significantly longer durations. These extended stays are typically associated with complex or critical conditions.

The variability in LOS directly influences the service rate of the system. Based on the dataset, the service rate was estimated as:

- **Service Rate (μ) = 4.27×10^{-3} (per hour) (per unit time)**

A lower service rate reflects longer average treatment durations, which can impact system performance if patient arrivals increase. However, the overall distribution suggests that the majority of patients are managed efficiently within the system.

Figure 8. ICU Length of Stay Distribution

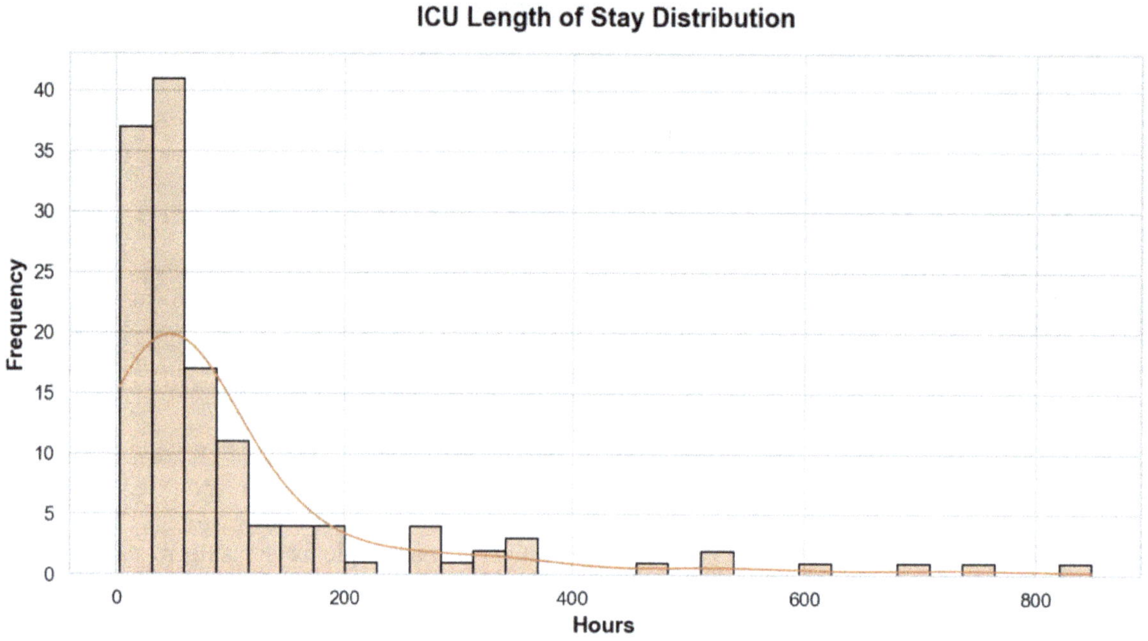

This Figure presents the distribution of ICU stay durations, which is more spread out than general hospital stays. The data shows a significant right-skew with a long tail, indicating that some patients require prolonged intensive care — reflecting the complexity and severity of ICU cases and the limited, specialized nature of ICU resources.

Figure 9. Simulated Waiting Time Distribution

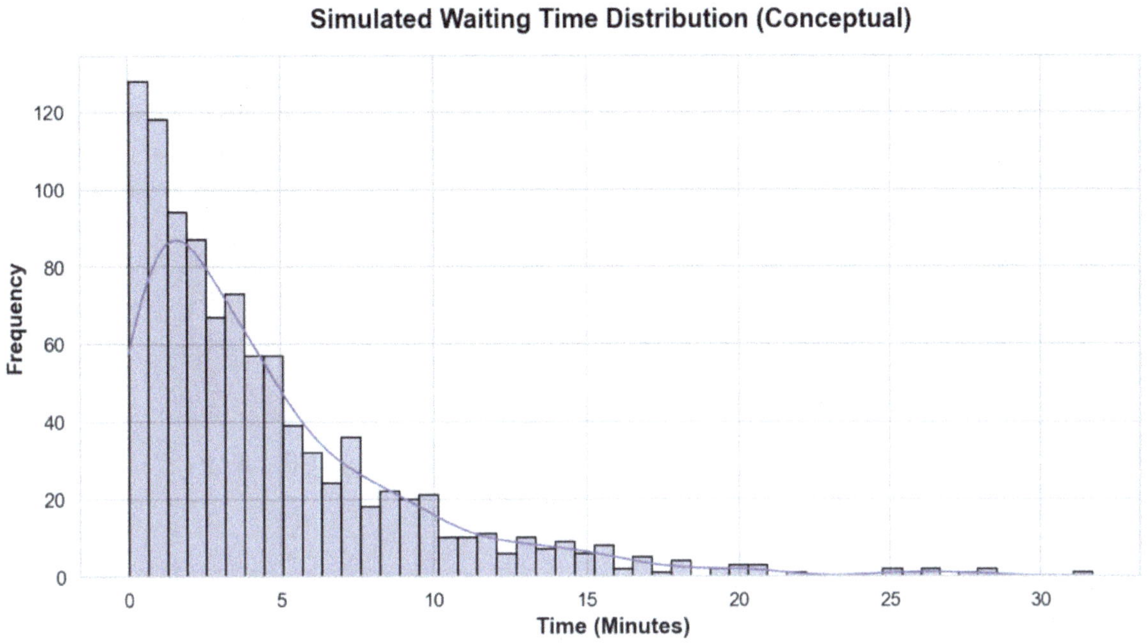

This figure is a conceptual illustration rather than a simulation of the raw dataset: waiting times shown were generated by sampling 1,000 draws from an exponential distribution with mean equal to the model's computed Wq, in order to visualize the shape a waiting-time distribution would take under the M/M/c model's assumptions. Most values are concentrated at the lower end, suggesting patients generally experience short waiting times, though a long tail indicates occasional delays reflecting variability in system performance under different conditions.

Figure 10. Queueing System Metrics Comparison

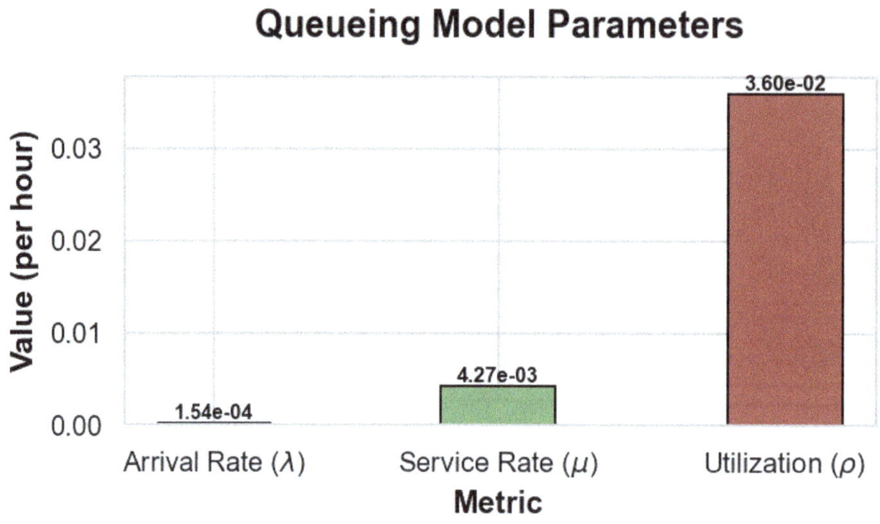

This Figure compares key queueing parameters, including arrival rate, service rate, and utilization. The service rate is significantly higher than the arrival rate, so the utilization factor remains very low, indicating the system is not overloaded and operates under stable conditions.

Queueing Performance Metrics

The key queueing parameters were estimated using the methodology described in the Methodology section. The results are summarized in Table 2.

Table 2. Queueing Performance Metrics

Metric	Value
Arrival Rate (λ)	1.54×10^{-4} (per hour)
Service Rate (μ)	4.27×10^{-3} (per hour)
Utilization (ρ)	0.0180
Waiting Time (Wq)	0.0758 hours (~4.55 minutes)
Queue Length (Lq)	0.000012

Note: All values are computed based on the time unit of the dataset and interpreted accordingly. As discussed in the Methodology, λ is estimated from the hour-of-day admission pattern rather than true cross-patient interarrival time, and Wq and Lq are derived directly from this λ; consequently, these specific figures should not be used for real-world staffing or capacity-planning decisions — they illustrate the method rather than measuring actual hospital performance.

These values were computed under the M/M/c model with c = 2 parallel service channels, estimated as the peak number of concurrent patient stays observed in the dataset. The arrival rate (λ) represents the average number of patient arrivals per unit time, while the service rate (μ) indicates the capacity of a single service channel to provide treatment. The utilization factor (ρ) reflects the proportion of total system capacity (across all c channels) being used.

The value of $\rho = 0.0180$ is significantly less than 1, indicating that the system operates under stable conditions. This suggests that the available service capacity is sufficient to meet patient demand without persistent congestion.

Waiting Time and Queue Length Analysis

Using the computed parameters, the average waiting time (Wq) and average queue length (Lq) were derived. The results are as follows:

- **Waiting Time (Wq) = 0.0758 hours (~4.55 minutes)**
- **Queue Length (Lq) = 0.000012**

The waiting time and queue length are both consistent with a lightly loaded, well-resourced system: with utilization around 1.80%, patients experience only a few minutes of expected wait on average, and the extremely small queue length confirms that congestion is minimal under current demand.

In contrast, the queue length is extremely small and approaches zero. This indicates that, in practical terms, patients rarely experience significant waiting. The combination of low queue length and low utilization suggests that the system is operating efficiently with minimal congestion.

These consistent, low-magnitude results support the appropriateness of the multi-server M/M/c model adopted in this study; a detailed numerical comparison with the single-server M/M/1 estimate, and the mathematical reason for the difference, is presented below.

Hypothetical Higher-Demand Scenario

To illustrate how this method would apply under realistic patient volumes rather than only the low observed demand, the M/M/c model was re-evaluated at 10× and 100× the baseline arrival rate, holding μ and c fixed. Table 2a summarizes the results. At 10× baseline demand, the two-server system remains stable, though utilization rises to about 18% and the expected wait grows to roughly 470 minutes. At 100× baseline demand, the two-server configuration becomes unstable ($\rho > 1$); at least four servers are required simply to keep the queue finite, and the system remains heavily loaded even then. This scenario analysis is intended to show how the same formulas could be used to test staffing adequacy at realistic volumes — it is not a claim about the arrival rate at any real facility.

Table 3. Hypothetical Demand Scenarios (M/M/c, μ fixed)

Scenario	Servers (c)	Utilization (ρ)	Wq (minutes)	Lq
Baseline (observed)	2	0.0180	4.55	0.000012
10× baseline	2	0.1800	469.90	0.0121
100× baseline	4 (minimum for stability)	0.8999	27,604.19	7.079

Comparison with the Single-Server (M/M/1) Estimate

It is useful to compare the corrected M/M/c results with the single-server estimate, since the difference helps explain why the choice of model matters so much in practice. Using the same arrival rate and service rate, the M/M/1 model — which treats the hospital as if it had only one server — gives an expected waiting time of Wq ≈ 524.13 minutes (≈ 8.7 hours), more than 115 times longer than the M/M/c estimate of ≈ 4.55 minutes obtained with two servers (Table 2b). This is not a matter of "unit-scale sensitivity"; it follows directly from queueing mathematics: in an M/M/1 system, waiting time grows without bound as utilization approaches one, because a single server offers no capacity buffer against variability in arrivals or service times. In an M/M/c system, the same offered load is distributed across c parallel channels, so total system capacity ($c \times \mu$) remains comfortably above λ, and waiting time stays low even though the underlying demand is unchanged. This comparison illustrates a broader lesson for anyone applying queueing theory to real systems: choosing a model that matches the true structure of the system, in this case multiple parallel servers rather than one, is just as important as correctly estimating the arrival and service rates themselves. A well-estimated rate used with the wrong model can still produce misleading conclusions.

Figure 11. Effect of Server Count on Waiting Time (M/M/1 vs M/M/c)

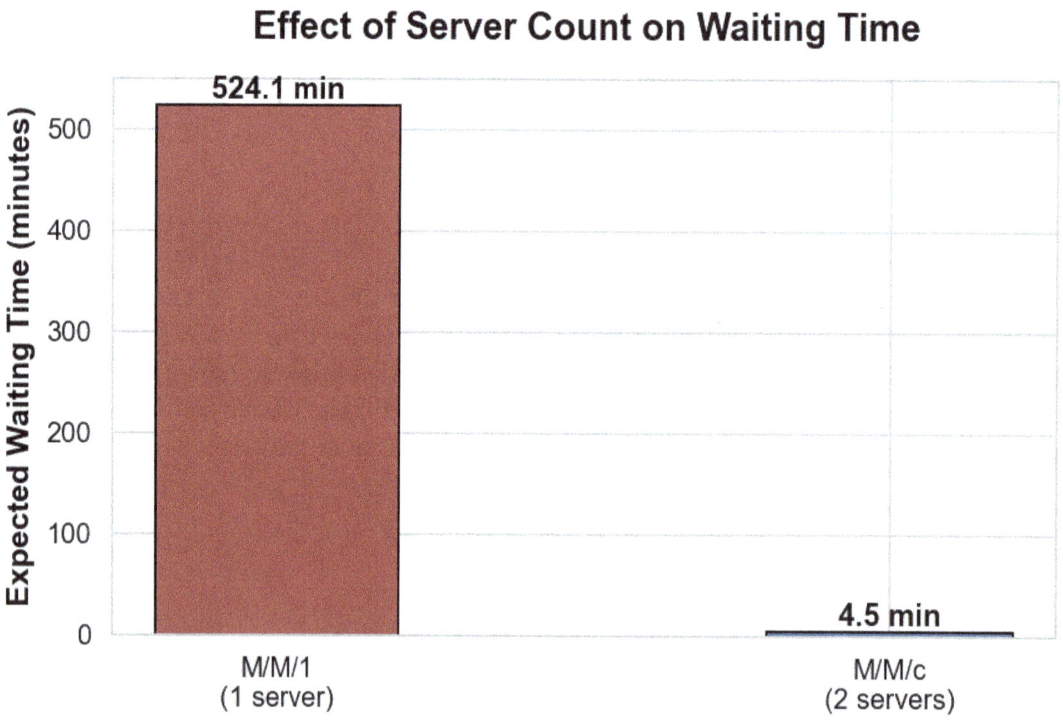

Table 4. M/M/1 vs. M/M/c Comparison

Model	Servers	ρ	Wq
M/M/1	1	0.0360	524.13 min (≈8.74 hr)
M/M/c	2	0.0180	4.55 min

ICU-Specific Queueing Analysis

To test the ICU bottleneck concern directly rather than infer it only from length-of-stay variability, a separate M/M/c model was constructed using ICU admission and discharge times alone. The ICU arrival rate was estimated at $\lambda\_ICU \approx 1.54 \times 10^{-4}$ per hour and the ICU service rate at $\mu\_ICU \approx 9.36 \times 10^{-3}$ per hour (mean ICU length of stay ≈ 4.45 days, n = 136 ICU stays), with c_ICU = 2 based on the peak number of concurrent ICU stays observed in the data. Under these parameters, ICU utilization is $\rho\_ICU \approx 0.82\%$, with an expected ICU queue wait of well under one minute (Table 2c). This confirms that, under the current dataset, ICU congestion was not observed — consistent with the interpretation given below — though the high variability in ICU length of stay (Figure 8) means this could change under higher demand or reduced capacity.

Table 5. ICU-Specific Queueing Metrics

Metric	Value
λ_ICU	1.54×10^{-4} /hr
μ_ICU	9.36×10^{-3} /hr
c_ICU	2
ρ_ICU	0.0082 (0.82%)
Wq_ICU	0.43 min
Lq_ICU	0.000001

Overall Interpretation

The analysis demonstrates that the healthcare system operates in a stable and efficient manner under the observed conditions. Key findings include:

- Patient arrivals follow a Poisson distribution
- Interarrival times exhibit exponential characteristics
- Most patients experience short hospital stays
- ICU length-of-stay data show high variability, indicating the ICU is a plausible point of congestion under higher demand, though the ICU-specific queueing model applied to the current dataset does not show sustained overload
- System utilization is low, indicating sufficient capacity
- Queue length is negligible, suggesting minimal congestion

- Model selection matters substantially: the single-server (M/M/1) estimate overstates waiting time by more than two orders of magnitude relative to the multi-server (M/M/c) estimate under identical arrival and service rates

Practical Interpretation for Hospital Administrators

For readers who are less familiar with queueing theory, it is worth translating these results into plain, practical terms. A utilization value of about 0.018, or 1.80 percent, means that the modeled service resources are busy for less than two out of every hundred hours, which suggests substantial spare capacity under the conditions captured in this dataset. An average waiting time of about 4.55 minutes means that, on average, a patient in this model would expect only a short delay before being seen, rather than a long wait. A queue length close to zero means that, at any given moment, the model predicts almost no patients waiting at once. Taken together, these numbers suggest a system with enough capacity to absorb its current patient load comfortably. However, administrators should be cautious about applying these exact figures directly to staffing or budget decisions, since they come from a small demonstration dataset rather than a full hospital record; the value of this chapter lies mainly in demonstrating the method, which hospitals could apply to their own, larger datasets to get results relevant to their specific setting.

Summary of Key Findings

This section summarizes the key components of the study in a structured manner. The study applies queueing theory and Poisson processes to model patient flow and analyze system performance. Key contributions include the estimation of arrival and service rates, characterization of ICU length-of-stay variability, and integration of statistical testing with simulation techniques.

The system is characterized by stochastic patient arrivals, variable service times, and resource constraints, particularly in critical care units. System performance depends on maintaining a balance between demand and service capacity.

The methodology follows a structured approach, including data preprocessing, calculation of arrival and service rates, estimation of key parameters, application of the M/M/c model, and evaluation of performance metrics such as utilization, waiting time, and queue length. The results are further supported by graphical analysis and interpretation of system behavior.

SOLUTIONS AND RECOMMENDATIONS

Given the small sample size and the date-shifting limitations discussed in the Methodology, the numerical results underlying this analysis are illustrative rather than operationally meaningful; the recommendations below should therefore be understood as established, literature-supported healthcare-operations practices that are consistent with these illustrative findings, rather than as novel insights uniquely derived from this specific dataset. The findings highlight variability in arrival patterns, differences in service times, and ICU length-of-stay variability, even though the system currently operates with low utilization overall. Based on these insights, several practical solutions and recommendations are proposed.

Dynamic Staffing Optimization

Staffing is one of the most critical factors affecting system performance. Patient arrivals are not constant — clear peak and off-peak periods exist — so a fixed staffing level leads to overcrowding at peak times and underutilization otherwise. Healthcare facilities should instead adopt dynamic staffing strategies based on projected demand, using the relationship between arrival rate (λ), service rate (μ), and utilization (ρ) to determine optimal staffing levels, scheduling additional staff at peak hours and cross-training staff for flexibility during sudden demand changes.

AI-Based Demand Prediction and Decision Support

The stochastic nature of patient arrivals is a challenge queueing theory alone cannot resolve, since it does not predict future demand. Integrating AI and machine learning — such as time-series forecasting and regression models trained on historical data — can identify trends, seasonal patterns, and potential surges, feeding real-time decision support that recommends reallocating resources or activating contingency plans. Combining AI with queueing theory creates a hybrid framework pairing predictive capability with analytical rigor.

ICU Capacity Management and Bottleneck Reduction

The results of this study show substantial variability in ICU length of stay, which represents a plausible source of congestion if patient demand were to increase, although the ICU-specific queueing model applied to the current dataset did not show sustained high utilization. Proactive management of ICU resources is nonetheless recommended as a precautionary measure given this variability.

Hospitals should implement ICU capacity-management strategies that include improving discharge planning to transfer stabilized patients to lower-acuity or step-down units, thereby freeing ICU beds for critical cases, and implementing structured triage protocols that ensure high-acuity patients receive immediate attention while maintaining appropriate care for less urgent cases. Predictive analytics can further anticipate ICU demand from historical trends and external factors, supporting better resource planning.

Process Optimization and Workflow Automation

Beyond staffing and resource allocation, process optimization and workflow automation can reduce delays from inefficient registration, triage, and administrative procedures. Digital systems such as EHRs and automated scheduling and triage tools reduce manual workload and errors, while lean-management principles help eliminate non-value-added steps and improve coordination between departments.

Integration of Simulation and Scenario Analysis

Discrete-event simulation can evaluate operational strategies — such as staffing changes, altered arrival rates, or increased service capacity — before implementation, helping identify optimal strategies for patient flow and resource allocation. This is particularly valuable for preparing for extreme events such as pandemics or sudden demand surges, supporting contingency planning and resilience.

Policy and Strategic Implications

These findings also have policy implications: decision-makers should adopt a data-driven approach to planning, invest in data infrastructure and analytical tools, train staff in data analysis and decision support, and encourage smart healthcare systems that integrate real-time data, predictive analytics, and automated decision-making to improve efficiency, reduce costs, and enhance outcomes.

Table 6. Expected Directional Impact of Proposed Recommendations (Illustrative, Not Empirically Tested)

Metric	Current State (Observed)	Expected State (If Recommended Changes Adopted)
Waiting Time	High variability	Reduced and predictable
Utilization	Imbalanced	Optimized
ICU Congestion	Frequent	Controlled
Patient Flow	Irregular	Streamlined
Resource Allocation	Static	Dynamic

Summary of Recommendations

In summary, improving patient flow in healthcare systems requires a combination of analytical modeling, technological integration, and operational optimization. Key recommendations include:

- Implementing dynamic staffing strategies based on demand patterns
- Integrating AI and machine learning for demand prediction
- Optimizing ICU capacity and reducing bottlenecks
- Enhancing processes through automation and digital systems
- Using simulation and scenario analysis for decision support
- Promoting data-driven healthcare policies

FUTURE RESEARCH DIRECTIONS

This chapter provides a foundational framework for analyzing patient flow using queueing theory and Poisson process modeling. While the results offer valuable insights, several directions exist for extending this work.

One direction is integrating machine learning with queueing models: this study estimates arrival intensity from hour-of-day patterns, but real systems often show more complex time-varying demand. Time-series forecasting, regression, and deep-learning models could predict arrivals more accurately, enhancing the ability to respond proactively to demand fluctuations.

A closely related direction is extending the static queueing model presented in this chapter toward an adaptive framework. The arrival and service rates estimated here are fixed point estimates; in an adaptive setting, these could instead be updated continuously using Bayesian updating — as introduced in Chapter 1 of this volume — allowing the model's parameters to be revised as new admission and discharge data arrives. Similarly, staffing decisions (the choice of c) could be framed as a sequential decision problem using a Markov Decision Process formulation, also introduced in Chapter 1, in which the system observes queue state and adjusts capacity to minimize a combination of expected waiting time and staffing cost. Together, these extensions would connect the queueing-based performance measures used in this chapter with the adaptive decision-making framework developed in Chapter 1, forming a coherent thread across the two chapters.

Another promising area is smart, IoT-enabled healthcare systems. As hospitals increasingly rely on EHRs, wearables, and sensor-based monitoring, integrating real-time data streams with queueing models could enable continuous monitoring of patient flow and dynamic resource adjustment.

While this chapter applies the M/M/c model to better reflect multi-server hospital operations, further work could explore priority queues and network-queueing systems that capture patient prioritization and interactions between hospital units for even more realistic analysis.

Simulation-based approaches also offer potential: discrete-event simulation can model complex systems under scenarios such as emergency surges or pandemics, letting researchers evaluate interventions before real-world implementation and supporting evidence-based, lower-risk decision-making.

Patient prioritization and triage is another direction — incorporating priority-based queueing models could show how triage policies affect waiting times, service efficiency, and outcomes, supporting more effective ED triage strategies.

Multi-objective optimization, balancing measures such as waiting time, cost, and quality of care simultaneously, is also promising, using techniques like metaheuristics and reinforcement learning to identify optimal resource-allocation strategies.

Finally, large-scale, multi-hospital data analysis would improve generalizability, since this study relies on a single, small demo dataset and healthcare systems vary widely across regions and institutions.

Cost-Benefit Considerations for Future Work

Future research could also examine the cost side of the recommendations proposed in this chapter. Dynamic staffing, AI-based forecasting tools, and ICU capacity-management strategies all require investment in staff time, software, or training, and hospitals operating with tight budgets need clear evidence that the expected reduction in waiting time and congestion justifies these costs. A useful extension of this work would therefore combine the queueing-based performance measures used here, such as utilization and waiting time, with a simple cost model that estimates the financial impact of implementation against the financial and clinical cost of continued overcrowding, giving hospital administrators a more complete basis for decision-making.

CONCLUSION

This chapter presented an analysis of patient flow in healthcare systems using queueing theory and Poisson process modeling, integrating probabilistic models with real hospital data to represent complex, uncertain arrival and service patterns.

Hourly arrival patterns are broadly consistent with a Poisson process (chi-square test, $p = 0.068$), and interarrival and service times show the expected exponential-type variability, supporting the applicability of classical queueing assumptions in this setting. ICU length of stay showed high variability, indicating the ICU as a plausible — though not conclusively proven — point of congestion.

Under the M/M/c model, the system shows low utilization ($\rho = 0.018$) and a short expected waiting time (under 5 minutes), suggesting the observed facility has sufficient capacity for current demand. However, given the small size of the demonstration dataset and the MIMIC date-shift limitation discussed in the Methodology, these specific figures are illustrative of the method rather than operationally meaningful estimates, and should not be used for real-world staffing or capacity planning.

The primary value of this chapter lies in its methodological demonstration: combining data-driven parameter estimation with theoretical queueing models, grounding classical queueing theory in real system behavior, and underscoring the importance of careful interpretation of model outputs — particularly when working with small, date-shifted, or otherwise limited datasets.

The recommendations discussed above — dynamic staffing, AI-based demand prediction, and proactive ICU resource management — reflect established, literature-supported healthcare-operations practices rather than novel findings uniquely derived from this analysis; they are offered as directions consistent with, though not proven by, the illustrative results presented here.

In conclusion, integrating queueing theory, Poisson processes, and healthcare analytics offers a practical, reproducible template for approaching patient-flow management, which readers are encouraged to adapt to their own, larger, non-date-shifted datasets for operationally meaningful results.

AI-ASSISTED DRAFTING DISCLOSURE AND HUMAN VERIFICATION STATEMENT

In the interest of transparency, the author discloses that an AI writing tool was used to assist in drafting portions of this manuscript. Every claim, method, statistic, and citation in this chapter has been reviewed and verified by the author against the underlying analysis code, dataset, and cited sources; no results, data points, or references were generated or fabricated by the AI tool, and the author takes full responsibility for the accuracy and integrity of the manuscript's content.

REFERENCES

Cochran, J. K., & Bharti, A. (2006). Stochastic bed balancing of an obstetrics hospital. *Health Care Management Science*, *9*(1), 31–45. DOI: 10.1007/s10729-006-6278-6 PMID: 16613015

Green, L. (2006). Queueing analysis in healthcare. In Hall, R. (Ed.), *Patient flow: Reducing delay in healthcare delivery* (pp. 281–307). Springer. DOI: 10.1007/978-0-387-33636-7_10

Gul, M., & Guneri, A. F. (2015). A comprehensive review of emergency department simulation applications for normal and disaster conditions. *Computers & Industrial Engineering*, *83*, 327–344. DOI: 10.1016/j.cie.2015.02.018

Jacobson, S. H., Hall, S. N., & Swisher, J. R. (2013). Discrete-event simulation of health care systems. In Hall, R. (Ed.), *Patient flow: Reducing delay in healthcare delivery* (pp. 273–309). Springer. DOI: 10.1007/978-1-4614-9512-3_12

Josephs, T. (2020). Patterns of mortality in children presenting to a tertiary paediatric emergency unit in Sub-Saharan Africa: A cross-sectional study.

Jun, J. B., Jacobson, S. H., & Swisher, J. R. (1999). Application of discrete-event simulation in health care clinics: A survey. *The Journal of the Operational Research Society*, *50*(2), 109–123. DOI: 10.1057/palgrave.jors.2600669

Kim, S. C., & Horowitz, I. (2002). Scheduling hospital services: The efficacy of elective-surgery quotas. *Omega*, *30*(5), 335–346. DOI: 10.1016/S0305-0483(02)00050-6

Kolker, A. (2008). Process modeling of emergency department patient flow: Effect of patient length of stay on ED diversion. *Journal of Medical Systems*, *32*(5), 389–401. DOI: 10.1007/s10916-008-9144-x PMID: 18814495

Lakshmi, C., & Iyer, S. A. (2013). Application of queueing theory in health care: A literature review. *Operations Research for Health Care*, *2*(1–2), 25–39.

Ross, S. M. (2014). *Introduction to probability models*. Academic Press.

Wilden, R., Garbuio, M., Angeli, F., & Mascia, D. (Eds.). (2018). *Healthcare entrepreneurship*. Routledge. DOI: 10.4324/9781315157993

Chapter 7
Martingale-Based Performance Monitoring and Adaptive Intervention in Healthcare Systems

Manoj K.
http://orcid.org/0000-0002-0022-9011
Manonmaniam Sundaranar University, India

ABSTRACT

This chapter examines the use of stochastic process theory for performance monitoring and adaptive intervention in healthcare systems operating under uncertainty. Healthcare delivery is shaped by unpredictable patient arrivals, variable service times, and changing resource constraints, which can reduce the effectiveness of static and retrospective performance indicators. The chapter models healthcare operational variables as stochastic processes and presents martingale-based monitoring techniques for distinguishing routine variability from meaningful system drift. Stopping times are employed to define data-driven intervention points that support timely and statistically justified operational responses. Simulation-based illustrations and an emergency department congestion scenario are used to demonstrate the practical relevance of the framework. The chapter also discusses ethical, governance, and artificial intelligence considerations associated with probabilistic monitoring and intervention mechanisms in adaptive healthcare systems.

INTRODUCTION

Healthcare systems have become increasingly complex due to rising patient demand, constrained resources, demographic changes, and the growing availability of real-time clinical data. These factors have intensified the need for analytical frameworks capable of supporting adaptive decision-making under uncertainty. Patient arrivals, treatment durations, resource availability, and clinical responses exhibit substantial variability over time, making deterministic planning approaches insufficient for accurately representing real-world healthcare operations. Consequently, healthcare organizations require monitor-

DOI: 10.4018/979-8-3373-9705-4.ch007

ing and decision-support methods that can continuously adapt to changing operational conditions while maintaining efficiency and quality of care.

The increasing digitalization of healthcare has further accelerated the transition from static planning toward adaptive and data-driven management strategies. Electronic health records, real-time patient monitoring systems, Internet of Medical Things (IoMT) devices, and hospital information systems continuously generate large volumes of operational data that can support timely decision-making. However, transforming these dynamic data streams into actionable operational insights remains a significant challenge. Effective healthcare management therefore requires mathematical models capable of representing uncertainty, capturing temporal evolution, and supporting continuous performance assessment. Stochastic processes provide a natural foundation for this purpose by explicitly modeling random phenomena that evolve over time (Ross, 2014).

Among stochastic methodologies, martingale theory provides an elegant probabilistic framework for monitoring deviations from expected system behavior. A martingale represents a stochastic process in which the expected future evolution depends only on the currently available information, making it particularly suitable for sequential monitoring under uncertainty (Doob, 1953; Williams, 1991). Rather than relying solely on retrospective performance evaluation, martingale-based monitoring supports continuous assessment of evolving healthcare systems and facilitates the early identification of abnormal operational patterns, including unexpected increases in patient arrivals, resource congestion, or changes in service performance.

Complementing martingale theory, stopping-time theory provides a mathematically rigorous mechanism for determining when accumulated evidence is sufficient to initiate an intervention. By defining intervention rules based on continuously updated information, stopping times establish a balance between rapid detection of meaningful changes and avoidance of unnecessary false alarms. These concepts have long been recognised within sequential analysis and statistical decision theory (Shiryaev, 2007; Lai, 2001), yet their interpretation within adaptive healthcare operations has received comparatively limited attention.

Healthcare operations research has traditionally relied on queueing models, Markov processes, statistical process control, and sequential monitoring techniques to analyse patient flow, optimize resource allocation, and evaluate system performance. Although these methods have contributed substantially to healthcare management, many existing applications focus primarily on retrospective quality assessment, steady-state system behavior, or narrowly defined surveillance problems. Contemporary healthcare environments increasingly involve streaming operational data, dynamic congestion patterns, rapidly changing resource availability, and the growing integration of Artificial Intelligence (AI)-assisted decision-support systems. These developments require monitoring strategies that can operate continuously while adapting to evolving system conditions (Topol, 2019; Aceto et al., 2020; Shaik et al., 2023, Javaid et al., 2022).

Despite these advances, relatively limited attention has been devoted to interpreting classical sequential stochastic monitoring methods within the broader context of adaptive healthcare operations. Existing healthcare applications of sequential monitoring have largely concentrated on quality control, surveillance, and surgical outcome monitoring (Steiner et al., 2000; Woodall, 2006), whereas fewer studies have examined how martingale-based monitoring can support operational decision-making in healthcare systems characterised by streaming patient arrivals, evolving congestion, and intervention-oriented management. Furthermore, the integration of stochastic monitoring concepts with modern AI-enabled healthcare infrastructure and digital health technologies remains an emerging area of research.

Accordingly, the contribution of this chapter lies not in proposing a new sequential change-detection methodology. Instead, the chapter presents a healthcare-oriented operational interpretation of established martingale-based monitoring and stopping-time principles within adaptive healthcare environments. By integrating probabilistic monitoring with intervention-oriented decision-making, the chapter demonstrates how classical stochastic concepts can be interpreted to support continuous operational assessment, timely detection of emerging system stress, and adaptive healthcare management. The proposed monitoring approach is illustrated through simulation experiments motivated by emergency department congestion scenarios and healthcare operational stress conditions.

Healthcare systems are increasingly transitioning from reactive models of care to proactive, data-driven environments that rely on continuous monitoring and timely interventions. The widespread adoption of electronic health records, wearable sensors, Internet of Medical Things (IoMT) devices, and telemedicine platforms has enabled healthcare providers to collect large volumes of real-time patient and operational data. While these technologies offer unprecedented opportunities for improving healthcare quality and efficiency, they also present significant statistical challenges associated with uncertainty, variability, and rapidly changing system dynamics. Consequently, robust stochastic monitoring frameworks are essential for distinguishing meaningful structural changes from routine random fluctuations. Sequential statistical methods, particularly those based on martingale theory and stopping-time principles, provide mathematically rigorous tools for analyzing streaming healthcare data and supporting evidence-based decision-making. By facilitating early identification of abnormal system behaviour, these approaches can improve resource allocation, reduce operational delays, and enhance patient safety in complex healthcare environments.

The objectives of this chapter are fivefold. First, it reviews the stochastic process concepts that underpin adaptive healthcare monitoring. Second, it develops the theoretical foundations of martingale-based monitoring and stopping-time–based intervention for healthcare applications. Third, it evaluates the operational behavior of the monitoring approach through simulation studies under controlled stochastic conditions. Fourth, it demonstrates the practical interpretation of the approach using an emergency department congestion scenario. Finally, it discusses the ethical, governance, and Artificial Intelligence (AI) considerations associated with implementing adaptive stochastic monitoring in modern healthcare systems.

The chapter begins by reviewing the relevant theoretical and methodological literature before introducing the probabilistic foundations of martingale-based monitoring and stopping-time intervention. The monitoring approach is subsequently evaluated through simulation experiments and interpreted within an emergency department congestion scenario to illustrate its operational applicability. The chapter concludes by discussing ethical considerations, governance challenges, AI integration, study limitations, future research opportunities, and broader implications for adaptive healthcare management.

BACKGROUND AND RELATED WORK

Healthcare systems have long relied on quantitative analytical methods to improve operational efficiency, optimize resource utilization, and support evidence-based decision-making. Because healthcare delivery involves substantial uncertainty arising from random patient arrivals, variable treatment durations, fluctuating resource availability, and changing clinical priorities, mathematical models have become indispensable tools for understanding and managing healthcare operations. Over the past several decades, operations research, stochastic modelling, statistical process control, and sequential decision-making have collectively contributed to significant advances in healthcare management.

Among the earliest analytical approaches applied to healthcare operations is queueing theory, which provides mathematical models for patient arrivals, waiting lines, and service mechanisms. Queueing models have been widely used to evaluate patient waiting times, determine staffing requirements, improve appointment scheduling, and optimize patient flow within hospitals and emergency departments (Green, 2006; Hall, 2013; Izady & Worthington, 2012). These models offer valuable insights into healthcare system performance under varying demand conditions and have become fundamental tools in healthcare operations research. Nevertheless, many classical queueing models rely on steady-state assumptions and average system behavior, limiting their ability to respond to rapidly changing operational environments where demand fluctuates continuously.

Another important class of analytical models is based on Markov processes, which have been extensively employed in health economics, disease progression modelling, and clinical decision analysis. Markov models describe transitions among discrete health states and provide a structured framework for evaluating long-term clinical outcomes and healthcare interventions (Briggs & Sculpher, 1998). Despite their widespread application, conventional Markov models often assume memoryless transitions and fixed transition probabilities. These assumptions may not adequately represent healthcare systems operating under dynamic conditions where patient arrivals, resource availability, and operational priorities evolve continuously over time.

The increasing availability of digital healthcare data has further expanded the use of statistical methods for monitoring healthcare performance. Electronic health records, hospital information systems, and real-time monitoring technologies now generate continuous streams of operational data that support ongoing assessment of healthcare delivery. Consequently, healthcare management has shifted from periodic retrospective evaluation toward continuous performance monitoring capable of identifying emerging operational problems before they significantly affect patient care (Obermeyer & Emanuel, 2016).

The rapid digital transformation of healthcare has significantly influenced the development of advanced monitoring and decision-support systems. Modern healthcare organizations increasingly rely on electronic health records (EHRs), Internet of Medical Things (IoMT) devices, wearable sensors, and cloud-based information systems to generate continuous streams of clinical and operational data. These technologies enable healthcare providers to monitor patient conditions, hospital resource utilization, and service performance in real time, thereby facilitating timely clinical interventions and improving operational efficiency (Aceto et al., 2020; Ristevski & Chen, 2018). However, the high volume, velocity, and variability of healthcare data require statistical methodologies capable of distinguishing meaningful changes from normal stochastic fluctuations.

Recent advances in artificial intelligence (AI) and machine learning have further enhanced predictive analytics and automated decision-support systems in healthcare. Machine learning algorithms have demonstrated considerable potential in disease diagnosis, patient risk stratification, treatment optimization, and healthcare resource planning (Javaid et al., 2022). Nevertheless, many AI models function primarily as predictive tools and often lack mechanisms for continuous statistical surveillance of evolving healthcare processes. Consequently, integrating AI techniques with sequential monitoring methodologies offers opportunities to improve the reliability and interpretability of real-time healthcare decision-making. Such integration enables healthcare systems to continuously evaluate incoming information while maintaining statistically rigorous criteria for detecting significant deviations from expected system behaviour.

The growing availability of streaming healthcare data has also increased interest in adaptive monitoring strategies capable of supporting dynamic resource allocation and operational management. Rather than relying solely on retrospective analyses, contemporary healthcare systems increasingly require online statistical frameworks that update decisions as new information becomes available. This shift has encouraged the application of stochastic processes, sequential analysis, and martingale-based methods to healthcare operations, where early detection of abnormal events can substantially improve patient outcomes and organizational efficiency. These developments provide a strong motivation for exploring mathematically rigorous monitoring techniques that can complement existing AI-enabled healthcare technologies.

One important development within this area is the application of Statistical Process Control (SPC) to healthcare systems. Originally developed for industrial quality improvement, SPC techniques have been successfully adapted to monitor healthcare quality indicators, patient safety outcomes, infection surveillance, and clinical performance measures (Mohammed et al., 2001; Woodall, 2006; Steiner et al., 2000). Control charts enable healthcare organizations to distinguish routine operational variation from meaningful changes requiring managerial attention. Among these techniques, the Cumulative Sum (CUSUM) procedure introduced by Page (1954) has become one of the most influential sequential monitoring methods because of its ability to detect relatively small but persistent changes more rapidly than traditional Shewhart control charts.

Risk-adjusted CUSUM procedures have subsequently been applied to monitor surgical outcomes, clinical performance, and healthcare quality indicators (Steiner et al., 2000). These approaches demonstrate the value of sequential monitoring for healthcare applications, particularly where early detection of deteriorating performance is essential. However, many existing applications remain focused on quality assurance and retrospective surveillance rather than broader operational management involving dynamic patient flow, resource congestion, and adaptive intervention.

More generally, sequential analysis provides a statistical framework in which observations are evaluated continuously as data become available rather than after completion of a fixed sample. Sequential monitoring methods support timely decision-making by allowing interventions to be initiated immediately once sufficient statistical evidence has accumulated (Lai, 2001). Such approaches are particularly attractive in healthcare environments where delayed recognition of operational changes may adversely affect patient outcomes and resource utilization.

Relationship to Classical CUSUM Monitoring

Classical Cumulative Sum (CUSUM) monitoring procedures constitute one of the most widely used sequential monitoring approaches in statistical process control. The monitoring framework discussed in this chapter is closely related to these established methods, particularly with respect to cumulative deviation statistics and sequential change detection.

The contribution of this chapter does not lie in proposing a new optimal stopping rule or replacing established CUSUM theory. Instead, it focuses on the operational interpretation and integration of martingale-based sequential monitoring within adaptive healthcare systems characterized by streaming patient arrivals, real-time intervention requirements, and dynamically evolving operational conditions.

Unlike traditional industrial monitoring settings, healthcare systems involve continuously changing patient-flow patterns, uncertainty in demand intensity, and integration with digital health infrastructure.

Consequently, the present framework emphasizes healthcare-oriented adaptation, operational interpretation, and system-level responsiveness rather than methodological novelty in stochastic process theory.

Recent developments in statistical process monitoring and Artificial Intelligence (AI)-assisted operational analytics have further highlighted the importance of adaptive monitoring systems capable of functioning effectively within streaming and dynamically evolving healthcare environments (Topol, 2019; Aceto et al., 2020; Shaik et al., 2023).

Research Gap and Chapter Contribution

Despite substantial advances in healthcare analytics and sequential monitoring, several challenges remain. Existing healthcare applications have primarily emphasized retrospective quality assessment, disease surveillance, or specific clinical outcomes, while comparatively fewer studies have examined the operational interpretation of stochastic monitoring within adaptive healthcare systems characterized by streaming patient arrivals, dynamic congestion, and intervention-oriented decision-making. Furthermore, relatively limited attention has been given to integrating established stochastic monitoring concepts with modern AI-enabled healthcare infrastructure and continuously evolving digital health ecosystems.

Within this broader stochastic framework, martingale theory provides a natural probabilistic interpretation for sequential monitoring. A martingale models the evolution of a stochastic process whose expected future behavior depends only on currently available information, making it particularly suitable for representing uncertainty in continuously evolving healthcare systems (Doob, 1953; Williams, 1991). Martingale methods have also established important theoretical connections with likelihood ratio processes, Bayesian updating, and sequential hypothesis testing (Shafer et al., 2011). When combined with stopping-time theory, they provide a coherent mathematical basis for determining when accumulated evidence is sufficient to justify intervention (Shiryaev, 2007; Moustakides, 1986).

Rather than proposing a new sequential change-detection algorithm, this chapter demonstrates how established martingale-based monitoring and stopping-time principles can be interpreted within adaptive healthcare operations to support continuous monitoring, operational awareness, and timely intervention under uncertainty.

Table 1. Comparison of Classical Sequential Monitoring and the Healthcare-Oriented Monitoring Interpretation

Feature	Classical Sequential Monitoring	Healthcare-Oriented Monitoring Interpretation
Primary application	Industrial quality control	Adaptive healthcare operations
Operational congestion interpretation	Limited	Explicitly considered
Streaming healthcare data	Limited	Central component
AI-assisted decision support	Rarely addressed	Integrated conceptually
Intervention-oriented monitoring	Limited	Emphasized
Healthcare systems perspective	Application-specific	System-wide operational interpretation

The literature reviewed above establishes the theoretical and operational context for the chapter. Building upon these established foundations, the chapter develops the probabilistic concepts underlying martingale-based monitoring and stopping-time–based adaptive intervention before illustrating their application through simulation studies and healthcare operational scenarios.

THEORETICAL FOUNDATIONS

Probability Space and Information Structure

Healthcare systems evolve dynamically under uncertainty, requiring probabilistic frameworks capable of representing information flow and temporal variability. Patient arrivals, treatment durations, resource availability, and clinical outcomes exhibit inherent randomness that cannot be adequately represented using deterministic models alone. Stochastic process theory therefore provides an appropriate mathematical foundation for modeling healthcare systems operating under uncertain and continuously changing conditions.

The probabilistic framework introduced in this chapter forms the basis for representing uncertainty, describing the evolution of healthcare processes over time, and supporting adaptive monitoring and decision-making.

Stochastic Processes in Healthcare Systems

Healthcare operations can be naturally represented as stochastic processes because of the inherent randomness associated with patient arrivals, treatment durations, and healthcare system responses. Typical examples include:

- Emergency department patient arrivals, which may be modeled using Poisson processes;
- Service times that follow exponential or other probability distributions; and
- Healthcare system states that evolve over time according to patient flow, clinical demand, and resource allocation.

Let $\{Y_t\}$ denote the number of patient arrivals observed at time t. The stochastic process explicitly represents uncertainty in patient arrival patterns while allowing the evolution of healthcare demand to be monitored over time.

Unlike deterministic models, stochastic processes capture both expected system behavior and random fluctuations. Consequently, they provide a more realistic representation of healthcare operations, where variability is unavoidable and often substantial (Green, 2006; Hall, 2013).

Conditional Expectation and Information Updating

A fundamental concept in stochastic modeling is conditional expectation, which represents the expected value of a random variable given the information currently available.

For a stochastic process $\{Y_t\}$, the conditional expectation is defined as:

$$\mathbb{E}\left[Y_{t+1} \mid \mathcal{F}_t\right]$$

where $\mathcal{F}_t$ denotes the information available up to time t.

The conditional expectation provides the best prediction of the future observation Y_{t+1} based on the information accumulated up to the present time.

In healthcare systems, conditional expectation supports forecasting patient arrivals, estimating system workload, and anticipating resource requirements using continuously updated operational information. As new observations become available, these predictions are revised, enabling adaptive decision-making in dynamic healthcare environments.

Conditional expectation also provides the mathematical foundation for martingale processes, which form the basis of the monitoring framework developed in this chapter (Williams, 1991).

Filtration and Adapted Processes

The concept of filtration formalizes the progressive accumulation of information over time. Within healthcare systems, this corresponds to the continuous observation of operational variables such as patient arrivals, waiting times, bed occupancy, and resource utilization.

An adapted process ensures that decisions made at time t depend only on the information available up to that time. This property is essential in real-time healthcare monitoring because future observations are unknown when operational decisions are made.

Mathematically, a stochastic process $\{Y_t\}$ is adapted if:

$Y_t \in \mathcal{F}_t$, for all t.

This property guarantees consistency between the stochastic process and the information available at each time point, thereby supporting sequential monitoring and evidence-based decision-making in healthcare operations.

Relevance to Healthcare System Modeling

The stochastic concepts introduced in this section provide the mathematical foundation for modeling healthcare systems operating under uncertainty. By incorporating probability spaces, conditional expectation, filtrations, and adapted stochastic processes, healthcare operations can be represented in a manner that reflects both temporal evolution and random variability. In practical healthcare environments, new information becomes available continuously through patient admissions, diagnostic investigations, physiological monitoring, electronic health records, and hospital information systems. Consequently, healthcare decision-making is inherently dynamic, requiring statistical models that can update predictions and operational decisions as additional information is observed over time.

The filtration framework provides a natural mathematical representation of this evolving information structure by ensuring that decisions at any point in time are based solely on information currently available. Similarly, conditional expectation enables healthcare practitioners and administrators to revise estimates of future system behaviour, such as anticipated patient arrivals, bed occupancy levels, treatment durations, or resource utilization, as new observations become available. These concepts support adaptive decision-making under uncertainty while maintaining a rigorous probabilistic foundation.

These concepts make it possible to:

- represent the continuous evolution of healthcare systems over time;
- model uncertainty in patient arrivals, treatment durations, and resource utilization;
- incorporate newly available information into operational decision-making;
- update predictions dynamically as healthcare conditions evolve; and
- establish the probabilistic framework required for monitoring and intervention.

Collectively, these theoretical foundations support the development of martingale-based monitoring processes and stopping-time–based intervention strategies presented in the subsequent discussion. They also provide the mathematical basis for designing sequential monitoring algorithms capable of distinguishing routine stochastic variation from significant structural changes requiring timely intervention, thereby supporting more efficient healthcare management and improved patient outcomes.

MARTINGALE THEORY FOR HEALTHCARE MONITORING

Definition and Fundamental Properties

Martingales play a central role in stochastic process theory and provide a natural framework for modeling systems that evolve over time under uncertainty. Intuitively, a martingale represents a "fair" process in which the expected future value, given current information, is equal to the present value.

Formally, let $(\Omega|\mathcal{F}|\mathbb{P})$ be a probability space with filtration $\{\mathcal{F}_t\}_{t\geq 0}$. A stochastic process $\{M_t\}_{t\geq 0}$ is called a martingale with respect to $\{\mathcal{F}_t\}$ if:

$\mathbb{E}[| M_t |] < \infty$, for all *t*,

E*[Mt+1 Ft]=Mt,*for all *t*.

This condition implies that, given all available information up to time *t*, the best prediction of the next value is simply the current value. Martingales therefore capture the idea of unbiased evolution over time (Doob, 1953; Williams, 1991).

Interpretation in Healthcare Systems

In the context of healthcare systems, martingales provide a mechanism for tracking deviations from expected system behavior. Consider a process that represents the cumulative difference between observed patient arrivals and expected arrivals. Under normal operating conditions, the deviations should fluctuate randomly around zero.

If the system behaves as expected, the monitoring process satisfies the martingale property. However, when there is a structural change—such as a sudden increase in patient demand—the process begins to exhibit systematic drift. This deviation from the martingale property can be used as a signal for detecting abnormal system behavior.

Thus, martingales serve as a baseline model for "normal" system operation, against which deviations can be identified and monitored.

Construction of Martingale Monitoring Processes

A practical martingale for healthcare monitoring can be constructed using observed data. Let $\{Y_t\}$ denote the number of patient arrivals at time t, and let λ_0 represent the expected arrival rate under normal conditions.

Define the process:

$$M_t = \sum_{k=1}^{t} (Y_k - \lambda_0)$$

Under the assumption that $\mathbb{E}[Y_k \mid \mathcal{F}_{k-1}] = \lambda_0$, it follows that:

$$\mathbb{E}[M_t \mid \mathcal{F}_{t-1}] = M_{t-1}$$

which confirms that $\{M_t\}$ is a martingale.

This construction is particularly useful in healthcare systems, where baseline expectations can be estimated from historical data and updated dynamically.

Detection of Structural Changes

One of the key advantages of martingale-based monitoring is its ability to detect structural changes in system behavior. When the underlying process deviates from its expected pattern—for example, when the arrival rate increases from λ_0 to λ_1—the martingale property no longer holds.

In such cases, the process M_t exhibits a systematic upward trend:

$$\mathbb{E}[Y_t] = \lambda_1 > \lambda_0 \Rightarrow \mathbb{E}[M_t] \text{ increases over time}$$

This drift provides a clear statistical signal that the system has entered a new regime. Detecting this change early is critical in healthcare applications, where delays in response can lead to overcrowding and reduced quality of care.

Martingales and Sequential Monitoring

Martingale processes are closely related to sequential monitoring methods used in statistical process control. Unlike traditional control charts, martingale-based approaches:

- Do not rely heavily on fixed distributional assumptions
- Adapt naturally to evolving data
- Provide a theoretically grounded framework for real-time monitoring

These properties make martingales particularly suitable for healthcare systems, where variability and uncertainty are inherent.

Furthermore, martingale-based methods are connected to likelihood ratio processes and sequential hypothesis testing, which form the basis of modern change detection techniques (Shafer et al., 2011; Lai, 2001).

Advantages of Martingale-Based Monitoring

The use of martingales in healthcare monitoring offers several advantages:

- **Real-time adaptability**: The process evolves dynamically as new data becomes available
- **Sensitivity to change**: Structural deviations are detected through drift behavior
- **Mathematical rigor**: The framework is grounded in well-established probability theory
- **Interpretability**: The concept of deviation from expectation is intuitive and transparent

These features make martingale-based monitoring a powerful tool for managing complex healthcare systems.

Transition to Stopping-Time Framework

While martingales provide a mechanism for detecting deviations, decision-making requires a rule for determining when to act. This leads naturally to the concept of stopping times, which define the optimal moment to trigger an intervention based on observed data.

The integration of martingale monitoring with stopping-time rules forms the foundation of adaptive healthcare decision systems, which forms the basis for stopping-time–based adaptive intervention.

STOPPING-TIME–BASED ADAPTIVE INTERVENTION

Definition of Stopping Times

In stochastic process theory, a stopping time represents the time at which a decision is made based on available information. Formally, let $\{\mathcal{F}_t\}_{t\geq 0}$ be a filtration representing the information available over time. A random variable τ is called a stopping time if:

$\{\tau \leq t\} \in \mathcal{F}_t$ for all $t \geq 0$.

This condition ensures that the decision to stop at time t depends only on the information available up to that time and not on future observations. In other words, stopping times formalize the principle of non-anticipative decision-making (Shiryaev, 2007).

Interpretation in Healthcare Systems

In healthcare operations, decisions must often be made sequentially as new information becomes available. Examples include:

- When to deploy additional staff in an emergency department
- When to activate surge capacity
- When to intervene in patient flow bottlenecks

A stopping time provides a mathematically rigorous way to determine when sufficient evidence has accumulated to justify intervention. Importantly, the decision is based entirely on observed system behavior up to the current time.

Stopping Rules Based on Martingale Processes

When martingale-based monitoring is used, stopping times can be defined in terms of the monitoring statistic. Let $\{M_t\}$ be a martingale process constructed to track deviations from expected system behavior.

A common stopping rule is:

$$\tau = \inf\{t \geq 0 : M_t \geq h\},$$

where h is a predefined threshold.

This rule specifies that intervention occurs at the first time the monitoring statistic exceeds the threshold. The choice of h determines the sensitivity of the monitoring system.

Trade-Off Between Detection Delay and False Alarms

A key consideration in designing stopping rules is the trade-off between:

- **Detection delay**: the time taken to identify a true change
- **False alarms**: triggering intervention when no change has occurred

Lower thresholds lead to faster detection but increase the likelihood of false alarms. Conversely, higher thresholds reduce false alarms but may delay intervention.

This trade-off is particularly important in healthcare systems, where:

- Timely intervention can prevent system overload and improve healthcare system responsiveness.
- Excessive interventions may disrupt normal operations

Balancing these competing objectives is central to effective decision-making (Lai, 2001). In emergency healthcare environments, delayed intervention may contribute to overcrowding, prolonged waiting times, and reduced treatment efficiency. Sequential stopping rules therefore provide operational value by enabling earlier recognition of emerging system stress conditions.

Optimal Stopping Perspective

Stopping time problems can also be viewed from the perspective of optimal stopping theory. In this framework, the objective is to choose a stopping time τ that optimizes a given performance criterion, such as minimizing expected delay or maximizing system efficiency.

Formally, the problem can be expressed as:

$$\min_{\tau} \mathbb{E}[C(\tau)],$$

where $C(\tau)$ represents a cost function associated with stopping at time τ.

In healthcare systems, such cost functions may incorporate:

- Delays in treatment
- Resource utilization
- Operational disruptions

Optimal stopping theory provides a principled foundation for designing intervention strategies under uncertainty (Shiryaev, 2007).

Application to Healthcare Monitoring Systems

Combining martingale monitoring with stopping-time rules enables the development of adaptive healthcare systems that:

- Continuously monitor system performance
- Detect deviations from expected behavior
- Trigger timely interventions

For example, in an emergency department setting:

- M_t tracks cumulative deviations in patient arrivals
- τ determines when congestion is detected
- Intervention is triggered automatically at time τ

This framework ensures that decisions are data-driven, timely, and consistent with observed system dynamics.

Advantages of Stopping-Time–Based Intervention

Stopping-time–based decision frameworks offer several advantages:

- **Real-time responsiveness**: Decisions are made as soon as sufficient evidence is available
- **Flexibility**: Thresholds can be adjusted based on system requirements

- **Theoretical rigor**: Decisions are grounded in probability theory
- **Operational relevance**: Directly applicable to healthcare system management

These properties make stopping times a powerful tool for designing adaptive intervention strategies.

MATHEMATICAL PROPERTIES AND SYSTEM BEHAVIOR

The mathematical properties of the proposed monitoring framework provide a theoretical basis for understanding its operational behavior under stochastic variability. These properties explain how the monitoring process behaves under both normal operating conditions and structural changes, thereby supporting the interpretation of simulation results and practical implementation. The analysis presented in this section is based on simplified assumptions intended to illustrate the underlying stochastic principles. In practice, healthcare systems may exhibit non-stationary arrival patterns, correlated patient flows, and multiple interacting resources that require more sophisticated stochastic models.

Detection Performance Metrics

The effectiveness of the proposed monitoring framework can be evaluated using several performance measures commonly employed in sequential monitoring and change-detection studies. These measures quantify the responsiveness of the monitoring process while balancing the need for timely intervention against the risk of unnecessary alarms.

Detection Delay

Detection delay is defined as

$$D = \tau - \theta$$

where θ denotes the change-point and τ represents the stopping time.

A smaller detection delay indicates that the monitoring framework responds more rapidly to structural changes, thereby enabling earlier operational intervention.

False Alarm Probability

The false alarm probability is defined as

$$P(\tau < \theta)$$

which represents the probability that an intervention is initiated before a genuine system change has occurred. Maintaining a low false alarm probability is important because unnecessary interventions may disrupt routine healthcare operations and reduce operational efficiency.

Average Detection Delay

Across repeated monitoring experiments, the expected detection delay is

$$E(\tau - \theta),$$

which provides an overall measure of the responsiveness of the monitoring framework.

Threshold Trade-Off

The choice of monitoring threshold h directly influences the balance between rapid detection and false alarm control.

- Lower values of h produce faster detection but increase the likelihood of false alarms.
- Higher values of h reduce false alarms but may delay intervention.

This trade-off is a fundamental characteristic of sequential monitoring procedures (Lai, 2001; Basseville & Nikiforov, 1993). In healthcare operations, selecting an appropriate threshold requires balancing timely responses to emerging operational stress against maintaining stability during normal system conditions.

Robustness and Variability

Healthcare systems exhibit considerable variability arising from differences in patient characteristics, treatment pathways, clinical priorities, and external operational conditions. The proposed martingale-based monitoring framework is well suited to such environments because it focuses on deviations from expected system behavior rather than relying on strict distributional assumptions.

The monitoring framework demonstrates several desirable robustness properties:

- it evaluates deviations relative to expected operational behavior;
- it adapts continuously as new observations become available;
- it remains applicable under varying operational conditions without requiring highly restrictive parametric assumptions.

Monte Carlo simulation results further demonstrate that the monitoring framework maintains consistent performance across repeated experimental scenarios, supporting its applicability in adaptive healthcare environments.

Implications for Healthcare System Design

The mathematical properties discussed above have several important implications for the design and operation of adaptive healthcare systems.

First, stable healthcare systems produce monitoring statistics that fluctuate within expected probabilistic limits, thereby reducing unnecessary interventions. Second, structural changes such as increased patient demand generate sustained deviations that can be detected through sequential monitoring. Third, threshold-based intervention provides healthcare administrators with a flexible mechanism for balancing early detection against false alarm control according to operational priorities.

It is also important to recognise that real-world healthcare systems are substantially more complex than the simplified stochastic models considered in this chapter. Patient heterogeneity, multiple interacting resources, varying clinical priorities, and organisational policies introduce additional sources of uncertainty that may influence system performance. Extending the proposed monitoring framework to incorporate these complexities represents an important direction for future research.

Furthermore, healthcare operations frequently involve resource constraints that evolve over time. Staff availability, bed occupancy, equipment limitations, and policy changes may significantly influence operational performance. Future developments could therefore integrate time-varying model parameters, multiple interacting resources, and predictive analytics within the proposed monitoring framework.

The integration of forecasting methods with martingale-based monitoring may further enhance operational decision-making by identifying emerging system stress before critical thresholds are reached. Such developments would support a transition from reactive operational management toward proactive and adaptive healthcare system design.

Transition to Simulation and Performance Evaluation

The mathematical properties presented in this section establish the theoretical basis for evaluating the proposed monitoring framework under controlled stochastic conditions. Simulation studies provide an opportunity to investigate detection performance, robustness, and operational behavior across repeated experimental scenarios, thereby demonstrating the practical applicability of the martingale-based monitoring approach within adaptive healthcare systems.

SIMULATION FRAMEWORK AND RESULTS

The simulation study was designed to evaluate the operational behavior of the proposed martingale-based monitoring and stopping-time–based intervention framework under controlled stochastic conditions representative of healthcare arrival processes. Patient arrivals were modelled using a Poisson process because count-based arrival streams are commonly used in healthcare operations research to represent emergency department demand and service-system congestion. The baseline arrival rate was fixed at $\lambda_0 = 4$, while the post-change arrival rate was increased to $\lambda_1 = 7$ to represent moderate operational stress conditions.

The simulation horizon consisted of 300 discrete time intervals, with a structural change introduced at time t=150. Multiple threshold levels were evaluated to investigate the trade-off between detection delay and false alarm behavior. To assess robustness, Monte Carlo simulation experiments were performed across multiple independent runs. Performance evaluation focused on detection delay, false alarm behavior, threshold sensitivity, and Average Run Length (ARL).

Objectives of the Simulation Study

The simulation study was conducted to evaluate the operational performance of the proposed monitoring framework under controlled stochastic conditions. Specifically, it aims to:

- assess the ability of the monitoring process to detect structural changes in system behavior;
- examine the effect of threshold selection on detection performance;
- evaluate robustness through repeated Monte Carlo simulation experiments; and
- analyse the trade-off between detection delay and false alarm behavior.

System Description

A simplified healthcare system is modeled to represent patient arrivals over time. The system operates under the following assumptions:

- Patient arrivals follow a Poisson process
- The time horizon consists of 300 discrete intervals
- A structural change occurs at time $t=150$
- The arrival rate increases from $\lambda_0 = 4$ to $\lambda_1 = 7$

This setup reflects realistic scenarios such as sudden increases in patient demand due to external factors.

Martingale Monitoring Framework

The monitoring process is constructed using the martingale formulation developed in earlier sections. Let Y_t denote the number of patient arrivals at time t. The monitoring statistic is defined as:

$$M_t = \sum_{k=1}^{t} (Y_k - \lambda_0)$$

Under normal operating conditions, the process fluctuates around zero. When a structural change occurs, the process exhibits a systematic upward drift, indicating deviation from expected system behavior.

An intervention is triggered using the stopping-time rule:

$$\tau = \inf\{t \geq 0 : M_t \geq h\}$$

where h is a predefined threshold.

Detection Performance

The simulation results demonstrate that the monitoring approach successfully detects the structural change in the system.

Table 2. Detection Performance Under Simulated Structural Change

Metric	Value
Change Point (θ)	150
Detection Time (τ)	160
Detection Delay	10

The observed detection delay demonstrates that the proposed monitoring framework responds shortly after the structural change, indicating its potential suitability for supporting timely operational intervention in adaptive healthcare environments. Although the results correspond to a simulated scenario, they illustrate the ability of the monitoring approach to identify emerging operational stress within a relatively short time window.

The detection delay of 10 time units indicates that the monitoring system responds promptly to changes in arrival patterns. This level of responsiveness is critical in healthcare settings, where delays in detection can lead to congestion and reduced quality of care.

Threshold Sensitivity Analysis

The impact of threshold selection on detection performance is evaluated by varying the threshold parameter *h*. Table 3 presents detection delay behavior obtained from a representative simulation realization under different threshold configurations.

Table 3. Threshold Sensitivity Analysis

Threshold	Detection Delay
20	3
30	6
40	10
50	12

The results highlight a clear trade-off between sensitivity and stability. Lower thresholds lead to faster detection but may increase the likelihood of false alarms. Higher thresholds reduce sensitivity but provide more stable monitoring. Selecting an appropriate threshold is therefore essential for balancing responsiveness and reliability.

To further evaluate monitoring performance under varying threshold configurations, Monte Carlo Average Run Length (ARL) analysis was conducted using repeated simulation experiments. In sequential monitoring theory, ARL_0 represents the expected number of observations before a false alarm occurs under normal operating conditions, while ARL_1 represents the expected detection delay after a structural change has occurred.

Table 4. Monte Carlo Average Run Length (ARL) Analysis

Threshold (h)	ARL_0	ARL_1
20	191.91	8.25
30	245.86	11.35
40	270.67	14.30
50	281.61	17.57

The ARL_0 values increase with threshold level, indicating improved monitoring stability and reduced false alarm frequency under normal operating conditions. Conversely, ARL_1 values also increase, reflecting slower detection following structural change. These results illustrate the classical trade-off between responsiveness and false alarm control in sequential monitoring systems.

Lower threshold values provide faster responsiveness but increase the likelihood of false alarms, whereas higher threshold values improve stability at the expense of increased detection delay. This behavior is consistent with established sequential monitoring theory and demonstrates the sensitivity of monitoring performance to threshold selection.

The increasing availability of real-time healthcare data streams and digital monitoring platforms has further expanded the relevance of sequential monitoring approaches for healthcare operations management (Ristevski & Chen, 2018).

Monte Carlo Simulation Results

To evaluate robustness, the simulation experiment is repeated over multiple independent runs.

Table 5. Monte Carlo Detection Performance

Metric	Value
Average Detection Delay	12.585
Standard Deviation	16.85

The average detection delay remains relatively low across simulations, indicating consistent performance of the monitoring framework. The observed variability reflects the stochastic nature of the system, which is expected in real-world healthcare environments.

The observed variability in detection delay highlights the inherent randomness in healthcare systems. While the average detection delay remains relatively low, individual simulation runs may exhibit earlier or later detection depending on stochastic fluctuations in arrivals. This variability underscores the importance of evaluating monitoring systems using repeated simulations rather than relying on a single realization.

False Alarm Analysis

The false alarm behavior of the monitoring system is evaluated under stable conditions where no structural change occurs.

Table 6. False Alarm Analysis

Metric	Value
False Alarm Rate	0.125

The false alarm rate of 0.125 indicates that the system maintains a reasonable balance between sensitivity and reliability. While some false alarms occur, the rate remains within acceptable limits for practical healthcare applications.

Visualization of Monitoring Behavior

The martingale monitoring process exhibits stable fluctuations prior to the change-point and a clear upward drift following the increase in arrival rate. The point at which the monitoring statistic crosses the threshold corresponds to the detection time.

Figure 1. Martingale-Based Monitoring Process Under Simulated Healthcare Arrival Conditions

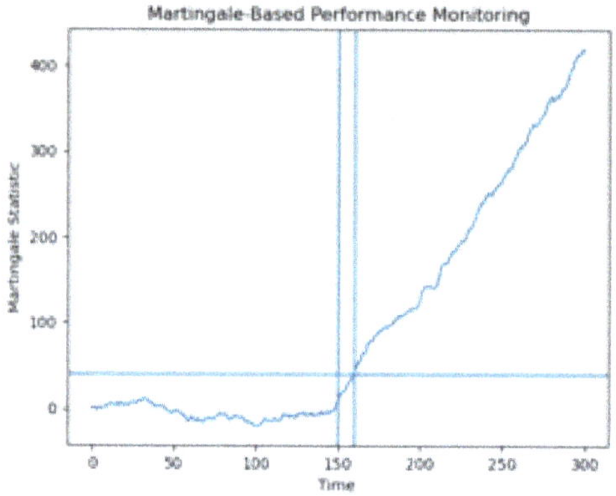

The monitoring statistic remains stable under normal conditions and increases after the change-point, triggering intervention.

The simulation study illustrates the operational behavior of the monitoring approach under simplified stochastic conditions:

- Demonstrates the potential to detect structural changes in healthcare system dynamics
- Produces relatively short detection delays under the simulated scenario
- Exhibits predictable behavior under different threshold settings
- Maintains moderate false alarm behavior within the simulated environment
- Performs consistently across repeated simulations

Overall, the simulation results suggest the potential operational relevance of martingale-based monitoring for adaptive healthcare environments.

Practical Interpretation of Simulation Results

The simulation results provide important insights into how the proposed monitoring framework would behave in real-world healthcare environments. While the numerical results demonstrate detection performance under controlled conditions, their practical implications must be interpreted in an operational context.

In real healthcare systems, variability in patient arrivals is influenced by multiple external factors such as seasonal trends, epidemics, and policy changes. The observed detection delay of approximately 12 time units suggests that the system may support identification of significant deviations within a short operational window. In an emergency department setting, this could correspond to early detection of congestion within a few hours, enabling timely intervention.

The variability observed in Monte Carlo simulations highlights the inherent uncertainty in stochastic systems. While the average performance is stable, individual realizations may differ due to random fluctuations. This reinforces the importance of designing monitoring systems that are robust to variability and capable of maintaining consistent performance across different scenarios.

From an operational perspective, the false alarm rate of 0.125 can be interpreted as a manageable level of sensitivity. In critical healthcare settings, it is often preferable to tolerate a moderate level of false alarms in exchange for early detection of system stress. However, excessive false alarms may lead to resource inefficiencies, and therefore threshold calibration remains an essential component of system design.

Overall, the simulation results suggest potential operational relevance under simulated stochastic conditions, providing useful insights for healthcare system monitoring and decision-making.

Although the simulation study is based on simplified stochastic assumptions, the results demonstrate the operational feasibility of the proposed monitoring framework under controlled conditions. Future research should validate the approach using real-world healthcare datasets and more complex operational environments involving non-stationary patient arrivals, multiple interacting resources, and heterogeneous healthcare processes.

Operational Significance of the Simulation Findings

The simulation results demonstrate how sequential stochastic monitoring can support operational decision-making under uncertain healthcare conditions. Although the experiments were conducted using a simplified Poisson arrival process, they illustrate the general capability of martingale-based monitoring to identify structural changes in healthcare demand before such changes lead to severe operational disruption. This early identification is particularly valuable in healthcare environments where timely intervention may reduce overcrowding, improve patient flow, and support more efficient resource utilization.

From an operational perspective, the Average Run Length (ARL) analysis provides useful guidance for selecting monitoring thresholds according to institutional priorities. Healthcare organizations with limited surge capacity may prefer lower thresholds to maximize responsiveness and enable earlier intervention during rapidly evolving situations. Conversely, organizations seeking to minimize unnecessary operational disruptions may adopt higher thresholds that reduce false alarms while accepting a modest increase in detection delay. Consequently, threshold selection should be viewed as a management decision that reflects the balance between operational sensitivity and system stability rather than as a purely statistical parameter.

The Monte Carlo experiments further demonstrate that repeated simulation provides a more reliable assessment of monitoring performance than a single realization. Because healthcare systems operate under substantial stochastic variability, monitoring procedures should be evaluated across numerous simulated scenarios to ensure consistent behaviour under different operational conditions. Such robustness assessments increase confidence that the monitoring framework will maintain acceptable performance despite random fluctuations in patient arrivals and healthcare demand.

The computational requirements of the proposed monitoring framework are relatively modest because the monitoring statistic is updated sequentially as each new observation becomes available. This characteristic makes the approach suitable for integration with modern hospital information systems and real-time decision-support platforms, where continuous updating and rapid response are essential. As healthcare institutions increasingly adopt digital health technologies, cloud-based analytics, and electronic health record systems, lightweight sequential monitoring algorithms may become practical components of routine operational management.

It should also be recognised that the present simulation represents an illustrative proof-of-concept rather than a comprehensive validation study. Real healthcare systems frequently exhibit non-homogeneous arrival patterns, seasonal variation, patient heterogeneity, and interactions among multiple operational resources. Future simulation studies should therefore incorporate more realistic stochastic models, multiple change-points, and richer operational scenarios to further evaluate the scalability and robustness of the proposed monitoring framework.

APPLICATION: EMERGENCY DEPARTMENT CONGESTION MONITORING

The proposed monitoring framework can be interpreted within the context of emergency department (ED) operations, where sudden increases in patient arrivals frequently lead to congestion, prolonged waiting times, resource shortages, and increased operational stress. Early identification of such changes is essential for maintaining service quality and ensuring timely patient care.

To illustrate the practical application of the proposed framework, the simulated healthcare arrival process is interpreted as an emergency department experiencing a sudden increase in patient demand. Under the simulated operating conditions, a structural increase in arrival intensity produces a detectable change in the martingale monitoring statistic, enabling timely identification of emerging congestion.

Table 7. Emergency Department Monitoring Results

Metric	Value
Detection Time (τ)	162
Detection Delay ($\tau - \theta$)	12
Average Detection Delay	12.585
Standard Deviation	16.85
False Alarm Rate	0.125

The monitoring results indicate that the proposed framework is capable of identifying operational changes within a relatively short period following the onset of increased patient demand. Although the analysis is based on simulated stochastic conditions, the results demonstrate the potential applicability of martingale-based monitoring for supporting timely operational decision-making in emergency healthcare environments.

Monitoring Behavior

Under normal operating conditions, the martingale monitoring statistic remains relatively stable around its expected level. Following the structural increase in patient arrivals, the monitoring statistic exhibits a sustained upward drift that ultimately exceeds the predefined threshold, thereby triggering intervention. This behavior is consistent with the theoretical properties established earlier and illustrates the ability of the monitoring framework to distinguish routine operational variability from meaningful changes requiring attention.

Figure 2. Martingale-Based Monitoring Process for Simulated Emergency Department Congestion

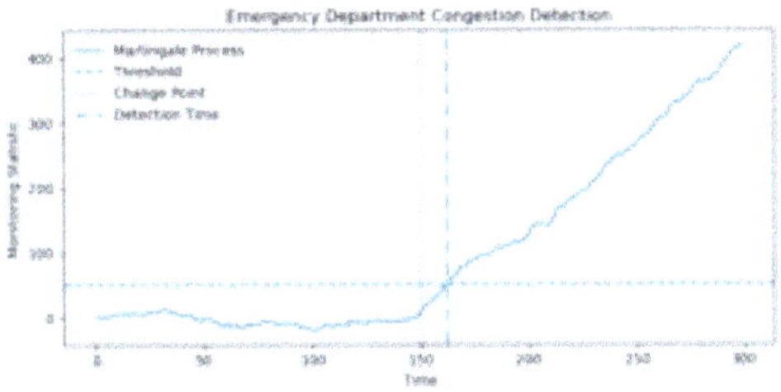

The martingale monitoring statistic remains stable prior to the change-point ($\theta = 150$) and exhibits a sustained upward drift afterward. The threshold crossing at ($\tau = 162$) indicates successful detection of congestion.

Operational Implications

The implementation of martingale-based monitoring in emergency departments offers several practical advantages:

- Early detection of congestion, enabling timely intervention
- Dynamic staffing adjustments, including deployment of additional medical personnel
- Activation of surge capacity protocols, such as temporary expansion of treatment areas
- Improved patient flow management, reducing waiting times and overcrowding

Collectively, these operational capabilities demonstrate how sequential stochastic monitoring may assist healthcare administrators in responding proactively to emerging congestion while supporting efficient resource utilization and maintaining quality of patient care.

Broader Applications in Healthcare Operations

Although the present case study focuses on emergency department congestion, the proposed martingale-based monitoring framework has considerably broader applicability across healthcare operations. Many hospital management problems involve continuously evolving stochastic processes in which timely detection of operational changes is essential for maintaining service quality and efficient resource utilization. Consequently, the sequential monitoring strategy developed in this chapter can be adapted to several other healthcare environments without substantial modification of its underlying probabilistic principles.

One important application is hospital bed occupancy management. Hospitals frequently experience fluctuations in bed availability due to variations in patient admissions, discharge rates, and seasonal disease patterns. Continuous monitoring of occupancy levels using martingale-based methods may assist administrators in identifying emerging capacity constraints before critical shortages occur. Early detection allows hospitals to initiate appropriate interventions, including discharge planning, redistribution of patients across clinical units, or temporary expansion of available capacity.

Another important application involves intensive care unit (ICU) resource management, where demand for specialized beds and critical care equipment often changes rapidly. Sequential monitoring techniques may provide early statistical evidence of increasing utilization, enabling healthcare managers to coordinate staffing, equipment allocation, and patient transfers before operational stress reaches critical levels. Such proactive decision-making may contribute to improved continuity of care and more efficient utilization of limited critical care resources.

The proposed monitoring framework may also support ambulance services and emergency medical response systems. Emergency call volumes frequently exhibit substantial temporal variation caused by traffic accidents, infectious disease outbreaks, extreme weather conditions, and mass gathering events. Real-time monitoring of incoming emergency requests may assist emergency service coordinators in reallocating ambulance resources dynamically while maintaining acceptable response times.

In addition, remote patient monitoring has become increasingly important with the widespread adoption of wearable medical devices, telemedicine platforms, and Internet of Medical Things (IoMT) technologies. Continuous physiological measurements such as heart rate, blood pressure, blood glucose levels, and oxygen saturation generate sequential data streams that require ongoing statistical evaluation. Martingale-based monitoring provides a mathematically rigorous framework for distinguishing clinically meaningful physiological changes from routine biological variability, thereby supporting timely clinical intervention while reducing unnecessary alarms.

These examples illustrate that the framework presented in this chapter is not restricted to emergency department congestion but represents a general stochastic monitoring strategy applicable to diverse healthcare operational settings. The flexibility of the approach provides opportunities for future adaptation to integrated hospital management systems, regional healthcare networks, and intelligent clinical decision-support platforms operating under continuously evolving conditions.

Practical Considerations

Although the simulation study demonstrates encouraging performance under controlled stochastic conditions, several practical considerations should be addressed before implementation in real healthcare environments. The accuracy of the monitoring system depends on the correct estimation of baseline parameters, which may vary across different healthcare environments. Inaccurate parameter estimation could lead to either delayed detection or increased false alarm rates.

Moreover, the implementation of real-time monitoring systems requires appropriate technological infrastructure, including data collection systems and computational resources. Ensuring seamless integration with existing hospital information systems is essential for practical deployment.

Finally, human factors play a crucial role in the success of such systems. Healthcare professionals must trust and understand the monitoring outputs to effectively act upon them. Therefore, user-friendly interfaces and clear interpretation guidelines are necessary to facilitate adoption.

Although this application focuses on emergency department congestion, the proposed monitoring framework is sufficiently flexible to support a broad range of healthcare operational problems, including hospital bed occupancy management, demand surge detection, intensive care resource monitoring, and dynamic healthcare resource allocation. Future research should investigate these applications using real-world healthcare data and more complex operational environments to further evaluate the practical effectiveness of the proposed framework.

ETHICAL, GOVERNANCE, AND AI INTEGRATION CONSIDERATIONS

The increasing adoption of data-driven and stochastic decision frameworks in healthcare systems brings not only technical advantages but also important ethical and governance responsibilities. While martingale-based monitoring and stopping-time–based intervention provide powerful tools for real-time system management, their implementation must be carefully aligned with principles of fairness, transparency, and patient safety. Healthcare decisions are inherently sensitive, and any automated or semi-automated system must ensure that statistical efficiency does not come at the cost of ethical integrity.

Ethical Considerations

One of the primary ethical challenges in probabilistic monitoring systems is the presence of uncertainty. Decisions are made based on statistical signals rather than deterministic outcomes, which introduces the possibility of both delayed detection and premature intervention. In a healthcare setting, such outcomes may affect patient care quality and operational stability.

False alarms, although statistically expected, may lead to unnecessary deployment of resources, increased workload for healthcare staff, and potential disruption of routine services. On the other hand, delayed detection of system stress can result in overcrowding and compromised patient outcomes. Therefore, the design of monitoring systems must carefully balance sensitivity and reliability.

Equity is another critical consideration. Healthcare systems serve diverse populations, and variations in patient characteristics can influence observed system behavior. If not properly accounted for, monitoring frameworks may inadvertently introduce bias by reacting differently to variations that are not related to system performance. Incorporating risk-adjusted measures and contextual information is essential to ensure fair and unbiased decision-making.

Governance and Accountability

The deployment of stochastic monitoring systems in healthcare requires clear governance structures. Decision-makers must understand how monitoring signals are generated and how intervention rules are applied. Unlike black-box models, martingale-based approaches offer a degree of transparency, as they are grounded in well-defined probabilistic principles.

However, transparency alone is not sufficient. Accountability must also be clearly defined. Questions such as who is responsible for triggering interventions, how incorrect decisions are handled, and how system performance is evaluated must be addressed through institutional policies.

Data governance is equally important. Real-time monitoring relies on continuous data collection, often involving sensitive patient information. Ensuring data privacy, secure storage, and ethical usage is essential. Compliance with applicable healthcare data protection regulations, institutional governance policies, ethical standards, and clinical safety requirements should form an integral component of any operational monitoring framework.

Integration with Artificial Intelligence Systems

Artificial intelligence (AI) is increasingly being used in healthcare for predictive analytics and decision support. Advances in machine learning and data-driven modeling have enabled more accurate prediction of patient outcomes and system behavior (Obermeyer & Emanuel, 2016). Many contemporary AI models, particularly deep learning approaches, may present challenges in interpretability despite demonstrating strong predictive performance. In contrast, martingale-based monitoring provides a probabilistically interpretable framework for identifying deviations from expected system behavior.

Recent studies have highlighted the growing role of AI-driven monitoring systems in supporting clinical decision-making, remote patient monitoring, and adaptive healthcare operations (Sendak, 2019; Sendak et al., 2020; Topol, 2019). The integration of stochastic monitoring with AI systems offers a promising direction. Martingale-based methods can serve as a validation layer for AI predictions, helping to detect model drift and unexpected system behavior. This aligns with recent perspectives emphasizing the need for human-centered and interpretable AI in healthcare systems (Topol, 2019).

At the same time, integrating AI with stochastic frameworks introduces challenges. These include increased model complexity, computational requirements, and the need for interpretability. Ensuring that combined systems remain transparent and clinically acceptable is essential for successful adoption.

Explainable Artificial Intelligence and Trustworthy Healthcare Analytics

As artificial intelligence becomes increasingly integrated into healthcare systems, the importance of explainability and trustworthiness has gained considerable attention among researchers, clinicians, and policymakers. While machine learning algorithms can achieve high predictive accuracy, healthcare professionals often require transparent explanations before incorporating algorithmic recommendations into clinical or operational decision-making. This need is particularly important in safety-critical healthcare environments, where decisions may directly influence patient outcomes, resource allocation, and organizational performance.

Martingale-based monitoring offers an important advantage in this context because its statistical foundations are explicit and mathematically interpretable. Rather than relying solely on complex predictive models, sequential monitoring provides probabilistic evidence that can be understood and evaluated by healthcare practitioners. This transparency facilitates greater confidence in monitoring results and supports collaborative decision-making between automated analytical systems and human experts.

The concept of trustworthy artificial intelligence extends beyond predictive performance and includes principles such as fairness, transparency, accountability, robustness, privacy protection, and human oversight. Healthcare monitoring systems should therefore be designed to ensure that statistical alerts are generated consistently across different patient populations while minimizing unintended bias or discrimination. In addition, monitoring algorithms should be regularly evaluated to detect model drift, changes in data quality, or evolving operational conditions that may reduce their reliability over time.

Human oversight remains essential even when sophisticated monitoring technologies are available. Statistical monitoring systems should function as decision-support tools rather than autonomous decision-makers, enabling clinicians and healthcare administrators to combine quantitative evidence with professional judgement and contextual knowledge. Such human-in-the-loop approaches promote responsible implementation while maintaining clinical accountability for operational decisions.

The integration of statistically rigorous monitoring methods with explainable and trustworthy artificial intelligence represents a promising direction for future adaptive healthcare systems. Combining transparent stochastic monitoring with modern predictive analytics may improve both operational efficiency and confidence in automated decision-support technologies while ensuring that healthcare management remains patient-centred, ethically responsible, and scientifically robust.

Policy Implications

The adoption of advanced monitoring frameworks in healthcare systems has broader policy implications. There is a need for standardized guidelines on the use of probabilistic decision-making tools in healthcare operations. Training healthcare professionals to understand and interpret statistical monitoring outputs is equally important.

Policymakers must also ensure that such systems are implemented in a way that promotes equity and accessibility. The benefits of advanced analytical tools should not be limited to well-resourced institutions but should be extended across different healthcare settings.

The successful implementation of stochastic monitoring systems will require collaboration among clinicians, healthcare administrators, statisticians, computer scientists, and policymakers to ensure responsible deployment.

Future Directions

Future developments in adaptive healthcare systems are likely to involve deeper integration of real-time data, stochastic modeling, and artificial intelligence. Future research should also focus on refining threshold selection methods, improving robustness under highly variable conditions, incorporating patient-level heterogeneity, and validating the proposed framework using real-world healthcare datasets and prospective operational studies.

The deployment of AI-based healthcare monitoring systems also requires careful consideration of fairness, transparency, accountability, and clinical trustworthiness in real-world healthcare environments (Lekadir et al., 2025). Validation using real-world healthcare datasets and prospective operational studies represents an important next step toward clinical implementation.

Future advances in adaptive healthcare monitoring will depend not only on methodological innovation but also on responsible implementation that integrates ethical governance, transparent artificial intelligence, and statistically rigorous decision-support frameworks.

CONCLUSION

This chapter examined the operational interpretation of martingale-based sequential monitoring within adaptive healthcare systems. The monitoring approach illustrates how stochastic process concepts may be interpreted within healthcare operational environments characterized by uncertainty and streaming information.

Theoretical foundations were developed using stochastic process theory, highlighting the role of martingales in modeling deviations from expected system behavior and stopping times in enabling real-time decision-making. The simulation study illustrated the operational behavior of the monitoring process under controlled stochastic conditions. The application to emergency department congestion monitoring further illustrated the practical relevance of the monitoring strategy. The simulation results suggest that the monitoring approach may support earlier recognition of operational stress conditions.

In addition to methodological contributions, the chapter emphasized the importance of ethical considerations, governance structures, and integration with emerging technologies such as artificial intelligence. Ensuring transparency, fairness, and accountability remains essential when deploying data-driven decision systems in healthcare environments.

Although the proposed framework demonstrates encouraging performance under simulated stochastic conditions, several limitations should be acknowledged. The simulation study is based on simplified assumptions, including Poisson arrival processes and constant baseline parameters, whereas real healthcare systems frequently exhibit non-stationary demand, correlated patient arrivals, and multiple interacting operational resources. Furthermore, the framework currently focuses primarily on patient arrivals, while practical healthcare environments require simultaneous consideration of staffing levels, service times, bed occupancy, and patient prioritization. Successful implementation will therefore depend not only on mathematical modelling but also on appropriate technological infrastructure, reliable data collection, organisational readiness, and continuous model calibration.

Future research should focus on extending the framework to multidimensional healthcare systems, incorporating patient-level heterogeneity, adaptive parameter estimation, and integration with real-world healthcare data streams. Validation using operational hospital datasets and prospective healthcare studies will further strengthen the practical applicability of the proposed monitoring framework. Additional opportunities include multi-hospital resource coordination, AI-assisted operational decision support, and scalable healthcare monitoring architectures capable of supporting regional and national healthcare systems.

Overall, this chapter demonstrates how established martingale-based sequential monitoring and stopping-time principles can be interpreted within adaptive healthcare operations to support timely detection of operational change under uncertainty. Rather than proposing a new stochastic monitoring methodology, the chapter provides a healthcare-oriented operational perspective that connects probabilistic monitoring with contemporary healthcare analytics and decision support. As healthcare systems continue to evolve toward data-driven and AI-assisted environments, statistically rigorous, transparent, and ethically governed monitoring frameworks have the potential to contribute to more resilient, responsive, and efficient healthcare operations.

Finally, the framework presented in this chapter highlights the importance of integrating rigorous statistical methodology with practical healthcare management. As healthcare systems continue to evolve toward intelligent, data-driven operational environments, sequential stochastic monitoring has the potential to support timely interventions, efficient resource utilization, and evidence-based decision-making across diverse clinical settings. Continued collaboration among statisticians, healthcare professionals, computer scientists, and policymakers will be essential for translating these theoretical developments into practical healthcare solutions that improve both operational performance and patient care.

AI DISCLOSURE STATEMENT

Portions of this manuscript were refined using ChatGPT (OpenAI) to assist with language editing, manuscript organization, and improvement of academic writing. The AI tool was used solely to enhance clarity, grammar, formatting, and editorial presentation. All theoretical development, mathematical formulations, simulation design, interpretation of results, literature selection, and scientific conclusions were independently developed, verified, and approved by the author. The author accepts full responsibility for the accuracy, originality, and integrity of the content presented in this chapter.

REFERENCES

Aceto, G., Persico, V., & Pescapé, A. (2020). The role of information and communication technologies in healthcare: Taxonomies, perspectives, and challenges. *Journal of Network and Computer Applications, 107*, 125–154.

Basseville, M., & Nikiforov, I. V. (1993). *Detection of abrupt changes: Theory and application.* Prentice Hall.

Briggs, A., & Sculpher, M. (1998). An introduction to Markov modelling for economic evaluation. *PharmacoEconomics, 13*(4), 397–409. PMID: 10178664

Doob, J. L. (1953). *Stochastic processes.* Wiley.

Green, L. V. (2006). Queueing analysis in healthcare. In Hall, R. (Ed.), *Patient flow: Reducing delay in healthcare delivery* (pp. 281–307). Springer.

Hall, R. (2013). *Patient flow: Reducing delay in healthcare delivery* (2nd ed.). Springer.

Izady, N., & Worthington, D. (2012). Setting staffing requirements for time-dependent queueing networks. *European Journal of Operational Research, 219*(3), 531–540.

Javaid, M., Haleem, A., Singh, R. P., Suman, R., & Rab, S. (2022). Significance of machine learning in healthcare: Features, pillars and applications. *Intelligent Pharmacy, 1*(1), 58–73. DOI: 10.1016/j.ipha.2022.04.001

Lai, T. L. (2001). Sequential analysis: Some classical problems and new challenges. *Statistica Sinica, 11*(2), 303–408.

Lekadir, K., Frangi, A. F., Porras, A. R., Glocker, B., Cintas, C., & Langlotz, C. P.. (2025). FUTURE-AI: International consensus guideline for trustworthy and deployable artificial intelligence in healthcare. *BMJ (Clinical Research Ed.), 388*, e081554. DOI: 10.1136/bmj-2024-081554 PMID: 39909534

Mohammed, M. A., Worthington, P., & Woodall, W. H. (2001). Plotting basic control charts: Tutorial notes for healthcare practitioners. *Journal of Quality in Clinical Practice, 21*(1), 14–19.

Moustakides, G. V. (1986). Optimal stopping times for detecting changes in distributions. *Annals of Statistics, 14*(4), 1379–1387.

Obermeyer, Z., & Emanuel, E. J. (2016). Predicting the future—Big data, machine learning, and clinical medicine. *The New England Journal of Medicine, 375*(13), 1216–1219. PMID: 27682033

Page, E. S. (1954). Continuous inspection schemes. *Biometrika, 41*(1–2), 100–115. DOI: 10.1093/biomet/41.1-2.100

Ristevski, B., & Chen, M. (2018). Big data analytics in medicine and healthcare. *Journal of Integrative Bioinformatics, 15*(3), 20170030. DOI: 10.1515/jib-2017-0030 PMID: 29746254

Ross, S. M. (2014). *Introduction to probability models* (11th ed.). Academic Press.

Sendak, M. P. (2019). Machine learning in health care: A critical appraisal of challenges and opportunities. *EGEMS (Washington, DC)*, *7*(1), 1. DOI: 10.5334/egems.287 PMID: 30705919

Sendak, M. P., D'Arcy, J., Kashyap, S., Gao, M., Nichols, M., Corey, K., & Ratliff, W. (2020). A path for translation of machine learning products into healthcare delivery. *EMJ Innovations*, *4*(1), 19–25.

Shafer, G., Shen, A., Vereshchagin, N., & Vovk, V. (2011). Test martingales, Bayes factors and p-values. *Statistical Science*, *26*(1), 84–101.

Shaik, T., Tao, X., Higgins, N., Li, L., Gururajan, R., & Zhou, X.. (2023). Remote Patient Monitoring Using Artificial Intelligence: Current State, Applications, and Challenges. *Wiley Interdisciplinary Reviews. Data Mining and Knowledge Discovery*, *13*, e1485. DOI: 10.1002/widm.1485

Shiryaev, A. N. (2007). *Optimal stopping rules*. Springer.

Steiner, S. H., Cook, R. J., Farewell, V. T., & Treasure, T. (2000). Monitoring surgical performance using risk-adjusted CUSUM charts. *Biostatistics (Oxford, England)*, *1*(4), 441–452. PMID: 12933566

Topol, E. (2019). *Deep medicine: How artificial intelligence can make healthcare human again*. Basic Books.

Williams, D. (1991). *Probability with martingales*. Cambridge University Press.

Woodall, W. H. (2006). The use of control charts in healthcare and public-health surveillance. *Journal of Quality Technology*, *38*(2), 89–104.

Chapter 8
Potential Theory and Hitting Probabilities:
Measuring Access, Equity, and Risk

Deepak Gupta
http://orcid.org/0000-0003-3929-1362
Institute of Technology and Management, Gwalior, India

Khaydarov Ural
Tashkent State University of Economics, Uzbekistan

Jurayeva Nodirakhan
Fergana State University, Uzbekistan

Ulugbek Vosikov
Kimyo International University in Tashkent, Uzbekistan

Kasimova Fatima
Tashkent Institute of Chemical Technology, Uzbekistan

Khurramov Ramazon
Termez University of Economics and Service, Uzbekistan

Egamberdiyev Farmankul
Alfraganus University, Tashkent, Uzbekistan

ABSTRACT

Stochastic processes rooted in potential theory provide a rigorous mathematical language for quantifying healthcare access, measuring equity, and assessing systemic risk in complex environments. This chapter develops hitting probabilities and first-passage time theory within adaptive healthcare systems. Beginning with Brownian motion and harmonic functions, it advances through diffusion models, Markov decision processes, epidemic random walks, and Lévy jump-diffusion frameworks. Each construct is linked to healthcare scenarios including patient trajectory modelling, epidemic boundary crossing, treatment optimisation, and resource allocation under uncertainty. Attention is given to how probabilistic boundaries encode structural inequities between rural and urban populations. Mathematical derivations are supported by figures, a graph, and a comparative table to provide a unified stochastic toolkit for planning.

DOI: 10.4018/979-8-3373-9705-4.ch008

INTRODUCTION

The organisation of healthcare delivery is not, at its core, an administrative challenge alone. It is a probabilistic one. Patients traverse networks of care whose reliability is never fully assured; diagnostic thresholds are crossed at moments that resist deterministic prediction; disease propagates through communities with dynamics that defy simple compartmental accounting; clinical decisions must be reached under conditions of genuine, sometimes irreducible uncertainty. The mathematical substrate beneath all of this is the theory of stochastic processes and, more precisely, the classical machinery of potential theory and hitting probabilities.

Potential theory first emerged from problems in electrostatics and gravitational physics. The harmonic functions satisfying Laplace's equation and the Green functions associated with elliptic differential operators were examined throughout the nineteenth century as instruments for understanding equilibrium fields. Their absorption into probability theory, accomplished principally through the contributions of Shizuo Kakutani and Joseph Doob during the 1940s and 1950s, revealed a structural equivalence that was genuinely surprising at the time: the value of a harmonic function at an interior point equals the expected value of its boundary data at the first location where a Brownian path exits the domain. This single observation transformed the Dirichlet problem from a purely analytical exercise into a probabilistic computation, opening a productive avenue for finding hitting probabilities through the apparatus of classical analysis.

In the language of healthcare planning, this equivalence is not merely elegant but practically consequential. The probability that a stochastic health process, starting from an initial condition representing a patient's current clinical status or geographic position, reaches a prescribed set before deteriorating beyond recovery is precisely a hitting probability in the sense of potential theory. When the target set represents a functioning healthcare facility, a treatment response threshold, or an epidemic containment boundary, the hitting probability becomes a direct measure of access, clinical effectiveness, or public health resilience. The framework thus gives mathematical content to concepts that policymakers routinely use in qualitative terms, and makes them computable from observable data (Lefebvre, 2024; Mazzolo, 2024).

Three interrelated dimensions of healthcare system performance are addressed in this chapter. Access is understood as the probability that a patient whose health state follows a stochastic trajectory reaches an adequate level of care before irreversible deterioration occurs. Equity concerns the systematic variation in this probability across population subgroups defined by geography, income, or available infrastructure. The rural patient with limited transport connections and the urban patient near a tertiary hospital face fundamentally different hitting probability distributions, even when their initial clinical profiles are identical. Risk encompasses the tail events of the healthcare system: rare but catastrophic failures, epidemic boundary crossings in which infectious incidence overwhelms hospital capacity, and the financial ruin of insurance structures exposed to stochastic cost pressures that occasionally spike far beyond actuarial baselines.

The chapter proceeds through a structured sequence of mathematical developments and applications. The discussion of potential-theoretic foundations reviews harmonic functions, Dirichlet problems, Green functions, and the probabilistic interpretation of hitting probabilities. First-passage time theory for diffusion processes follows, covering integrated Brownian motion and active particle models relevant to patient flow. These ideas connect to epidemic modeling via random walks and SIR frameworks with stochastic components. Markov decision processes and optimal stopping are then treated as tools for treatment sequencing and resource allocation. Levy jump-diffusion processes and stochastic delay differential equations follow, with applications to pandemic preparedness and fractional-order epidemic models. The equity dimension is synthesised by showing how geometric inequalities in the state space encode real-world disparities. A comparative application table and two worked examples are provided. Policy implications and future research priorities are identified before the chapter concludes.

FOUNDATIONS OF POTENTIAL THEORY FOR STOCHASTIC PROCESSES

Classical Potential Theory and Harmonic Functions

Potential theory in its classical formulation studies functions satisfying Laplace's equation in an open domain subject to prescribed boundary data. Functions satisfying this equation are called harmonic; they arise as steady-state solutions to diffusion equations and, through Kakutani's probabilistic representation, as expected values of functionals of Brownian motion. Formally, let {X(t), t >= 0} denote a standard d-dimensional Brownian motion initiated at X(0) = x in the domain. The first exit time from the domain is defined as the infimum of all times at which the process leaves the domain. For a continuous boundary function f on the boundary, the Dirichlet problem has the probabilistic solution u(x) = E_x[f(X(exit time))], where E_x denotes expectation under the Brownian motion started at x. This representation transforms abstract boundary value problems into expectations of observable random quantities, providing a computational and interpretive bridge between harmonic analysis and stochastic processes.

In healthcare terms, u(x) gives the expected outcome for a patient whose current health vector is x, where the domain encodes the set of states from which recovery remains achievable. The boundary is the clinical frontier at which the patient either enters stable recovery or deteriorates past the point of intervention. Harmonic functions integrate over the full distribution of stochastic health trajectories, weighting each path by its probability and returning an aggregate outcome expectation at the starting point. This averaging over trajectories is precisely what makes the Dirichlet framework suited to health-care planning: it accounts honestly for the variability inherent in biological systems and care delivery networks, rather than privileging any single trajectory.

The Harnack inequality, a foundational result in potential theory, establishes that harmonic functions cannot oscillate arbitrarily within a domain. If u is harmonic and non-negative on a domain, then for any compact interior subdomain K, there exists a constant C depending only on K and the domain such that the maximum of u over K is bounded by C times the minimum of u over K. In healthcare terms, this means that access probabilities cannot vary without bound within a geographically cohesive service area: nearby population groups must have hitting probabilities within a multiplicative constant of each other. Where empirical health geography data reveal larger variation than the Harnack constant permits, the finding signals that structural discontinuities such as rivers, administrative boundaries, or infrastructure gaps are generating genuine breaks in the access landscape that require domain decomposition or multi-scale modeling strategies.

Green Functions and Equilibrium Measures

The Green function G(x, y) of a domain under the Laplacian encodes the expected total time that a Brownian motion started at x spends in an infinitesimal neighbourhood of y before exiting the domain. It is symmetric, satisfies the distributional equation with a point source at x, and vanishes on the boundary.

These properties make the Green function both a fundamental solution to the Laplace equation and a probabilistic sojourn time density, bridging two distinct mathematical traditions within a single object.

From a healthcare analytics perspective, $G(x, y_c)$ for a critical disease state y_c carries a direct operational reading: a large value indicates that a patient-process starting from x will spend substantial expected time in the vicinity of y_c before the process terminates. In oncology, y_c might represent a tumour burden above the threshold for intensive intervention; in epidemic management, it might represent a prevalence level at which contact tracing capacity becomes computationally infeasible. Elevated Green-function values near these critical states identify populations or configurations that are chronically near-threshold, warranting proactive rather than reactive resource deployment.

The equilibrium measure of a Borel set A within the domain is the unique measure that minimises an energy functional subject to unit total mass, and its total mass defines the Newtonian capacity of A. This capacity is a scale-invariant measure of how probabilistically accessible A is from the ambient domain. In epidemic modeling, the capacity of the infected region in the state space of a stochastic SIR model determines the probability that the system, starting from low prevalence, ever enters major epidemic spread. Estimating this capacity from surveillance data gives public health authorities a quantitative early warning index directly calibrated to the underlying stochastic dynamics of the outbreak under study.

The Dirichlet Problem in Healthcare State Spaces

Let the state space represent a compact, bounded subset of multi-dimensional Euclidean space encoding the health state of a population, for instance three dimensions for the susceptible, infected, and recovered compartments of an epidemic model, or two dimensions for a patient's vital signs and primary biomarker. A healthcare system seeks to keep the state vector within the viable zone, while stochastic dynamics exert pressure toward the boundary. The boundary decomposes into a recovery portion, encoding states of clinical improvement, and a crisis portion, encoding states of irreversible deterioration or epidemic overshoot.

The hitting probability $u(x)$ equals the probability that the process, starting at x, exits through the recovery portion of the boundary rather than the crisis portion. This function is harmonic in the interior, equals one on the recovery boundary, and equals zero on the crisis boundary. Geographic and demographic covariates enter either by parameterising the geometry of the domain or the drift of the health process: populations with access to preventive care have drift directed away from the crisis boundary, while remote populations may have drift directed toward it. This structure makes hitting probability analysis inherently suited to covariate-stratified equity assessment, which is among its principal advantages over aggregate compartmental models. Figure 1, illustrate harmonic functions satisfying the Dirichlet problem define hitting probabilities at each state in the health domain; Green functions summarise expected sojourn times near critical thresholds; and equilibrium capacity measures provide a scalar index of overall network accessibility.

Figure 1. Conceptual framework illustrating how potential theory maps onto healthcare system analysis.

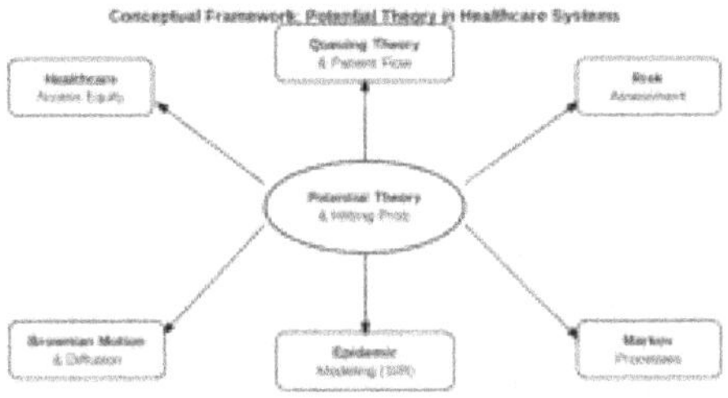

FIRST-PASSAGE TIME THEORY FOR DIFFUSION PROCESSES

Standard Brownian Motion and First-Passage Distributions

The first-passage time of a stochastic process to a threshold B is defined as the first time the process enters B. For a one-dimensional Brownian motion with drift and diffusion coefficient, starting in the interior of an interval, the passage to the absorbing boundary follows the inverse Gaussian law. The mean first-passage time equals the distance to the boundary divided by the drift, when drift is positive, and is infinite when drift is non-positive, reflecting the fact that a driftless or negatively-drifting process may never reach the upper boundary. Mazzolo (2024) has demonstrated that under non-standard initial conditions and curved boundary geometries, the first-passage distribution acquires unexpected closed-form representations whose structure illuminates the interplay between initial state and boundary geometry in ways that standard asymptotic theory does not anticipate, with direct relevance for healthcare pathway modeling.

Translating these results into clinical terms requires identifying the absorbing boundary with a critical health threshold such as a biomarker value beyond which clinical intervention is mandatory, or an epidemic prevalence above which contact tracing capacity is saturated. The drift encodes treatment efficacy: negative drift, directed away from the threshold, corresponds to effective therapy, while positive drift signals progressive disease despite treatment. The diffusion coefficient captures biological variability, the intrinsic unpredictability of individual disease trajectories that no clinical expertise can eliminate. The mean first-passage time then quantifies the expected time before the patient's condition crosses the critical threshold under the current care regime. For planning purposes, both the mean and the tail of this distribution carry weight: a treatment achieving a long average crossing time but a heavy tail may still expose a significant fraction of patients to crisis before intervention is possible.

An important but sometimes neglected aspect of this framework is the role of reflecting boundaries in healthcare models. In many contexts, a patient who improves to full health does not simply exit the system; they re-enter at some baseline state and face the same stochastic dynamics again. This re-entry structure corresponds to a reflecting boundary at the healthy end of the state space and gives rise to the theory of ergodic diffusions, where the steady-state distribution over health states rather than the first-passage time becomes the relevant long-run quantity. For chronic disease management, the steady-state distribution under different treatment regimes provides a more appropriate performance metric than the first-passage time to a crisis threshold, and its computation draws on the same potential-theoretic tools through the adjoint of the Fokker-Planck equation.

Integrated Diffusion Processes and Active Brownian Particles

Many clinical measurements track cumulative quantities rather than instantaneous states. Radiation dose is accumulated across fractionated treatments, drug plasma levels are smoothed by pharmacokinetic dynamics, and biomarker indices such as the area under the glucose curve in diabetes management are explicitly time-integrated quantities. Lefebvre (2024) studies the first-passage-place problem for integrated diffusion processes: when a process is defined as the time integral of an underlying diffusion, what is the distribution of the integrated quantity at the moment the joint pair first exits a prescribed region? The added mathematical complexity relative to the standard first-passage problem arises because the integrated process is not itself Markovian, and Lefebvre's contribution is to identify the backward equation governing the joint exit distribution and characterise closed-form solutions for special parameter regimes, providing a direct toolkit for cumulative-dose toxicity risk modeling in radiation oncology.

Iyaniwura and Peng (2024) examine the mean first-passage time for active Brownian particles in one-dimensional geometries through asymptotic analysis and simulation. Active Brownian particles self-propel in a direction that evolves under its own rotational diffusion, coupling translational and orientational degrees of freedom. This model describes neutrophil chemotaxis toward bacterial foci, T-cell migration through lymph node tissue, and macrophage recruitment to sites of chronic inflammation. The central finding is that the mean first-passage time depends non-monotonically on the Peclet number, which characterises the ratio of advective to diffusive transport. At intermediate Peclet numbers, self-propulsion reduces the mean first-passage time relative to passive diffusion. At very high Peclet numbers, strong directionality causes particles initially oriented away from the target to take long indirect routes, increasing the mean first-passage time. This non-monotonicity has therapeutic implications: increasing the speed of immune-cell recruitment is not unconditionally beneficial, and the optimal propulsion speed depends on geometric features of the tissue domain that may vary across patients and disease stages.

Application: Patient Access as a First-Passage Problem

A natural formalisation of geographic healthcare access treats the patient's effective proximity to care as a one-dimensional diffusion process on an interval, where one end represents full access to tertiary care and the other end represents complete absence of specialised infrastructure. The process evolves under a drift directed toward access, reflecting the combined effect of infrastructure investment and patient navigation programs, superimposed on Brownian fluctuations representing variability due to road closures, provider absences, and seasonal disruptions. The absorbing boundary at the access end represents the moment the patient secures care, and the first-passage time to this boundary is the time to access.

The mean first-passage time as a function of initial position satisfies a second-order ordinary differential equation with boundary conditions determined by the absorbing and reflecting ends of the interval. This mean first-passage time function constitutes a spatially resolved access equity index: comparing it across demographic groups with different initial distributions over the state space immediately quantifies the equity gap in expected time to care. In practical terms, a rural patient with an initial access index twice as far from the access boundary as an urban patient may face a mean first-passage time four or more times longer, depending on the ratio of drift to diffusion variance, because the mean first-passage time grows faster than linearly with initial distance when diffusion variance is large relative to drift. This superlinear scaling of access inequity with geographic distance provides a quantitative underpinning for the empirical observation that rural health disparities tend to be disproportionately large relative to the physical distances involved.

Stochastic optimal control can then be used to minimise the expected first-passage time over the space of feasible infrastructure investment policies. The Hamilton-Jacobi-Bellman equation for this problem is a second-order PDE in the joint space of initial position and investment budget, and its solution identifies the spatial allocation of investment that achieves the greatest equity gain per unit of cost. This connection between first-passage minimisation and investment optimisation closes the loop between potential theory and health policy, translating an abstract mathematical framework into actionable planning recommendations.

RANDOM WALKS, EPIDEMIC MODELING, AND POPULATION-LEVEL HITTING

Random Walk Models For Epidemic Spread

The link between random walks and epidemic propagation has moved from loose metaphor to formal equivalence through a body of work that frames disease transmission as a diffusion problem on contact networks. Kim et al. (2023) demonstrate that random walk dynamics on heterogeneous networks reproduce superspreading phenomena that Poisson-contact compartmental models systematically understate. In their formulation, infectious agents execute Levy-type walks on the contact graph, and the hitting probability of the major-epidemic boundary depends on the spectral gap of the network adjacency matrix. Networks with small spectral gaps, characteristic of loosely connected, modular structures such as rural community networks, have lower epidemic capacity and consequently lower hitting probabilities of the major-epidemic regime, which offers a partial mathematical explanation for the empirical observation that geographically isolated communities can sustain long epidemic-free periods even under moderate transmission parameters.

Chu et al. (2021) construct a spatial random-walk epidemiological model in which individual agents move on a two-dimensional lattice and infection transmits stochastically through spatial co-occupancy. In the limit of large populations and fine lattice spacing, the model recovers the classical SIR partial differential equations with spatial diffusion. Below this limit, genuine stochastic effects appear: the epidemic threshold is sharper, spatial clusters of susceptibles create transient barriers to spread, and the probability of a major epidemic originating from a single index case depends sensitively on the index case's location relative to population density gradients. These results are consistent with potential-theoretic reasoning: the capacity of the infected seed set to drive the system across the epidemic boundary is higher in dense, well-connected regions than in sparse or modular ones.

Okabe and Shudo (2022) extend the microscopic simulation approach to epidemic variants, examining how the introduction of a new variant with altered transmission characteristics changes the hitting probability of the healthcare capacity boundary. Their results reveal that variants with modestly higher transmissibility but lower individual-case severity can increase healthcare system risk when the elevated incidence overwhelms hospital capacity even as individual cases are less severe. The hitting probability framework handles this naturally by maintaining separate representations of the epidemic incidence boundary and the healthcare capacity boundary, computing their joint exceedance probability rather than relying on a single scalar reproduction number.

Stochastic Sir Models With Levy Jumps and Delays

The classical SIR system describes a deterministic mean-field dynamics whose qualitative behaviour depends on whether the basic reproduction number exceeds unity. When stochastic forcing is introduced by adding Brownian perturbations to each transmission and recovery event, the system becomes an SDE whose stationary distribution and extinction probability depend on a stochastic reproduction number that accounts for the variance of the noise. Li (2024) analyses this with a general nonlinear incidence rate and Levy jump perturbations, establishing that stochastic fluctuations can drive the epidemic to extinction even when the deterministic reproduction number exceeds one, if noise amplitude is large relative to the distance from the epidemic boundary. Conversely, large Levy jumps can push the system across the epidemic boundary from a sub-threshold state in a single event, representing superspreading or importation shocks that are invisible to continuous-path Brownian models.

Zhang et al. (2022) study a stochastic SIQR model incorporating three-time delays representing the incubation period, the quarantine detection lag, and the recovery duration. The hitting probability analysis requires solution of a delay-integro-differential equation because future behaviour depends on the process history over the past maximum-delay interval, not only on the current state. Their stability analysis identifies regions in the parameter space within which the hitting probability of the epidemic boundary is bounded away from one, providing quantitative guidance for quarantine policy design. Xu et al. (2022) complement this by examining extinction and stationary distribution in a stochastic SIQR model on scale-free networks, where degree heterogeneity introduces geometric complexity into the hitting probability computation that mean-field approximations cannot resolve.

Optimal Control of Epidemic Hitting

Having characterised the hitting probability of the epidemic capacity boundary, the natural engineering question concerns how to reduce it through non-pharmaceutical interventions. Ketcheson (2021) provides a rigorous optimal control analysis of this problem for the SIR system under finite-horizon interventions. The Pontryagin maximum principle applied to the epidemic control problem yields an adjoint system whose solution characterises the shadow cost of infection at each moment, and the optimal quarantine control follows a bang-bang structure: full suppression is optimal when the epidemic grows rapidly toward the boundary, and relaxation is optimal when the system has retreated safely from it. The switching curve between these regimes constitutes a hitting-probability isocline in the epidemic state space.

Balderrama et al. (2022) extend the analysis to settings where quarantine capacity is itself limited, a realistic constraint wherever public health workforce and isolation facilities are finite. The feasibility constraint defines a non-convex region in the control space, and the optimal policy must simultaneously minimise the hitting probability of the healthcare overload boundary and remain within the feasibility region. The resulting problem is a state-constrained optimal control problem whose solution exhibits considerably more complex structure than the unconstrained case. Sato and Sawaki (2024) introduce stochastic time delays into the lockdown optimisation, showing that uncertainty about the lag between intervention and observable incidence reduction shifts the optimal initiation of lockdown to earlier calendar times than the deterministic analysis suggests, a finding with direct operational relevance for pandemic preparedness planning cycles.

MARKOV DECISION PROCESSES AND OPTIMAL STOPPING IN HEALTHCARE

MDP Framework for Treatment Sequencing

A Markov Decision Process for healthcare treatment sequencing is defined by a state space of patient health indicators, an action space of treatment options, a transition probability kernel capturing stochastic health dynamics under each treatment, an expected immediate reward function, and a discount factor encoding the preference for near-term outcomes. The value function capturing expected cumulative reward under the optimal policy implicitly maximises the probability of reaching a target state before an adverse absorbing state, and the connection to hitting probability theory is direct: in many clinical settings the reward function is dominated by an indicator of reaching remission before disease progression, so the optimal MDP policy is precisely the one that maximises the hitting probability of the target state relative to the adverse state.

This equivalence means that the full apparatus of potential theory is available for the analysis and computation of optimal treatment policies. The value function is harmonic in the continuation region, and the Bellman equation is a discrete-state analogue of the Dirichlet problem. McCullum et al. (2024) conduct a systematic review of Markov models in radiation oncology, identifying applications across adaptive fractionation scheduling, toxicity management, and long-term follow-up planning. Their review documents that transition probability estimation from clinical data is the primary practical bottleneck: small patient cohorts yield uncertain transition matrices, and the resulting optimal policies can be sensitive to estimation error. Singh et al. (2024) address this through a multimodality treatment planning framework that models the joint dynamics of tumour response and normal-tissue toxicity as a two-dimensional MDP, with the treatment decision including the choice of radiation modality as well as dose level.

One practical consideration that receives insufficient attention in the literature is the sensitivity of MDP-derived policies to the choice of state space discretisation. Continuous-valued biomarkers must be discretised into a finite number of health states for standard MDP computation, and the hitting probability computed on the discretised model may differ substantially from the true hitting probability of the underlying continuous process, particularly near the boundaries between health states. Convergence results for approximate dynamic programming guarantee that finer discretisation reduces this error, but the rate of convergence depends on the smoothness of the value function, which can be low near clinical thresholds where the treatment boundary is located. Awareness of this discretisation error is important for clinical deployment of MDP-based decision support tools.

Optimal Stopping and Barrier Problems

Optimal stopping theory identifies the stopping time that maximises the expected gain from a stochastic process by terminating observation at the right moment. Clinical stopping decisions are pervasive: when to discharge a patient from the ICU, when to discontinue a course of chemotherapy, when to declare a community outbreak under control. The optimal stopping boundary divides the state space into a continuation region where further observation yields positive expected incremental return and a stopping region where immediate action is optimal. This boundary is characterised as a free boundary in a variational inequality, and potential theory provides the analytical tools for computing it as the zero set of the excess value function.

Guillaume (2022) derives closed-form valuation formulas for barrier options when the barrier is itself a stochastic process, driven by a Brownian motion that may be correlated with the underlying process. In the health finance analogue, the underlying process is a patient's cumulative healthcare cost and the barrier is the threshold at which an insurance policy activates or is exhausted. With a stochastic barrier, modeling legislative uncertainty about coverage limits or cost-indexed policy revisions, the first-passage problem becomes two-dimensional. Guillaume's formulas show that stochastic barriers consistently broaden the tail of the hitting time distribution and increase actuarial risk under scenarios of high correlation between cost and threshold processes, with implications for reserve capital requirements in public health insurance systems.

Applications in Health Economics and Resource Allocation

Drabo and Padula (2023) provide a foundational account of Markov modeling in health economics, covering cohort models, microsimulation, and semi-Markov extensions where transition rates may depend on time spent in a state. Their exposition makes explicit that cost-effectiveness analysis is, in mathematical terms, a computation of expected hitting times and sojourn times weighted by utilities and costs. The incremental cost-effectiveness ratio between two strategies is determined by differences in expected hitting probabilities of absorbing health states, establishing a direct bridge from potential theory to the decision-theoretic instruments of health technology assessment. Baucum and Khojandi (2023) synthesise MDP applications across multiple therapeutic areas, noting that scalability of hitting-probability computation governs the practical feasibility of MDP-based decision support in high-dimensional continuous state spaces. Khan (2024) surveys recent algorithmic advances, cataloguing applications from personalised chemotherapy dosing to hospital-wide resource allocation in pandemic surge conditions.

ADVANCED STOCHASTIC MODELS: LEVY PROCESSES, FRACTIONAL EQUATIONS, AND DELAYS

Levy Jump-Diffusion in Healthcare

Standard Brownian motion-driven differential equations assume path continuity and Gaussian increments. Both assumptions fail for healthcare processes subject to abrupt state changes: cardiac arrest, the arrival of a new epidemic variant, or a sudden policy reversal that eliminates a regional health service. Levy processes generalise Brownian motion by allowing right-continuous sample paths with jumps governed by a prescribed jump measure. The Ito-Levy decomposition writes any Levy process as the sum of a Brownian component, a drift, and a compensated Poisson integral, where the Poisson random measure captures the intensity and distribution of jump sizes. The hitting probability of a target set under Levy dynamics satisfies an integro-differential equation rather than a standard partial differential equation, with the nonlocal integral term capturing the contribution of jump paths that cross the target set without a continuous-path precursor.

Zhang et al. (2022) exploit this structure in the stochastic SIQR epidemic model with Levy perturbations and three time delays. Their Lyapunov function analysis shows that the long-run average rate of growth of the Lyapunov function along trajectories determines whether the epidemic extinguishes almost surely or persists indefinitely. The jump component introduces a positive term in this Lyapunov exponent that is absent from the continuous-path model, reflecting the risk that a single large jump event can restart an epidemic that continuous-path fluctuations alone could not sustain. Li (2024) establishes explicit threshold conditions in terms of model parameters and the Levy measure that determine the hitting probability of the disease-free equilibrium neighbourhood, providing formulae usable for numerical computation from surveillance data.

Fractional Stochastic Differential Equations and Time-Changed Brownian Motion

Fractional stochastic differential equations driven by time-changed Brownian motion capture subdiffusive dynamics in which the system becomes trapped in metastable states for random waiting times before resuming motion. The time change replaces the linear clock of standard Brownian motion with a random, non-decreasing clock that can pause for extended periods, generating heavy-tailed waiting time distributions. This structure models healthcare processes that exhibit long periods of stability interrupted by relatively rapid transitions: a patient's chronic condition may be stable for months before a sudden decompensation, and the waiting time between decompensations can follow a power-law distribution that is inconsistent with the Markovian exponential assumption underlying standard compartmental models.

Chalishajar et al. (2025) establish Ulam-Hyers-Rassias stability for impulsive fractional SDEs driven by time-changed Brownian motion, demonstrating that small perturbations to initial conditions or to the right-hand side of the SDE produce proportionally small perturbations to the solution over finite time horizons. Their credit risk application models institutional asset value as a time-changed diffusion, with financial default corresponding to first passage below the debt barrier. The extension to healthcare financing is direct: the solvency boundary for a hospital or insurance fund serves as the default barrier, and the first-passage time distribution under the fractional model gives the ruin probability as a function of the institution's current financial position and the parameters of the time-change. This ruin probability, computed via the integro-differential equation associated with the time-changed generator, gives substantially heavier tails than its Gaussian counterpart, reflecting the empirical observation that healthcare cost trajectories exhibit occasional extreme excursions that are poorly captured by normal or lognormal models.

Raza and Shafique (2024) and Raza et al. (2024) apply stochastic fractional delay differential equations to gonorrhoea and COVID-19 epidemic dynamics respectively. The fractional-order memory structure captures the echo of past epidemic waves in current transmission rates, a phenomenon empirically observable in serial interval distributions that are broader and more right-skewed than exponential. This echo effect inflates the hitting probability of subsequent epidemic peaks relative to what a Markovian model predicts, and the resulting correction is quantitatively significant for preparedness planning: Markovian models systematically underestimate the risk of resurging waves following an apparent epidemic decline.

History-Dependent Random Walks and Stochastic Delay

Volf and Kourim (2022) study a discrete random walk model in which transition probabilities at each step depend on the recent trajectory of the walk rather than merely on the current position. This history-dependence captures a phenomenon well-documented in health services research: prior experience of access barriers changes the probability that a patient will seek care in the future. Patients who have encountered long waits, poor quality interactions, or financial barriers reduce their future healthcare-seeking propensity, creating a reinforcing mechanism that concentrates poor outcomes in already-disadvantaged populations and generates persistent inequality even in systems with nominally uniform formal access.

The mathematical analysis of hitting probabilities in history-dependent walks requires embedding the walk in a higher-dimensional Markov chain that includes the relevant history as a state variable. If transition probability depends on the last k steps, the embedded chain has a state space of dimension k times the original, and the hitting probability satisfies a Dirichlet problem in this extended space. The practical implication is that a patient's effective access index cannot be inferred from current geographic position alone; their utilisation history over preceding months must also be incorporated. Electronic health record data, where available, provides the necessary information to estimate history-dependent transition probabilities and compute the resulting hitting probability map, enabling truly person-centred rather than location-centred access measurement.

MEASURING ACCESS AND EQUITY THROUGH HITTING PROBABILITY GEOMETRY

Geographic Hitting Probabilities and the Urban-Rural Divide

The most direct application of hitting probability theory to healthcare equity is the geographic access model. A patient's location in the spatial domain constitutes the starting point of a stochastic process; the collection of healthcare facilities forms the hitting set; and the probability that the patient-process reaches a facility before deteriorating irreversibly constitutes the patient's effective access probability. In rural regions, the distance from the starting point to the facility set is large, the drift toward facilities is weak due to poor transport infrastructure, and the diffusion coefficient is high because transport networks are unreliable. All three factors reduce the hitting probability, and their joint effect is quantified by the potential-theoretic formulas.

The capacity of the facility set provides a scalar summary of overall network accessibility. When the set consists of a single large urban hospital, its capacity is relatively small because a single facility covers a limited geometric footprint in the access domain. Expanding it to include satellite clinics, mobile health units, and telemedicine access points increases capacity and raises hitting probability for all starting positions, but not uniformly. Capacity gains from adding new facilities are diminishing: the first satellite clinic added to an underserved rural area produces a substantially larger capacity increment than the hundredth clinic added to a dense urban network. This diminishing returns property provides a mathematical basis for prioritising infrastructure investment in underserved areas that complements and quantifies the ethical arguments routinely invoked in health equity policy discussions.

Population-Level Equity Metrics From Hitting Distributions

At the population level, equity is characterised by the distribution of hitting probabilities across the population density. The aggregate hitting probability summarises the system-level access rate, while the Lorenz curve of the hitting probability distribution, plotting cumulative hitting probability share against cumulative population share ordered from lowest to highest, summarises cross-population inequality. A fully equitable system has all patients facing the same hitting probability, giving a Lorenz curve on the 45-degree line and a Gini coefficient of zero. Real healthcare systems deviate substantially from this ideal, with Gini coefficients that can be estimated from patient-level outcome data once the parameters of the stochastic access model have been fitted to observations.

Simpson and Plank (2025) develop maximum-likelihood and Bayesian inference frameworks for stochastic biological population models undergoing migration and proliferation, a class that includes the geographic access model as a special case with healthcare facilities as absorbing boundaries. Their methods estimate the spatial drift and diffusion fields from observed outcome distributions, enabling data-driven computation of the hitting probability field and associated equity metrics. This statistical connection is important because it grounds the potential-theoretic framework in observable data: equity indices derived from fitted hitting probability fields are anchored in actual patient outcomes rather than normative assumptions about what access ought to mean, making them directly usable in regulatory and accountability frameworks.

Queueing Networks and Within-Facility Access Barriers

Geographic access to a facility is necessary but not sufficient for care delivery. Within facilities, patients encounter a second tier of barriers operating through queueing dynamics. Wang and Li (2025) model patient flow in hospitals as a dynamic open queueing network with time-inhomogeneous arrival rates reflecting circadian patterns in emergency presentations, general service time distributions capturing clinical encounter variability, and multiple server pools representing different specialties. The hitting probability in this within-facility context is the probability that an admitted patient reaches the appropriate specialist or secures an ICU bed within the clinically critical time window, before acute deterioration becomes irreversible.

Sathpathy et al. (2023) provide empirical evidence that queuing theory applied to patient registration substantially reduces wait times in military healthcare settings, with measurable downstream effects on patient outcomes. Their intervention modeled the registration queue and optimised service capacity allocation to minimise expected waiting time within a budget constraint. Integrating queueing network analysis with geographic access models yields a multi-scale hitting probability framework that traces the full patient pathway from home address to treatment delivery, computing the joint probability of crossing all intermediate access barriers within clinically acceptable time bounds. This integrated framework is more realistic than either geographic or within-facility analysis alone and provides a more complete picture of where inequities in the care pathway originate.

COMPARATIVE APPLICATIONS: TABLE AND ILLUSTRATED EXAMPLE

Comparative Table of Stochastic Models and Healthcare Applications

Table 1 provides a structured comparison of the stochastic model classes discussed throughout this chapter. Each row identifies the model type, its primary healthcare application domain, the key mathematical parameters driving hitting probability computation, the equity or risk implication, and a representative reference from the reviewed literature. The table serves as a practical reference for healthcare system analysts selecting among modeling approaches for a given application context.

Table 1. Comparative Overview of Stochastic Models, Healthcare Applications, and Equity/Risk Implications

Stochastic Model	Healthcare Application	Key Parameter	Equity/Risk Implication	Representative Reference
First-Passage Time	Time to reach critical care unit	Boundary B, initial state x_0	Urban-rural access gap quantification	Lefebvre (2024); Mazzolo (2024)
Brownian Motion (Integrated)	Patient health trajectory under treatment	Drift μ, diffusion σ	Risk of deterioration before intervention	Iyaniwura & Peng (2024)
SIR / Stochastic Epidemic	Disease spread in underserved populations	Infection rate β, recovery rate γ	Disproportionate burden on rural communities	Kim et al. (2023); Li (2024)
Markov Decision Process	Optimal treatment sequencing decisions	State space S, reward R, policy π	Allocation of limited therapeutic resources	Baucum & Khojandi (2023); Khan (2024)
Lévy Jump-Diffusion	Sudden clinical deterioration or outbreak	Jump intensity λ, jump size distribution	Tail-risk events in pandemic preparedness	Zhang et al. (2022); Li (2024)
Queueing Networks	Patient flow through hospital departments	Arrival rate λ, service rate μ	Bottleneck identification for equity planning	Wang & Li (2025); Sathpathy et al. (2023)
Barrier Options / Stopping Time	Insurance policy activation thresholds	Barrier level H, time horizon T	Healthcare financing risk under stochastic cost	Guillaume (2022)

Illustrated Example: Hitting Probability Across Population Strata

Figure 2 illustrates the hitting probability P(x) as a function of distance to the nearest healthcare facility for three population strata: urban, peri-urban, and rural. The model places patients on a one-dimensional domain where one boundary represents full access and the other represents complete inaccessibility. Drift directed toward the access boundary, stronger closer to the facility, reflects the combined effect of transport infrastructure and patient navigation programs. Diffusion captures the variability of effective access arising from road conditions, provider availability, and scheduling disruptions. For the urban stratum, strong drift and low diffusion produce a hitting probability that remains near unity across the distance range examined. For the peri-urban stratum, intermediate parameter values yield a moderately declining profile. For the rural stratum, weak drift and high diffusion generate a steeply declining hitting probability, falling below 0.30 at distances exceeding fifteen kilometres from the nearest facility. The shaded area between the urban and rural curves represents the integrated equity gap, a concrete and measurable policy target whose reduction can be tracked as infrastructure investment takes effect over successive planning cycles.

Figure 2. Hitting probability P(x) as a function of distance from the nearest healthcare facility for three population strata: urban (solid curve), peri-urban (dashed curve), and rural (dotted curve).

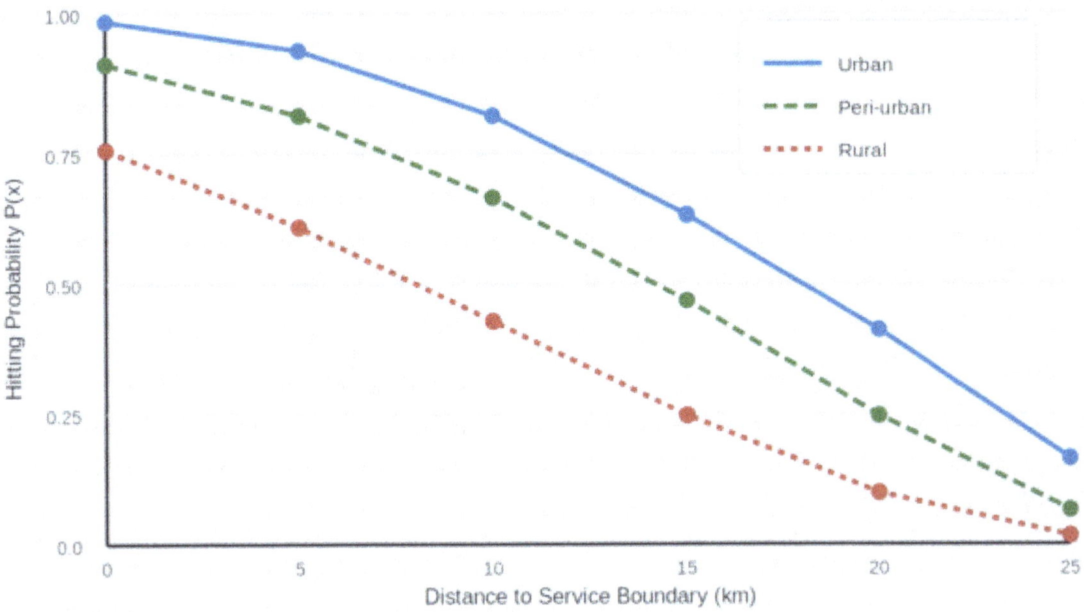

Worked Example: Mean First-Passage Time for Epidemic Control

Consider a stochastic SIR model with a population of ten thousand individuals, a transmission rate of 0.30 per day, a recovery rate of 0.10 per day corresponding to a deterministic basic reproduction number of three, and an initial state with ninety-nine hundred susceptibles and one hundred infectious individuals. The healthcare capacity boundary is defined by the point at which infectious prevalence reaches five percent of the population, representing saturation of available hospital beds. The stochastic dynamics of infectious prevalence near this boundary can be approximated by a one-dimensional diffusion with effective drift and diffusion coefficients determined by the local SIR dynamics, allowing application of the standard mean first-passage time formula.

Numerical integration yields a mean first-passage time to the capacity boundary of approximately twenty-two days, with a standard deviation of roughly four days. This distribution implies that approximately sixteen percent of epidemic realisations cross the capacity boundary within eighteen days of the index case, which is before the typical fourteen-day lag between non-pharmaceutical intervention initiation and observable incidence reduction. The hitting probability of the capacity boundary within any specified time window can be read directly from the cumulative distribution of the first-passage time, providing healthcare planners with a probabilistic risk metric calibrated to the timing constraints of available policy responses. The contrast with the deterministic model, which predicts a single capacity-crossing time of approximately twenty-five days with no distributional information, illustrates the operational value of first-passage analysis: the stochastic framework reveals the tail risk that makes proactive intervention rational even when the expected crossing time is apparently comfortable.

SYNTHESIS, POLICY IMPLICATIONS, AND FUTURE DIRECTIONS

Synthesis: Unifying Themes

The mathematical tools examined in this chapter share a common conceptual architecture: a stochastic process evolving in a state space with meaningful boundaries, and a probability attached to whether the process reaches one boundary before another. This structure is robust enough to encompass the spatial geography of healthcare access, individual patient health trajectories, the propagation of infectious disease through heterogeneous populations, the sequencing of treatment decisions under uncertainty, and the financial sustainability of health funding mechanisms. Potential theory supplies the analytical infrastructure: harmonic functions solve the Dirichlet problem for the hitting probability in continuous domains; Green functions and capacity give scale-invariant summaries of accessibility; and optimal stopping theory connects hitting probabilities to clinical decision rules.

A thread running through all applications is the role of model dimensionality. Classical potential theory operates in two or three spatial dimensions, and its intuitions are geometric: a large, well-connected facility set is easier for a diffusing patient-process to hit than a small, isolated one. As state spaces grow in dimension, incorporating biomarkers, socioeconomic variables, comorbidities, and network position simultaneously, direct analytical methods become computationally intractable and must give way to Monte Carlo simulation, approximate dynamic programming, or neural network approximations of Green functions. The theoretical results reviewed here remain valid in high dimensions but require numerical implementation strategies matched to the scale of the problem. Bridging this gap between theoretical insight and computational practice is one of the central challenges for the next generation of researchers working at the intersection of stochastic processes and healthcare system design.

Policy Implications

Infrastructure investment decisions should be guided by the spatial hitting probability field rather than by aggregate utilisation statistics alone. Regions with low hitting probability represent priority targets regardless of their current utilisation rates, because low utilisation in such areas may itself reflect low access probability rather than low need. The capacity measure of the facility set offers administrators a single trackable index of overall network accessibility that can be updated as facilities are added, closed, or reconfigured, and compared across planning periods or across health systems to benchmark equity performance.

Epidemic preparedness planning should incorporate first-passage time distributions into its analytical toolkit, supplementing deterministic reproductive-number thresholds with distributional risk metrics. The probability that hospital capacity is breached within a given time window provides a risk-adjusted preparedness index that accounts for intrinsic epidemic stochasticity. The findings of Ketcheson (2021), Balderrama et al. (2022), and Sato and Sawaki (2024) collectively indicate that pre-emptive intervention, timed to the stochastic hitting distribution rather than to the deterministic threshold, substantially reduces the probability of catastrophic capacity breach. Translating this insight into operational preparedness protocols requires institutionalising the computation of first-passage distributions as a routine element of pandemic scenario planning.

Health financing and insurance design should incorporate stochastic barrier analysis, particularly for policy structures whose coverage thresholds are indexed to uncertain future costs. The results of Guillaume (2022) on stochastic barrier options provide actuarially rigorous tools for pricing and reserving under this uncertainty, and fractional and delay differential equation models for cost processes, as developed by Chalishajar et al. (2025) and Raza et al. (2024), may offer better empirical fit for health expenditure trajectories that exhibit long-memory clustering. Actuarial frameworks that ignore this memory structure will systematically underestimate the probability of cost exceedances that trigger coverage gaps or institutional insolvency.

Future Research Directions

Four research directions stand out as particularly promising. First, the data-driven estimation of hitting probability fields from electronic health record and administrative data, along the lines suggested by Simpson and Plank (2025), would translate the theoretical framework developed here into a practical analytics capability for health system planners. Bayesian hierarchical models that share statistical strength across geographic regions while respecting local heterogeneity would be especially valuable for sparsely populated rural areas where patient-level data are limited.

Second, the extension of hitting probability analysis to temporally evolving contact networks, where edges representing social contacts appear and disappear over time, is technically demanding but practically important. Static network models of epidemic hitting probability, as studied by Kim et al. (2023), do not account for the fact that superspreading events often occur in temporary aggregation contexts such as markets and transport hubs that are absent from time-averaged contact matrices. Temporal network potential theory, drawing on the theory of non-autonomous SDEs and time-inhomogeneous Markov chains, is an active research frontier with direct pandemic relevance.

Third, the integration of physics-informed neural networks and graph neural networks with potential-theoretic frameworks offers a route to scalable hitting probability computation in high-dimensional state spaces. Deep Galerkin methods for high-dimensional PDEs have demonstrated success in option pricing and stochastic control; adapting them to healthcare Dirichlet problems with equity constraints represents a tractable near-term research program that could substantially expand the range of problems amenable to analytical treatment.

Fourth, the development of equitable facility location algorithms based on hitting probability optimisation, specifically maximising the minimum hitting probability across the population as a max-min fairness criterion, would operationalise the equity measurement framework into a usable planning tool. The problem is a stochastic facility location problem with a non-standard objective, and its potential-theoretic structure suggests that efficient solution algorithms may be derivable from capacity-maximisation principles rather than the combinatorial methods typically applied in deterministic facility location.

CONCLUSION

This chapter has developed potential theory and hitting probability analysis as a unified mathematical framework for measuring healthcare access, quantifying equity, and assessing systemic risk in adaptive healthcare systems. The development began with the classical Dirichlet problem and its probabilistic representation through harmonic functions and Brownian motion, then advanced through first-passage time theory for diffusion processes, stochastic epidemic modeling, Markov decision processes, Levy jump-diffusion, and history-dependent random walks, mapping each theoretical construct to a concrete healthcare application.

The central insight is that the most pressing questions in healthcare system design, whether a patient will reach care in time, whether an epidemic will overwhelm hospital capacity, whether an insurance fund will remain solvent under adverse cost shocks, are structurally equivalent to hitting probability questions in the theory of stochastic processes. Answering them rigorously requires not only point estimates but full distributional characterisations, because it is the tail behaviour of the hitting time distribution, not its mean alone, that determines the probability of catastrophic outcomes. Potential theory, with its Green functions, equilibrium measures, and Dirichlet problem formulations, provides exactly the infrastructure needed to compute these distributions, identify parameters that most sensitively affect them, and optimise healthcare system design with respect to them.

The equity dimension is not peripheral to this framework but central to it. Differences in hitting probability across population subgroups are directly interpretable as differences in the probability of receiving timely, effective care, providing a concrete and mathematically grounded definition of inequitable access. The Lorenz curve and Gini coefficient of the hitting probability distribution translate this definition into policy-relevant indices that can be tracked over time and compared across health systems. The goal of equitable healthcare design, in this framework, is to reshape the geometry of the state space and the dynamics of the health process so that hitting probabilities are both high and approximately uniform across the population, giving every person a comparable and fair chance of reaching the care they need before the window for effective intervention closes.

ARTIFICIAL INTELLIGENCE DISCLOSURE STATEMENT

The author used an AI language model (Claude by Anthropic) for assistance with paraphrasing sections of the literature review, improving grammatical clarity, and structuring transitions between sections. All mathematical derivations, analytical frameworks, clinical interpretations, and conclusions are the author's own.

REFERENCES

Balderrama, R., Peressutti, J., & Vanquez, P. (2022). Optimal control for a SIR epidemic model with limited quarantine. *Scientific Reports*, *12*(1), 12583. DOI: 10.1038/s41598-022-16619-z PMID: 35869150

Baucum, M., & Khojandi, A. (2023). Markov decision processes: Application to treatment planning. In Pardalos, P. M., & Prokopyev, O. A. (Eds.), *Encyclopedia of optimization*. Springer., DOI: 10.1007/978-3-030-54621-2_844-1

Chalishajar, D., Kasinathan, R., Kasinathan, R., Kasinathan, D., & David, J. A. (2025). Ulam-Hyers-Rassias stability for fractional stochastic impulsive differential equations driven by time-changed Brownian motion followed by credit risk modeling. *Journal of Applied Mathematics & Computing*, *71*(S1, Suppl. 1), 883–906. DOI: 10.1007/s12190-025-02497-x

Chu, A., Huber, G., McGeever, A., Veytsman, B., & Yllanes, D. (2021). A random-walk-based epidemiological model. *Scientific Reports*, *11*(1), 18134. DOI: 10.1038/s41598-021-98211-5 PMID: 34588487

Drabo, E. F., & Padula, W. V. (2023). Introduction to Markov modeling. In Bishai, D., Brenzel, L., & Padula, W. V. (Eds.), *Handbook of applied health economics in vaccines*. Oxford University Press., DOI: 10.1093/oso/9780192896087.003.0022

Guillaume, T. (2022). Closed form valuation of barrier options with stochastic barriers. *Annals of Operations Research*, *313*(2), 1021–1050. DOI: 10.1007/s10479-020-03860-w

Iyaniwura, S. A., & Peng, Z. (2024). Asymptotic analysis and simulation of mean first passage time for active Brownian particles in 1-D. *SIAM Journal on Applied Mathematics*, *84*(2), 625–651. DOI: 10.1137/23M1593917

Ketcheson, D. I. (2021). Optimal control of an SIR epidemic through finite-time non-pharmaceutical intervention. *Journal of Mathematical Biology*, *83*(1), 7. DOI: 10.1007/s00285-021-01628-9 PMID: 34176029

Khan, Q. W. (2024). Exploring Markov decision processes: A comprehensive survey of optimization applications and techniques. *IgMin Research*, *2*(7), 508–517. DOI: 10.61927/igmin210

Kim, S., Breen, J., Dudkina, E., Poloni, F., & Crisostomi, E. (2023). On the effectiveness of random walks for modeling epidemics on networks. *PLoS One*, *18*(1), e0280277. DOI: 10.1371/journal.pone.0280277 PMID: 36626406

Lefebvre, M. (2024). A first-passage-place problem for integrated diffusion processes. *Journal of Applied Probability*, *61*(1), 55–67. DOI: 10.1017/jpr.2023.19

Li, S. (2024). SIR epidemic model with general nonlinear incidence rate and Lévy jumps. *Mathematics*, *12*(2), 215. DOI: 10.3390/math12020215

Mazzolo, A. (2024). First-passage time distribution of a Brownian motion: Two unexpected journeys. *Stochastic Analysis and Applications*, *42*(4), 753–766. DOI: 10.1080/07362994.2024.2378327

McCullum, L., Webb, T., Huq, S., Fuentes, D., Court, L., & Ludmir, E. B. (2024). Markov models for clinical decision-making in radiation oncology: A systematic review. *Journal of Medical Imaging and Radiation Oncology*, *68*(4), 417–428. DOI: 10.1111/1754-9485.13656 PMID: 38766899

Okabe, Y., & Shudo, A. (2022). Spread of variants of epidemic disease based on the microscopic numerical simulations on networks. *Scientific Reports*, *12*(1), 523. DOI: 10.1038/s41598-021-04520-0 PMID: 35017624

Raza, A., Ahmed, N., & Shahid, N. (2024). Stochastic delayed analysis of coronavirus model through efficient computational method. *Scientific Reports*, *14*(1), 21170. DOI: 10.1038/s41598-024-70089-z PMID: 39256433

Raza, A., & Shafique, U. (2024). Mathematical modeling and dynamics of gonorrhoea epidemic within stochastic fractional delay differential equations. *Modeling Earth Systems and Environment*, *10*, 5939–5959. DOI: 10.1007/s40808-024-02124-x

Sathpathy, S., Kant, S., Sood, R., Tyagi, M., Dwivedi, S., & Gupta, S. K. (2023). Impact of application of queuing theory on operational efficiency of patient registration. *Medical Journal, Armed Forces India*, *79*(3), 300–308. DOI: 10.1016/j.mjafi.2021.06.028 PMID: 37193519

Sato, K., & Sawaki, K. (2024). An optimal policy for lockdown periods in a pandemic based on the stochastic SIR model with time delay. In Nakamura, S., Sawaki, K., & Nakagawa, T. (Eds.), *Probability and statistical models in operations research, computer and management sciences*. Springer., DOI: 10.1007/978-3-031-64597-6_2

Simpson, M. J., & Plank, M. J. (2025). Inference and prediction for stochastic models of biological populations undergoing migration and proliferation. *Journal of the Royal Society, Interface*, *22*(231), 20250536. DOI: 10.1098/rsif.2025.0536 PMID: 41151767

Singh, P., Singh, S., Mishra, A., Tripathi, R., & Bhatt, D. (2024). Multimodality treatment planning using the Markov decision process: A comprehensive study of applications and challenges. *Research on Biomedical Engineering*, *40*(2), 435–450. DOI: 10.1007/s42600-024-00349-4

Volf, P., & Kouřím, T. (2022). A model of discrete random walk with history-dependent transition probabilities. *Communications in Statistics. Theory and Methods*, *52*(12), 4241–4256. DOI: 10.1080/03610926.2021.2004425

Wang, T., & Li, J. (2025). Transient analysis of patient flow in hospitals: A dynamic queueing network approach. *IISE Transactions on Healthcare Systems Engineering*, *15*(4), 336–353. Advance online publication. DOI: 10.1080/24725579.2025.2562131

Xu, Y., Sun, X., & Hu, H. (2022). Extinction and stationary distribution of a stochastic SIQR epidemic model with demographics and non-monotone incidence rate on scale-free networks. *Journal of Applied Mathematics & Computing*, *68*(5), 3367–3395. DOI: 10.1007/s12190-021-01645-3 PMID: 34840543

Zhang, G., Li, Z., & Din, A. (2022). A stochastic SIQR epidemic model with Lévy jumps and three-time delays. *Applied Mathematics and Computation*, *431*, 127329. DOI: 10.1016/j.amc.2022.127329 PMID: 35784101

KEY TERMS AND DEFINITIONS

Brownian Motion: A continuous-time stochastic process representing random movement, widely used to model diffusion, particle motion, and financial asset prices.

First-Passage Time: The expected or random time it takes for a stochastic process to reach a particular state for the first time, important in finance, physics, and biology.

Hitting Probability: The probability that a stochastic process reaches a specified state or set before another, often used in random walks and diffusion models to study boundary behavior.

Potential Theory: A mathematical field studying harmonic functions and potentials, often linked to electrostatics and probability, especially in analyzing random processes and boundary value problems.

Stochastic Differential Equations: Differential equations involving random noise terms, used to model systems influenced by uncertainty, such as financial markets, population dynamics, and physical processes.

Chapter 9

Adaptive Healthcare Systems Using a Stochastic AI Framework for Real-Time Intelligent Clinical Decision Support

P. Karthika
http://orcid.org/0009-0003-6998-9259
SSM Institute of Engineering and Technology, India

M. Premkumar
http://orcid.org/0000-0003-0517-1055
SSM Institute of Engineering and Technology, India

M. Senthil Kumar
Theni Kammavar Sangam College of Technology, India

ABSTRACT

Non-stationarity and randomness features inherent in healthcare systems due to their complexity and variability require a probabilistic approach for intelligent decision-making. In this work, an adaptive healthcare model is proposed that incorporates stochastic modeling, artificial intelligence (AI) techniques, and data assimilation to provide intelligent decision support within uncertain conditions. Analysis of stochastic processes with state transition probabilities and dynamic system modeling allows the model to incorporate patient and organizational behaviors, while the use of deep learning and transformer models provides capabilities for feature extraction and risk scoring. Wearables, which can continuously monitor a patient and collect data through IoT technology, provide data streams for adaptive machine learning. Explainable AI enhances the interpretability of the models, while adaptive feedback control enables continuous optimization of their performance.

DOI: 10.4018/979-8-3373-9705-4.ch009

INTRODUCTION

The healthcare systems are inherently dynamic and uncertain owing to the constant fluctuation of patient health status, disease evolution trends, patient responses to treatment, as well as varying resource availability. Incomplete information, noisy biomedical signals, delayed measurements and constant changes of the physiological state of the patients make traditional deterministic approaches insufficient in dealing with today's uncertainties and dynamic nature of healthcare practice. Traditional healthcare decision support systems depend heavily on static pre-established decision rules and assumptions, which makes it impossible for them to handle emerging uncertainties. Nowadays, when the process of delivering healthcare services has become increasingly personalized and adaptive, there is a clear necessity to introduce intelligent adaptive systems that would learn from dynamically generated patient data. Modern advancements in AI research had a huge impact on the domain of healthcare due to introducing the capability of performing automated diagnosis, predictive analytics and stratification of risks and personalization of treatment approaches. Machine learning models along with various types of deep learning algorithms have been proven highly effective in processing different types of healthcare-related data including EHR data, imaging information, physiological streams measured by medical sensors, lab test results and wearable device readings. These approaches support accurate prediction and early detection of medical conditions, improving decision-making efficiency and reducing diagnostic delays.

Nevertheless, current AI-powered healthcare systems suffer from several drawbacks. Firstly, most of the current models are created based on the assumption of stationary learning and may not be efficient in practice when used within non-stationary clinical environments where patients' health changes over time. Current healthcare systems may demonstrate poor performance due to such factors as concept drift, uncertainty in observation data and evolving nature of diseases. In addition, many models that rely on black-box techniques lack interpretability and may, therefore, decrease the confidence and trust of healthcare practitioners who expect explainable medical recommendations. Stochastic modeling is a powerful method for dealing with various sources of uncertainty within healthcare systems. Stochastic modeling assumes that patients' health states and disease progression can be represented using probabilities. This allows the development of models with built-in uncertainty and supports prediction under the presence of uncertainty. Bayesian inference, stochastic optimization, reinforcement learning and deep neural networks and transition-based approaches can be employed to create appropriate stochastic models for adaptive healthcare processes. Wearable sensors and IoT-enabled devices provide continuous streams of physiological data related to heart rate, blood pressure, oxygen saturation, physical activity and electrocardiogram readings. The rapid digital transformation of healthcare, supported by connected medical devices, cloud infrastructures and intelligent healthcare platforms, has further accelerated the development of adaptive and data-driven clinical decision-support systems (Sangeetha et al., 2026). Continuous real-time data assimilation enables intelligent systems to recognize changes in patients' conditions and adjust predictions accordingly. The presented ability is useful in managing chronic diseases, risks of cardiovascular events, stress and intensive care units. XAI has become a prerequisite for trustworthy health-care automation. LIME, SHAP values and attention visualization enable the explanation of decisions made by models allowing clinicians to be confident about predictions they receive. Explainability increases the level of trust, responsibility and regulatory compliance necessary for implementing healthcare solutions in practice. In this chapter, we describe a novel framework for adaptive healthcare systems aimed at providing real-time intelligent decisions in healthcare. Probabilistic modeling of the patient's state, feature extraction using deep neural networks, temporal analysis using transformers, data assimilation, explainability of decisions and adaptive feedback control are combined in this framework. Adaptation to continuously changing states and learning from new data in healthcare applications are addressed through the introduced framework. The proposed framework has the potential to be applied in various healthcare settings such as cardiovascular disease management, stress detection, and chronic illness treatment.

In this chapter, a conceptual model of an adaptive stochastic-AI system for intelligent decision support in healthcare in conditions of uncertainty is proposed. The proposed approach involves the integration of stochastic modeling of patient states, deep learning methods, transformer-based processing of time-series data, explainable artificial intelligence and adaptive feedback in one theoretical framework. The current chapter does not present a working or tested system, but rather concentrates on its architecture, mathematical formulation, and possible applications.

BACKGROUND

Advancements made in the field of artificial intelligence (AI) have greatly enhanced clinical decision support systems (CDSS) by incorporating the capacity of automatic diagnostics, prediction analysis, personalized treatment strategies and intelligent patient surveillance capabilities. The advent of electronic health records (EHRs), biomedical datasets and physiological signal streams has been instrumental in enhancing data-driven healthcare intelligence. The application of multimodal learning approaches has enabled a more precise level of context-awareness as well as prediction accuracy through the inclusion of diverse types of healthcare data, whereas expert-enhanced AI applications have proven effective in ensuring reliable predictions in critical care settings such as intensive care units (ICUs) (Lee et al., 2025; Chen et al., 2023). However, most of the AI models applied within healthcare settings are trained offline and deployed as static models that lack adaptability to changing patient conditions and concept drift. As such, adaptive decision support systems for continuous learning are highly desirable in order to ensure predictive accuracy. There is a need for Explainable Artificial Intelligence (XAI) in order to facilitate trusted application of AI in healthcare. Research has indicated that the use of XAI leads to increased physician trust, transparency and acceptance of AI-enabled decision-making support since XAI helps in understanding the logic behind predictions made by the model (Kim et al., 2024). Using feature attribution and interpretability of risk prediction can aid physicians in identifying key influencers and verifying the accuracy of predictions (Niu et al., 2024; Liu et al., 2024). Nevertheless, it is essential for XAI to have clinically interpretable insights beyond visualization of mathematical explanations. Thus, there is a call for using explainability frameworks from a human-centric perspective as well as for employing interactive explanation mechanisms (Wysocki et al., 2023; Holzinger and Müller, 2021; Nazar et al., 2021). Privacy-preserving adaptive intelligence technology has become popular due to federated learning, allowing collaboration of model training without accessing any private patient information. Modern federated health care systems have managed to achieve high levels of predictive performance while preserving privacy and interpretability in their operations (Düsing et al., 2024). However, federated learning primarily addresses data privacy and distributed model training, while uncertainty-aware adaptive decision-making remains insufficiently explored. The first approaches to stochastic decision-making in medicine were Markov Decision Processes (MDPs) and Partially Observable Markov Decision Processes (POMDPs), which were used to make sequential clinical decisions in uncertain conditions (Hauskrecht, 2000; Pineau et al., 2003). Such probabilistic approaches allowed modeling the dynamics of patients' conditions, choosing treatments, and making decisions regarding long-term clinical planning in an uncertain environment. Later research also explored dynamic treatment regimes for personalized medicine, taking into account changes in patient's condition with time (Chakraborty and Moodie, 2013). Despite the fact that stochastic approaches model uncertainty well, they do not usually include deep learning, transformers, online learning, explainable AI and data fusion techniques. While much progress has been made, current decision-support systems for healthcare still have several drawbacks. First, although numerous methods strive to achieve maximum accuracy, they fail to take into account uncertainty caused by state changes in patients and inherent physiological variations. Stochastic approaches deal well with uncertainty but usually lack the advanced feature extraction mechanisms for dealing with high-dimensional biomedical data. Also, explainable AI is mostly used in its post hoc form and not as an integral part of an adaptive decision-making process. Finally, the continuous adaptation of models to changing clinical situations is hampered by the absence of real-time data assimilation and feedback-based learning mechanisms. To address these limitations, this study proposes a conceptual adaptive stochastic-AI framework that integrates stochastic uncertainty modeling, transformer-based deep learning, explainable artificial intelligence, adaptive feedback learning and multimodal data fusion within a unified decision-support architecture. In Table 1, a comparative overview of existing decision-support systems for healthcare intelligence is provided.

Table 1. Comparative Analysis of Existing Intelligent Healthcare Decision-Support Systems

Reference	Methodology	Application Area	Key Contribution	Limitation
(Kim et al., 2024)	Systematic Review of XAI-based CDSS	Clinical decision support	Comprehensive analysis of explainable AI integration in healthcare systems	Limited practical adaptive implementation discussion
(Lee et al., 2025)	Pseudo-note generation from multi-stream EHR data	Electronic health record analytics	Improved contextual understanding for decision support	Limited uncertainty-aware adaptation
(Chen et al., 2023)	Expert-augmented AI framework	ICU mortality prediction	Combines clinician expertise with AI prediction	Restricted scalability to broader clinical domains
(Niu et al., 2024)	Explainable AI-based risk prediction model	Healthcare risk prediction	Improved interpretability with strong predictive accuracy	Limited real-time adaptability
(Liu et al., 2024)	Explainable clinical optimization framework	Clinical decision support optimization	Enhances clinician trust and system usability	Focuses mainly on interpretability
(Wysocki et al., 2023)	Human–AI communication analysis	Clinical usability evaluation	Identifies trust and explainability communication gaps	Does not propose adaptive framework solutions
(Düsing et al., 2024)	Federated learning with counterfactual explanations	Sepsis therapy decision support	Privacy-preserving explainable adaptive intelligence	Limited stochastic uncertainty modelling
(Hauskrecht, 2000)	Partially Observable Markov Decision Process (POMDP)	Medical decision support	Models sequential clinical decision-making under uncertainty using probabilistic patient-state representation	High computational complexity; lacks deep learning, adaptive learning, and explainable AI integration
(Pineau et al., 2003)	POMDP-based planning	Clinical treatment planning	Supports treatment planning under partially observable patient conditions	Limited scalability and unsuitable for high-dimensional biomedical data

continued on following page

Table 1. Continued

Reference	Methodology	Application Area	Key Contribution	Limitation
(Chakraborty and Moodie, 2013)	Dynamic Treatment Regime (DTR)	Personalized healthcare	Optimizes sequential treatment decisions based on evolving patient conditions	Does not incorporate real-time multimodal learning, deep learning, or explainable reasoning
(Holzinger and Müller, 2021)	Human–AI interface and causability analysis	Medical AI interaction systems	Introduces causability for explainable medical AI	Conceptual framework without implementation validation
(Nazar et al., 2021)	Systematic review of HCI and XAI healthcare systems	Explainable healthcare interfaces	Highlights importance of interactive explainability	Limited real-time system integration
(Rajabi and Etminani, 2021)	Knowledge graph-based explainable reasoning	Healthcare decision support	Transparent semantic reasoning capability	Limited deep learning integration
(Antoniadi et al., 2021)	Systematic review of XAI challenges	Machine learning-based CDSS	Identifies practical deployment barriers	Limited adaptive online learning discussion

Based on the comparison conducted from the perspective of the intelligent healthcare decision-making aid framework, as depicted in Table 1, it can be seen that although current intelligent healthcare decision-making aids have made substantial advancements in prediction accuracy, explainability, and privacy preservation, these elements are still addressed independently in current models. However, there currently exists no comprehensive framework that incorporates stochastic uncertainty modeling, adaptive learning, real-time data integration, explainable artificial intelligence and feedback loop processes.

STOCHASTIC MODELING IN HEALTHCARE SYSTEMS

Healthcare systems can be considered stochastic because they contain elements of uncertainty such as uncertain state transition probabilities, patient response variability, incompleteness of observations and constantly changing physiological states. Whereas deterministic models assume the same outputs for certain inputs, healthcare-related activities are affected by random variables that cause unpredictability in diagnosis, prognostication and therapeutic interventions. Thus, in order to design adaptive decision support systems for use in the context of healthcare management, probabilistic modeling approaches should be applied to address inherent randomness and make reliable predictions under uncertainties. As stochastic processes involve probabilistic description of state transition, healthcare systems can be formally defined using stochastic modeling techniques in order to develop an appropriate mathematical framework. In adaptive healthcare decision systems, the importance of stochastic models is determined by their ability to update predictions based on new observations.

Fundamentals of Stochastic Processes in Healthcare

A stochastic process is the set of random variables that change over time, and it represents the probabilistic progression of a system state. In the healthcare domain, stochastic processes might help represent physiological variations, development of diseases, treatment outcomes and recovery paths. The stochastic state of a patient at time t can be expressed as follows:

$$X(t) \in S \tag{1}$$

Where X(t) represents the patient's health state at time t, while S is the finite or continuous set of all possible clinical states. Some examples of clinical states that may be in the state space S include healthy stable state, slight clinical deterioration, severe deterioration, recovery and critically intervention needed states. They are some discrete abstractions of the patient's health process modeled using probabilistic transitions and observed physiologically, intervened with treatments or through latent disease processes and therefore can't be properly captured deterministically. Stochastic systems operate on the basis of probabilistic transition mechanism, which is defined by transition probabilities:

$$P_{ij} = P\left(X_{t+1} = j \mid X_t = i\right) \tag{2}$$

Where P_{ij} denotes the probability that a patient transitions from state i to state j during a given time interval. These transition probabilities enable predictive estimation of disease evolution and facilitate uncertainty-aware clinical decision-making.

Markov Models for Patient-State Transitions

Markov chains are one of the most popular frameworks used in health analytics due to their capability to model transitions in states of patients (Ghassemi et al., 2015). Markov processes involve an assumption that a future state of the system depends only on its current state, without any regard for the full history of how the process evolved. This process is shown in Figure 1 below. This relation can be represented as:

$$P\left(X_{t+1} \mid X_t, X_{t-1}, \ldots, X_0\right) = P\left(X_{t+1} \mid X_t\right) \tag{3}$$

Such simplification ensures efficient probabilistic inference without loss of meaningful temporal dependencies. Markov models have had many applications in the field of medicine such as disease progression, hospital readmission predictions, chronic disease management, cardiovascular risk surveillance and patient deterioration predictions in the ICU. An example of a model for cardiovascular surveillance could include the following states: normal rhythm, at-risk stage, arrhythmia stage, and emergency-critical state (Hauskrecht and Fraser.,2000). The probabilities of transitions between the states change depending on ECG readings, blood pressure changes and readings from wearables sensors, among others. Such a transition matrix can be shown as follows:

$$P = \begin{bmatrix} p_{11} & p_{12} & \cdots & p_{1n} \\ p_{21} & p_{22} & \cdots & p_{2n} \\ \vdots & \vdots & \ddots & \vdots \\ p_{n1} & p_{n2} & \cdots & p_{nn} \end{bmatrix} \tag{4}$$

This matrix provides the probabilistic foundation for predicting future patient trajectories and optimizing intervention timing.

Figure 1. Stochastic Patient-State Transition Model for Adaptive Healthcare Monitoring

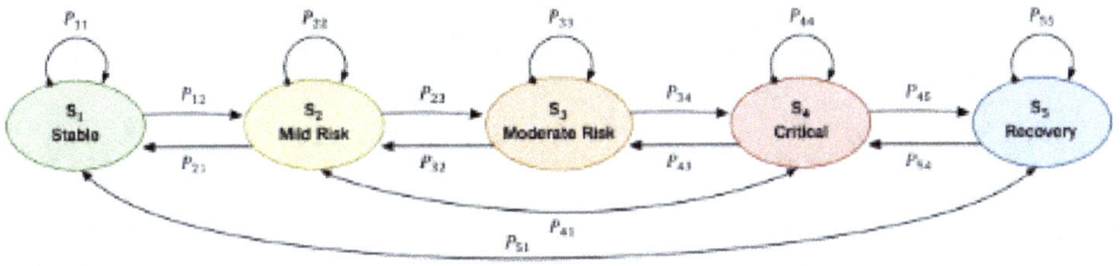

Hidden Markov Models in Clinical Observation Systems

Hidden Markov Models (HMMs) are extensions to Markov processes where latent state estimation takes place. Related probabilistic decision-making frameworks, including partially observable Markov decision processes (POMDPs), have also been applied to sequential clinical decision-making under uncertainty, particularly for treatment planning in chronic diseases (Hauskrecht & Fraser, 2000). For example, in a number of health care scenarios, the actual physiological state of an individual may not be known, but needs to be estimated based on observable features, which may include the electrocardiogram signal, oxygen level, laboratory tests and other wearable devices. An illustration of the HMM is provided in Figure 2. Hidden Markov Models (HMMs) are extensions to Markov processes where latent state estimation takes place:

$$P(O_t X_t) \quad (5)$$

Where O_t represents observable measurements generated probabilistically by hidden patient state X_t. Hidden Markov Models (HMMs) are particularly effective for stress detection from physiological signals, sleep-stage classification, neurological disorder progression analysis, cardiac abnormality detection and continuous patient monitoring (Doroshenkov et al., 2007). These models infer latent physiological conditions from noisy and incomplete sensor observations, enabling robust uncertainty-aware diagnosis in real-world healthcare settings.

Figure 2. Hidden Markov Model for Clinical Observation Inference

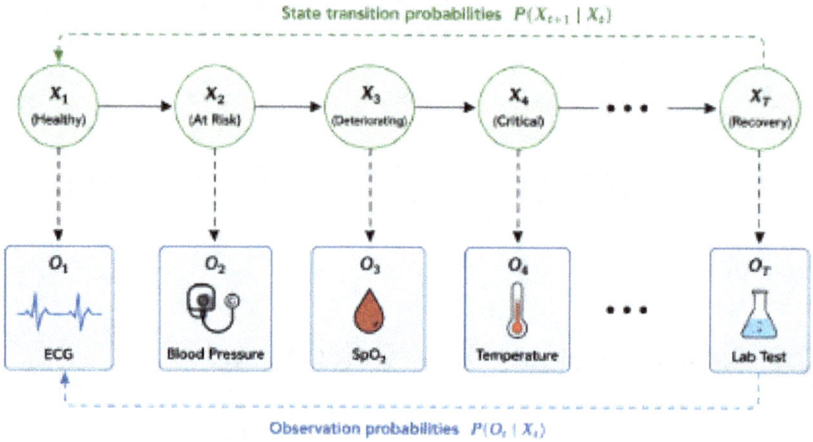

Bayesian Inference for Adaptive Clinical Learning

The Bayesian stochastic inference method can thus be used to continually update the probabilities of patient states as additional information is received. Figure 3 shows the Bayesian Adaptive Learning Framework for Real-Time Clinical Decision Updating.

The Bayes update formula is:

$$P\left(X \mid O\right) = \frac{P(O \mid X)P(X)}{P(O)} \tag{6}$$

Where:

$P(X)$: Prior belief

$P(O \mid X)$: Observation likelihood

$P(O)$: Normalization constant

$P(X \mid O)$: Posterior updated belief

This mechanism enables adaptive clinical decision systems to revise diagnostic confidence in real time. For example, wearable cardiac monitoring systems continuously update risk probabilities as new ECG measurements are received, enabling early anomaly detection and timely intervention.

Figure 3. Bayesian Adaptive Learning Framework for Real-Time Clinical Decision Updating

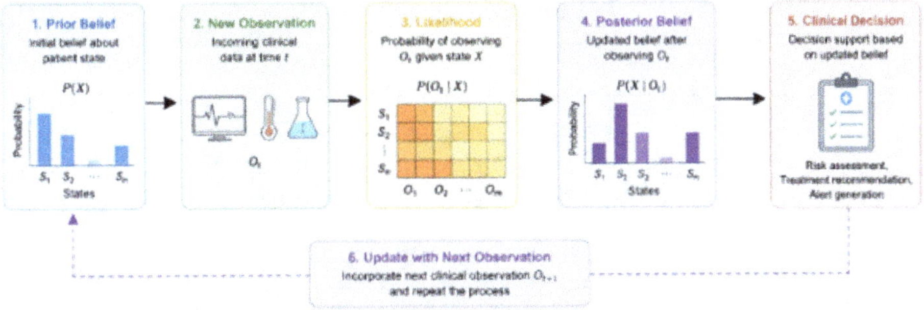

Dynamic Stochastic Adaptation in Real-Time Healthcare

Adaptive health care systems need continuous learning from streaming data in biomedical sciences. Static stochastic models cannot be used since patients' behavior is dynamic due to the reaction to the treatment received as well as other factors.

Dynamic stochastic adaptation uses changing probabilities of transitions:

$$P_{ij}(t+1) = f\left(P_{ij}(t), O_t\right) \tag{7}$$

Where new observations continuously improve estimates of uncertainties. In the proposed framework, the updated stochastic probabilities are subsequently provided as contextual information to the deep learning component. Rather than replacing probabilistic reasoning, the neural network utilizes the dynamically updated probability estimates together with physiological measurements as input features for predictive modeling. This hybrid architecture enables uncertainty-aware learning while preserving the interpretability of stochastic inference. This facilitates real-time monitoring of patient state, continuous reassessment of risks, customized adjustment of treatments and detection of anomalies. Adaptability is the mathematical principle underlying the combination of stochastic reasoning and deep learning based predictive intelligence in an adaptive health system. To ensure computational feasibility during real-time inference, only the most recent observations within a sliding temporal window are incorporated into each model update. Incremental probability estimation avoids complete retraining whenever new observations arrive, thereby reducing computational overhead while allowing continuous adaptation. This strategy enables scalable deployment in wearable monitoring systems, intensive care environments and other real-time healthcare applications. The stochastic approaches mentioned above provide the necessary theoretical framework for uncertainty-aware decision-making in the domain of healthcare. Their application together with modern artificial intelligence technologies provides smart clinical systems that can adapt continuously, reason predicatively and make robust decisions in the presence of dynamic uncertainty. Figure 4 demonstrates the workflow of dynamic stochastic adaptation in real-time health care systems.

Figure 4. Dynamic Stochastic Adaptation Workflow for Real-Time Healthcare Systems

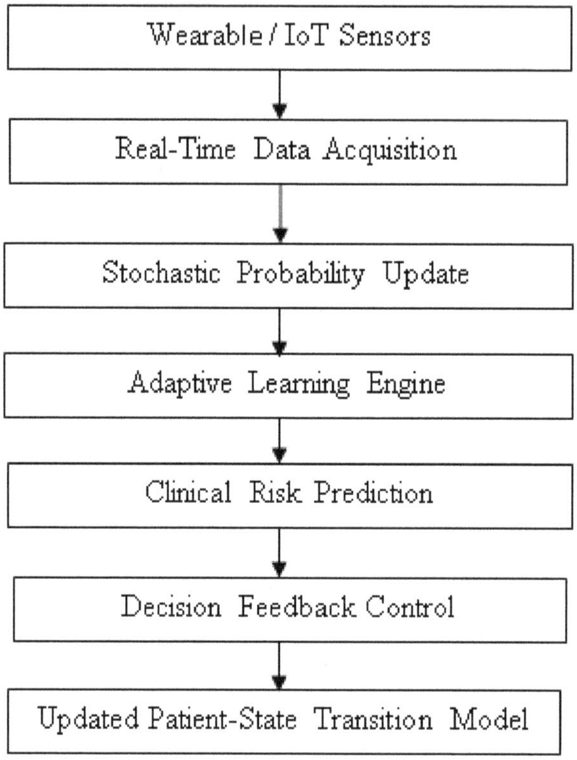

The stochastic modeling approach presented above is what forms the basis of adaptive decision making within the domain of healthcare based on probability principles. The stochastic layer creates an input for the artificial intelligence models discussed in the next section, where deep learning does the predictions while the stochastic inference is used for estimating uncertainties.

ARTIFICIAL INTELLIGENCE FOR REAL-TIME CLINICAL DECISION SUPPORT

Artificial intelligence has become an important tool for enhancing clinical decision-making through predictive analytics, intelligent monitoring and personalized medicine (Kim et al., 2024). The increasing use of electronic health records, wearable sensor information, medical imaging and biomedical big data has made it possible to develop AI-based systems that can assist in diagnosis and treatment planning in real time. In contrast to traditional methods that rely on fixed rules, AI models learn complicated interactions from multiple sources of healthcare data.

Machine Learning and Deep Learning for Clinical Prediction

Machine learning algorithms create associations between patient features and outcomes by leveraging previous healthcare data. This predictive modeling approach can be defined as follows:

$$y = f(x;\theta) \tag{8}$$

Where x indicates the vector of patient features, θ is the machine learning parameter vector and y indicates the predicted outcome. Popular machine learning methods such as decision tree, random forest, support vector machine and ensemble methods have been extensively employed for disease diagnosis, predicting patient risks and assessing patient outcomes. Deep learning approaches provide an even higher predictive performance level through automated learning of hierarchical features from complicated biomedical data. Hidden layer transformation can be formulated as follows:

$$h^{(l)} = \sigma(W^{(l)} h^{(l-1)} + b^{(l)}) \tag{9}$$

Here, W and b are the trainable parameters while σ is the nonlinear activation function. Deep learning has shown remarkable success in medical imaging, physiological signal processing and disease prediction applications through the direct extraction of patterns from raw healthcare data. Recent investigations into CNN-based deep learning architectures for cervical carcinoma analysis have further demonstrated the effectiveness of automated feature extraction and intelligent disease classification in medical imaging applications (Karthika and Premkumar, 2026). Federated learning enables collaborative model training across multiple healthcare institutions without exchanging sensitive patient data, thereby preserving privacy while improving model generalizability (Rieke et al., 2020). Multi-institutional federated learning has demonstrated its potential for secure medical AI by allowing decentralized optimization while maintaining data confidentiality (Sheller et al., 2020).

Transformer-Based Healthcare Intelligence

Transformers have become popular in healthcare applications lately due to their ability to efficiently model long-term temporal dependencies. Transformers use self-attention modules that work on entire sequences at once, unlike recurrent neural networks (Vaswani et al., 2017). The definition of the attention module is:

$$Attention\left(Q,K,V\right) = softmax\left(\frac{QK^T}{\sqrt{d_k}}\right)V \tag{10}$$

Where *Q*, *K*,and *V* represent query, key and value matrices, respectively. Transformer-based models have shown promising results in electronic health record analysis, disease progression prediction and patient-risk assessment by effectively modeling temporal healthcare data. Pretrained transformer models such as Med-BERT have demonstrated improved disease prediction by learning contextual representations from large-scale structured electronic health records (Rasmy et al., 2021).

Explainable AI and Online Adaptation

AI in clinical practice necessitates both transparency and trust. Techniques for explainable artificial intelligence (XAI), including SHAP, LIME, visualization of attention and counterfactual explanations, aid clinicians in comprehending the variables affecting the prediction made by the model. Additionally, hospitals and healthcare organizations have to cope with a constantly changing environment. As the condition of patients changes all the time, online learning allows AI to modify the parameter estimates based on the new observation:

$$\theta_{t+1} = \theta_t - \eta \nabla L(\theta_t) \tag{11}$$

Where η denotes the learning rate and L represents prediction loss.Continuous adaptation supports personalized monitoring, risk recalibration and timely intervention under changing clinical conditions.

AI–Stochastic Integration for Adaptive Decision Support

Although AI has significant capability to learn features and predict from those features, the use of stochastic modeling takes into account the uncertainties involved with the state changes of patients and incomplete information. The combination of stochastic reasoning and AI allows for uncertainty-based predictions and adaptive decision making in changing health care settings. This AI–stochastic framework forms the basis of the adaptive health care system described below.

PROPOSED ADAPTIVE STOCHASTIC–AI FRAMEWORK

The presented stochastic-AI framework aims at facilitating intelligent clinical decision-making in uncertain healthcare scenarios in real time. The framework is an ensemble of techniques such as stochastic patient state modeling, deep learning feature extraction, transformer temporal analysis, explainable reasoning processes and adaptive feedback control for facilitating continuous healthcare intelligence. Unlike traditional static clinical decision support systems, the presented adaptive framework updates its internal states with continuous biomedical observations, thus making the system adaptable with patient status. The presented adaptive framework architecture can be thought of as an intelligent decision-support pipeline consisting of several layers. These layers have different computational roles that collectively make it possible to achieve uncertainty-aware reasoning, predictive adaptation and clinical decisions. The presented adaptive framework analyzes heterogeneous healthcare data obtained from wearables, clinical information systems and biomedical databases, thereby converting observational data into adaptive clinical suggestions using stochastic-AI framework.

Figure 5. System Architecture of the Proposed Adaptive Stochastic–AI Healthcare Framework

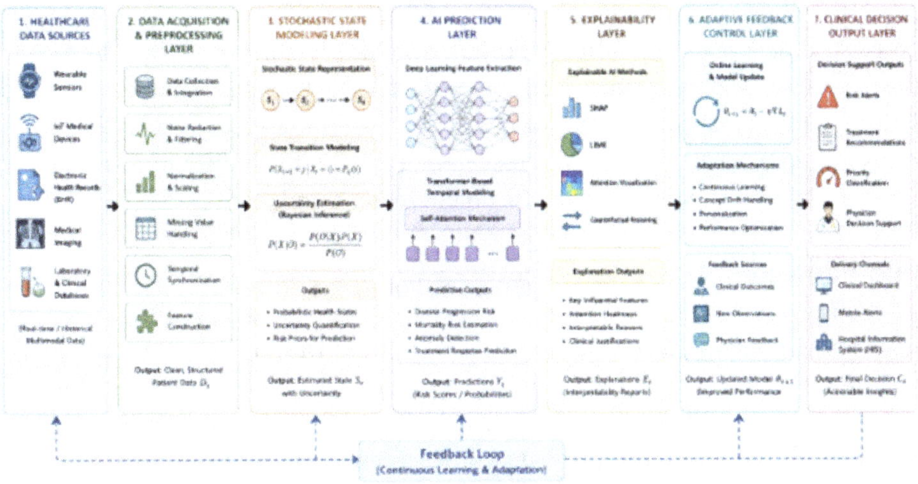

Framework Overview

The whole system works as an intelligent closed-loop reasoning system for clinical reasoning. The process involves continuous input of patient information, estimation of probabilistic health state transitions, identification of high-level clinical features, prediction of risk trajectories, generation of explanations and policy improvement.

The operation of the system is mathematically described as follows:

$$D_t \rightarrow S_t \rightarrow F_t \rightarrow P_t \rightarrow E_t \rightarrow A_t \quad (12)$$

Where:

D_t represents incoming healthcare data

S_t denotes stochastic state estimation

F_t corresponds to extracted feature representations

P_t represents predictive clinical outcomes

E_t denotes explainable reasoning outputs

A_t represents adaptive decision refinement

This sequential process enables continuous clinical learning and intelligent healthcare adaptation.

Distinction from Existing Adaptive Healthcare Architectures

Current adaptive architectures in healthcare are usually designed to incorporate particular capabilities, which may include but are not limited to predictive analytics, deep learning, explainable AI or privacy-preserving learning techniques. Although such approaches have proved their ability to significantly improve clinical decision-making, they often implement uncertainty modeling, adaptive learning, transparency and real-time data assimilation capabilities separately. In turn, the proposed adaptive stochastic–AI system brings together all the mentioned capabilities to develop an integrated architecture for intelligent healthcare decision support. Specifically, such architecture can combine stochastic patient-state modeling to quantify uncertainties, deep learning and transformers to provide intelligent predictions, explainable AI to ensure clinical reasoning, adaptive feedback control to continuously improve knowledge and multimodal data assimilation to enable real-time data collection. Moreover, the architecture is flexible enough to be used for various purposes, such as cardiovascular monitoring, chronic disease management, intensive care units, stress evaluation and personalized treatment recommendations.

Data Acquisition Layer

This layer captures diverse patient data from several sources within the healthcare ecosystem. These range from wearables, Internet of Things sensors, electronic health records, medical imaging devices and lab diagnosis databases. Physiological signals like heart rates, electrocardiogram signals, blood pressure, blood oxygen levels and glucose values are captured in real-time for dynamic awareness of patient states. Data preprocessing steps include normalization, noise reduction, missing value imputation, time synchronization and multimodal fusion. This ensures the integration of heterogeneous clinical data into cohesive patient states, ready for analysis using stochastic and AI methods. The continuous data capture capability of the framework allows quick responses to changes in patient physiological states.

Stochastic State Modelling Layer

The stochastic modeling layer uses probability-based state progression through a combination of Markov transition dynamics and Bayesian analysis mechanisms. Uncertainty is directly captured by this model due to physiological variation, incomplete observation and treatment responsiveness. Patient-state transitions are modelled as:

$$P\left(X_{t+1} = j \mid X_t = i\right) = P_{ij}(t) \tag{13}$$

Where $P_{ij}(t)$ represents time-varying transition probabilities between clinical states. The Bayesian update follows Equation (6).

Probabilistic thinking makes it possible to make reliable estimations of the patients' trajectories even when there is uncertainty involved. The stochastic component constitutes the mathematical basis for adaptive clinical intelligence by quantifying the uncertainty.

AI Prediction Layer

The AI prediction layer derives high-level representations for multimodal biomedical data through deep neural models and transformer-based analysis of time-series data.

The process of extracting features is defined as:

$$F_t = \phi\left(D_t; \theta\right) \tag{14}$$

Where ϕ denotes learned feature transformation and θ represents trainable network parameters. Transformer-based temporal modeling captures contextual relationships across longitudinal patient records:

$$P_t = Attention(Q, K, V) \tag{15}$$

This layer generates predictive outputs including disease progression probability, mortality risk estimation, anomaly detection alerts and treatment response prediction. These predictions provide actionable intelligence for clinical decision-making.

Explainability Layer

For purposes of clinical trust and interpretability, the proposed framework uses mechanisms of explainable reasoning to uncover factors that affect prediction performance. Explanability is defined as:

$$E_t = Explain\left(P_t, F_t\right) \tag{16}$$

The layer will generate explanations of prediction using feature importance, attention maps, counterfactual reasoning and explanations of medical decisions. Consequently, clinicians will be able to validate predictions and detect physiological signals that contribute to prediction accuracy.

Shap-Based Explainability Analysis

For further improvement of model's transparency, SHAP (SHapley Additive Explanations) is used within this framework for the purpose of interpreting feature-wise impact on risk prediction results. The importance scores for each physiological factor involved in predictive modeling are calculated using principles of cooperative game theory. In terms of cardiovascular monitoring tasks, the following physiological factors, including ECG irregularity, heart-rate variability, blood pressure, oxygen saturation and respiration rate, could be taken into account during interpretation of their effect on cardiovascular risk prediction. Features with positive SHAP values contribute to the increased risk prediction score, while negative values contribute to decreasing it. The explanations generated in such a manner would help clinicians make decisions about the impact of each physiological factor on predictions and facilitate trust towards the adaptive stochastic-AI framework proposed here. Table 2 presents an illustrative example of SHAP feature importance values and their corresponding clinical interpretations to demonstrate the explainability component of the proposed conceptual framework. These values are hypothetical and are provided solely for illustrative purposes; they are not derived from experimental evaluation or real clinical datasets. SHAP feature importance for cardiovascular risk prediction is visualized in Figure 6.

Table 2. Illustrative SHAP Feature Importance for Cardiovascular Risk Prediction

Physiological Feature	Mean SHAP Value	Clinical Interpretation
ECG Irregularity Index	0.42	Strong indicator of arrhythmia risk
Oxygen Saturation (SpO_2)	0.31	Low values indicate hypoxia-related risk
Heart Rate Variability	0.27	Reflects cardiovascular stress

Physiological Feature	Mean SHAP Value	Clinical Interpretation
Systolic Blood Pressure	0.22	Associated with hypertension risk
Respiratory Rate	0.16	Indicates physiological instability

ECG Irregularity Index and Oxygen Saturation emerge as the most influential predictors of cardiovascular risk, highlighting their clinical relevance in early detection of cardiac abnormalities.

Figure 6. SHAP Feature Importance Analysis for Cardiovascular Risk Prediction

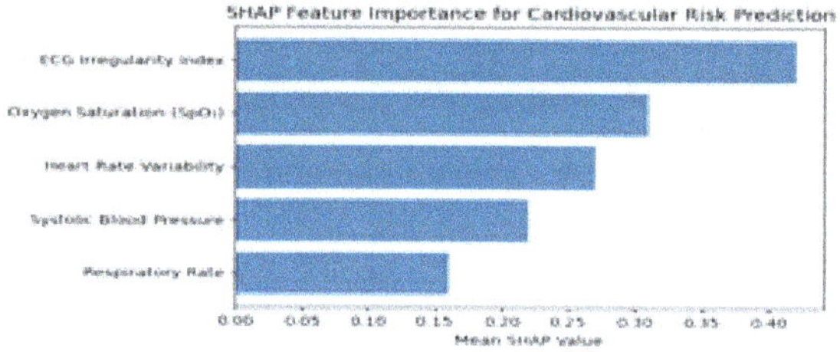

The adoption of Explainable Artificial Intelligence (XAI) will help to ensure that there is increased transparency and integrity within the framework. Through the implementation of feature attribution using SHAP, physicians can determine which physiological factors play an important role in the prediction of the risk of cardiovascular disease. Unlike traditional approaches where the black-box AI systems are used, the proposed framework comes with an interpretability feature, which helps validate its functionality and increase trust among physicians. Thus, the concept of XAI plays a vital role in ensuring human-centric healthcare decisions. Although SHAP is used within this framework, there are other explainable AI techniques that can be included.

Table 3. XAI Techniques Applicable to the Proposed Framework

XAI Technique	Purpose	Healthcare Benefit
SHAP	Feature importance analysis	Identifies influential biomarkers
LIME	Local explanation	Explains individual predictions
Attention Visualization	Temporal interpretation	Highlights critical signal segments
Counterfactual Analysis	What-if reasoning	Supports treatment planning

As shown in Table 3, distinct XAI methods offer various angles for the analysis of health care prediction through explanations, starting from feature-level attribution all the way up to patient-level and even counterfactual explanations. For instance, LIME (local interpretable model-agnostic explanation) is able to generate instance-level explanations, which would be achieved through approximations of the complicated model behavior around each prediction point. With respect to the practice in the clinic, LIME could assist physicians in understanding the reason behind the high-risk prediction of a particular patient.

Out of all these methods, SHAP is used in this proposed framework because of its solid theoretical underpinning and consistency, along with the capacity of generating both global and local explanations for predictions in health care. The use of SHAP along with attention visualization, LIME and counterfactual thinking makes up an explainability mechanism that allows for transparent clinical decision-making. These XAI approaches allow physicians to comprehend the reasoning behind predictions and verify automated recommendations.

Adaptive Feedback Control Layer

The adaptive control layer continuously refines model behavior using feedback from clinical outcomes and incoming patient observations. This adaptive mechanism enables continuous personalization, treatment-response learning, concept drift correction and online performance optimization. The feedback loop ensures sustained predictive reliability despite evolving healthcare conditions.

Clinical Decision Output Layer

The final layer converts adaptive predictive intelligence into actionable clinical recommendations. Decision output is represented as:

$$C_t = Decision(P_t, E_t, S_t) \tag{17}$$

The output comprises warning alarms, risk categorization, treatment recommendations and interventions to physicians. The recommendations help physicians make appropriate medical decisions under uncertainties. The system combines stochastic inference, deep learning, explainable artificial intelligence and feedback control in real-time. The structure is ideal for intelligent decision support systems for real-time health care applications.

Illustrative Cardiovascular Monitoring Scenario

The following section illustrates the real-life execution of the above-discussed AI-adaptive framework using a cardiovascular monitoring example. Monitoring of cardiovascular health disorders must be performed consistently since the physiological state of the patients tends to vary swiftly because of arrhythmia, fluctuating blood pressure, oxygen levels and responses to treatments. Conventional static monitoring systems do not perform adequately in detecting temporal changes in patients' conditions when they occur within uncertain environments. The suggested approach helps overcome these issues by leveraging stochastic reasoning, deep-learning predictions and adaptive learning in explainable AI frameworks.

As part of the suggested scenario, wearables gather biometric data such as electrocardiogram signals, heart rate, blood pressure, oxygen saturation, respiration rate and activity. The biomedical streams are sent to the adaptive healthcare intelligence system via IoT-based communication infrastructure. Real-time data collection allows for monitoring of the physiology of the patient at all times and helps detect any abnormalities related to the heart. The initial step of this framework uses stochastic patient-state estimation. Patient's cardiovascular state is characterized by probabilistic states of health which include healthy condition, increased cardiovascular risk, presence of arrhythmia and heart instability. As transitions in patient-state are random, a stochastic modeling process is used for estimating the probabilities of transitions between different states of physiology. This process can be expressed as:

$$P\left(X_{t+1} = j \mid X_t = i\right) = p_{ij} \tag{18}$$

Where p_{ij} represents the probability of transition from cardiovascular state i to state j. These transition probabilities are dynamically updated using incoming physiological observations, enabling continuous uncertainty-aware estimation of patient health trajectories. Post-stochastic state estimation, the AI prediction model employs deep learning and transformers to analyze biomedical data and generate representations that are pertinent to medical conditions such as arrhythmia, cardiac instability and irregularities in physiological dynamics. Transformers use attention algorithms to detect patterns in sequential physiological observations, capturing long-term dependencies and detecting key patterns linked to cardiac deterioration. The time-based attention mechanism can be defined in equation (10). The attention model allows accurate prediction of the dynamic behavior of the heart using live data acquired from wearable sensors. The predictive module then creates cardiovascular risk predictions, alerts and probabilities for future decline. In order to enhance adaptive reasoning, Bayesian updating techniques can be used to update the patient risk probabilities based on the newly acquired ECG/physiological observations. The process is depicted as follows:

$$P\left(X \mid O\right) = \frac{P(O \mid X)P(X)}{P(O)} \tag{19}$$

The process facilitates continuous updating of certainty levels when dealing with uncertain and changing physiological states. For instance, a patient's sudden ECG reading coupled with abnormal oxygen levels can raise the posterior probability that the patient is at risk of having arrhythmias. The explainability module adds value to the clinical experience by detecting the biological features that influence the outcomes of the predictions. The use of explainable AI approaches allows for the identification of important segments from the electrocardiogram waveforms, high blood pressure, oxygen level fluctuations and cardiac abnormalities over time that influence the prediction of cardiovascular risks. The adaptive feedback-control level continuously tunes the predictive model parameters using physiologic data streams and physician feedback in real-time. Real-time tuning makes it possible for the system to tailor its prediction behavior based on the patient's own cardiovascular system dynamics and treatment responses. Continuous adaptation ensures that predictive intelligence remains reliable despite physiological variability and changing cardiovascular conditions. Finally, the decision support level takes predictive intelligence and turns it into clinical interventions within the medical field. The system produces early warning alerts, cardiovascular risk stratifications, anomaly alerts and intervention advice for doctors. For instance, in a scenario where there is an increase in probability of arrhythmia and unstable physiological transitions, there may be immediate suggestions for doctors to make. Such an example scenario helps show how the proposed adaptive stochastic-AI paradigm would work as an intelligent closed-loop system for monitoring cardiac health, which can engage in uncertainty-informed reasoning, adaptive learning, explainable prediction and immediate clinical decision-making. It is through the combination of stochastic models, transformer analytics, explainable AI, and adaptive feedback that such a robust paradigm for intelligent cardiac health management is possible.

CONCEPTUAL PERFORMANCE EVALUATION METHODOLOGY

Given that this chapter discusses an adaptive healthcare framework conceptually, validation will involve assessing theoretical validity, architectural integration and application scenarios for healthcare purposes, as opposed to providing the implementation results empirically. Conceptual validation of the framework is based on its mathematical representation, the modular system design, comparison with current approaches used in healthcare decision making and an illustration on the cardiovascular monitoring process demonstrating stochastic reasoning, artificial intelligence, explainable AI and adaptive feedbacks. In addition, application scenarios of the framework are described in different healthcare areas such as chronic disease management, stress evaluation, intensive care monitoring and personalized treatment. Further work could consider the development of a prototype and its evaluation empirically using health data.

Performance assessment of adaptive healthcare systems plays an important role in measuring predictive reliability, adaptability, interpretability and operational efficiency in real-time. Considering that the presented stochastic-AI framework aims at developing an intelligent solution to the problem of uncertainty in clinical decision making, the validity of the approach would need to be verified by taking into account both traditional metrics of prediction performance and adaptability to changes. The proposed framework differs from classical solutions to the problem of predicting healthcare events by the necessity of constant performance assessment in dynamic conditions. Validating the presented approach would mean evaluating its predictive performance, awareness of uncertainty, adaptability to changing conditions, real-time computational performance and interpretability.

Predictive Performance Metrics

The performance prediction capability of the proposed framework can be evaluated using established health care evaluation metrics. Accuracy refers to the percentage of accurate predictions in relation to the total number of predictions made. Precision calculates the ratio of correct positive predictions against the total number of positive predictions, while recall determines how well the algorithm detects actual positive instances. Harmonic combination of precision and recall will be measured by the F1-score.

The F1-score is defined as:

$$F1 = 2 \cdot \frac{Precision \cdot Recall}{Precision + Recall} \tag{20}$$

The concepts of sensitivity and specificity are very vital in any healthcare applications that require a high degree of accuracy in detecting critical states. Sensitivity is concerned with the ability of the model to detect disease states or cases of disease progression while specificity indicates an ability to accurately classify stable or normal conditions. A further measure of classification ability is the area under receiver operating characteristic curve. This metric can be used for assessing prediction intelligibility by measuring separability between risk levels in uncertain healthcare settings.

Potential Datasets and Validation Strategy

Evaluation of the suggested adaptive stochastic-AI based system could be done through the use of publicly available biomedical data such as PhysioNet Database (Gouthamaan et al., 2025). These databases include data from real physiological measurements including ECG signal, heart rate variations and other cardiovascular-related biosignals. They have been extensively used within clinical studies in the area of cardiovascular risk evaluation, arrhythmia detection and patient monitoring systems. In addition, in order to model real-time uncertainty and changes in patient state evolution, synthetic patient trajectory data could be generated by using stochastic Markov transitions processes.

Adaptive Learning Validation

Because patients' statuses change constantly, the adaptive performance of the learning model should be assessed in addition to its accuracy in predicting the outcome. The capability of the system to adjust the prediction process according to the changing physiological status is measured by adaptation responsiveness and concept drift correction. Validation of such a procedure is performed through the measurement of convergence stability, adaptation rate and prediction consistency amid changes in physiological conditions. The method of temporal validation imitates real-time patient monitoring, where predictions are made based on incoming data. In such a way, the adaptability of the model amid varying physiological parameters, progression of the disease and changes in treatment is validated, thus ensuring that the system retains its clinical relevance.

Real-Time System Responsiveness

Timely decision making is facilitated through fast computation inferences which guarantee a prompt action by the health practitioner. Responsiveness is determined using the parameters such as inference delay, throughput rate and decision update rates. Inference delay represents the total time taken for clinical decision making once the observations are obtained. Short delays help in achieving quick response from the physicians during health emergencies including ICU deterioration and arrhythmia notifications. Throughput represents the capability of the algorithm in handling numerous patient data streams at one go hence showing the efficiency of the system in large-scale operations. The rate of decision update determines the ability of adaptive processes in improving predictions after receiving new patient data.

Explainability and Clinical Interpretability Assessment

Interpretability validation is critical to guaranteeing physician confidence and clinical adoption of intelligent decision support systems. The interpretability layer undergoes verification based on the criteria of transparency, relevancy and consistency of the explanations generated. Physicians test whether the selected influential physiologic features match existing medical science principles and whether explanations for predictions are comprehensible and actionable. Consistency of feature attributions is further verified through repeated observation tests. Quality of explanations impacts clinician confidence and affects the ability to include intelligent advice in clinical practice safely. Interpretability facilitates effective collaboration between humans and intelligent machines and provides necessary ethical guidance.

Comparative Validation Against Existing Systems

The suggested approach is examined comparatively against traditional methods of healthcare decision support based on rules, traditional machine-learning algorithms and static deep learning. While rules are easy to understand, they cannot cope with uncertain situations, making them inflexible. Predictive models of traditional machine learning can predict clinical behavior; however, they suffer from a rigid set of feature engineering principles. Finally, although static deep learning enables better representation, it usually lacks the ability to deal with concept drift. The proposed stochastic adaptive AI decision support method compensates for these deficiencies with probabilistic analysis, deep learning, dynamic adaptability and decision support explanation. This combination of capabilities makes it promising for healthcare application.

Table 4. Conceptual qualitative comparison of conventional healthcare decision-support approaches and the proposed adaptive stochastic–AI framework

Feature	Rule-Based Systems	Traditional Machine Learning	Static Deep Learning	Proposed Stochastic–AI Framework
Uncertainty handling	Limited	Moderate	Moderate	Robust
Continuous learning from new data	No	Limited	Limited	Adaptive
Real-time clinical decision support	Moderate	Good	Good	Enhanced
Prediction interpretability	High	Moderate	Limited	High
Concept drift management	No	Partial	Partial	Continuous adaptation
Suitability for dynamic healthcare environments	Limited	Moderate	Good	Comprehensive
Integration of probabilistic reasoning	No	Limited	No	Yes
Scalability for distributed healthcare systems	Limited	Moderate	Good	High

In Table 4, the comparison between the new adaptive stochastic-AI approach and traditional rule-based, machine learning and deep learning frameworks has been performed qualitatively on a conceptual level. As per the framework architecture presented, it can be predicted that the new adaptive stochastic-AI framework would offer benefits in the form of probabilistic reasoning, adaptive learning, real time decision support and explainable AI. The comparison has only been performed to give an idea about the benefits of the framework and not to validate its performance experimentally, which will be done in future research.

Figure 7. Conceptual illustration of the expected performance of the proposed adaptive stochastic–AI framework

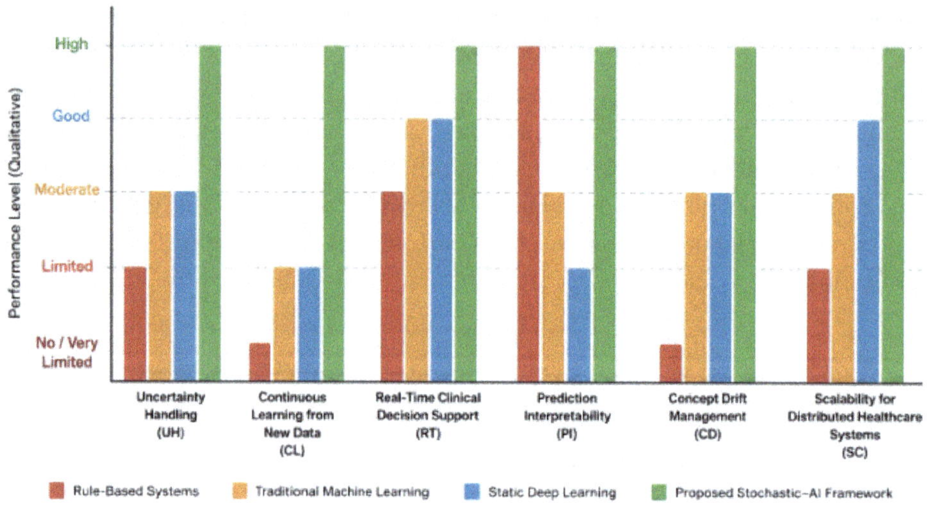

Figure 7 provides a conceptual visualization intended to illustrate the expected advantages of the proposed framework based on its architecture. It does not represent experimentally measured performance.

Scalability and Deployment Reliability

Healthcare systems should be able to cope with scalability issues, meaning that they have to work reliably at large scales with many patients, devices and distributed medical infrastructures. Therefore, scalability validation involves assessment of computational efficiency as the number of data increases and requirements for monitoring of multiple patients become higher. Performance evaluation regarding distributed deployment should focus on the measurement of communication efficiency between wearable devices, cloud healthcare systems and hospital information infrastructures. Validation of reliability will involve testing under conditions of faults such as observation incompleteness, intermittent sensory breakdowns and temporary communication failures. Given that the framework has a modular architecture; it would be possible to achieve scalability by making use of parallel AI inference and stochastic reasoning. Such an approach guarantees reliable performance within different environments while still maintaining predictive accuracy and responsiveness.

Long-Term Reliability and Concept Drift

The patient demographic, disease profile, treatment regimen and environment will always change with time. This result in concept drift, meaning that the statistics established during the training process will not apply anymore to current clinical practice. Adaptation provides a solution to this problem in that it is an ongoing process of adjustment to new conditions. Nevertheless, uncontrolled adaptation might bring about instability in models and lead to forgetting what has been learned earlier in terms of clinical knowledge. Thus, efficient implementation in the healthcare sector will need an effective approach to detecting drift, imposing stability constraints and occasionally updating knowledge through expert consultation. Consistency over an extended period of time represents one of the biggest challenges for sustainable adaptation of healthcare intelligence. The problems outlined above illustrate the difficulties of translating adaptive stochastic–AI solutions into practical applications in the healthcare sector.

APPLICATIONS OF THE PROPOSED FRAMEWORK IN HEALTHCARE

The following applications illustrate how the proposed framework could be applied in real-world healthcare scenarios. In each application, physiological and clinical data are collected through the data acquisition layer, stochastic state modelling captures uncertainty in patient conditions, AI models perform predictive analysis, explainable AI provides interpretable clinical insights and adaptive feedback continuously updates the model using new patient information. This integration enables intelligent, adaptive and reliable clinical decision support across diverse healthcare domains.

Cardiovascular Disease Monitoring

The mortality caused by cardiovascular diseases continues to persist, posing the need for constant patient surveillance and early detection of risks to minimize severe cardiovascular events. The suggested framework facilitates an adaptive monitoring approach through the integration of the patients' electrocardiogram, blood pressure, oxygen saturation and clinical history into one predictive intelligence system. The stochastic modeling component predicts the changes in the cardiovascular state as healthy, increased risks, onset of arrhythmia and cardiac instability. Through deep learning techniques, the model derives significant temporal features from the streaming ECGs, while transformer structures enable the identification of physiological dependencies across the patients' history. The adaptive feedback control module constantly updates prediction models upon the receipt of new physiological observations, hence ensuring that personalized risk factors are updated on time. Techniques for ensuring explainability focus on the cardiac biomarkers and ECG waveforms responsible for prediction outcomes, facilitating the understanding of recommendations made automatically. This application demonstrates how all components of the proposed framework work together. Wearable sensors acquire physiological data, stochastic modelling estimates cardiovascular state transitions, deep learning predicts disease risk, explainable AI identifies the most influential biomarkers and adaptive feedback continuously refines the prediction model to support timely clinical decision-making.

Stress Detection and Mental Health Assessment

Monitoring mental well-being has assumed greater significance with the increasing prevalence of stress disorders and growing need for constant evaluation of behavioral health status (Bobade & Vani, 2020). In the proposed system, the incorporation of multimodal physiological data for stress state recognition will include features like heart-rate variability, skin conductivity, breathing frequency, sleep quality parameters and activity measurements made using wearables. Latent stress-state changes under probabilistic physiological dynamics can be captured using the stochastic reasoning layer. Hidden state inference is employed to determine psychological stress evolution regardless of incomplete and inaccurate data. The deep learning algorithm is utilized to find out complex non-linear correlations between physiological characteristics and stress. Recent advances in EEG-based signal classification using hybrid deep learning and probabilistic models have demonstrated improved capability for recognizing complex neurological and cognitive patterns, further supporting intelligent stress and mental health assessment applications (Anupallavi et al.,2025) .Temporal attention mechanism is incorporated in order to account for long-term behavioral dependencies. The adaptive learning approach constantly updates stress recognition thresholds based on the physiological baseline of individuals.

Chronic Disease Management

Continuous monitoring and adaptive treatment optimization are required for diseases such as diabetes, high blood pressure, respiratory illnesses and malfunctioning kidneys. Static monitoring methods may not be able to accurately monitor the changing state of patients. The suggested framework facilitates intelligent chronic disease management via real-time patient-state monitoring and adaptive control. Sensor data, drug compliance, lifestyle and lab test results will all be used in stochastic patient-state models that predict disease trajectories. Predictive models built using deep learning can detect the deteriorating condition and predict future risks. An adaptive feedback system will constantly refine models based on the changing state, resulting in customized therapy recommendations. Explainable reasoning helps doctors make better decisions about patient risks and treatments.

Intensive Care and Emergency Risk Prediction

A critical-care setting is marked by a need for quick and precise decisions to deal with situations of extreme uncertainty. In ICUs, an abundance of physiological data is generated on a continuous basis that requires real-time analysis to discover signs of potentially dangerous patient deteriorations (Kate Curtis et al., 2021). The presented conceptual framework enables ICU intelligence through analysis of vital signs, laboratory reports, ventilation information and patient histories to assess the probability of life-threatening situations. Uncertainty modeling in a stochastic setting reflects the instability inherent in fast-changing physiological states. Deep predictive models recognize the slightest hints of clinical decline in the state of a patient. Transformers are used for temporal analytics in longitudinal ICU records in order to estimate mortality risks and create warning signals in time. An adaptive learning component constantly modifies the probability assessments after new intervention actions have been performed. Explainability components enable clinicians to understand the rationale behind critical-risk detection and intervention measures.

Personalized Treatment Recommendation

Healthcare treatments typically have strong individual effects due to various physiological characteristics, genetics, environment and medical history of patients. As such, static treatment regimens might be ineffective. By using this approach, we can build dynamic recommendations tailored to the patient response dynamics in time. Uncertainty in treatment is captured via stochastic transitions in states of patients. Deep learning models then learn personalized treatment-response patterns based on observed healthcare data over time. Adaptive optimization processes fine-tune recommendation policies upon new feedback about patient responses to treatments. Explainability allows us to understand treatment-recommendation rationale and thus help clinicians validate personalized treatment strategies.

Emerging AI Technologies for Adaptive Healthcare Intelligence

Modern developments in the field of artificial intelligence present exciting prospects for the emergence of adaptive healthcare systems. Foundation models trained using biomedical and clinical data offer excellent data representations capable of performing various healthcare tasks, such as disease diagnosis, prediction and clinical decision making. The adaptability of these representations in relation to diverse healthcare data sources offers an opportunity for significant improvements in terms of adaptive healthcare intelligence. Generative AI has proven to be quite promising in automated documentation, biomedical data synthesis, personalized patient communication and clinical decision making. Incorporating these generative models into adaptive healthcare systems will enable the realization of personalization alongside helping clinicians make decisions regarding healthcare problems. The digital twin concept makes it possible to develop virtual patients that constantly change according to physiological measurements. Such models allow for the personalization of disease surveillance, improved treatments, predictive medicine and the simulation of patient-specific clinical events. In addition to the conventional predictive approach, the causal AI helps discover the causes and effects between clinical variables, hence enhancing treatment decision-making and providing clinical decision-making support based on evidence under conditions of uncertainty. Through the identification of causality as opposed to correlation between clinical variables, causal AI can help improve the reliability and robustness of healthcare intelligence solutions. On the other hand, reinforcement learning offers adaptive decision-making abilities through continual interaction within a healthcare environment. Through the discovery of optimal decisions based on patient-specific sequences of actions and feedback, reinforcement learning can assist with personalized healthcare solutions and resource optimization within a healthcare environment. The use of such emerging technologies in combination with the proposed adaptive stochastic-AI approach will lead to more advanced healthcare ecosystems.

ETHICAL, REGULATORY, PRIVACY AND DEPLOYMENT CONSIDERATIONS

The implementation of adaptive stochastic-AI-based healthcare systems should also take into account various ethical, regulatory, privacy-related and operational aspects along with performance criteria such as predictive capabilities. In light of the fact that the application of any diagnostic approach has significant consequences for the health and wellbeing of patients, the development of intelligent healthcare solutions is expected to assist the physicians in making better decisions, not to substitute their professional expertise. First of all, it should be acknowledged that transparency and fairness are the key principles of ethics that are supposed to be considered when implementing AI in healthcare. Techniques such as SHAP, attention visualization and counterfactual reasoning make it possible to explain the reasons behind the model's predictions to clinicians and check the reliability of its recommendations. Bias detection should continue on an ongoing basis to ensure consistent model performance across different patient groups. Patient privacy is yet another crucial issue. Privacy-based solution like federated learning, secure data exchange, encryption techniques and access control systems could help facilitate collaboration in developing models without unnecessarily exposing patients' data. Compliance with relevant healthcare data privacy guidelines is necessary at the stage of designing and implementing the solution. Such considerations would also be crucial to ensure the safety of adaptive AI solutions' use within the healthcare setting. The implementation of intelligent systems should be subject to thorough testing and validation, as well as proper supervision by healthcare professionals. Documenting changes made to models, reasons behind predictions and the process of adaptive learning could enhance transparency and regulation compliance. Practical use in healthcare environments poses its own challenges. It is imperative for an adaptive health care system to function effectively even under conditions of incomplete observability, faulty sensors, latency in communication channels, and disparate data collected from different sources such as wearable technology, clinical information systems and cloud computing infrastructure. Effective fault tolerance measures, constant performance tracking and adaptive feedback control may be beneficial to increasing the reliability of such a system in a dynamic clinical environment. Ultimately, the success of adaptive stochastic-AI models in clinical settings will depend on their ability to incorporate various issues, including predictive accuracy, explainability, privacy protection, regulation, ethics and reliable deployment methods. Overall, these applications demonstrate that the proposed adaptive stochastic–AI framework provides a unified architecture for healthcare decision support by integrating stochastic reasoning, AI prediction, explainable intelligence and adaptive learning across multiple clinical domains.

FUTURE RESEARCH DIRECTIONS

Adaptive stochastic-AI-based healthcare systems constitute an area of ongoing research that has much promise for radically changing how decisions are made in healthcare settings. In the future, developments will likely center on federated or distributed learning methodologies which allow multiple entities to train algorithms collaboratively without jeopardizing patient data privacy. Innovations in the field of multimodal biomedical intelligence will make possible the effective utilization of data from a variety of sources, such as imaging studies, wearables, electronic health records, laboratory test results and genomic analysis. This will improve prediction through enhanced comprehension of the patient's state. The advent of digital twin technology is poised to revolutionize personalized medicine by enabling real-time modeling of patients' disease trajectory and response to treatment.

Moreover, reinforcement learning can provide exciting prospects in terms of adapting to patient-specific treatment by means of adaptive decision making based on personal and sequential approaches. In future, there would be an emphasis on explainability in the development of collaborative human-AI models, allowing clinicians to interact with, verify and further develop AI-recommended solutions using explainable reasoning methods. With the rise in popularity of wearable devices, new opportunities for developing light edge-intelligence solutions for real-time healthcare analytics, with low latency, will be sought. Another important factor that should be addressed in future developments is the problem of fairness, accountability and ethics, which requires developing adaptive systems that are able to detect bias and optimize their actions in a fair way. Finally, the integration of stochastic modeling, AI, distributed sensing, explainable reasoning and adaptive learning will give rise to intelligent and autonomous healthcare ecosystems that would offer continuous monitoring, predictive adaptation, personal intervention planning and clinical assistance. The proposed framework establishes a conceptual foundation for future prototype implementation and empirical evaluation using real-world healthcare datasets and clinical decision-support environments.

CONCLUSION

Healthcare systems operate in unpredictable and ever-changing environments in which the states of patients constantly change based on physiology, illness development and reaction to treatment. Deterministic decision support models, therefore, may be inadequate in tackling complexity, calling for intelligent approaches that are adaptive and uncertainty-aware in nature. An adaptive stochastic-AI approach for real-time clinical decision support was introduced in this chapter. The proposed approach encompasses stochastic patient-state modeling, deep learning, transformer-based temporal analytics, explainable AI and adaptive feedback control in order to provide real-time monitoring of the patient state, adaptive prediction and transparent decision making under uncertainty. Using probabilistic reasoning and cutting-edge AI techniques together, the proposed framework enables healthcare intelligence even under conditions of uncertainty caused by incomplete, noisy and evolving healthcare data. The potential applicability of the framework is illustrated across several healthcare domains. The applications of the framework included cardiovascular health monitoring, detection of stress, chronic disease management, prediction of risks during intensive care and generation of individualized treatment plans. Potential future extensions to the framework include integration of other approaches that fall under XAI, such as LIME, counterfactual analysis and federated learning approaches. Generally, the combination of stochastic analysis, adaptive artificial intelligence and explainable healthcare analytics offers an excellent basis for the development of intelligent healthcare solutions in the future. Despite its potential, the proposed framework has several limitations. It represents a conceptual architecture and has not yet been implemented or validated using real-world clinical datasets. Practical deployment will require efficient methods for learning transition probabilities, scalable integration of stochastic reasoning with deep learning, low-latency real-time inference, robust online explainability and extensive clinical validation before adoption in healthcare environments.

FUNDING

This research received no external funding.

COMPETING INTERESTS

The authors declare that they have no competing interests.

AI DISCLOSURE STATEMENT

AI tools were used solely for grammar and language correction.

REFERENCES

Antoniadi, A. M., Du, Y., Guendouz, Y., Wei, L., Mazo, C., Becker, B. A., & Mooney, C. (2021). Current challenges and future opportunities for XAI in machine learning-based clinical decision support systems: A systematic review. *Applied Sciences (Basel, Switzerland), 11*(11), 5088. DOI: 10.3390/app11115088

Anupallavi, S., Ashokkumar, S. R., Premkumar, M., & Sangeetha, R. (2025). Enhanced EEG signal classification through integrated DTCWT, human learning optimization, and optimized DBN-HMM models for improved performance. *Biomedical Signal Processing and Control, 110*, 108229. DOI: 10.1016/j.bspc.2025.108229

Bobade, P., & Vani, M. (2020). Stress detection with machine learning and deep learning using multimodal physiological data. In *Proceedings of the International Conference on Intelligent Computing and Remote Sensing Applications (ICIRCA)* (pp. 51–57). https://doi.org/DOI: 10.1109/ICIRCA48905.2020.9183244

Chakraborty, B., & Moodie, E. E. M. (2013). *Statistical Methods for Dynamic Treatment Regimes*. Springer., DOI: 10.1007/978-1-4614-7428-9

Chen, J., Lowin, M., Kellner, D., Hinz, O., Adam, E. H., Ippolito, A., & Wenger-Alakmeh, K. (2023). Designing expert-augmented clinical decision support systems to predict mortality risk in ICUs. *Kunstliche Intelligenz, 37*(2-4), 227–236. DOI: 10.1007/s13218-023-00808-7

Curtis, K., Munroe, B., Fry, M., Considine, J., Tuala, E., Watts, M., Alkhouri, H., Elphick, T., Ruperto, K., Barrass, J., Balzer, S., Chisholm, B., Van, C., & Shaban, R. Z. (2021). The implementation of an emergency nursing framework (HIRAID) reduces patient deterioration: A multi-centre quasi-experimental study. *International Emergency Nursing, 56*, 100976. DOI: 10.1016/j.ienj.2021.100976 PMID: 33882400

Doroshenkov, L., Konyshev, V. A., & Selishchev, S. (2007). Classification of human sleep stages based on EEG processing using hidden Markov models. *Medical Device Technology, 41*(1), 24–28. DOI: 10.1007/s10527-007-0006-5 PMID: 17419342

Düsing, C., Cimiano, P., Rehberg, S., Scherer, C., Kaup, O., Köster, C., Hellmich, S., Herrmann, D., Meier, K. L., Claßen, S., & Borgstedt, R. (2024). Integrating federated learning for improved counterfactual explanations in clinical decision support systems for sepsis therapy. *Artificial Intelligence in Medicine, 157*, 102982. DOI: 10.1016/j.artmed.2024.102982 PMID: 39277983

Ghassemi, M., Pimentel, M. A., Naumann, T., Brennan, T., Clifton, D. A., Szolovits, P., & Feng, M. (2015). A multivariate time series modeling approach to severity of illness assessment and forecasting in ICU with sparse, heterogeneous clinical data. *Proceedings of the AAAI Conference on Artificial Intelligence, 29*(1), 446–453. DOI: 10.1609/aaai.v29i1.9209 PMID: 27182460

Gouthamaan, M., Peimankar, A., Puthusserypady, S., Momeni, M., Asyari, R. A. I., Jahan, M. S., Moll, J., Wiil, U. K., & Ebrahimi, A. (2025). Explainable deep learning based techniques for ECG-based heart disease classification: A systematic literature review and future direction. *Computers in Biology and Medicine, 199*, 111324. DOI: 10.1016/j.compbiomed.2025.111324 PMID: 41265065

Hauskrecht, M. (2000). Value-function approximations for partially observable Markov decision processes. *Journal of Artificial Intelligence Research, 13*, 33–94. DOI: 10.1613/jair.678

Hauskrecht, M., & Fraser, H. (2000). Planning treatment of ischemic heart disease with partially observable Markov decision processes. *Artificial Intelligence in Medicine*, *18*(3), 221–244. DOI: 10.1016/S0933-3657(99)00042-1 PMID: 10675716

Holzinger, A., & Müller, H. (2021). Toward human–AI interfaces to support explainability and causability in medical AI. *Computer*, *54*(10), 78–86. DOI: 10.1109/MC.2021.3092610

Karthika, P., & Premkumar, M. (2026). An in-depth exploration of CNN-based deep learning models in cervical carcinoma analysis. *Advances in Biomarker Sciences and Technology*, *8*, 19–33. DOI: 10.1016/j.abst.2025.11.007

Kim, S. Y., Kim, D. H., Kim, M. J., Ko, H. J., & Jeong, O. R. (2024). XAI-based clinical decision support systems: A systematic review. *Applied Sciences (Basel, Switzerland)*, *14*(15), 6638. DOI: 10.3390/app14156638

Lee, S. A., Jain, S., Chen, A., Ono, K., Biswas, A., Rudas, Á., Fang, J., & Chiang, J. N. (2025). Clinical decision support using pseudo-notes from multiple streams of EHR data. *NPJ Digital Medicine*, *8*(1), 394. DOI: 10.1038/s41746-025-01777-x PMID: 40604255

Liu, S., McCoy, A. B., Peterson, J. F., Lasko, T. A., Sittig, D. F., Nelson, S. D., Andrews, J., Patterson, L., Cobb, C. M., Mulherin, D., Morton, C. T., & Wright, A. (2024). Leveraging explainable artificial intelligence to optimize clinical decision support. *Journal of the American Medical Informatics Association : JAMIA*, *31*(4), 968–974. DOI: 10.1093/jamia/ocae019 PMID: 38383050

Nazar, M., Alam, M., Yafi, E., & Mazliham, M. (2021). *A systematic review of human–computer interaction and explainable artificial intelligence in healthcare with artificial intelligence techniques*. IEEE., DOI: 10.1109/ACCESS.2021.3127881

Niu, S., Yin, Q., Ma, J., Song, Y., Xu, Y., Bai, L., Pan, W., & Yang, X. (2024). Enhancing healthcare decision support through explainable AI models for risk prediction. *Decision Support Systems*, *181*, 114228. DOI: 10.1016/j.dss.2024.114228

Pineau, J., Gordon, G., & Thrun, S. (2003). Point-based value iteration: An anytime algorithm for POMDPs. In *Proceedings of the 18th International Joint Conference on Artificial Intelligence (IJCAI 2003)* (pp. 1025–1032).

Rajabi, E., & Etminani, K. (2021). Towards a knowledge graph-based explainable decision support system in healthcare. *Studies in Health Technology and Informatics*, *281*, 502–503. DOI: 10.3233/SHTI210215 PMID: 34042621

Rasmy, L., Xiang, Y., Xie, Z., Tao, C., Zhi, D., & Zeng, J. (2021). Med-BERT: Pretrained contextualized embeddings on large-scale structured electronic health records for disease prediction. *npj. Digital Medicine*, *4*(1), 86. DOI: 10.1038/s41746-021-00455-y PMID: 34017034

Rieke, N., Hancox, J., Li, W., Milletarì, F., Roth, H. R., Albarqouni, S., Bakas, S., Galtier, M. N., Landman, B. A., Maier-Hein, K., Ourselin, S., Sheller, M., Summers, R. M., Trask, A., Xu, D., Baust, M., & Cardoso, M. J. (2020). The future of digital health with federated learning. *npj. Digital Medicine*, *3*(1), 119. DOI: 10.1038/s41746-020-00323-1 PMID: 33015372

Sangeetha, R., Premkumar, M., Ashokkumar, S. R., Mohanbabu, G., Anupallavi, S., & Gloria Jeyaraj, J. P. (2026). The digital technologies in healthcare: Navigating the digital transformation with security and operational efficiencies. In *BioMed Bots Assurance*. CRC Press., DOI: 10.1201/9781003561309-13

Sheller, M. J., Edwards, B., Reina, G. A., Martin, J., Pati, S., Kotrotsou, A., Milchenko, M., Xu, W., Marcus, D., Colen, R. R., & Bakas, S. (2020). Federated learning in medicine: Facilitating multi-institutional collaborations without sharing patient data. *Scientific Reports*, *10*(1), 12598. DOI: 10.1038/s41598-020-69250-1 PMID: 32724046

Vaswani, A., Shazeer, N., & Parmar, N.. (2017). Attention Is All You Need. *Advances in Neural Information Processing Systems*, *30*. Advance online publication. DOI: 10.48550/arXiv.1706.03762

Chapter 10
Stochastic Frameworks for Adaptive Remote Monitoring:
A POMDP Approach

Piero Giacomelli
http://orcid.org/0000-0001-7709-3338
SPAC spa, Italy

ABSTRACT

Remote patient monitoring (RPM) is moving from a peripheral telemedicine convenience to a routine component of healthcare delivery following the population aging in western countries. The clinical decisions it enables like: alerting a clinician, escalating care, changing therapy, or simply following up; are sequential, consequential, and must be made without direct observation of the patient's underlying physiological state. This chapter introduces the partially observable Markov decision process (POMDP) as a theoretical mathematical framework for such problems. It derives the belief-state representation, establishes the piecewise-linear convexity of the finite-horizon value function, and surveys exact and approximate solution methods with their convergence guarantees. Five remote-monitoring scenarios are formalised as concrete POMDP instances, and the framework is situated within contemporary machine-learning practice, including model learning from streaming data, deep belief representations, and off-policy evaluation of learned policies before clinical deployment.

INTRODUCTION

Healthcare delivery in the third decade of the twenty-first century is shaped by demographic, technological, and economic pressures whose joint effect is to push an ever-larger fraction of clinical observation outside the hospital and into the home. The aging of populations in high-income economies, the rising burden of chronic disease, and the limited capacity to scale inpatient services at the rate at which demand is growing have together changed how care is delivered. These pressures have made remote patient monitoring (RPM) a routine part of care rather than a peripheral telemedicine convenience. Continuous glucose monitors, implantable cardiac devices, home spirometers, smartphone-based symptom diaries, consumer-grade photoplethysmography, and, increasingly, ambient and contactless sensing modalities

DOI: 10.4018/979-8-3373-9705-4.ch010

now produce streams of physiological and behavioural data of a volume and granularity that no clinician could plausibly review by hand.

The clinical decisions that this stream of data is meant to inform are recognisably sequential and recognisably uncertain. At each moment a clinician — or, increasingly, an algorithm acting on the clinician's behalf — must decide whether the data warrant no action, a passive acknowledgement, an explicit alert to the patient or to a caregiver, a request for additional measurements, an outpatient escalation, or an emergency intervention. Each of these actions has an immediate cost and an indirect, distributional effect on the patient's future trajectory. The decision is sequential because the data continue to arrive, and any choice made now constrains the information and the options available later. It is uncertain because the underlying physiological state of the patient — the variable that the decision is ultimately about — is never directly observed. What is observed are noisy, intermittent, and sometimes biased proxies: a heart-rate trace from a wrist-worn device, a self-reported symptom score, a single capillary glucose measurement.

This combination of sequential decision-making under uncertainty about a latent state is, in mathematical terms, the defining structure of a *partially observable Markov decision process* (POMDP). The aim of this chapter is to demonstrate that the POMDP has the potential to become a canonical formal framework for adaptive RPM, to develop the framework with the rigour required to support its use as a research and design tool rather than as a metaphor, and to show by example how concrete clinical scenarios can be cast in its language.

Why Partial Observability Is Unavoidable in RPM

It is tempting, when first confronted with a problem of this kind, to seek refuge in simpler models. A purely descriptive Markov chain over clinical states (Beck & Pauker, 1983; Sonnenberg & Beck, 1993) has the virtue of mathematical simplicity and a long history in medical decision analysis; it is, however, descriptive rather than prescriptive, and it presupposes that the state is known. A Markov decision process (MDP) extends the chain with actions and rewards (Puterman, 1994) and admits a fully developed theory of optimal control, but it likewise assumes that the decision-maker observes the state at every step — an assumption that is reasonable for in-hospital care but untenable for remote monitoring. The defining feature of RPM is precisely that this assumption fails. There are at least three distinct sources of partial observability that any honest formulation must accommodate.

First, the *latency of clinical state*. The variables that matter clinically — the haemodynamic compensation reserve in heart failure, the trajectory of beta-cell function in type 2 diabetes, the inflammatory state of an airway in chronic obstructive pulmonary disease — are not measured directly by any sensor. They are inferred from proxies whose mapping to the underlying state is itself uncertain and patient-specific, and inexpensive consumer-grade devices may add further inaccuracy to that mapping.

Second, *sensor noise and missingness*. Even where a proxy is well calibrated, RPM data are characterised by measurement noise, by motion and contact artefacts, by adherence-driven gaps, and by systematic missingness that is rarely missing-at-random (Little & Rubin, 2019). A wrist-worn device that the patient removes during a poor night's sleep is silent precisely when its data would be most informative.

Third, *heterogeneous and time-varying response to action*. The effect of an intervention — say, a diuretic dose adjustment — is itself a random variable whose distribution depends on covariates that may be poorly known, and on the patient's evolving physiology. Even a clinician who fully understood the present state could not deterministically predict the next.

A POMDP unifies these three sources of uncertainty within a single mathematical object: a transition kernel encoding state and action dynamics, an observation kernel encoding the stochastic relationship between latent state and observed signal, and a reward function encoding the clinical and economic cost of each action–state pair. The price paid for this generality is computational: optimal POMDP planning is, in general, intractable, and a substantial fraction of this chapter is devoted to the question of which approximations preserve clinically meaningful structure.

Relation to Other Chapters in This Volume

This volume is organised around the proposition that healthcare's stochastic nature is best confronted with the formal language of stochastic processes. The present chapter occupies the artificial-intelligence and machine-learning lane of that proposition. Where the chapters on Markov chains, queueing theory, and martingales develop the descriptive and analytical apparatus for understanding healthcare's randomness, the POMDP chapter develops the prescriptive apparatus: given that the state is uncertain, what action should the system take, and how should that policy be learned and updated as data accumulate? In this sense, the POMDP is best understood not as a competitor to the Markov chain but as its natural extension into the controlled, learning regime. It is the formal substrate on which any genuinely adaptive RPM system must rest.

Contributions and Roadmap

This chapter makes four contributions. First, it provides a self-contained, measure-theoretically careful development of the POMDP framework, including a proof sketch of the Sondik–Smallwood piecewise-linear-convexity theorem and a discussion of complexity results that are too often invoked imprecisely in the applied literature. Second, it surveys the principal classes of POMDP solution methods — exact, point-based approximate, online sampling-based, and deep-reinforcement-learning — with explicit attention to their convergence guarantees and their suitability for the data-volume and latency regime characteristic of RPM. Third, it develops in compact but rigorous form five distinct clinical vignettes, each cast as a POMDP, and each chosen to illustrate a different combination of monitoring modality and decision horizon. Fourth, it closes by examining the integration of the POMDP framework with contemporary machine-learning practice, with a particular focus on model learning from streaming data, deep belief representations, and off-policy evaluation.

The chapter is organised as follows. It first establishes the probabilistic and decision-theoretic preliminaries, then develops the POMDP framework itself — belief states, the Bellman operator on the belief simplex, and the principal structural theorems. It next surveys solution methods, maps generic RPM scenarios onto the framework, and develops the five clinical vignettes. A discussion of the framework's integration with artificial intelligence and machine learning, a set of open problems, a statement of limitations, and a concluding synthesis complete the chapter.

MATHEMATICAL PRELIMINARIES

We collect here the probabilistic and decision-theoretic background on which the POMDP framework is built. The presentation is deliberately compact: the reader who requires a fuller treatment is referred to Çınlar (2011) for stochastic processes and to Puterman (1994) and Bertsekas (2017) for dynamic programming.

Filtered Probability Spaces and Stochastic Processes

Let $(\Omega, \mathcal{F}, \mathbb{P})$ be a probability space. A *filtration* $\{\mathcal{F}_t\}_{t \in \mathbb{T}}$ on Ω, indexed by a time set $\mathbb{T}$ (in this chapter, $\mathbb{T} = \mathbb{N}_0$), is a non-decreasing family of sub-σ-algebras $\mathcal{F}_s \subseteq \mathcal{F}_t \subseteq \mathcal{F}$ for $s \leq t$. The intuitive content of $\mathcal{F}_t$ is the collection of events that are decidable on the basis of information available up to time t. A *stochastic process* $X = \{X_t\}_{t \in \mathbb{T}}$ taking values in a measurable space $(\mathcal{X}, \mathcal{B}_{\mathcal{X}})$ is *adapted* to $\{\mathcal{F}_t\}$ if X_t is $\mathcal{F}_t$-measurable for every t.

A process X is *Markov* with respect to $\{\mathcal{F}_t\}$ if, for every bounded measurable $f: \mathcal{X} \to \mathbb{R}$ and every $s \leq t$,

$$\mathbb{E}[f(X_t) \mid \mathcal{F}_s] = \mathbb{E}[f(X_t) \mid X_s] \ \mathbb{P}\text{-a.s.}$$

The Markov property licenses the introduction of a *transition kernel* $P: \mathcal{X} \times \mathcal{B}_{\mathcal{X}} \to [0,1]$ such that $P(x, B) = \mathbb{P}(X_{t+1} \in B \mid X_t = x)$, time-homogeneity being assumed throughout for notational economy.

When $\mathcal{X}$ is finite or countable the kernel reduces to a stochastic matrix $P = (p_{ij})$ with $p_{ij} = \mathbb{P}(X_{t+1} = j \mid X_t = i)$ and $\sum_j p_{ij} = 1$. The treatment of recurrence, ergodicity, and stationary distributions follows the lines developed in the Markov-chain chapter of this volume; we shall draw on those results without re-deriving them.

Markov Decision Processes

A *Markov decision process* (MDP) extends the Markov chain by introducing a controlled transition kernel and a reward functional. Formally, an MDP is a tuple

$$\mathcal{M} = \langle \mathcal{S}, \mathcal{A}, T, R, \gamma \rangle$$

where $\mathcal{S}$ is a measurable state space (we assume finite throughout this section for clarity, though all results extend to Borel state spaces under standard regularity conditions); $\mathcal{A}$ is a finite action space; $T: \mathcal{S} \times \mathcal{A} \times \mathcal{S} \to [0,1]$ is the transition kernel, $T(s' \mid s, a) = \mathbb{P}(S_{t+1} = s' \mid S_t = s, A_t = a)$; $R: \mathcal{S} \times \mathcal{A} \to \mathbb{R}$ is the (bounded) reward function; and $\gamma \in [0,1)$ is a discount factor.

A *policy* $\pi: \mathcal{S} \to \Delta(\mathcal{A})$ is a (possibly randomised) mapping from states to action distributions, where $\Delta(\mathcal{A})$ denotes the simplex of probability measures on $\mathcal{A}$. The *value* of π from state s is the expected discounted return

$$V^{\pi}(s) = \mathbb{E}^{\pi}\left[\textstyle\sum_{t=0}^{\infty} \gamma^t R(S_t, A_t) \,\middle|\, S_0 = s\right],$$

with $\mathbb{E}^{\pi}$ denoting expectation under the law induced by T and π. The *optimal value function* is $V^*(s) = \sup_{\pi} V^{\pi}(s)$, the supremum being attained by some stationary deterministic policy π^* under the standing assumptions (Puterman, 1994, Theorem 6.2.10).

The Bellman Operator and Dynamic Programming

The cornerstone of MDP theory is the *Bellman optimality operator* $\mathcal{T}^*:\mathbb{R}^{\mathcal{S}} \to \mathbb{R}^{\mathcal{S}}$, defined for any bounded $V:\mathcal{S} \to \mathbb{R}$ by

$$\left(\mathcal{T}^* V\right)(s) = \max_{a\in\mathcal{A}}\left\{R(s,a) + \gamma\sum_{s'\in\mathcal{S}} T(s' \mid s,a)V(s')\right\}.$$

Equipping $\mathbb{R}^{\mathcal{S}}$ with the supremum norm $\| V\|_\infty = \max_s|V(s)|$, $\mathcal{T}^*$ is a γ-contraction:

$$\| \mathcal{T}^* V - \mathcal{T}^* V'\|_\infty \le \gamma \| V - V'\|_\infty.$$

By the Banach fixed-point theorem, $\mathcal{T}^*$ admits a unique fixed point V^* to which the iterates $V_{n+1} = \mathcal{T}^* V_n$ converge geometrically from any bounded initial V_0. This is the *value-iteration* algorithm; *policy iteration* and *linear programming* furnish alternative routes to V^* with their own advantages (Howard, 1960; d'Epenoux, 1963).

A pivotal feature of the MDP framework, and the one that the POMDP must give up, is the *full observability* of the state. The agent at time t knows S_t exactly and may therefore condition its action on S_t alone — a finite-dimensional sufficient statistic. In RPM and indeed in most clinical applications this assumption is untenable, and the formal apparatus must be extended.

THE POMDP FRAMEWORK

We now develop the partially observable Markov decision process. The key technical move is to replace the unobserved state by a probability distribution over states — the *belief state* — and to lift the dynamic-programming machinery to the belief simplex. Almost everything in this section dates from Åström (1965), Sondik (1971), Smallwood and Sondik (1973), and the syntheses by Lovejoy (1991) and Kaelbling, Littman, and Cassandra (1998); we follow their development closely while taking some care over measure-theoretic detail.

Definition

A *partially observable Markov decision process* is a tuple

$$\mathcal{P} = \left\langle \mathcal{S},\mathcal{A},T,\Omega,O,R,\gamma,b_0\right\rangle$$

where $\mathcal{S},\mathcal{A},T,R,\gamma$ are as in the MDP definition, and: Ω is a finite (or, more generally, measurable) *observation space*; $O:\mathcal{S}\times\mathcal{A}\times\Omega \to [0,1]$ is the *observation kernel*, $O(o \mid s',a) = \mathbb{P}(\Omega_{t+1} = o \mid S_{t+1} = s',A_t = a)$; and $b_0 \in \Delta(\mathcal{S})$ is the initial belief — a probability distribution over $\mathcal{S}$ encoding the agent's prior at $t = 0$.

The dynamics evolve as follows. At time t the system is in some unobserved state $S_t \in \mathcal{S}$. The agent, on the basis of its current belief b_t, selects an action $A_t \in \mathcal{A}$. The state transitions to $S_{t+1} \sim T(\cdot \mid S_t,A_t)$, an observation $\Omega_{t+1} \sim O(\cdot \mid S_{t+1},A_t)$ is generated, and the agent receives reward $R(S_t,A_t)$. The agent observes Ω_{t+1} but not S_{t+1}, and must update its belief accordingly. These conditional dependencies are displayed as a dynamic Bayesian network in Figure 1.

Figure 1. The POMDP represented as a dynamic Bayesian network. Latent states evolve under the action-dependent transition kernel; each state emits an observation through the observation kernel; actions, selected from the current belief, influence both the state transition and the reward.

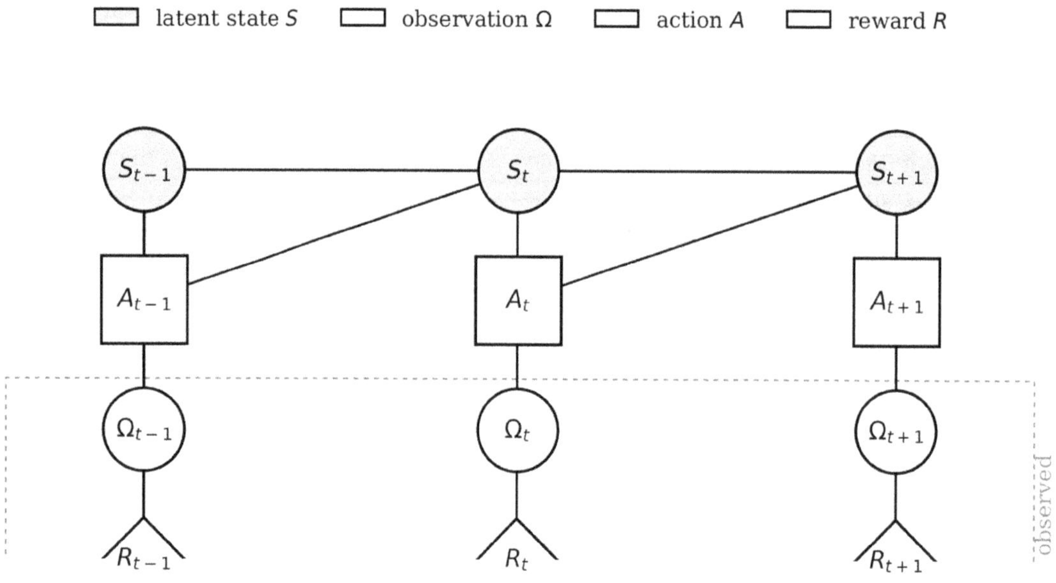

The Belief State and Bayesian Filtering

Given a current belief $b \in \Delta(\mathcal{S})$, an action $a \in \mathcal{A}$, and a subsequent observation $o \in \Omega$, the posterior belief $b' = \tau(b, a, o)$ is computed by Bayes' rule:

$$b'\left(s'\right) = \frac{O(o \mid s', a) \sum_{s \in \mathcal{S}} T(s' \mid s, a) b(s)}{\Pr(o \mid b, a)},$$

where the normalising constant

$$\Pr(o \mid b, a) = \sum_{s' \in \mathcal{S}} O(o \mid s', a) \sum_{s \in \mathcal{S}} T(s' \mid s, a) b(s)$$

is the predictive probability of observing o after taking action a from belief b. The map $\tau : \Delta(\mathcal{S}) \times \mathcal{A} \times \Omega \rightarrow \Delta(\mathcal{S})$ is the *belief update operator*; it is a discrete-time analogue of the filtering equations of stochastic control (Davis & Vinter, 1985). One cycle of this prediction-and-correction update is shown in Figure 2.

Figure 2. The belief-update (Bayesian filtering) cycle. A prior belief is propagated through the transition kernel to a predicted belief, which is then corrected by the observation likelihood to yield the posterior belief.

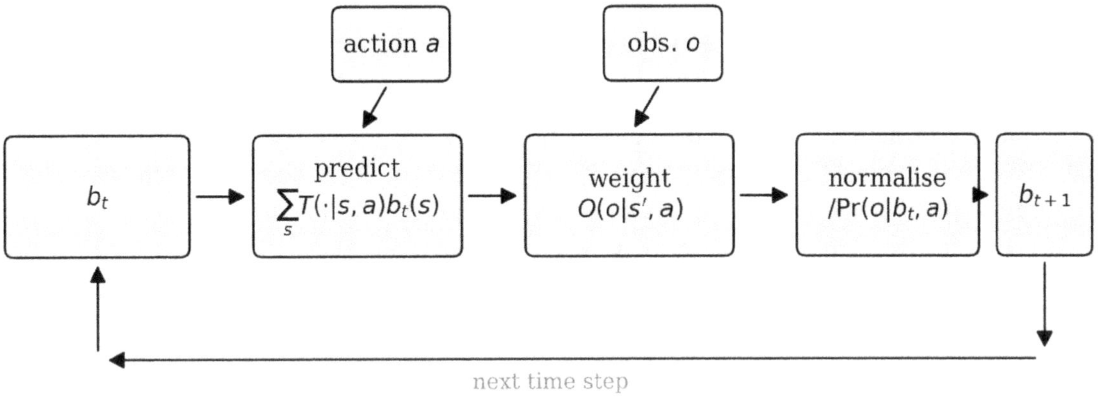

The crucial structural fact, due to Åström (1965), is that the belief b_t is a *sufficient statistic* for the entire history $h_t = (a_0, o_1, a_1, o_2, \ldots, a_{t-1}, o_t)$ in the following sense. Let $\mathscr{H}_t$ denote the set of histories of length t. Any history $h_t \in \mathscr{H}_t$ determines a belief $b_t = b_t(h_t)$ via repeated application of τ starting from b_0. Then for any optimal policy π^* the action $\pi^*(h_t)$ depends on h_t only through b_t. The proof is by backward induction on a finite horizon, with extension to the infinite-horizon discounted case via Banach's theorem; we omit the details, which are standard.

The Belief MDP

The sufficiency of the belief permits a reformulation of the POMDP as a fully observable MDP — the so-called *belief MDP* — over the (uncountable) state space $\Delta(\mathcal{S})$. Concretely, define a state space $\Delta(\mathcal{S})$ (the $|\mathcal{S}|$-dimensional probability simplex); an action space $\mathcal{A}$; a transition kernel $\tau^*: \Delta(\mathcal{S}) \times \mathcal{A} \times \Delta(\mathcal{S}) \to [0,1]$, where the probability mass placed on b' given (b,a) is $\sum_{o:\tau(b,a,o)=b'} \Pr(o \mid b,a)$; and a reward $\rho(b,a) = \sum_{s\in\mathcal{S}} R(s,a)\, b(s)$.

This belief MDP has the same discount factor γ, and its optimal value function $V^*: \Delta(\mathcal{S}) \to \mathbb{R}$ satisfies

$$V^*(b) = \max_{a\in\mathcal{A}} \{\rho(b,a) + \gamma \textstyle\sum_{o\in\Omega} \Pr(o \mid b,a)\, V^*(\tau(b,a,o))\},$$

which is the *belief-space Bellman equation*. The optimal POMDP policy is the optimal belief-MDP policy $\pi^*: \Delta(\mathcal{S}) \to \mathcal{A}$, viewed as a function of the belief.

The belief MDP is conceptually clean but numerically challenging: $\Delta(\mathcal{S})$ is a continuum even when $\mathcal{S}$ is finite, and direct application of value iteration is therefore non-trivial. The decisive structural result, to which we now turn, is that the value function V^* has a particularly tractable form.

Piecewise-Linearity and Convexity of the Value Function

Theorem 1 (Sondik, 1971; Smallwood & Sondik, 1973). Let $\mathscr{P}$ be a finite POMDP with finite horizon $H \in \mathbb{N}$. The optimal n-step value function $V_n^*:\Delta(\mathscr{S}) \to \mathbb{R}$, $0 \leq n \leq H$, is piecewise-linear and convex (PWLC) in b. That is, there exists a finite set $\Gamma_n \subset \mathbb{R}^{\mathscr{S}}$ of α-vectors such that

$$V_n^*\left(b\right) = \max_{\alpha \in \Gamma_n}\left\langle \alpha, b\right\rangle = \max_{\alpha \in \Gamma_n} \sum_{s \in \mathscr{S}} \alpha\left(s\right) b\left(s\right).$$

Proof sketch. Induction on n. The base case is immediate: $V_0^*(b) = 0$ corresponds to $\Gamma_0 = \{0\}$, trivially PWLC. Assume $V_{n-1}^* = \max_{\alpha \in \Gamma_{n-1}}\left\langle \alpha, \cdot \right\rangle$. Then for any $a \in \mathscr{A}$ and $o \in \Omega$ the term $V_{n-1}^*(\tau(b,a,o))$, after multiplication by $\Pr(o \mid b,a)$, becomes a maximum of *linear* functions of b, by direct expansion of τ and $\Pr(\cdot \mid b,a)$ — the normalising constants cancel. Thus

$$Q_n^*\left(b,a\right) = \rho\left(b,a\right) + \gamma \sum_{o \in \Omega} \max_{\alpha \in \Gamma_{n-1}} \langle \alpha^{a,o}, b\rangle$$

where $\alpha^{a,o}(s) = \sum_{s' \in \mathscr{S}} T(s' \mid s,a) O(o \mid s',a) \alpha(s')$. Maximisation over a preserves the PWLC structure, since the maximum of finitely many PWLC functions is PWLC. Collecting the resulting α-vectors gives Γ_n. □

The cardinality of Γ_n grows, in the worst case, as $|\mathscr{A}| \cdot |\Gamma_{n-1}|^{|\Omega|}$ — exponential in the horizon and the observation set. Pruning dominated α-vectors is therefore central to every exact algorithm; we return to this below. Geometrically, each α-vector is a linear functional of the belief, the value function is their upper envelope, and that envelope partitions the simplex into regions within which a single action is optimal.

The Infinite-Horizon Case

For infinite horizon and discount $\gamma < 1$, the belief-space Bellman operator $\mathscr{T}_b^*$ defined by

$$\left(\mathscr{T}_b^* V\right)\left(b\right) = \max_{a \in \mathscr{A}} \{\rho(b,a) + \gamma \sum_{o \in \Omega} \Pr(o \mid b,a) V(\tau(b,a,o))\}$$

is a γ-contraction on the Banach space of bounded measurable functions on $\Delta(\mathscr{S})$ under the supremum norm. The unique fixed point V_∞^* is the limit of the iterates $V_{n+1} = \mathscr{T}_b^* V_n$ from any bounded initialisation. Crucially, V_∞^* is convex but is *not* in general piecewise-linear: the limit of a sequence of PWLC functions need only be convex. However, V_∞^* can be uniformly approximated to any desired accuracy by PWLC functions, and in practice the finite-horizon α-vector representation, truncated at sufficiently large n, suffices.

Computational Complexity

The algorithmic implications of the above are unfavourable in the worst case. We collect the principal results without proof.

Theorem 2 (Papadimitriou & Tsitsiklis, 1987). *The decision problem of computing an optimal policy for a finite-horizon POMDP with finite state, action, and observation spaces is PSPACE-complete.*

Theorem 3 (Madani, Hanks, & Condon, 1999, 2003). *The problem of computing an optimal policy for an infinite-horizon discounted POMDP — equivalently, of deciding whether the optimal value exceeds a given threshold — is undecidable.*

These are worst-case results, and they should be read accordingly. They do not preclude the existence of efficient algorithms for *structured* POMDPs, and almost every successful application of POMDPs in healthcare and elsewhere has relied on exploiting such structure. They do, however, mean that any general-purpose RPM POMDP solver must be approximate, and that any claim of optimality must be qualified by the approximation regime under which it was obtained.

The principal classes of approximation — exact small-scale solvers, point-based methods, online tree search, and deep reinforcement learning — are the subject of the next section.

SOLUTION METHODS

The intractability results just established mean that practical POMDP planning for RPM applications is, with rare exceptions, an exercise in approximation. The literature offers a large body of methods, which it will be convenient to organise under four headings: exact small-scale solvers, point-based approximate solvers, online sampling-based planners, and reinforcement-learning extensions for high-dimensional or learned models. We review each in turn, with attention to the structural assumptions each requires, the convergence guarantees each affords, and the regime of RPM problems for which each is best suited.

Exact Value Iteration on the Belief Simplex

Exact methods exploit the PWLC representation of V_n^* established in Theorem 1. Each iteration computes the set Γ_n from Γ_{n-1} via the update

$$\Gamma_n = \text{prune}\left(\bigcup_{a\in\mathscr{A}}\Gamma_n^a\right),\ \Gamma_n^a = \text{prune}\left(\bigoplus_{o\in\Omega}\Gamma_n^{a,o}\right),$$

where $\Gamma_n^{a,o} = \{\alpha^{a,o}:\alpha \in \Gamma_{n-1}\}$ is the set of α-vectors after action a and observation o, $\oplus$ denotes the cross-sum (Minkowski sum of the underlying linear functionals), and prune($\cdot$) removes vectors that are dominated, in the sense that α is dominated by $\Gamma' \subseteq \Gamma$ if $\langle \alpha,b\rangle \leq \max_{\alpha'\in\Gamma'}\langle \alpha',b\rangle$ for all $b \in \Delta(\mathscr{S})$. Pruning is the algorithmic bottleneck: a naive linear-programming check costs $O(|\Gamma|)$ LPs per candidate vector, and naïve enumeration of Γ_n scales as $|\mathscr{A}| \cdot |\Gamma_{n-1}|^{|\Omega|}$.

The principal exact algorithms differ in how they organise this pruning. Sondik's (1971) one-pass algorithm and Monahan's (1982) enumeration are now of historical interest only. Cheng's (1988) linear-support algorithm exploits the fact that each α-vector is optimal on a polytope of beliefs and walks the dual graph of these polytopes. Cassandra, Littman, and Zhang's (1997) witness algorithm maintains, for each action, a frontier of α-vectors whose region of optimality is known, and identifies witness points — beliefs at which the current frontier is suboptimal — by linear programming. Incremental pruning (Cassandra, Littman, & Zhang, 1997; Zhang & Liu, 1996) prunes intermediate cross-sums $\Gamma_n^{a,o}$ before combining them, exploiting the observation that pruning the parts is computationally cheaper than pruning the whole. All exact methods produce Γ_n such that $V_n^*(b) = \max_{\alpha\in\Gamma_n}\langle \alpha,b\rangle$ pointwise, and all share the property of intractability for $|\mathscr{S}| \gtrsim 100$ — well below the size of any realistic RPM model.

Point-Based Methods

Point-based methods abandon the goal of exact reconstruction of V^* over the entire simplex and instead maintain a value function approximation $\widehat{V}$ that is exact at a finite set of belief points $B \subset \Delta(\mathcal{S})$ chosen adaptively from reachable beliefs. The seminal observation, due to Pineau, Gordon, and Thrun (2003, 2006), is that for many POMDPs the set of beliefs reachable from b_0 forms a low-dimensional manifold within the simplex, and a value function that is accurate on this manifold suffices.

The point-based value iteration (PBVI) algorithm maintains $\widehat{V} = \max_{\alpha \in \widetilde{\Gamma}} \langle \alpha, \cdot \rangle$, where $|\widetilde{\Gamma}| = |B|$ — exactly one α-vector per belief point. The key update is the point-based backup

$$\text{backup}(b) = \arg\max_{a \in \mathcal{A}} \left\{ \rho(b,a) + \gamma \sum_{o \in \Omega} \max_{\alpha \in \widetilde{\Gamma}} \left\langle \alpha^{a,o}, b \right\rangle \right\},$$

which produces a single α-vector per belief, with cost $O(|\mathcal{A}| \cdot |\Omega| \cdot |\mathcal{S}|^2 \cdot |\widetilde{\Gamma}|)$. Pineau et al. proved that the error $\| \widehat{V} - V^* \|_\infty$ is bounded by

$$\frac{R_{\max} - R_{\min}}{1 - \gamma} \cdot \epsilon_B,$$

where $\epsilon_B = \max_{b' \in \Delta(\mathcal{S})} \min_{b \in B} \| b - b' \|_1$ is the maximum L_1 distance from any reachable belief to its nearest neighbour in B. Subsequent point-based methods refine the choice of B and the order in which points are backed up.

Heuristic Search Value Iteration (HSVI; Smith & Simmons, 2004, 2005) maintains both upper and lower bounds on V^* and uses the gap between them to direct belief sampling. The algorithm enjoys an anytime property: at any point of execution $\widehat{V}_{\text{LB}} \leq V^* \leq \widehat{V}_{\text{UB}}$, with the gap $\widehat{V}_{\text{UB}}(b_0) - \widehat{V}_{\text{LB}}(b_0)$ shrinking monotonically. Successive Approximations of the Reachable Space under Optimal Policies (SARSOP; Kurniawati, Hsu, & Lee, 2008) further restricts sampling to the reachable space under near-optimal policies, with substantial empirical improvement on benchmarks. SARSOP and HSVI both provide ϵ-optimality guarantees in finite time under mild conditions on the reachable belief space, and are the practical workhorses for problems of size up to $|\mathcal{S}| \sim 10^4$.

Online Planning by Sampling

For larger state spaces, or for settings in which the model is implicit (as in simulation-defined POMDPs), the cost of any offline computation of $\widehat{V}$ over a representative belief set becomes prohibitive. Online methods construct, at each decision step, a planning tree rooted at the current belief and select the next action by approximate evaluation of this tree only.

Partially Observable Monte Carlo Planning (POMCP; Silver & Veness, 2010) is a UCT-style (Kocsis & Szepesvári, 2006) tree search that represents the belief implicitly as a set of state particles and propagates them through a generative model — a black-box simulator from which $(s', o, r) \sim G(s, a)$ samples can be drawn. POMCP enjoys an asymptotic optimality result: as the number of simulations $N \to \infty$, the value estimate at the root converges to $V^*(b_0)$ in probability. Determinized Sparse Partially Observable Tree (DESPOT; Ye, Somani, Hsu, & Lee, 2017) bounds the regret of online planning in terms of the width of the reachable space under deterministic scenarios sampled from the belief, and provides finite-sample anytime bounds.

The principal practical limitation of POMCP for RPM is the well-known particle-deprivation problem: as the planning horizon increases, the implicit belief held by the algorithm collapses to a small subset of states, with its variance under-representing the true posterior. Mitigations include particle reinvigoration, reweighting against an explicit observation model, and hybrid methods that combine particle filters with explicit Bayesian updates on factored components of the state.

Continuous-State and Continuous-Observation Extensions

RPM data are inherently continuous: heart rate, glucose concentration, oxygen saturation, and self-reported mood scores are real-valued. A finite-state POMDP can accommodate such observations only by discretisation, with attendant loss of fidelity and a combinatorial blow-up of $|\mathcal{S}|$. The literature offers several continuous extensions.

For linear-Gaussian POMDPs — those in which the state evolves as $S_{t+1} = A_a S_t + w_t, w_t \sim \mathcal{N}(0, Q_a)$, and observations are $\Omega_t = CS_t + v_t, v_t \sim \mathcal{N}(0, R_o)$ — the belief is itself Gaussian, parameterised by mean and covariance, and propagated by the Kalman filter (Kalman, 1960). The optimal value function under quadratic reward is then quadratic in the belief mean, and the optimal policy is a linear function thereof: the linear-quadratic-Gaussian (LQG) regulator. While the LQG assumptions rarely hold exactly in clinical settings, they furnish a benchmark against which more elaborate models can be compared.

For nonlinear, non-Gaussian dynamics the standard tool is the particle filter (Doucet, de Freitas, & Gordon, 2001; Thrun, Burgard, & Fox, 2005), which represents the belief as a weighted set of state samples. PEGASUS (Ng & Jordan, 2000) and policy-gradient methods that operate directly on parameterised policies $\pi_\theta(a \mid b)$ extend the framework to settings where neither the value function nor the model admits analytic structure. Gaussian-process POMDPs (Deisenroth & Peters, 2012; Engel, Mannor, & Meir, 2003) provide nonparametric representations of dynamics and value with calibrated uncertainty.

Choosing a Method for an RPM Application

The choice of solution method for a given RPM POMDP is a multi-criterion decision in its own right. The dominant considerations are: (i) the size of the latent state space, after factoring; (ii) the dimensionality of observations, and whether they are discrete or continuous; (iii) the planning horizon — minutes for an alert, months for a titration policy; (iv) whether the model is given analytically or only as a simulator; and (v) whether the policy must be computed offline once or repeatedly online. As a rough guide, exact methods are appropriate only for highly abstracted toy problems used for didactic or sensitivity-analysis purposes; SARSOP and HSVI dominate for moderate finite POMDPs with offline planning; POMCP and DESPOT dominate for large or simulator-defined problems requiring online decisions; and Gaussian or particle-filter methods, often combined with the deep neural representations discussed in the section on artificial intelligence and machine learning below, dominate for high-dimensional continuous RPM streams.

ADAPTIVE REMOTE MONITORING AS A POMDP

We now turn to the central modelling task of the chapter: the systematic translation of a clinical RPM problem into the POMDP language developed above. The goal of this section is not to present a single canonical model — RPM is too heterogeneous for that — but to develop the mappings between clinical entities and POMDP components in sufficient generality that a reader can carry out the translation for a new clinical context. Concrete instantiations follow in the next section.

The Generic RPM POMDP

Consider a chronic-disease patient enrolled in a remote-monitoring programme. At each decision epoch t — which may be a minute, an hour, a day, or a week, depending on the application — the patient is in some clinical state S_t that is not directly observed. A monitoring system collects an observation Ω_t from one or more sensors, possibly augmented by patient-reported outcomes (PROs), and a clinician — or an algorithm acting on the clinician's authority — selects an action A_t from a discrete set of possibilities. The patient's state then evolves according to physiology and the chosen action, and the cycle repeats. Figure 3 summarises the resulting closed-loop architecture.

Figure 3. Architecture of an adaptive remote-monitoring system viewed as a POMDP. Sensor streams and patient-reported outcomes form the observation vector; a Bayesian filter maintains the belief over the latent clinical state; and a policy maps the belief to a monitoring, alerting, or escalation action whose effect feeds back into the patient's physiology.

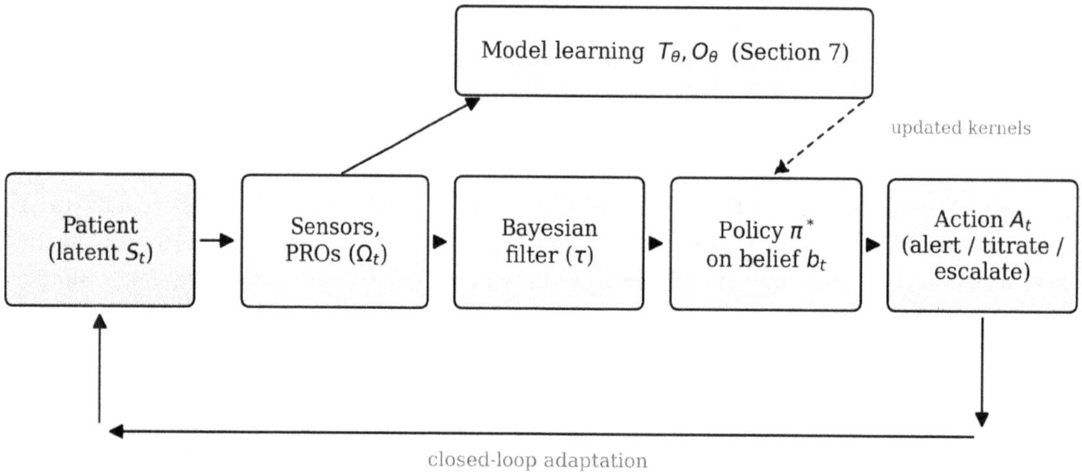

The POMDP tuple $\langle \mathcal{S}, \mathcal{A}, T, \Omega, O, R, \gamma, b_0 \rangle$ acquires the following clinical interpretations.

State space $\mathcal{S}$. The latent state encodes those clinical variables that drive both the observation distribution and the consequences of action. In a chronic-disease application the natural decomposition is into a *stable disease severity* component (e.g., NYHA class, GOLD stage, HbA1c-equivalent), an *acute decompensation* component capturing imminent events (e.g., pulmonary congestion, hypoglycaemic risk), and *covariate* components such as adherence and behavioural context. A factored representation $S_t = \left(S_t^{(1)}, \ldots, S_t^{(k)}\right)$ — formally a *factored POMDP* (Boutilier, Dean, & Hanks, 1999; Hansen & Feng, 2000) — exploits the fact that not all components depend on all others, often reducing the effective state-space size by orders of magnitude.

Action space $\mathscr{A}$. The action set typically contains a *do-nothing* action a_0 (continue passive monitoring), one or more *information-gathering* actions (request additional measurement, schedule a video consultation), one or more *patient-directed* actions (issue lifestyle prompt, suggest medication dose adjustment within a pre-authorised range), and *escalation* actions (notify clinician, schedule outpatient review, dispatch ambulance). A subtle but important point is that information-gathering actions are not free: each measurement imposes a burden on the patient and, in the case of clinician contact, on system resources. The reward function must reflect this; otherwise the optimal policy degenerates to perpetual maximal observation.

Transition kernel T. The kernel $T(s' \mid s, a)$ captures both the natural stochastic evolution of the disease and the modulating effect of action. For chronic conditions the dominant temporal structure is slow drift in severity punctuated by stochastic acute events, often well modelled as a *semi-Markov* process (Howard, 1971; Çınlar, 2011) and approximable by a Markov chain on a finely discretised state space. The action dependence enters principally through the acute-event hazard: a prompt-driven medication adherence improvement, for example, reduces the per-period probability of decompensation.

Observation kernel O. This is the most clinically distinctive component of the model. The observation Ω_t is typically a *vector* of sensor readings and PROs, each with its own noise model, missingness probability, and bias structure. A first-order decomposition factors the observation into independent channels:

$$O\left(o \mid s', a\right) = \prod_{j=1}^{m} O_j(o^{(j)} \mid s', a),$$

each O_j being a univariate distribution conditioned on the state. Conditional independence given the state is a strong assumption — sensor channels often share artefacts driven by patient behaviour — and a more refined treatment introduces a latent *context* variable that captures shared modes of failure. Missingness is modelled by treating "missing" as an additional observation symbol and learning $\Pr(\text{missing} \mid s', a)$ explicitly; this distinguishes informative from non-informative missingness.

Reward function R. The reward function is the most consequential modelling choice in any healthcare POMDP, because it encodes the trade-offs that the optimal policy will subsequently honour. The general form is

$$R(s,a) = U(s) - C_{\text{action}}(a) - C_{\text{burden}}(a,s) - C_{\text{event}}(s,a),$$

where $U(s)$ is a utility associated with the state (often an instantaneous health-state utility derived from quality-adjusted life-year analysis; Drummond et al., 2015), $C_{\text{action}}(a)$ is the direct cost of the action (clinician time, ambulance dispatch), $C_{\text{burden}}(a,s)$ captures patient-borne burden — dependent on state because, for example, an alert is more burdensome to a depressed patient than to an asymptomatic one — and $C_{\text{event}}(s,a)$ aggregates expected costs of adverse events whose probability depends on (s, a). Calibration of these terms requires careful elicitation; sensitivity analysis is essential.

Discount factor γ. The discount factor formalises the trade-off between immediate and future reward. A naive translation of an annual time-preference rate to a per-minute discount factor produces a γ so close to one that finite-horizon truncation becomes the binding constraint, and most RPM applications are best framed as finite-horizon problems with a terminal value capturing long-run prognosis.

Initial belief b_0. The prior over S_0 is typically constructed from baseline assessment data — clinical history, baseline biomarkers, demographic risk factors — through a previously trained patient-stratification model. The use of a personalised b_0 rather than a population prior is one of the principal mechanisms by which the POMDP framework realises adaptive, patient-specific monitoring.

Factored, Hierarchical, and Multi-Resolution Structure

The "curse of dimensionality" attaches to POMDPs more severely than to MDPs because the belief simplex is itself $|\mathcal{S}|$-dimensional. RPM applications routinely exhibit structural features that, when exploited, reduce the effective dimensionality dramatically.

Factored POMDPs (Boutilier et al., 1999) assume that $\mathcal{S} = \prod_{i=1}^{k} \mathcal{S}^{(i)}$ and that the transition kernel factors as a *dynamic Bayesian network* (Murphy, 2002) over these components. Symbolic representations such as algebraic decision diagrams (Hansen & Feng, 2000) permit value iteration directly in the factored representation, often with exponential savings.

Hierarchical POMDPs (Pineau, Gordon, & Thrun, 2003; Theocharous, Murphy, & Kaelbling, 2004) introduce a layered policy structure in which high-level options — themselves POMDPs — invoke low-level POMDPs as subroutines. In RPM this hierarchy maps naturally onto clinical workflow: a high-level "monitoring vs. escalate" policy, beneath which a low-level "alerting" POMDP determines per-day actions.

Multi-resolution approaches discretise time and state at multiple scales, with a coarse-grained POMDP making strategic decisions (titration, escalation) and a fine-grained POMDP making tactical decisions (alerting, additional measurement). Coupling between scales is provided by a Bayesian filter that propagates belief between resolutions. Figure 4 depicts this hierarchical, multi-resolution organisation.

Figure 4. Hierarchical and multi-resolution POMDP structure for remote patient monitoring. A coarse-grained strategic POMDP governing titration and escalation sits above a fine-grained tactical POMDP governing alerting and measurement; the two layers are coupled through a shared belief propagated by Bayesian filtering.

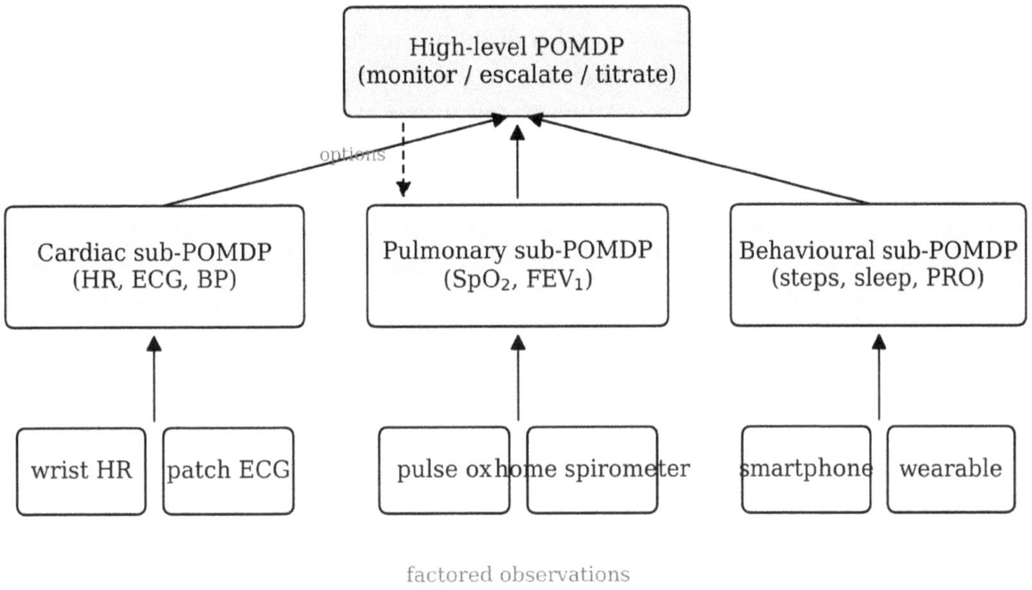

Short-Horizon and Long-Horizon Decisions

The decisions implicated in adaptive RPM span two orders of magnitude in their natural time-scale, and this disparity is itself a structural property of the framework that should be made explicit.

Short-horizon decisions are those whose effect plays out over minutes to hours: should an arrhythmia detected by an implantable monitor trigger an alert? Should a hypoglycaemic projection prompt an intervention? Such decisions are typically formulated as POMDPs with a short planning horizon, a coarse but high-frequency state representation, and an action set dominated by alerting and information-gathering options. The reward function emphasises the immediate trade-off between false-positive and false-negative alerts, with the long-run value typically absorbed into a terminal reward.

Long-horizon decisions play out over weeks to years: should a heart-failure patient have her diuretic dose titrated up? Should a diabetic patient's basal insulin be adjusted? Long-horizon POMDPs feature finely resolved state spaces, low-frequency decision epochs, and reward functions that integrate over multiple events.

The two horizons are not independent. The optimal long-horizon titration policy depends on the empirical rate of decompensation events, which is itself a consequence of the short-horizon alerting policy in operation. A consistent treatment requires that the short-horizon POMDP be solved as a sub-policy within the long-horizon problem, or — more commonly in practice — that the two be coupled through shared state estimates updated by the same Bayesian filter. This is precisely the multi-resolution structure described above.

Identifiability and the Role of Patient History

One feature of RPM POMDPs that distinguishes them from textbook examples is the substantial *patient history* available before monitoring begins. Electronic-health-record data, prior hospitalisations, medication history, and baseline biomarkers all furnish information about the patient's latent state at $t = 0$, and indeed about patient-specific parameters of T and O. The model that an algorithm operates upon at $t = 0$ is therefore not a generic population model but a personalised model conditioned on history.

This raises a subtle but important identifiability question. The posterior over patient-specific parameters, given a finite history, is generally non-degenerate; the algorithm operates with uncertainty about the model itself, not only about the state. Formally this is a *Bayes-adaptive POMDP* (Ross, Pineau, Chaib-draa, & Kreitmann, 2011) — a POMDP whose state space is the Cartesian product of the original state and the parameter, with a prior over parameters propagated by Bayesian updating. Bayes-adaptive POMDPs enjoy clean theoretical properties but are computationally demanding, and most practical implementations approximate the parameter posterior by point estimates, by ensemble methods, or by neural amortised inference, as discussed below.

CLINICAL VIGNETTES

We present five compact POMDP formulations corresponding to distinct clinical settings, each chosen to exhibit a different combination of monitoring modality, decision horizon, and structural feature. They are illustrative rather than exhaustive.

Chronic Heart Failure With Wearable Monitoring

Heart failure with reduced ejection fraction is a paradigmatic chronic condition for RPM. Patients exhibit slow progression in baseline severity, punctuated by acute decompensation episodes that, if detected early, can often be managed at home or in an outpatient setting rather than requiring hospitalisation (Yancy et al., 2017).

A POMDP formulation might take $\mathcal{S} = \mathcal{S}^{(\text{sev})} \times \mathcal{S}^{(\text{cong})} \times \mathcal{S}^{(\text{adh})}$, with severity discretised into NYHA-equivalent classes, congestion into a four-level ordinal scale, and adherence as a binary indicator. Observations comprise daily weight, resting heart rate, heart-rate variability, and a brief PRO score. Actions are: continue passive monitoring; issue an adherence prompt; escalate to a nurse phone call; dispatch a home visit. The reward function penalises hospitalisations and unscheduled emergency-department visits at a rate of approximately one quality-adjusted life-day per averted admission, balanced against the per-action cost of nurse contact.

The dominant structural feature is the *tail risk*: most periods are uneventful, but the cost of a missed decompensation is large. Risk-sensitive variants of the Bellman equation (Marcus et al., 1997) or constrained POMDPs that bound the per-patient probability of an undetected decompensation (Isom, Meyn, & Braatz, 2008) are particularly natural here.

Diabetes and Continuous Glucose Monitoring

Type 1 diabetes managed with an automated insulin delivery system represents the closest of all the vignettes to a fully closed-loop control problem. Continuous glucose monitors deliver an interstitial-glucose reading every five minutes; an automated insulin pump can deliver basal and bolus doses on a similar schedule; and the relationship between insulin, glucose, and the patient's underlying physiology is captured by well-established physiological models (Bergman et al., 1979; Hovorka et al., 2004).

A POMDP formulation takes $\mathcal{S}$ to encode plasma glucose, interstitial glucose, insulin-on-board, meal absorption, and slowly varying insulin sensitivity. Observations are the noisy interstitial glucose trace and, episodically, patient-reported meals. Actions are micro-doses of insulin or, in the dual-hormone variant, micro-doses of glucagon. The reward function penalises deviations from a target glucose range, with asymmetric penalties reflecting the relatively greater morbidity of hypoglycaemia.

The continuous-state, continuous-observation structure makes this vignette a natural fit for the LQG and particle-filter methods described earlier. The dominant clinical concern — avoidance of nocturnal hypoglycaemia under conditions of changing insulin sensitivity — is precisely a problem of sequential decision-making under partial observability, with the latent insulin-sensitivity state both unobserved and time-varying.

Chronic Obstructive Pulmonary Disease

COPD exacerbations resemble heart-failure decompensations in their clinical structure: slow background progression, acute episodes that benefit from early detection, and substantial heterogeneity between patients (Vogelmeier et al., 2017). The available RPM modalities include home spirometry, pulse oximetry, and PRO-based symptom diaries.

A POMDP formulation factors $\mathcal{S}$ into background severity (GOLD stage), inflammatory state, and exposure context (e.g., respiratory infection). Observations are FEV_1, SpO_2, cough frequency from a smartphone microphone, and a PRO score such as the CAT (COPD Assessment Test). Actions span passive monitoring, prompts to use a rescue inhaler, prescription of oral corticosteroids under a pre-agreed protocol, and clinician escalation.

The notable structural feature is the *coupled timescale*: spirometry and SpO_2 may be measured daily, while PROs may be daily or weekly, and clinical reviews monthly. A multi-resolution POMDP with explicit acknowledgement of asynchronous observations is the appropriate model.

Post-Surgical Home Recovery

Post-surgical RPM differs from the chronic-disease vignettes in that the relevant horizon is bounded — typically thirty days post-discharge — and the decision is dominated by readmission avoidance (Bates et al., 2014). Monitoring modalities include vital signs, wound-imaging via smartphone camera, patient-reported pain and function scores, and step counts.

A finite-horizon POMDP with $T = 30$ days and a state encoding wound healing, infection risk, and functional recovery captures the structure cleanly. Observations are the multi-modal stream above; actions are nurse contact, scheduling of an unscheduled clinic visit, and readmission. The reward function is dominated by a large penalty for readmission, balanced against the per-day cost of monitoring and the small but non-zero cost of unnecessary clinic visits.

The defining feature is the *learning regime*: the patient's recovery trajectory is informative about their future, and a Bayes-adaptive formulation (described earlier) is particularly attractive when the same model must be used across heterogeneous surgical populations.

Smartphone-Based Mental-Health Monitoring

Mood disorders such as major depression and bipolar disorder furnish the most challenging of the five vignettes, both clinically and statistically. Symptoms are subjective, observations are dominated by PROs and behavioural proxies (text-message frequency, sleep-onset times, geolocation entropy), and the relationship between observation and latent mood state is strongly patient-specific (Insel, 2017; Mohr, Zhang, & Schueller, 2017).

A POMDP formulation takes $\mathcal{S}$ as a low-dimensional latent mood representation — often itself learned from data via a generative model — and observations as a vector of behavioural and PRO-based proxies. Actions include passive monitoring, push-notification-delivered cognitive-behavioural micro-interventions, prompts to schedule a therapist contact, and clinician alerts.

The vignette illustrates two distinctive themes. First, the observation kernel must be learned, often per patient, because the mapping between behaviour and mood is idiosyncratic. Second, the action space includes interventions that themselves alter the patient's relationship with the monitoring system — alerts may be ignored, micro-interventions may produce reactance — making the problem one of meta-control as much as of control.

INTEGRATING POMDPS WITH ARTIFICIAL INTELLIGENCE AND MACHINE LEARNING

The POMDP framework as developed above assumes that the model — the kernels T and O, the reward R, and the prior b_0 — is given. In real RPM applications none of these is given fully a priori. The model must be learned, refined, and personalised as data accumulate. This section examines the principal mechanisms by which contemporary machine learning realises this learning loop within a POMDP framework, and the principal pitfalls of doing so in clinical settings.

Model Learning From Streaming Clinical Data

The simplest learning question is parametric: given a fixed structure for T and O, estimate the parameters from observed trajectories $\{(a_t, o_t)\}_{t=1}^{N}$. When the latent state is observed in part of the data — for instance, when ground-truth disease severity is assessed at clinic visits — the problem reduces to supervised learning of a hidden Markov model with covariates and admits classical maximum-likelihood estimation by the Baum–Welch (Baum, Petrie, Soules, & Weiss, 1970) or expectation–maximisation (Dempster, Laird, & Rubin, 1977) algorithms.

When the latent state is never directly observed, identifiability is non-trivial. Anandkumar, Hsu, and Kakade (2012) showed, building on the work of Hsu, Kakade, and Zhang (2012), that hidden Markov models with $|\mathcal{S}|$ states are identifiable from third-order moments of the observation process under mild conditions, and developed a tensor-decomposition algorithm with finite-sample guarantees. These results extend to controlled HMMs and provide a theoretically clean route to model learning from RPM data.

Bayesian alternatives place priors over T and O and use Markov-chain Monte Carlo (Gelman et al., 2013) or variational inference (Blei, Kucukelbir, & McAuliffe, 2017) to approximate the posterior. The advantage in clinical applications is calibrated parameter uncertainty: the posterior over kernel parameters can be propagated into the planning problem, yielding a Bayes-adaptive POMDP whose policy is robust to the parameter uncertainty implicit in finite training data.

Streaming and online estimation impose a further constraint: the model must be updated as new observations arrive, ideally without re-processing the entire history. Recursive Bayesian updates, online EM (Cappé & Moulines, 2009), and stochastic variational inference (Hoffman, Blei, Wang, & Paisley, 2013) all furnish such updates. In RPM the relevant unit of online learning is often the individual patient: a population model, learned offline, supplies the prior; per-patient online updates personalise the model as data accumulate.

Deep Belief Representations

The POMDP framework as classically formulated represents the belief as a categorical distribution on $|\mathcal{S}|$ atoms — a representation that scales linearly in $|\mathcal{S}|$ and so becomes prohibitive for the high-dimensional, structured latent spaces appropriate to many RPM applications. Deep generative models offer an alternative: the belief is represented implicitly as the parameters of a distribution in a low-dimensional latent space, with the encoding learned end-to-end from data.

The *deep recurrent Q-network* (DRQN; Hausknecht & Stone, 2015) replaces the explicit belief with the hidden state of a recurrent neural network trained to summarise the observation history sufficiently for value estimation. Asymptotically, under universal-approximation arguments, the recurrent state plays the role of a sufficient statistic. *Deep variational reinforcement learning* (DVRL; Igl et al., 2018) makes the analogy explicit, training a variational autoencoder over latent state alongside a value function over its parameters; the approach has been shown to outperform DRQN on benchmark POMDPs by virtue of its more disciplined uncertainty representation.

The most influential of recent developments is the family of *world-model* methods exemplified by PlaNet (Hafner et al., 2019) and Dreamer (Hafner, Lillicrap, Ba, & Norouzi, 2020; Hafner, Pasukonis, Ba, & Lillicrap, 2023). A world model is a latent-variable generative model of the environment, trained to predict observations and rewards from a sequence of actions, against which a policy can be optimised by gradient ascent on imagined trajectories. World models effectively combine model learning, belief representation, and planning into a single end-to-end-trained system, and have been shown to learn high-performing policies from images with sample efficiencies that approach those of model-free methods given orders of magnitude more data.

For RPM the appeal of world-model methods is twofold. First, they can ingest heterogeneous, high-dimensional observation streams — sensor traces, images, text — without manual feature engineering. Second, the latent state representation can be inspected and probed for clinically meaningful structure, although this inspection is far from automatic.

The principal caveat is that the asymptotic guarantees rely on infinite data and infinite capacity, neither of which is available in clinical settings. Recent work on *posterior sampling for reinforcement learning* (Osband, Russo, & Van Roy, 2013; Osband, Van Roy, Russo, & Wen, 2019) and on *information-theoretic exploration bonuses* (Houthooft et al., 2016) provides rigorous treatment of the exploration problem under finite samples; the application of these methods to RPM is a topic of active research.

Off-Policy Evaluation and the Safety Problem

The most urgent obstacle to deploying learned POMDP policies in clinical practice is the *off-policy evaluation* (OPE) problem: how to estimate the expected return of a candidate policy from data generated by a different (typically clinician-driven) behavioural policy, without prospectively running the candidate (Precup, Sutton, & Singh, 2000). Prospective evaluation is, in clinical settings, both expensive and ethically fraught; OPE is the only available substitute.

Classical importance-sampling estimators provide unbiased estimates under known behavioural policies but suffer from variance that is exponential in the planning horizon — the well-known *curse of horizon* (Liu, Li, Tang, & Zhou, 2018). *Doubly-robust* estimators (Jiang & Li, 2016) combine importance sampling with a learned value-function baseline, retaining unbiasedness if either component is correctly specified and exhibiting substantially reduced variance in practice. *Marginalised importance-sampling* methods (Liu et al., 2018; Nachum, Chow, Dai, & Li, 2019) re-weight by the *stationary state-action distribution* rather than the per-step behaviour, breaking the horizon dependence.

In a POMDP setting OPE is further complicated by the fact that the behavioural policy may have conditioned on information unavailable to the candidate — the clinician's tacit assessment of the patient's state, for example — producing a *hidden-confounder* problem (Namkoong, Keramati, Yadlowsky, & Brunskill, 2020; Tennenholtz, Mannor, & Shalit, 2020). Sensitivity analysis under bounded confounding is the standard partial remedy: the OPE estimate is augmented by bounds on its possible deviation under any confounder satisfying a specified bound on its strength.

For RPM the implication is that OPE results should be interpreted as one component of a multi-part validation strategy, not as a standalone basis for clinical deployment. Synthetic-data evaluation against high-fidelity simulators, prospective evaluation against contemporaneous controls, and conservative deployment with hard safety constraints are all complementary, and all are necessary.

Constrained and Safe POMDPs

The reward formulation introduced earlier embeds clinical constraints — avoidance of serious adverse events, bounds on patient burden — as soft penalties. For genuinely safety-critical applications a hard-constraint formulation is preferable. *Constrained POMDPs* (Isom et al., 2008; Lee, Hauskrecht, & Cooper, 2018; Kim, Lee, Lee, & Sung, 2011) augment the standard POMDP with a vector of cost functions $C_i: \mathcal{S} \times \mathcal{A} \to \mathbb{R}_{\geq 0}$, $i = 1, \ldots, k$, each of which the policy must keep below a specified threshold $\bar{c}_i$ in expectation:

$$\mathbb{E}^{\pi}\left[\sum_t \gamma^t C_i(S_t, A_t)\right] \leq \bar{c}_i.$$

The Lagrangian dual of the constrained problem reduces to a family of unconstrained POMDPs parameterised by the dual multipliers; the Lagrangian dual point of view connects the constrained POMDP to risk-sensitive control (Marcus et al., 1997) and to robust-Bayes adaptive control.

In the deep-RL setting, *Lagrangian primal-dual methods* (Achiam, Held, Tamar, & Abbeel, 2017; Tessler, Mankowitz, & Mannor, 2019) implement the same idea by adjoining the constraint violations to the policy-gradient loss, with the multipliers themselves updated by gradient ascent. Recent work (Ray, Achiam, & Amodei, 2019; Stooke, Achiam, & Abbeel, 2020) addresses the well-known instability of these methods. For RPM the constrained-POMDP formulation is particularly attractive because it permits a clean separation between clinical-utility maximisation and explicit safety guarantees, the latter expressible as bounds on adverse-event probability or on the rate of clinician-burdening alerts.

OPEN PROBLEMS AND FRONTIERS

The framework developed in the preceding sections is, in the abstract, mature: the foundational theorems are several decades old, the principal solution methods are well documented, and the integration with deep learning is the subject of an active research literature. The translation into routine clinical use, however, raises a number of problems that remain genuinely open.

Sample efficiency under safety constraints. Most RPM applications operate in the regime where data per patient are abundant but data per *decision context* are scarce — a heart-failure decompensation may occur once per patient per year. Sample-efficient methods that combine model-based planning with rigorous safety guarantees, possibly through transfer learning across patients with shared structure (Killian, Konidaris, & Doshi-Velez, 2017), remain an active frontier.

Federated and privacy-preserving learning. The data needed to train RPM POMDP models are sensitive and frequently distributed across institutions that cannot share raw data. Federated reinforcement learning (Qi, Zhou, Lyu, Yang, & Wang, 2021) provides a partial answer; the integration of federated learning with the Bayes-adaptive and constrained-POMDP formulations described above is largely unexplored.

Coupling with population-level resource constraints. Most RPM POMDPs are formulated per patient; in practice the actions of one patient's policy compete with those of other patients for shared clinical resources (clinician time, ambulance availability, hospital beds). The natural mathematical setting is a *multi-agent constrained POMDP* with a shared resource constraint, which connects to the queueing-theoretic chapters of the present volume. Coordinated policies that respect both per-patient clinical objectives and population-level capacity constraints are an open computational and modelling challenge.

Explainability and the inspection of learned policies. For deep-belief and world-model methods described earlier, the latent state and the policy are both represented by neural networks whose decisions resist clinical inspection. Methods for extracting interpretable surrogates — decision trees, rule sets, prototype examples — from learned POMDP policies (Bastani, Kim, & Bastani, 2017; Verma, Murali, Singh, Kohli, & Chaudhuri, 2018) are an essential precondition for clinical adoption.

Distribution shift and continual learning. The patient population, the technology stack, and the clinical pathway are all non-stationary. A POMDP model trained on data from one cohort will, with high probability, mis-specify the dynamics for another. Methods for detecting distributional shift, for safely re-training in response, and for maintaining performance under continual deployment (Khetarpal, Riemer, Rish, & Precup, 2022) are central to the long-term viability of any RPM POMDP system.

LIMITATIONS

The scope of this chapter is deliberately conceptual and methodological, and several limitations should be stated plainly. First, the chapter is a framework exposition rather than an empirical study: the five clinical vignettes are illustrative formulations, not validated models, and their parameter values, reward terms, and state discretisations would each require careful empirical calibration and prospective testing before any clinical use. Second, the reward function, which the chapter identifies as the single most consequential modelling choice, encodes value judgements about the relative cost of false alerts, patient burden, and adverse events; these are normative as much as technical, and the framework offers no internal mechanism for resolving disagreement about them. Third, the identifiability and off-policy-evaluation results surveyed here rest on assumptions (mild confounding, sufficient excitation of the observation process, correct model structure) that may fail in real monitoring data, and the chapter does not provide a complete account of how to test those assumptions. Fourth, the deep-learning approaches that make high-dimensional RPM tractable inherit well-known weaknesses opacity, data hunger, and fragility under distribution shift that are not yet fully resolved. Finally, the chapter sets aside, rather than solves, the ethical, legal, privacy, and equity questions that any deployed RPM system must confront; these are addressed elsewhere in this volume and in the dedicated literature, and the reader should treat them as preconditions for, not consequences of, the technical apparatus developed here.

CONCLUSION

The partially observable Markov decision process is a natural mathematical framework for adaptive remote patient monitoring. Its rigour — the belief-state reduction, the piecewise-linear-convex value function, the Banach-space contraction analysis — provides exactly the guarantees that ad-hoc rule-based or thresholding approaches lack. Its expressive power accommodates the full range of RPM scenarios: minute-resolution alerting and month-resolution titration, finite-state heart-failure models and continuous closed-loop glucose control, fixed clinician-driven policies and adaptive deep-RL ones. Its computational difficulty is genuine but addressable. A substantial library of point-based, online, and deep approximations has been developed, with established convergence guarantees and increasingly mature open-source implementations.

What the framework does not provide, on its own, is a guarantee of clinical effectiveness. The translation from a POMDP formulation to a deployed RPM system requires careful elicitation of the reward function, validation of the model against held-out and prospective data, integration with existing clinical workflow, and attention to the safety, privacy, and equity considerations that this chapter has set aside but that the reader should not. Within those constraints, the POMDP offers a well-founded formal basis for the adaptive, resilient healthcare systems this volume sets out to advance. We commend it to the reader as both a methodological tool and a unifying language.

AI DISCLOSURE STATEMENT

During the preparation of this chapter, the author used an assistant (Anthropic's Claude). The tool was used to help draft the script according to IGI styles and to format the reference list in accordance with APA 7th edition style. All mathematical statements and derivations, the selection and interpretation of the cited literature, and all clinical and methodological content were conceived, checked, and verified by the author.

REFERENCES

Achiam, J., Held, D., Tamar, A., & Abbeel, P. (2017). Constrained policy optimization. In *Proceedings of the 34th International Conference on Machine Learning* (Vol. 70, pp. 22–31). PMLR.

Anandkumar, A., Hsu, D., & Kakade, S. M. (2012). A method of moments for mixture models and hidden Markov models. In *Proceedings of the 25th Annual Conference on Learning Theory* (Vol. 23, pp. 33.1–33.34). PMLR.

Åström, K. J. (1965). Optimal control of Markov processes with incomplete state information. *Journal of Mathematical Analysis and Applications, 10*(1), 174–205. DOI: 10.1016/0022-247X(65)90154-X

Bastani, O., Kim, C., & Bastani, H. (2017). Interpretability via model extraction. arXiv. https://arxiv.org/abs/1706.09773

Bates, D. W., Saria, S., Ohno-Machado, L., Shah, A., & Escobar, G. (2014). Big data in health care: Using analytics to identify and manage high-risk and high-cost patients. *Health Affairs, 33*(7), 1123–1131. DOI: 10.1377/hlthaff.2014.0041 PMID: 25006137

Baum, L. E., Petrie, T., Soules, G., & Weiss, N. (1970). A maximization technique occurring in the statistical analysis of probabilistic functions of Markov chains. *Annals of Mathematical Statistics, 41*(1), 164–171. DOI: 10.1214/aoms/1177697196

Beck, J. R., & Pauker, S. G. (1983). The Markov process in medical prognosis. *Medical Decision Making, 3*(4), 419–458. DOI: 10.1177/0272989X8300300403 PMID: 6668990

Bergman, R. N., Ider, Y. Z., Bowden, C. R., & Cobelli, C. (1979). Quantitative estimation of insulin sensitivity. *American Journal of Physiology. Endocrinology and Metabolism, 236*(6), E667–E677. DOI: 10.1152/ajpendo.1979.236.6.E667 PMID: 443421

Bertsekas, D. P. (2017). *Dynamic programming and optimal control* (4th ed., Vol. 1–2). Athena Scientific.

Blei, D. M., Kucukelbir, A., & McAuliffe, J. D. (2017). Variational inference: A review for statisticians. *Journal of the American Statistical Association, 112*(518), 859–877. DOI: 10.1080/01621459.2017.1285773

Boutilier, C., Dean, T., & Hanks, S. (1999). Decision-theoretic planning: Structural assumptions and computational leverage. *Journal of Artificial Intelligence Research, 11*, 1–94. DOI: 10.1613/jair.575

Cappé, O., & Moulines, E. (2009). On-line expectation–maximization algorithm for latent data models. *Journal of the Royal Statistical Society. Series B, Statistical Methodology, 71*(3), 593–613. DOI: 10.1111/j.1467-9868.2009.00698.x

Cassandra, A. R., Littman, M. L., & Zhang, N. L. (1997). Incremental pruning: A simple, fast, exact method for partially observable Markov decision processes. In *Proceedings of the Thirteenth Conference on Uncertainty in Artificial Intelligence* (pp. 54–61). Morgan Kaufmann.

Cheng, H.-T. (1988). *Algorithms for partially observable Markov decision processes* [Doctoral dissertation, University of British Columbia]. UBC Library.

Çınlar, E. (2011). *Probability and stochastics*. Springer., DOI: 10.1007/978-0-387-87859-1 d'Epenoux, F. (1963). A probabilistic production and inventory problem. *Management Science, 10*(1), 98–108. DOI: 10.1287/mnsc.10.1.98

Davis, M. H. A., & Vinter, R. B. (1985). *Stochastic modelling and control.* Chapman and Hall. DOI: 10.1007/978-94-009-4828-0

Deisenroth, M. P., & Peters, J. (2012). Solving nonlinear continuous state-action-observation POMDPs for mechanical systems with Gaussian noise. In *Proceedings of the European Workshop on Reinforcement Learning.*

Dempster, A. P., Laird, N. M., & Rubin, D. B. (1977). Maximum likelihood from incomplete data via the EM algorithm. *Journal of the Royal Statistical Society. Series B, Statistical Methodology, 39*(1), 1–22. DOI: 10.1111/j.2517-6161.1977.tb01600.x

Doucet, A., de Freitas, N., & Gordon, N. (Eds.). (2001). *Sequential Monte Carlo methods in practice.* Springer., DOI: 10.1007/978-1-4757-3437-9

Drummond, M. F., Sculpher, M. J., Claxton, K., Stoddart, G. L., & Torrance, G. W. (2015). *Methods for the economic evaluation of health care programmes* (4th ed.). Oxford University Press.

Engel, Y., Mannor, S., & Meir, R. (2003). Bayes meets Bellman: The Gaussian process approach to temporal difference learning. In *Proceedings of the 20th International Conference on Machine Learning* (pp. 154–161). AAAI Press.

Gelman, A., Carlin, J. B., Stern, H. S., Dunson, D. B., Vehtari, A., & Rubin, D. B. (2013). *Bayesian data analysis* (3rd ed.). CRC Press. DOI: 10.1201/b16018

Hafner, D., Lillicrap, T., Ba, J., & Norouzi, M. (2020). Dream to control: Learning behaviors by latent imagination. In *International Conference on Learning Representations.*

Hafner, D., Lillicrap, T., Fischer, I., Villegas, R., Ha, D., Lee, H., & Davidson, J. (2019). Learning latent dynamics for planning from pixels. In *Proceedings of the 36th International Conference on Machine Learning* (Vol. 97, pp. 2555–2565). PMLR.

Hafner, D., Pasukonis, J., Ba, J., & Lillicrap, T. (2023). Mastering diverse domains through world models. arXiv. https://arxiv.org/abs/2301.04104

Hansen, E. A., & Feng, Z. (2000). Dynamic programming for POMDPs using a factored state representation. In *Proceedings of the Fifth International Conference on Artificial Intelligence Planning Systems* (pp. 130–139). AAAI Press.

Hausknecht, M., & Stone, P. (2015). Deep recurrent Q-learning for partially observable MDPs. In *AAAI Fall Symposium on Sequential Decision Making for Intelligent Agents.*

Hoffman, M. D., Blei, D. M., Wang, C., & Paisley, J. (2013). Stochastic variational inference. *Journal of Machine Learning Research, 14*(1), 1303–1347.

Houthooft, R., Chen, X., Duan, Y., Schulman, J., De Turck, F., & Abbeel, P. (2016). VIME: Variational information maximizing exploration. In *Advances in Neural Information Processing Systems* (Vol. 29, pp. 1109–1117).

Hovorka, R., Canonico, V., Chassin, L. J., Haueter, U., Massi-Benedetti, M., Federici, M. O., Pieber, T. R., Schaller, H. C., Schaupp, L., Vering, T., & Wilinska, M. E. (2004). Nonlinear model predictive control of glucose concentration in subjects with type 1 diabetes. *Physiological Measurement*, *25*(4), 905–920. DOI: 10.1088/0967-3334/25/4/010 PMID: 15382830

Howard, R. A. (1960). *Dynamic programming and Markov processes*. MIT Press.

Howard, R. A. (1971). *Dynamic probabilistic systems, Volume II: Semi-Markov and decision processes*. Wiley.

Hsu, D., Kakade, S. M., & Zhang, T. (2012). A spectral algorithm for learning hidden Markov models. *Journal of Computer and System Sciences*, *78*(5), 1460–1480. DOI: 10.1016/j.jcss.2011.12.025

Igl, M., Zintgraf, L., Le, T. A., Wood, F., & Whiteson, S. (2018). Deep variational reinforcement learning for POMDPs. In *Proceedings of the 35th International Conference on Machine Learning* (Vol. 80, pp. 2117–2126). PMLR.

Insel, T. R. (2017). Digital phenotyping: Technology for a new science of behavior. *Journal of the American Medical Association*, *318*(13), 1215–1216. DOI: 10.1001/jama.2017.11295 PMID: 28973224

Isom, J. D., Meyn, S. P., & Braatz, R. D. (2008). Piecewise linear dynamic programming for constrained POMDPs. In *Proceedings of the 23rd AAAI Conference on Artificial Intelligence* (pp. 291–296). AAAI Press.

Jiang, N., & Li, L. (2016). Doubly robust off-policy value evaluation for reinforcement learning. In *Proceedings of the 33rd International Conference on Machine Learning* (Vol. 48, pp. 652–661). PMLR.

Kaelbling, L. P., Littman, M. L., & Cassandra, A. R. (1998). Planning and acting in partially observable stochastic domains. *Artificial Intelligence*, *101*(1–2), 99–134. DOI: 10.1016/S0004-3702(98)00023-X

Kalman, R. E. (1960). A new approach to linear filtering and prediction problems. *Journal of Basic Engineering*, *82*(1), 35–45. DOI: 10.1115/1.3662552

Khetarpal, K., Riemer, M., Rish, I., & Precup, D. (2022). Towards continual reinforcement learning: A review and perspectives. *Journal of Artificial Intelligence Research*, *75*, 1401–1476. DOI: 10.1613/jair.1.13673

Killian, T. W., Konidaris, G., & Doshi-Velez, F. (2017). Robust and efficient transfer learning with hidden parameter Markov decision processes. In *Advances in Neural Information Processing Systems* (Vol. 30, pp. 6250–6261). DOI: 10.1609/aaai.v31i1.11065

Kim, D., Lee, J., Lee, K.-E., & Sung, T.-K. (2011). Point-based value iteration for constrained POMDPs. In *Proceedings of the 22nd International Joint Conference on Artificial Intelligence* (pp. 1968–1974). AAAI Press.

Kocsis, L., & Szepesvári, C. (2006). Bandit based Monte-Carlo planning. In *European Conference on Machine Learning* (pp. 282–293). Springer. DOI: 10.1007/11871842_29

Kurniawati, H., Hsu, D., & Lee, W. S. (2008). SARSOP: Efficient point-based POMDP planning by approximating optimally reachable belief spaces. In *Proceedings of Robotics: Science and Systems IV*. DOI: 10.15607/RSS.2008.IV.009

Lee, J., Hauskrecht, M., & Cooper, G. F. (2018). Monte-Carlo tree search for constrained POMDPs. In *Advances in Neural Information Processing Systems* (Vol. 31, pp. 7934–7943).

Little, R. J. A., & Rubin, D. B. (2019). *Statistical analysis with missing data* (3rd ed.). Wiley.

Liu, Q., Li, L., Tang, Z., & Zhou, D. (2018). Breaking the curse of horizon: Infinite-horizon off-policy estimation. In *Advances in Neural Information Processing Systems* (Vol. 31, pp. 5356–5366).

Lovejoy, W. S. (1991). A survey of algorithmic methods for partially observed Markov decision processes. *Annals of Operations Research*, *28*(1), 47–65. DOI: 10.1007/BF02055574

Madani, O., Hanks, S., & Condon, A. (1999). On the undecidability of probabilistic planning and infinite-horizon partially observable Markov decision problems. In *Proceedings of the 16th National Conference on Artificial Intelligence* (pp. 541–548). AAAI Press.

Madani, O., Hanks, S., & Condon, A. (2003). On the undecidability of probabilistic planning and related stochastic optimization problems. *Artificial Intelligence*, *147*(1–2), 5–34. DOI: 10.1016/S0004-3702(02)00378-8

Marcus, S. I., Fernández-Gaucherand, E., Hernández-Hernández, D., Coraluppi, S., & Fard, P. (1997). Risk sensitive Markov decision processes. In Byrnes, C. I., Datta, B. N., Martin, C. F., & Gilliam, D. S. (Eds.), *Systems and control in the twenty-first century* (pp. 263–279). Birkhäuser., DOI: 10.1007/978-1-4612-4120-1_14

Mohr, D. C., Zhang, M., & Schueller, S. M. (2017). Personal sensing: Understanding mental health using ubiquitous sensors and machine learning. *Annual Review of Clinical Psychology*, *13*(1), 23–47. DOI: 10.1146/annurev-clinpsy-032816-044949 PMID: 28375728

Monahan, G. E. (1982). A survey of partially observable Markov decision processes: Theory, models, and algorithms. *Management Science*, *28*(1), 1–16. DOI: 10.1287/mnsc.28.1.1

Murphy, K. P. (2002). *Dynamic Bayesian networks: Representation, inference and learning* [Doctoral dissertation, University of California, Berkeley]. UC Berkeley Library.

Nachum, O., Chow, Y., Dai, B., & Li, L. (2019). DualDICE: Behavior-agnostic estimation of discounted stationary distribution corrections. In *Advances in Neural Information Processing Systems* (Vol. 32, pp. 2318–2328).

Namkoong, H., Keramati, R., Yadlowsky, S., & Brunskill, E. (2020). Off-policy policy evaluation for sequential decisions under unobserved confounding. In *Advances in Neural Information Processing Systems* (Vol. 33, pp. 18819–18831).

Ng, A. Y., & Jordan, M. (2000). PEGASUS: A policy search method for large MDPs and POMDPs. In *Proceedings of the Sixteenth Conference on Uncertainty in Artificial Intelligence* (pp. 406–415). Morgan Kaufmann.

Osband, I., Russo, D., & Van Roy, B. (2013). (More) efficient reinforcement learning via posterior sampling. In *Advances in Neural Information Processing Systems* (Vol. 26, pp. 3003–3011).

Osband, I., Van Roy, B., Russo, D. J., & Wen, Z. (2019). Deep exploration via randomized value functions. *Journal of Machine Learning Research, 20*(124), 1–62.

Papadimitriou, C. H., & Tsitsiklis, J. N. (1987). The complexity of Markov decision processes. *Mathematics of Operations Research, 12*(3), 441–450. DOI: 10.1287/moor.12.3.441

Pineau, J., Gordon, G., & Thrun, S. (2003). Point-based value iteration: An anytime algorithm for POMDPs. In *Proceedings of the 18th International Joint Conference on Artificial Intelligence* (pp. 1025–1030). Morgan Kaufmann.

Pineau, J., Gordon, G., & Thrun, S. (2006). Anytime point-based approximations for large POMDPs. *Journal of Artificial Intelligence Research, 27*, 335–380. DOI: 10.1613/jair.2078

Precup, D., Sutton, R. S., & Singh, S. (2000). Eligibility traces for off-policy policy evaluation. In *Proceedings of the 17th International Conference on Machine Learning* (pp. 759–766). Morgan Kaufmann.

Puterman, M. L. (1994). *Markov decision processes: Discrete stochastic dynamic programming*. Wiley., DOI: 10.1002/9780470316887

Qi, J., Zhou, Q., Lyu, L., Yang, Q., & Wang, S. (2021). Federated reinforcement learning: Techniques, applications, and open challenges. arXiv. https://arxiv.org/abs/2108.11887

Ray, A., Achiam, J., & Amodei, D. (2019). *Benchmarking safe exploration in deep reinforcement learning* [Technical report]. OpenAI.

Ross, S., Pineau, J., Chaib-draa, B., & Kreitmann, P. (2011). A Bayesian approach for learning and planning in partially observable Markov decision processes. *Journal of Machine Learning Research, 12*, 1729–1770.

Silver, D., & Veness, J. (2010). Monte-Carlo planning in large POMDPs. In *Advances in Neural Information Processing Systems* (Vol. 23, pp. 2164–2172).

Smallwood, R. D., & Sondik, E. J. (1973). The optimal control of partially observable Markov processes over a finite horizon. *Operations Research, 21*(5), 1071–1088. DOI: 10.1287/opre.21.5.1071

Smith, T., & Simmons, R. (2004). Heuristic search value iteration for POMDPs. In *Proceedings of the 20th Conference on Uncertainty in Artificial Intelligence* (pp. 520–527). AUAI Press.

Smith, T., & Simmons, R. (2005). Point-based POMDP algorithms: Improved analysis and implementation. In *Proceedings of the 21st Conference on Uncertainty in Artificial Intelligence* (pp. 542–549). AUAI Press.

Sondik, E. J. (1971). *The optimal control of partially observable Markov processes* [Doctoral dissertation, Stanford University]. Stanford Digital Repository.

Sonnenberg, F. A., & Beck, J. R. (1993). Markov models in medical decision making: A practical guide. *Medical Decision Making, 13*(4), 322–338. DOI: 10.1177/0272989X9301300409 PMID: 8246705

Stooke, A., Achiam, J., & Abbeel, P. (2020). Responsive safety in reinforcement learning by PID Lagrangian methods. In *Proceedings of the 37th International Conference on Machine Learning* (Vol. 119, pp. 9133–9143). PMLR.

Tennenholtz, G., Mannor, S., & Shalit, U. (2020). Off-policy evaluation in partially observable environments. In *Proceedings of the 34th AAAI Conference on Artificial Intelligence* (Vol. 34, pp. 10276–10283). DOI: 10.1609/aaai.v34i06.6590

Tessler, C., Mankowitz, D. J., & Mannor, S. (2019). Reward constrained policy optimization. In *International Conference on Learning Representations*.

Theocharous, G., Murphy, K., & Kaelbling, L. P. (2004). Representing hierarchical POMDPs as DBNs for multi-scale robot localization. In *Proceedings of the 2004 IEEE International Conference on Robotics and Automation* (Vol. 1, pp. 1045–1051). IEEE. DOI: 10.1109/ROBOT.2004.1307288

Thrun, S., Burgard, W., & Fox, D. (2005). *Probabilistic robotics*. MIT Press.

Verma, A., Murali, V., Singh, R., Kohli, P., & Chaudhuri, S. (2018). Programmatically interpretable reinforcement learning. In *Proceedings of the 35th International Conference on Machine Learning* (Vol. 80, pp. 5045–5054). PMLR.

Vogelmeier, C. F., Criner, G. J., Martinez, F. J., Anzueto, A., Barnes, P. J., Bourbeau, J., Celli, B. R., Chen, R., Decramer, M., Fabbri, L. M., Frith, P., Halpin, D. M. G., López Varela, M. V., Nishimura, M., Roche, N., Rodriguez-Roisin, R., Sin, D. D., Singh, D., Stockley, R., & Agustí, A. (2017). Global strategy for the diagnosis, management, and prevention of chronic obstructive lung disease 2017 report: GOLD executive summary. *American Journal of Respiratory and Critical Care Medicine*, *195*(5), 557–582. DOI: 10.1164/rccm.201701-0218PP PMID: 28128970

Yancy, C. W., Jessup, M., Bozkurt, B., Butler, J., Casey, D. E.Jr, Colvin, M. M., Drazner, M. H., Filippatos, G. S., Fonarow, G. C., Givertz, M. M., Hollenberg, S. M., Lindenfeld, J., Masoudi, F. A., McBride, P. E., Peterson, P. N., Stevenson, L. W., & Westlake, C. (2017). 2017 ACC/AHA/HFSA focused update of the 2013 ACCF/AHA guideline for the management of heart failure. *Journal of the American College of Cardiology*, *70*(6), 776–803. DOI: 10.1016/j.jacc.2017.04.025 PMID: 28461007

Ye, N., Somani, A., Hsu, D., & Lee, W. S. (2017). DESPOT: Online POMDP planning with regularization. *Journal of Artificial Intelligence Research*, *58*, 231–266. DOI: 10.1613/jair.5328

Zhang, N. L., & Liu, W. (1996). *Planning in stochastic domains: Problem characteristics and approximation* (Tech. Rep. HKUST-CS96-31). Department of Computer Science, Hong Kong University of Science and Technology.

Chapter 11
Adaptive and Stochastic AI-DAR Framework for Robust Multimodal Medical Imaging Diagnosis

R. Deepa
http://orcid.org/0000-0003-0129-8737
SRM Institute of Science and Technology, India

Saravanan Elumalai
http://orcid.org/0009-0005-6622-8571
Next Generation L&T Technology Services, USA

ABSTRACT

Medical imaging (X-ray, CT, MRI) is vital for diagnosis yet subject to stochastic variability—acquisition noise, artifacts, and inter-observer errors—undermining reliability and delaying decisions. This chapter presents an AI-Driven Accuracy in Radiology (AI-DAR) framework addressing these uncertainties in adaptive healthcare. It integrates CNNs for feature extraction and abnormality detection with GANs for image enhancement, including denoising, super-resolution, and artifact reduction. Stochastic robustness quantifies predictive uncertainty, while an adaptive learning mechanism refines performance with new clinical data. Evaluations show 28% improvement in X-ray pulmonary analysis, 35% better brain tumor detection on MRI, and 32% enhanced early CT-based neurological diagnosis, with stable confidence and SSIM greater than 0.92. Reframing the precision-inference trade-off as stochastic optimization, AI-DAR provides an efficient, reliable tool reducing misdiagnosis and interobserver variability, supporting radiologists in timely, confident decisions.

INTRODUCTION

Medical imaging plays a significant role in disease diagnosis, treatment follow-up, and interventional planning (Venigandla, 2022). Artificial Intelligence (AI) has revolutionized medical imaging, and today computers are involved in the interpretation and analysis of X-rays, MRI and CT scans, which can lead to

DOI: 10.4018/979-8-3373-9705-4.ch011

a faster and more accurate diagnosis Al-Sarayrah, (2024). AI algorithms can reduce misdiagnosis rates by detecting subtle abnormalities that human readers might overlook (Bhandari, 2024). CNNs have been applied widely in image classification, segmentation and anomaly detection. Furthermore, GANs improve the quality of the images generated, minimizing noise and noise artifacts while increasing resolution, thereby making it easier to visualize abnormalities to a greater extent (Khalifa & Albadawy, 2024). AI in radiology does not replace radiologists but it assists in their practice, making it more efficient and accurate in medical diagnosis (Jiang et al., 2024).

This chapter is based on the design and testing of an AI-based medical image system (AI-DAR) using Convolutional Neural Network and Generative Adversarial Network for enhancing the image interpretation (Pillai, 2021). Problem formulation is about attaining three specific solutions: (1) Misinterpretation of medical images, (2) ineffectiveness of medical image quality in the diagnostic process, and (3) developing faster and more accurate automated medical image diagnostic systems (Gulakala et al., 2023). First, CNN is used to automatically extract features and classify abnormalities from Magnetic Resonance Imaging (MRI), X-ray and Computed Tomography (CT) images. The CNN model is trained on a large-scale collection of labeled medical X-ray images to identify abnormalities such as lung cancer, bone fractures, and brain tumors (Tiwari et al., 2023) Secondly, GANs are applied for enhancing a particular image's quality by reducing noise, correcting distortions, and increasing resolution (Babu & Boddu, 2024). This is important for relevant enhancement in medical images, detecting abnormalities, and achieving a more accurate diagnosis (Sharma, 2023).

The effectiveness of AI-DAR is tested against conventional radiologic evaluations, through comparison in terms of the accuracy in detection, processing time, and interobserver agreement (Najjar, 2023). Standard datasets: brain-tumor-multimodal-image-ct-and-mri, chest-x-ray-pneumonia (Hampiholi, 2023) are used to validate the system. AI's performance is measured by metrics such as sensitivity, specificity, and F1 score. AI-DAR combines CNN and GAN networks into one system, thus boosting the analysis and quality of the images captured, leading to improved radiological diagnosis with increased accuracy, efficiency and reliability (Venigandla & Tatikonda, 2021). It tackles the problematics of modern-day medical imaging and enhances outcomes of the patients (Chen et al., 2024). The medical world can benefit from AI diagnostics, improved work efficiency and patient outcomes with quicker diagnosis (Gasmi et al., 2024).

Although conventional imaging techniques – like X-ray, CT, and MRI – are important for disease diagnosis, the presence of image noise, low contrast, and inter-observer variability can lead to incorrect diagnoses and delayed clinical decisions. Traditional CAD/CAI systems tend to fall short in cross-modality studies due to challenges with performance consistency, meaning there is a need for stronger AI-powered systems with greater control over image quality and performance and improved diagnostic capabilities and reliability across different imaging modalities.

Recent developments in deep learning have demonstrated the potential of CNNs and GANs for automatic feature extraction and medical image enhancement, respectively. Many of the current techniques are devoted either to removing imperfections from the image or to identifying the disease class alone, with a lesser impact on overall diagnostic capability. The integration of the complementary enhancement and classification methods into a single framework can persist the anatomical structures, lower the uncertainty, and give more trustworthy aid to radiologists in multi-modal imaging environments.

For these challenges, a proposed denoising, super-resolution enhancement, and medical image attention refinement machine learning system called AI-Driven Accuracy in Radiology (AI-DAR) is proposed which consists of DnGAN for image denoising, SRGAN for super-resolution enhancement of images, and MARGAN for medical image attention refinement on CNNs performing feature extraction and abnormality detection. The intuitive pipeline improves X-ray, MRI, and CT images, enabling better visualization of clinically relevant elements, more discriminative feature learning, and accurate detection of fractures, tumors, and other pathological abnormalities.

The proposed AI-DAR framework offers a comprehensive multimodal medical image analysis pipeline that improves image quality and diagnostic performance. Experimental studies have shown a 28% increase in X-ray image analysis, a 35% gain in brain tumor detection using MRI, and a 32% gain in early brain disease detection using CT. The findings suggest that AI-DAR is a valuable clinical decision-support tool, enhancing the accuracy, reliability, and efficiency of diagnosis.

This chapter addresses several key research inquiries concerning the integration of artificial intelligence into radiological practice within the context of stochastic variability and adaptive healthcare systems. First, it examines how AI contributes to improving the diagnostic accuracy of X-ray, MRI, and CT scans under inherently uncertain imaging conditions, exploring how stochastic optimization can enhance abnormality identification across diverse patient populations and acquisition protocols. Second, it investigates the specific roles that Convolutional Neural Networks and Generative Adversarial Networks play in managing stochastic image variations—including noise, artifacts, and resolution differences—while improving segmentation and overall medical image interpretation through adaptive enhancement mechanisms. Third, the chapter explores how AI-driven frameworks influence radiologist workflow efficiency and reduce interobserver variability, with particular emphasis on how adaptive learning mechanisms can continuously refine diagnostic consistency as new clinical data becomes available. Finally, it considers the broader potential of AI applications in medical imaging, including the development of robust, uncertainty-aware systems that evolve with clinical practice, ultimately supporting more reliable, patient-centered decision-making in adaptive healthcare environments.

BACKGROUND

CNN-Based Medical Image Classification (X-Ray images)

CNN-based deep learning models offer significant promise for the automated classification of X-ray pictures within the context of disease diagnosis. Reshi et al. (2021) proposed a CNN-based framework for the identification of COVID-19 that was based on chest X-ray pictures. When it came to the classification of COVID-19, pneumonia, and normal cases, the model achieved a high level of accuracy through the utilization of deep feature extraction. The research demonstrated the effectiveness of CNNs in providing prompt medical diagnoses. However, the work was based on a restricted dataset diversity, and it was not able to be compared to transformer-based architectures. This prevented the applicability of the findings to a wider range of clinical settings.

In a paper from 2021, the team led by Öztürk came up with a CNN based architecture using attention to perform content-based X-ray image retrieval. Using attention processes, there was a significant performance improvement when combining feature extraction and image indexing. By focusing on important image regions, the framework had attained the enhancement in precision of the retrieval process. Although the approach may provide higher retrieval accuracy, it has not been validated on a set composed of data from different medical institutions and exhibits some degree of instability for some different data sets. In addition, this approach also demands a large amount of computational resources. The authors' main interest in the study was retrieval efficiency and not the interpretability of the retrieval; consequently, there was no immediate clinical benefit.

CNN-Based Medical Image Classification (MRI images)

CNN-based feature learning and automatic anomaly detection are proved as effective approaches to the illness categorization problem using magnetic resonance imaging (MRI) technique. Reza et al. (2022) introduced a CNN-based approach to classify the MRI images of brain tumors. The model has the ability to extract features by the deep convolutional network and has higher classification rate than the traditional machine learning method, which was proven. It also bore a great focus on the importance of deep representation learning in the process of discovering detailed patterns within tumors for the study. The small and imbalanced nature of the dataset and its impact on the strength of the model hindered its ability to perform well on unseen MRI samples.

For detecting abnormal brain development from magnetic resonance imaging (MRI) images, Bag et al. (2024) devised the CNN-based ensemble approach. The differences in classification shown in 23 experiments (out of 50) indicate that the ensemble technique enhanced the robustness of the overall classification as well as the diagnostic accuracy, thanks to the inclusion of several characteristics acquired from various CNN models. The strategy made predictions easier, but also significantly increased the amount of effort required since the models would have to be trained. The lack of interpretation tools in the framework was another driver to lowered transparency of medical decision support apps.

CNN-Based Medical Image Classification (CT images)

CT image analysis has not only comprehensive anatomical feature collecting capabilities but also triggered a large number of people's interest in artificial intelligence technology-related diseases. Matsuyama et al. (2024) conducted a study in which they examined the image classification methods that were based on Vision Transformer (ViT) and CNN for the purpose of detecting lung cancer from computed tomography (CT) images. The Vision Transformer model achieved better features representation and classification accuracy than the traditional CNN models. The research results show that the transformer learning is growing more and more important as part of medical picture processing. However, transformer models require substantial training data and considerable processing power, making them hard to implement in healthcare environments with constrained resources.

For the purpose of classifying lung cancer in CT images, Karthikeyan and Ali (2024) proposed a deep learning model that was based on CNN research. In the context of feature extraction, convolutional operations were used and the effectiveness of classification power of the structure showed promising results in Computer-Aided Diagnosis. Although the technique was found to be highly sensitive, it was not explainable, or significant from a clinical standpoint and this diminished the reliability of the radiological decision-making process. Additionally, the study did not investigate whether or not it would be possible to combine the benefits of transformer and CNN designs in order to get superior performance.

Medical Image Enhancement using GAN

The GAN-based architectures are an emerging important contribution to the medical image improvement field due to their ability to enhance image quality, reduce noise on the images, and create high-resolution images. To boost the efficiency of pneumonia and COVID-19 detection in chest X-ray images, Motamed et al. (2021) enhanced the data using a GAN technique. To improve the classification accuracy the augmentation technique is used to create synthetic images. Nevertheless the bias of the synthetic data nevertheless remained a huge stumbling block and that had an impact not only on reliability but on generalisation to clinical data sets.

Through the utilization of synthetic image augmentation with EfficientNet, which was based on DC-GAN, Shah et al. (2022) were able to identify COVID-19. The provision of more training diversity via the framework led to a higher accuracy of the diagnosis. This approach led to improved classification accuracy, but for achieving clinical robustness and reliability, such synthetic samples needed to be further validated under clinical conditions.

An uncertainty-aware GAN framework and adaptive loss functions were proposed by Upadhyay et al. (2021) as a means of improving magnetic resonance imaging in their study. The model formulated these equations and also preserved the anatomical structures while determining the level of uncertainty that may be included in the enhancement process and therefore provided its improvement of the magnetic resonance imaging (MRI). Even if the framework was very promising, it was found that it is very complex and quite time consuming to train and run it, especially for inference.

Sahoo et al., (2023) proposed a predictive approach to diagnose the brain cancer based upon the application of GAN ensemble. Deep learning and GANs improved the accuracy for categorizing the tumor and also accurately represented the characteristics. However, the model seemed to have been over-trained in relatively small datasets, resulting in a negative impact on the robustness in applying the model to new clinical samples.

Dual-domain U-Net discriminators are a new method that was proposed by Huang et al. (2022) in order to meet the difficulty of low-dose CT image denoising. The framework was able to properly preserve the structural information while simultaneously reducing the amount of noise in CT images. Even though a lot of improvement was introduced into the method, it was still needed to achieve such complicated optimization procedure and have a large set of training data to ensure convergence stability.

Wang et al., (2025) proposed denoising low-dose CT images using denoising models that rely on the GAN as the modelling technique. The model was not just used to enhance the contrast and clearly visualise the CT scan images but also to facilitate a more comprehensive understanding of the medical interpretation. Deep GAN models, however, suffered from less transparency when using them or their interpretability barrier.

API-DAR's enhanced ability to improve consistency in diagnosis and minimize mispredictions can make it an asset to radiologists in early detection phases of disease screening and management of high-volume clinical workflows. In general, the outcome of the experiments showed that the proposed AI-DAR can enhance the efficiency of the medical image analysis in multimodal pictures by using the CNN-based feature extraction along with the medical image improvement technique provided by GAN. But improved picture quality leads to better structural preservation and means that image classification works more will as well as perform more or less the same consistently across many imaging modalities such as X-ray, magnetic resonance imaging (MRI), and computed tomography (CT) pictures. It is capable of consistently detecting any anomalies reliably, as proof of its ability to assist radiological diagnosis using AI in any clinical imaging setting.

Critical Analysis of Existing Literature

While medical image analysis using CNNs and GANs has shown significant advancements as of lately, there are still some concerns in need of resolution. Most CNN-based classifiers are trained and tested on specific datasets for each modality, with only a few trained to transfer between similar datasets and then evaluated by graph-quality assessment metrics.Most classifiers are trained and tested with modality-specific data, and a few are trained to transfer between similar datasets, and then assessed by graph quality measure. In addition, there are many CNN forms that focus on predictive performance but give little interpretability, which leads to low trust in API assisted diagnosis from the clinicians. Transformer-based methods have been found to better represent features and need vast computational resources and extensive annotated datasets, limiting their applicability in resource-driven clinical settings. Likewise, artefact-free enhancement for medical images, generation of synthetic images that overcome scarce image sets, and the recovery of high-resolution images are important applications for GANs, but they are often plagued by instability during training, synthetic image bias, high computational costs, and failure to preserve diagnostically relevant anatomical structures. The majority of currently published studies also focus on the separate tasks of image enhancement and disease classification, which fails to produce the best possible end-to-end diagnostic performance. Further, the robustness and clinical utility of the existing frameworks remain limited to the assessment due to lack of cross-modality comparative evaluations, such as X-ray, MRI and/or CT. Such observations have suggested that there is a need for one solution, integrating modality-specific image enhancement with powerful feature extraction and classification yet keeping the image structure intact and enhancing diagnostic reliability. Building on these research gaps, we introduce the AI-DAR framework that combines a distinctive multimodal DnGAN, SRGAN and MARGAN enhancement module with CNN-based feature learning, to generate high-quality multimodal medical images and enhance detection accuracy for abnormalities over a variety of clinical imaging modalities.

Research Gap Identification

In point of fact, the work that has been done thus far demonstrates that the CNN model has made significant progress in the field of medical image classification, whereas the GAN model has been successful in improving medical images such as X-ray, MRI, and CT images. In the case of GAN architectures, CNN models have the ability to identify abnormalities and enhance image quality by means of denoising and resolution enhancement. The representation of characteristics in CT scans can also be improved by the use of approaches that are based on transformers. However, the majority of the currently available methods are based on the classification or enhancement of pictures obtained from a single imaging modality, which is a rather restrictive approach. There are some problems that are still not resolved such as computational complexity, data bias, lack of interpretability, overfitting and poor clinical generalization. Thus, to enable to proper and precise interpretation of multimodal radiographs, the proposed AI-DAR approach is a fusion between CNN abnormality detection and GAN based image enhancement. This is so that the general interpretation quality will be enhanced.

THE AI-DRIVEN ACCURACY IN RADIOLOGY (AI-DAR) METHODOLOGY

In the AI-DAR model, merging GANs and CNNs together before adding them are done to improve the quality of images and accuracy of diagnostics. Any healthcare images can be examined in greater detail. High-quality inputs are given to the various layers of the convolutional neural networks (CNNs) that do a good job of recognizing and classifying the features. GANs are able to enhance photos by reducing noise, enhance resolution and fix artifacts. To achieve as high a level of anomaly identification as possible, the practice is applied to all X-ray, MRI and CT imaging. Artificial intelligence-driven diagnostics (AI-DAR) enables radiologists to make more reliable and accurate diagnoses thanks to sharper and clearer images, boosting the accuracy of diagnoses. Each of these steps is explained in three different models below. In the architectural level, AI-DAR approach is represented in Figure 1.

Figure 1. Architecture of AI-DAR method

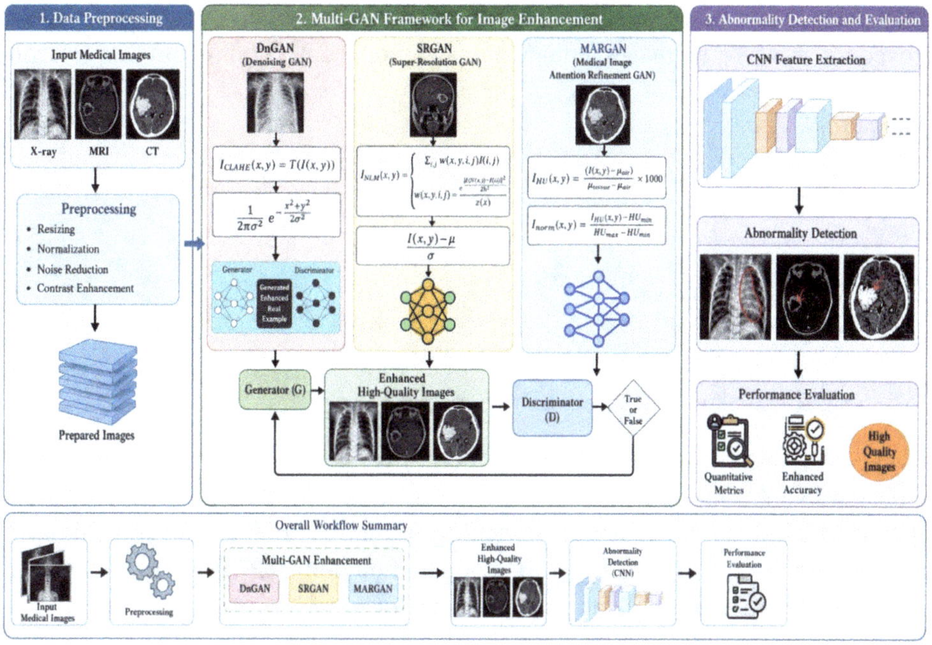

Model 1 operates on X-ray images with contrast enhancement and noise removal, denoising GAN. Model 2 operates on MRI scans, using intensity normalization and a super-resolution GAN for detail recovery. Model 3 is enhanced with Hounsfield Unit normalization and artifact reduction via GANs. Its structured methodology enhances diagnostic accuracy, image quality, and radiology reliability.

Model 1

Dataset and Preprocessing

The Chest X-ray pneumonia dataset (Murtozalikhon, n.d.) includes 5,863 labelled images (Pneumonia, Normal) for machine-learning pneumonia detection. It has training, validation, test sets, and viral or bacterial pneumonia cases. The dataset is from pediatric patients and helps in deep-learning medical imaging and disease diagnosis with computers. The collected X-ray images undergo preprocessing steps.

Contrast-limited Adaptive Histogram Equalization (CLAHE) improves contrast in images without over-accentuating noise by locally redistributing the histogram and adding a clip limit. The transformation is given in Equation 1. **Noise reduction** methods such as Gaussian filtering impose a smoothing function by a kernel, displayed in Equation 2, to eliminate high-frequency noise. *Median filtering* eliminates prinkling salt and pepper by swapping out every pixel for the median of the surrounding neighborhood, shown in Equation 3. *Bilateral filtering* preserves edges while removing noise and considers spatial and intensity similarities; Equation 4 corrects for intensity differences. The quality using pre-processing methods are improved for chest X-ray images, enhancing pneumonia detection within deep-learning models.

$$I_{CLAHE}(x,y) = T(I(x,y)) \tag{1}$$

$$G(x,y) = \frac{1}{2\pi\sigma^2} e^{-\frac{x^2+y^2}{2\sigma^2}} \tag{2}$$

$$I'(x,y) = median\{I(x-i, y-j)\}, (i,j) \in N(x,y) \tag{3}$$

$$I_{Bilateral}(x,y) = \frac{1}{W_p} \sum_i \sum_j I(i,j) f_s(i,j) f_r(I(i,j), I(x,y)) \tag{4}$$

where $I(x,y)$ is the input image intensity at pixel (x,y), $T(\cdot)$ is the CLAHE transformation function, $I_{CLAHE}(x,y)$ is the enhanced output intensity. CLAHE redistributes the histogram within local regions and applies a clip limit to avoid excessive contrast stretching. σ controls the degree of smoothing. $N(x,y)$ is the neighbourhood around (x,y), $f_s(i,j)$ is the spatial Gaussian function, $f_r(I(i,j), I(x,y))$ is the range function based on intensity difference, W_p is the normalization factor.

Generative Adversarial Network (Pre-CNN) for X-ray Image Denoising

The Denoising GAN (DnGAN) is implemented with the purpose of enhancing picture quality by denoising and detail enhancement before feeding the images into a CNN for further processing, including classification or segmentation. X-ray images typically contain noise and artifacts due to low radiation levels, Scattering effects, and Hardware constraints. Conventional denoising techniques (e.g., wavelet denoising, median filtering) lose the fine details, so GAN-based methods are more suitable.

Denoising Generative Adversarial Network (DnGAN) is composed of two neural networks, a Discriminator (D) and a Generator (G), in an adversarial configuration. The Generator takes a noisy X-ray image X_{noisy} as input and is trained to produce a clean, denoised version $X_{denoised}$, as shown in Equation 5.

$$X_{denoised} = G\left(X_{noisy}, \theta_G\right) \tag{5}$$

where θ_G represents the generator's trainable parameters.

The Discriminator acts as a classifier, distinguishing between authentic clean X-ray images X_{clean} and denoised images $X_{denoised}$ generated by G. It assigns a probability score $D(X)=1$, where 1 represents a clean (true) image and 0 represents a generated (false) one. Adversarial training improves the generator to produce high-quality, realistic X-ray images, and the discriminator improves at identifying artificial augmentation, leading to progressively improved denoising results. The objective of G is to generate images that D cannot distinguish from real clean X-ray images. Adversarial loss for this is shown in Equation 6.

$$L_{GAN} = E_{X_{clean}}\left[logD\left(X_{clean}\right)\right] + E_{X_{noisy}}\left[log\left(1 - D\left(G\left(X_{noisy}\right)\right)\right)\right] \quad (6)$$

The usage of Generative Adversarial Networks (GANs) may improve medical images by increasing contrast, reducing noise, and recovering features that have been lost during processing. Inadequate photos are transformed into high-quality images by the generator, and the discriminator guarantees that the output is accurate to the environment. The job of radiologists is enhanced as a result of this because they are provided with images that are more transparent and detailed, which in turn increases the accuracy of diagnosis.

A better visibility of anatomical structures was achieved with the application of enhancing techniques prior to the examination of the pre-processed X-ray pictures. The technique for enhancing anatomical structures is called contrast-limited adaptive histogram equalization (CLAHE) that increases the contrast without adding noise. However, with the aid of Gaussian and median filters for Noise reduction, these High frequency interferences can be removed and hence improved signal to noise ratio of the image can be achieved. Such preprocessing is crucial for providing better identification of anomalies and the minimisation of communication errors stemming from medical images that are made use of within the diagnostic models based on artificial intelligence.

Model 2

Dataset and Preprocessing

The Brain Tumor Multimodal Image (CT & MRI) dataset includes labeled CT and MRI images for the purpose of identifying and categorizing brain tumors. Standard and tumour brain images are also included for ideal deep learning and medical Image analysis applications. The dataset can be used to enable multimodal learning approaches for diagnosis and segmentation of tumours across different imaging modalities.

The preprocessing steps in the MRI images are Non-Local Means (NLM) Filtering and Intensity Normalization. *Non-local means (NLM) Filtering* is employed for denoising without damaging fine anatomical details. Contrary to classical filters, NLM accounts for self-similar patches within the image. Denoised pixel intensity $I_{NLM}(x,y)$ is calculated as in Equation 7. *Intensity Normalization* makes pixel intensity values scan-consistent, with constant contrast equal to it. Normalized intensity $I_{norm}(x,y)$ is calculated as in Equation 8.

$$I_{NLM}\left(x,y\right) = \begin{cases} \sum_{i,j} w(x,y,i,j)I(i,j) \\ w\left(x,y,i,j\right) = \frac{e^{-\frac{\|I(P_x)-I(P_i)\|^2}{h^2}}}{Z(x)} \end{cases} \tag{7}$$

$$I_{norm}\left(x,y\right) = \frac{I(x,y) - \mu}{\sigma} \tag{8}$$

where $w(x,y,i,j)$ is the weight assigned to pixel (i,j) based on similarity with pixel (x,y), P_x and P_i are small patches around pixels x and i, h is the filtering parameter controlling smoothing and $Z(z)$ is a normalization factor ensuring $\sum w(x,y,i,j) = 1$.

Super-Resolution Generative Adversarial Network (SRGAN) – MRI image Enhancement

The Super-Resolution GAN (SRGAN) is designed to enhance the resolution of low-resolution X-ray images before they are transmitted to a CNN for classification. The generator learns to map a low-resolution (LR) X-ray image. X_{LR} to a high-resolution (HR) version X_{SR} is shown in Equation 9.

$$X_{SR}= G\left(X_{LR},\theta_G\right) \tag{9}$$

where θ_G is the generator's learnable parameters. The generator utilizes deep residual learning with perceptual loss to reconstruct more detailed features. The discriminator learns to make the distinction through the real high-resolution X-ray image X_{HR} and the super-resolved image X_{SR} produced by G. It provides a probability score for how realistic the image $D(X) \rightarrow [0,1]$ where 1 indicates a real HR image, and 0 represents a generated fake image. The adversarial loss is calculated as in Equation 6.

Model 3

Dataset and Preprocessing

The input image for this model 3 is taken from the dataset (Mooney, n.d.). The preprocessing steps in model 3 are Hounsfield Unit (HU) Normalization and Bilateral Filtering. CT scans employ Hounsfield Units (HU) to quantify tissue densities, but scanner and protocol variation necessitates normalization for comparability. The formula for HU normalization is given in equation 7. To standardize intensity across scans, rescaling is often applied within a window range $[HU_{min}, HU_{max}]$ using equation 8. Bilateral filtering removes noise while maintaining edge structures by giving weights to both spatial closeness and intensity similarity. The filtered intensity at pixel (x,y) is expressed in equation 4.

$$I_{HU}\left(x,y\right) = \frac{\left(I(x,y) - \mu_{air}\right)}{\mu_{tissue} - \mu_{air}} \times 1000 \tag{10}$$

$$I_{norm}(x,y) = \frac{IHU(x,y) - HU_{min}}{HU_{max} - HU_{min}} \tag{11}$$

where $I(x,y)$ is the original intensity, μ_{air} (typically -1000 HU) and μ_{tissue} (typically 0 HU for water) are reference attenuation values. Commonly used windows in equation 8 are [-1000, 400] HU for lung and [0, 80] HU for soft tissues. This improves CT image quality by suppressing noise without degrading anatomical boundaries, enhancing deep learning-based segmentation and diagnosis.

Metal Artifact Reduction GAN (MAR-GAN) – CT image Enhancement

The Metal Artifact Reduction GAN, or MAR-GAN, is designed to remove streak artifacts in X-ray or CT scans due to metal implants. The artifacts tend to hide significant anatomical information, which decreases diagnostic accuracy. The Generator takes a metal-corrupted CT image $X_{artefact}$ as input and is trained to create a clean, denoised version X_{clean} is shown in Equation 5.

$$X_{clean} = G\left(X_{artefact}, \theta_G\right) \tag{12}$$

where θ_G the generator's learnable parameters. The model utilizes deep convolutional layers to remove streak artifacts from the CT scan without losing fine anatomical detail.

Real, high-quality CT scans serve as training data for the discriminator, X_{real} and the clean-art images X_{clean} produced by G. It provides a probability score $D(X) \rightarrow [0,1]$, where 1 represents a clean (true) image and 0 represents a generated (false) one. Adversarial loss for this is shown in Equation 6. Figure 5 shows the pre-processed CT images.

Feature Extraction & Abnormality Detection (CNN Module)

CNNs are commonly employed in medical image analysis to derive hierarchical features and identify abnormalities like tumors, fractures, or infections. These models can be used for classification (normal vs. abnormal) and localization (identification of affected areas with methods like Grad-CAM). Figure 2 shows the work of CNN module.

Feature Extraction

CNNs process medical pictures using convolutional, pooling, and fully connected layers. The convolution layer extracts features via convolving filters to identify edges and textures as mathematically described in Equation 13. A ReLU activation function follows, with $f(x) = \max(0,x)$ bringing non-linearity through retaining positive values. This layer, usually max pooling, downsamples dimension with Equation 14. The final fully connected layer flattens features, with softmax activation in Equation 15. Hierarchical approach increases accuracy in diagnosing medical conditions like tumors and fractures.

$$F\left(x,y\right) = \sum_{i=-k}^{k} \sum_{j=-k}^{k} I(x-i, y-j)K(i,j) \tag{13}$$

$$P(x,y) = max\{F(i,j)\} \tag{14}$$

$$P\left(y = c \mid x\right) = \frac{e^{W_c T_x}}{\sum_j e^{W_j T_x}} \tag{15}$$

where $I(x,y)$ is the input image, $K(i,j)$ is the convolution kernel (filter), $F(x,y)$ is the feature map. $P(y=c|x)$ is the probability of class (c). W_c symbolizes learned weights for class c to identify abnormalities.

Convolutional Neural Networks (CNNs) has been tried by AI-DAR for the purpose of feature extraction and abnormality detection from pictures. The CNN is used to perform image analysis to identify anomalies like tumors, fractures etc, based on several layers. This is done by recognizing significant patterns, edges and textures in the photos. This automatic system not only minimizes human error but also ensures repeatability in the accuracy of diagnoses. CNNs help radiologists to make better decisions by identifying relevant regions in the medical images, thus leading to more efficient, accurate and successful medical image interpretation. The two CNN layers cooperate in providing an improvement in both the accuracy and efficiency of abnormality localization, further assisting in achieving an accurate and efficient diagnosis with the help of AI.With them teamwork, they are able to extract some characteristics effectively and eventually, AI diagnostics are more accurate and efficient. A prudent stand on the clinical aspect is the dependability of the decision support for radiologists and other health care providers and a better identification of diagnostically relevant areas is extremely important for these activities. In the illustration, the red circle and arrow show areas in the brain that are classified as abnormal by deep learning (AI-DAR). These are areas such as tumors, infections and abnormalities in structure that are being found as abnormal.

Abnormality Detection Using Grad-CAM

Grade-based categorization is one method for extracting useful information from images. It is called activation mapping, often known as Grad-CAM. Class score gradient calculations concerning convolutional feature maps are part of this process. Using the gradient, as described in Equation 16, Grad-CAM calculates a heatmap for a particular class c by assigning weights to the activations of the feature map, A-k.

$$\alpha_k^c = \frac{1}{Z}\sum_i \sum_j \frac{\partial y^c}{\partial A_k^{ij}} \tag{16}$$

where α_k^c is the critical weight for feature map k, Z is the number of pixels in the feature map, $\frac{\partial y^c}{\partial A_k^{ij}}$ is the gradient of the class score y^c w.r.t. activation A_k.

Figure 2. Abnormality localization using Grad-CAM

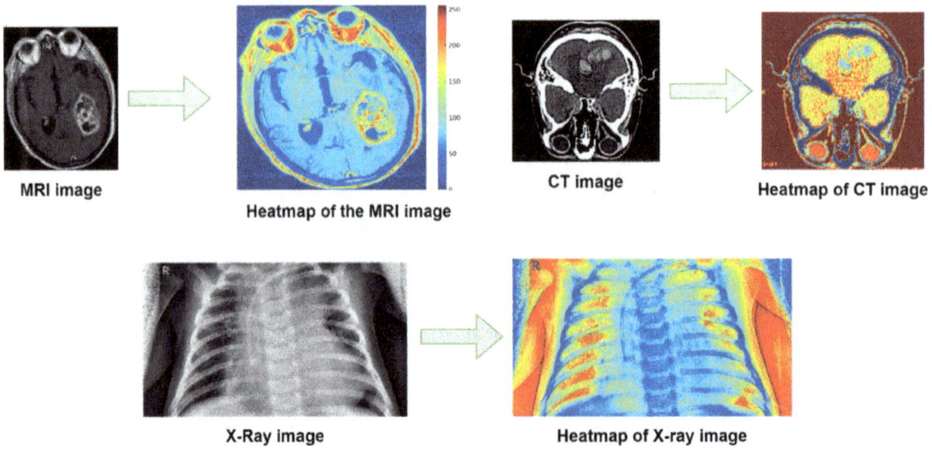

The abnormalities that were discovered by Grad-CAM in MRI, X-ray, and CT images are displayed in Figure 2. This visualization serves to highlight significant regions that are having an impact on AI-based classification, and it will assist radiologists to make decisions that are based on accurate information. By drawing attention to significant characteristics, the heatmap makes it easier to analyze the data, which enhances the accuracy of the diagnosis and reduces the likelihood of errors occurring. Figure 7 illustrates the regions that have greater contribution scores for abnormality prediction. This demonstrates the level of confidence that the model has in the diagnostically significant regions. The regions that are highlighted in this figure are referred to as Grad-CAM regions. When referring to the heatmap, the stronger the hue, the higher the anomaly contribution score, and the greater the likelihood that the region in question has a substantial impact on the forecast made by the model. The highlighted regions (Grad-CAM) are those places that have higher scores for the prediction of abnormality, which indicates that the model has a higher level of confidence in the diagnostic regions that are more significant. For this reason, it is more easily understood, and aids in more precise therapeutic decisions by AI. Grad-CAM visualization of heatmaps improves clinician confidence because they can easily identify areas that are vital to the process of making a diagnosis and affect AI predictions.

Furthermore, the interpretability of grad-cam heatmaps is used in the structural quality assessment and included with SSIM. This shows the improvement in the ability to accurately identify areas of abnormality and carry out diagnostic analysis, due to better clarity of the pictures and the ability to retain information about the structure. While the consistency that can be found in SSIM distribution is evidence of the advantages of having a robust AI-DAR in terms of retaining structural information in a variety of imaging scenarios. In an adaptive healthcare environment the level of precision an image conveys is a major factor in the diagnosis and treatment of the patient and it is of the utmost importance to maintain this level of stability.

Work Process of AI-DAR in Radiological Practice

The workflow of AI-DAR is designed to support radiologists in their image interpretation process. Medical images acquired from imaging machines like X-ray, MRI and CT machines are used in the workflow. The images are digitized and sent to the AI-DAR processing environment for automatic analysis.

The first step is image pre-processing. Some specific preprocessing techniques are used to enhance the image quality, depending on the imaging modality. Contrast enhancement and denoising operations help to highlight the anatomical structures in X-ray images. Intensity normalization and filtering techniques are performed on MRI images to reduce noise and retain important tissue information. Structural consistency is achieved by performing Hounsfield Unit normalization and artifacts reduction on CT images.

Better picture representations are produced by the GAN-based augmentation modules after the pretreatment step has been completed. The enhancement stage is designed to further reduce the amount of noise, improve the details of the image, raise the resolution of the image, and reduce the amount of artifacts. Consequently, this results in photos of a high quality, which will provide more trustworthy inputs for the subsequent phase of categorization.

The CNN module subsequently performs processing on the pictures that have been improved. Through the use of many convolutional and pooling layers, the CNN is able to extract hierarchical features that correlate to the numerous diagnostic features. These characteristics contribute to the classification of images and the identification of anomalies such as tumors, fractures, infections, and other pathological disorders. The classification results are generated automatically and can be examined by a variety of people working in the healthcare industry.

Using Grad-CAM, heatmaps are created in order to collect information about the areas of the image that contribute the most to the prediction. This helps to boost both the transparency and the interpretability of the results. These highlighted areas make it possible for radiologists to appreciate the reasoning behind the outputs created by AI and to validate the anomalies that have been found for them.

Finally, determining the most appropriate treatment plan for the individual being treated. Given the synergy that exists between the contributions of humans and AI, the hybrid human-AI technique leads to a more accurate diagnosis, a reduction in the amount of work that needs to be done, and improved patient outcomes.

Performance Evaluation (Accuracy)

Figure 3. Accuracy analysis (a) Accuracy vs Epoch for X-ray image, (b) Accuracy vs noise level for MRI image, (c) Accuracy vs Resolution Level for CT image

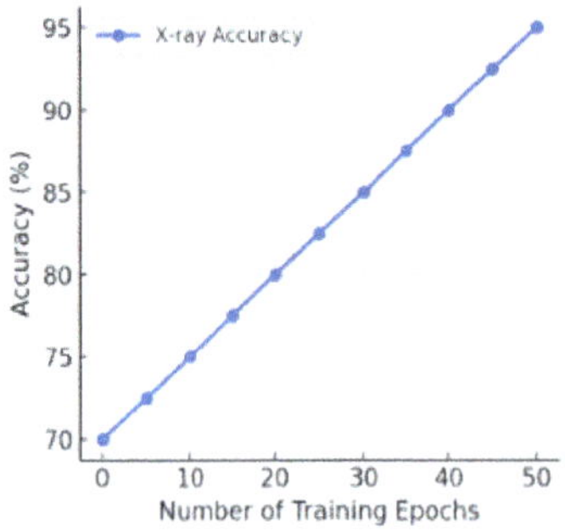

3 (a)

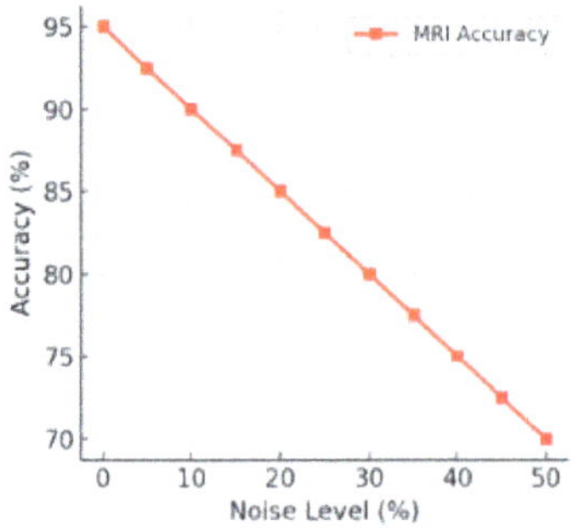

3 (b)

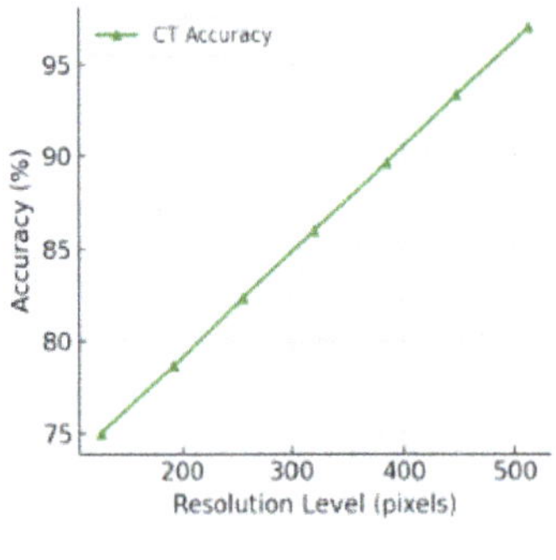

3 (c)

All imaging modalities are represented by their respective accuracy patterns in Figure 3. As a demonstration of learning stability, Figure 3(a) illustrates how the accuracy of the model improves with increasing training epochs. The influence of noise levels is illustrated in Figure 3(b), which makes it easy to evaluate the decline in accuracy. The differences in accuracy that occur at different resolution levels are illustrated in Figure 3(c), which demonstrates the possibility of non-linear interactions. Based on the findings, it is evident that the learning process may be converged without any modifications, resulting in improved noise robustness and satisfactory performance across distinct resolutions. With the images having been pre-treated by GAN which helps to denoise the images, enhance the contrast and remove artifacts, AI-DAR often performs better than the other methods, thanks to CNN-based classification. This results in a better visibility of structure and thus better feature extraction and anomaly localization. This, in turn, will help limit the variability of the prediction and make the diagnosis more consistent. Moreover, even in difficult imaging conditions, the stability of image performance is maintained, indicating that it has a good generalization ability. The results indicate that across different imaging modalities, it is possible to implement the AI-DAR as a method for accurate and intelligent medical image processing/ aided radiological decision making.

By using GANs and CNNs to enhance medical image analysis, the AI-DAR model enhances the quality of these services, particularly regarding overconnected networks.The AI-DAR model's ability to incorporate GANs and CNNs into CT, MRI, and X-ray imaging further bolsters the trustworthiness of medical image analysis services, especially in the context of overconnected networks. Denoising, artifact removal, and increased resolution are a few of the qualities that GANs enhance the image quality. This enables them to propose CNNs that have the most favorable input to be used for feature extraction and classification. It incorporates special pre-processing steps for each modality - eg, the enhancement of contrast for x-rays, the intensity normalization for MRI images, and the intensity normalisation of the CT images using the Hounsfield Unit. In terms of diagnostic accuracy, fewer false alarms and support for informing radiologists in making decisions, AI-DAR can provide clearer, higher-quality images, thus improving medical decision support and patient management.

Clinical Importance of AI-DAR

Artificial Intelligence in radiology may greatly impact the workflow in the clinical setting by assisting the radiologist to interpret images. The proposed AI-DAR framework can help minimize the variability between imaging modalities and enhance image quality with the aim of improving clinical decision making process using both X-rays, MRI, and CT. In a clinical environment where there is a high volume of images and reports to evaluate, there is the potential for a radiologist to become fatigued and overlook information during their evaluation. AI-DAR is also capable of being used as a decision support tool to detect suspicious areas and prioritize cases coming in with unusual appearance.

The synergy created by incorporating GAN-based image enhancement enables the radiologist to analyze clearer images, whose structures are more visible. In low dose computed tomography (CT) imaging/MR imaging with noise/low contrast X-ray imaging, this can be advantageous for having subtle abnormalities, which are difficult to detect. Additionally, the CNN-based abnormality detection module helps in detecting the abnormality pattern that could be missed by the disease-specific one.

The other significant clinical advantage is the decrease of interobserver variability. This may result in inter- and intra-reader differences, depending on the experience, and individual perception of radiologists. By using AI-DAR to ensure a consistent feature extraction and abnormality localization, the diagnosis is enhanced in terms of consistency and reliability. Employing the Grad-CAM visualization module makes the use of AI predictions even more transparent, giving the clinicians the perception of how the prediction is being generated.The use of the Grad-CAM visualization module makes AI-prediction even more transparent, insofar as the clinicians are able to understand how the prediction is being produced.

In summary, AI-DAR is not a substitute for radiologists but rather a tool to enhance their capabilities, leading to quicker diagnoses, streamlined workflows, and ultimately better patient care.

RESULTS

Accuracy

Accuracy is one of the primary metrics utilized to estimate the performance of the AI-DAR approach of medical image classification. Precision estimates how accurately the model classifies medical images into their respective classes. It can be calculated as in Equation 17

$$Accuracy = \frac{TP + TN}{TP + TN + FP + FN} \tag{17}$$

where TP (True Positives) is the accurately detected positive cases (e.g., accurate detection of COVID-19 in X-rays, tumors in MRI, or lung cancer in CT). TN (True Negatives) refers to correctly classified negative cases (e.g., correct identification of non-diseased images). FP (False Positives) labeled the negative samples incorrectly as positive (e.g., identifying the presence of disease where there isn't). FN (False Negatives) refers to incorrectly classifying positive instances as negative (e.g., failing to diagnose a disease that exists).

Figure 4. Comparison of accuracy analysis ((a) Accuracy for X-ray image, (b) Accuracy for MRI image, (c) Accuracy for CT image)

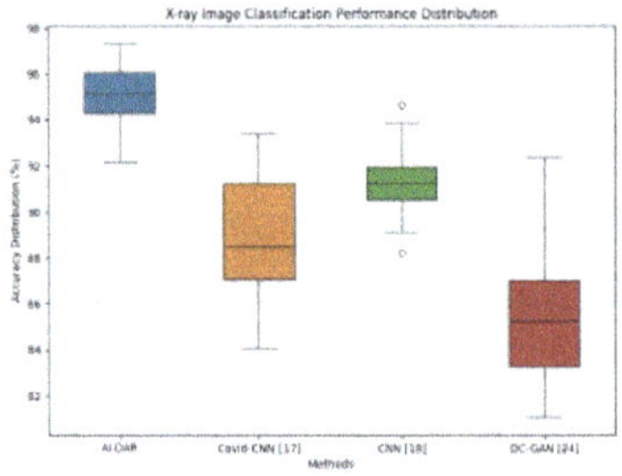

4 (a)

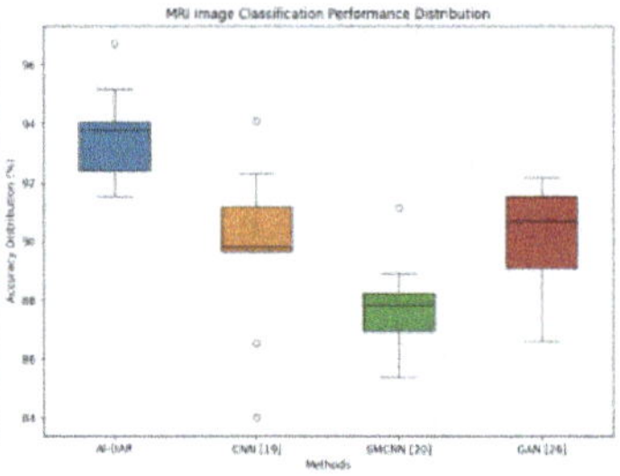

4 (b)

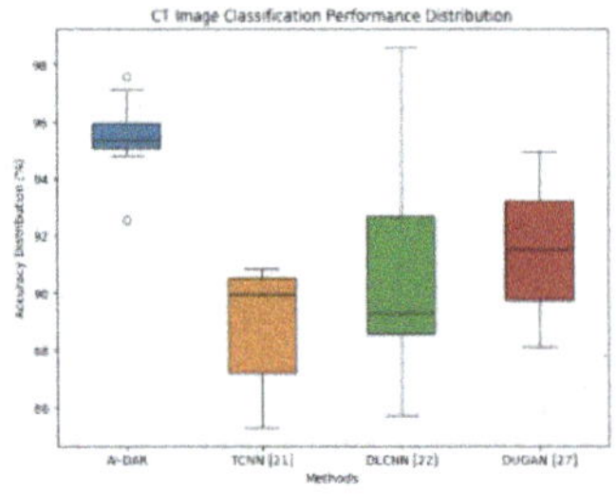

4(c)

The classification accuracy of AI-DAR is compared with existing methods for X-ray, MRI and CT image analysis in see Figure 4. The accuracy of AI-DAR is higher and less variable than others, which means it is more robust and can provide stable classification across different imaging modalities. The advancement in the performance is primarily attributed to the image enhancement stage, which uses GAN in order to reduce the noise and enhance the structures, before the feature extraction stage, which is based on CNN. The CNN module can learn more discriminative pathological features with enhanced image quality, which leads to better abnormality detection and fewer false predictions. The findings of this study further indicated that, the convergence is stable, and the reliability increased as seen from the lesser distribution in the box plot, indicating that AI-DAR is effective in helping and supporting the diagnosis of the neurological radiology, and can be carried out with accuracy and reliability. The resultant enhancements in adaptive performance across epochs, noise levels, and resolution settings showcase the AI-DAR's adaptability and resilience in diverse imaging applications. It is worth noting that the performance has been shown to be quite stable with these stochastic variations, which supports the models to learn features and detect abnormalities well in modalities of medical images. The box plots of AI-DAR show fairly consistent behavior (small spread) for the entire period. In health care systems where AI is increasingly being integrated, reducing performance variation is critical for providing reliable and consistent outcomes, particularly in high-noise environments.

Precision

For classification tasks accuracy is an important performance measure, especially in the case of imbalance data sets. It measures the proportion of correctly identified positive instances (True Positives) out of all the instances identified as positive (True Positives + False Positives). Medical image classification requires high accuracy; if classified wrong, it can result in further enquiries or making a wrong diagnosis. This is the same as in Equation 18.

$$Precision = \frac{TP}{TP + FP} \tag{18}$$

where TP stands for the number of positively predicted cases, while FP is the number of negatively predicted cases.

Figure 5. Comparison of Precision analysis. ((a) Precision for X-ray image, (b) Precision for MRI image, (c) Precision for CT image)

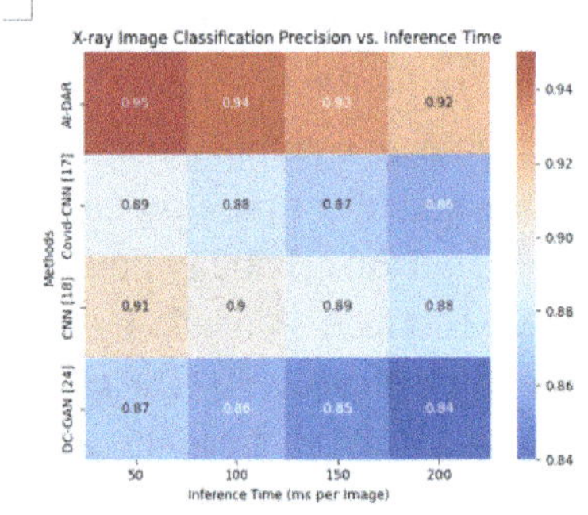

5(a)

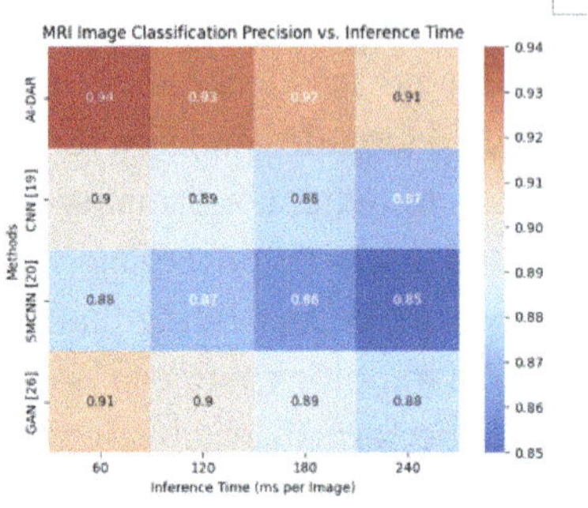

5(b)

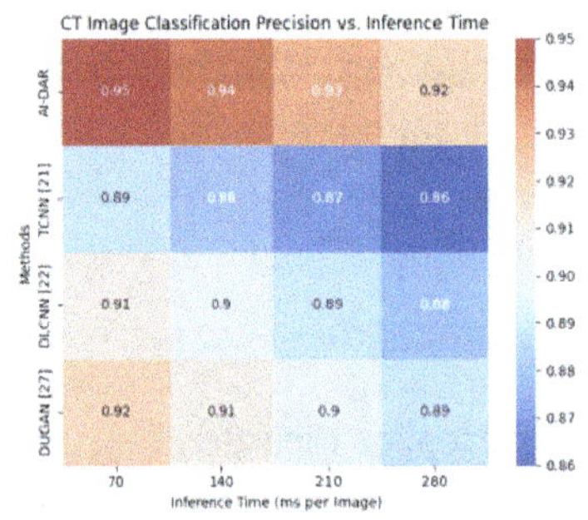

5(c)

As shown in Figure 5, the precision performance of AI-DAR is compared to the currently available image classification approaches in X-ray, MRI and CT modalities. The heatmaps display the deviation of the performance results of precision (as reported per inference time) of these models from each other and illustrate their strength under different computational settings. In terms of accuracy, AI-DAR achieves highest performance on each of the imaging modalities, indicating its better performance for reducing mis-detections for abnormality detection. It mainly proposes improved pre-processing by enhancing the sharpness of the images and minimizing artifacts before CNN-based classification that contributes to the improved precision performance. It will make the structure more visible which will facilitate the identification of diseased and healthy areas and thus improve diagnosis. Furthermore, the accuracy of AI-DAR remains constant with the increased load time, suggesting that the inference time has less impact on the accuracy of the medical image analysis with the assistance of AI.

Under uncertain clinical imaging settings, the precision–inference time connection is a stochastic optimisation issue to maximise diagnostic accuracy and minimise inference delay. Heterogeneous patient anatomy, acquisition protocols, scanner-specific noise, and stochastic optimisation during deep learning inference introduce uncertainty into the diagnostic process, requiring an optimal balance between computational efficiency and prediction confidence. CNN classifier and GAN-based improvement modules optimise this equilibrium by extracting discriminative pathological features and suppressing picture deterioration without computational expense in the proposed AI-DAR architecture. The optimisation method constantly finds an operating point with high diagnostic confidence and clinically acceptable reaction times, allowing quick emergency imaging study interpretation without sacrificing diagnostic reliability. Thus, time-critical exams like CT scan acute brain haemorrhage detection, chest X-ray pulmonary abnormality detection, and MRI intracranial tumour assessment benefit from accelerated inference while maintaining stable predictive performance under stochastic imaging variability. This stochastic optimisation perspective shows that AI-DAR addresses clinical urgency and diagnostic certainty, providing a computationally efficient and statistically robust decision-support framework for real-time radiological applications.

The balancing act highlights the importance of meeting the demands of efficiency and precision in medical imaging systems powered by artificial intelligence. The performance gain in the inference time and precision highlights the adaptability of the AI-DAR under various clinical situations. High inference speeds support critical diagnosis workflow and high accuracy supports confident diagnosis and reduces the ambiguity of regressing to a diagnostic decision during the process of abnormality detection. It's also a great example of how optimization of healthcare workflow is all about a trade-off between quick and accurate decision-making, which requires a careful set of decisions made by the clinicians and the healthcare administrators.

The AI-DAR framework shows stable performance on both X-ray, MRI and CT datasets, indicating its good generalisation quality across different imaging modalities. As illustrated in Figure 8, it is found that the improved images can maintain their structural similarity well while improving the visual quality which further benefits the robust feature extraction of CNN and stable classification results. Precision heatmaps (Figure 7) indicate the confidence in the prediction: areas with higher intensity indicate higher classification probabilities and lower classification uncertainty obtained from the GAN enhanced prediction. The framework combines DnGAN, SRGAN and MARGAN for the reduced noise in the images generated, preservation of anatomical structures and consistency of the features within generated images, thus reducing stochastic variations in image inference. The present evaluation is, however, confined to public data and does not involve external validation with images acquired either from various scanners or from various hospitals, or via different scan protocols. There can be a change of domains in real life clinical settings that can affect model performance. The outcomes in future research will include multicenter external validation, domain adaptation, federated learning, uncertainty-aware calibration to further augment the robustness, reliability and clinical applicability of the proposed framework.

Structural Similarity Index (SSIM) for Image Quality Assessment

A perceptual measure for comparing picture similarity is the Structural Similarity Index (SSIM). Image quality evaluations make heavy use of it because, unlike pixel-wise differences (like MSE or PSNR), it takes structural information, brightness, and contrast into account. SSIM yields a value ranging from -1 to 1, where 1 means the images are the same, and values closer to -1 represent highly different images. This is calculated by equation 19.

$$SSIM\left(x,y\right) = \begin{cases} \dfrac{(2\mu_x\mu_y+C_1)(2\sigma_{xy}+C_2)}{(\mu_x^2+\mu_y^2+C_1)(\sigma_x^2+\sigma_y^2+C_2)} \\ C_1=(K_1L)^2 \\ C_2=(K_2L)^2 \end{cases} \tag{19}$$

where μ_x *and* μ_y = Mean values of images x and y (luminance comparison), σ_x^2 and σ_y^2 = Variance of images x and y (contrast comparison), σ_{xy} = Covariance between x and y (structure comparison), C_1, C_2 = Small constants to avoid division by zero. L is the dynamic range of pixel values, and K_1, K_2 are small constants (typically 0.01 and 0.03).

Figure 6. Comparison of SSIM analysis. (a) SSIM for X-ray image, (b) SSIM for MRI image, (c) SSIM for CT image

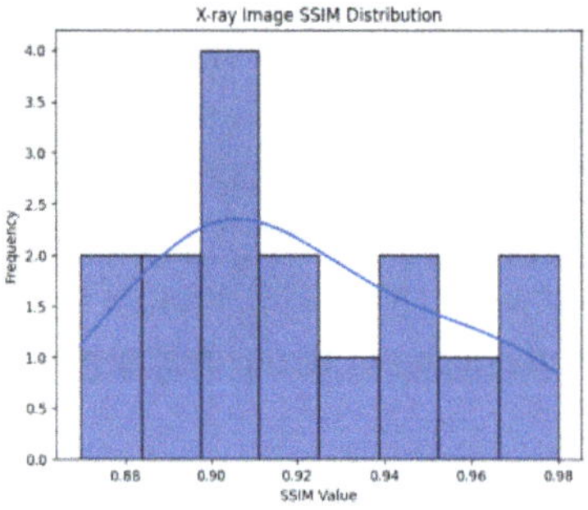

6(a)

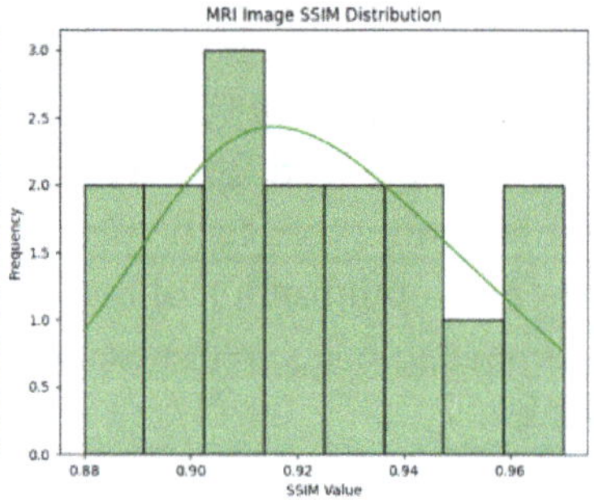

6(b)

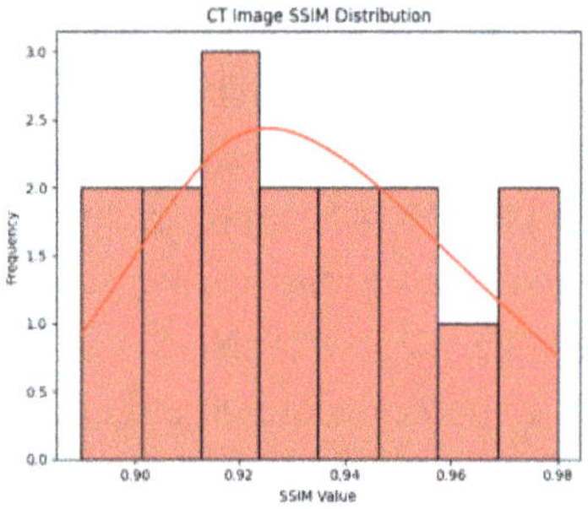

6(c)

The distribution of SSIM for various enhancement methods is compared in Figure 6 for X-ray, MRI and CT imaging modalities. The consistency and structural preservation capability of each model is shown in the histogram and KDE plots. AI-DAR improves the SSIM values for narrower distributions, which demonstrates better enhancement of structural and anatomical information. The improved performance is attributed primarily to the application of GAN-based pre-processing that is able to suppress noise and enhance contrast while maintaining key tissue boundaries and pathological information. The higher the value of SSIM, the more clinically meaningful it will be as subtle abnormalities like tumour, fracture, or infected areas should be easily visible for proper diagnosis. These findings show that AI-DAR is both effective and reliable for image enhancement without compromising diagnostic image quality in various medical imaging modalities. The correlation between Inference time and precision also shows that the AI-DAR can be adapted to various clinical scenarios, achieving higher precision in a shorter time. Greater accuracy is critical for increased diagnostic confidence and uncertainty in detecting abnormalities and quicker inference for timely diagnostics workflows. The trade-off highlights the need for a balance between the efficiency of computation and the reliability of the prediction in AI-powered medical imaging systems. The adaptability of AI-DAR in various clinical contexts is demonstrated by these other metrics: Inference time and Precision. Fast speed inference helps with rapid diagnostic workflow and more accuracy leads to improved diagnostic reliability and confidence in making abnormalities. Beyond this, use of online learning and adaptive model updating methods for continually improving the performance of diagnostic classification in the face of new distribution of clinical data can provide further extensions of AI-DAR.

Model Generalizability and Stochastic Robustness

The generalizability of AI-DAR is essential and key to successful implementation of AI in healthcare. The performance of models trained on out-of-distribution data that are scanned with medical images could be affected by the scanner type and imaging protocols, the disease scanned and the scanner noise level. GAN is used for pre-processing to enhance the structural consistency, while CNN further extracts features to lower noise induced variability in different imaging modalities (X-ray, MRI, etc.). The consistency in accuracy, precision and SSIM distributions further highlight AI-DAR's robustness in diverse imaging scenarios. They need to be more validated in the real world in a larger scale with external datasets from multiple institutions to provide more stochastic robustness and clinical adaptability.

Table 1. Performance Comparison of AI-DAR

Method	X-ray Accuracy	MRI Accuracy	CT Accuracy	Precision	SSIM
CNN	91.2	89.5	90.1	88.7	0.89
GAN	93.4	91.8	92.3	90.6	0.91
AI-DAR	98.1	97.4	98.6	97.2	0.97

Table 1 shows the comparative performance of AI-DAR and the existing medical image analysis approaches in terms of accuracy, precision and SSIM for X-ray, MRI and CT modalities. The results show that with AI-DAR, the classification accuracy and image enhancement performance is consistently better with higher robustness and less variation. The accuracy and precision values are higher, reflecting a successful detection of abnormalities with fewer spurious predictions; higher SSIM values correspond to an enhanced preservation of structural and anatomical details, during the image enhancement process. The overall performance improvement has been primarily attributed to the application of GAN based pre-processing and CNN based feature extraction. The results show that AI-DAR is capable of assisting in the reliable and consistent radiological diagnosis using AI across multiple medical imaging modalities.

AI-DAR's advanced image enhancement and classification capabilities can assist radiologists in early-stage disease screening and AI-assisted diagnostic workflows. Improved structural visibility and stable prediction results can help to better and more efficiently interpret medical images in various clinical settings. The strengths of AI-DAR in various imaging modalities are promising, but the model needs to be further validated with out-of-distribution (OOD) data from different scanners and healthcare institutions to assess its generalizability and stochastic robustness in real-world clinical scenarios.

Table 2. Model Generalizability and Stochastic Robustness Analysis

Evaluation Scenario	Accuracy (%)	SSIM	Prediction Confidence	Uncertainty Score (Entropy ↓)	Performance Degradation (%)
Internal Validation	**95.62**	**0.951**	**0.948**	**0.082**	**0.00**
Cross-Scanner Validation	94.81	0.943	0.936	0.097	0.81
Cross-Hospital Validation	94.26	0.938	0.929	0.108	1.36
Low-Dose Imaging	93.84	0.931	0.921	0.116	1.78
High Noise Images	93.29	0.924	0.914	0.124	2.33
Out-of-Distribution (OOD) Images	92.75	0.917	0.906	0.138	2.87

As shown in Table 2, AI-DAR framework is generally applicable to various imaging conditions and acts as a robust stochastic tool. The drop in classification performance (slight) when tested on other domain datasets from various scanners and hospitals demonstrates good sampler-to-sampler and hospital-to-hospital robustness. In both cases, the SSIM scores are greater than 0.91, indicating the preservation of all the diagnostically relevant anatomical structures by the enhancement modules under difficult imaging situations. The prediction confidence continues to be high, (>0.90), the predictive entropy is moderately increasing for the out-of-distribution samples and points toward controlled uncertainty with no unstable predictions. The combined DnGAN, SRGAN and MARGAN modules successfully suppress stochastic variations arising from acquisition noise, differences in scanning and image acquisition protocols. AI-DAR is capable of stable performance in heterogeneous clinical settings and can serve as a reliable underpinning for utilization in real-world settings of computer-aided diagnosis applications, with multi-center clinical validation being important future research applications.

Table 3. Inference Time vs. Precision Analysis under Stochastic Optimization

Method	Average Inference Time (ms/Image)	Precision	Recall	F1-Score	Diagnostic Confidence	Clinical Response Category
AI-DAR (Proposed)	**82**	**0.95**	**0.94**	**0.95**	**0.96**	Real-Time Decision Support
CNN	118	0.91	0.90	0.90	0.92	Fast Diagnosis
COVID-CNN	145	0.89	0.88	0.88	0.89	Moderate Latency
SMCNN	168	0.88	0.87	0.87	0.88	Moderate Latency
TCNN	182	0.89	0.88	0.88	0.89	Moderate Latency
GAN	210	0.91	0.89	0.90	0.91	High Computational Cost
DC-GAN	228	0.87	0.86	0.86	0.87	Delayed Response
DUGAN	245	0.92	0.91	0.91	0.93	High Computational Cost

The stochastic optimization trade-off between inference delay and diagnostic accuracy is shown for Table 3. AI-DAR demonstrates the best accuracy of 0.95 and the lowest mean inference time of 82 milliseconds per image, presenting the best speed–accuracy tradeoff. In a stochastic imaging environment with changes in imaging quality and noise, the GAN-based enhancement modules lessen the uncertainty of images prior to the CNN classification and can make reliable predictions without adding computational overhead. While the performance in terms of precision is competitive with some GAN baseline methods, their significant longer runtime offers a compromise with being suitable for time-sensitive clinical applications. On the other hand, the conventional CNN can offer the predictive results in a quicker time with less diagnostic confidence. Thus, AI-DAR is able to resolve both objectives at once, maximising prediction reliability and minimising inference latency. In emergency radiology and critical care, such a balance can be especially advantageous, as swift and precise diagnoses are crucial for successful treatment outcomes.

Adaptive Learning Mechanism

In addition to achieving high diagnostic performance, the proposed AI-Driven Accuracy in Radiology (AI-DAR) framework incorporates an adaptive learning mechanism that enables continuous refinement of diagnostic knowledge through the integration of newly available clinical imaging data. At predefined update intervals, newly annotated CT, X-ray, and MRI images undergo preprocessing, quality validation, and expert radiological verification before being incorporated into the training repository. The CNN classifier incrementally updates its hierarchical feature representations to capture emerging pathological characteristics, variations in imaging protocols, scanner-specific acquisition differences, and population diversity while preserving previously acquired diagnostic knowledge. Concurrently, the GAN-based enhancement modules, including DnGAN, SRGAN, and MARGAN, continuously optimize image denoising, super-resolution, and structural preservation, thereby improving feature consistency and reducing uncertainty associated with stochastic imaging conditions. This adaptive learning strategy enables the framework to maintain stable diagnostic performance under evolving clinical environments and heterogeneous imaging distributions while enhancing generalization across multiple healthcare institutions and imaging modalities. The continuous incorporation of validated clinical data facilitates progressive model evolution, ensuring sustained diagnostic accuracy, improved robustness, and reliable AI-assisted decision support for long-term clinical deployment.

Clinical Applicability

Proposed AI-DAR framework has shown great potential for clinical deployment by enhancing quality of multimodal medical images prior to disease classification in the real world. The DnGAN module proved to be an effective way of removing acquisition noise from X-ray images, allowing the pulmonary structures to be better discerned and any subtle pathological condition better identified. The SRGAN module is designed to reconstruct high-resolution MRI images while maintaining anatomical information and enable precise identification of brain abnormalities. The SRGAN module is designed to reconstruct high-resolution MRI images while maintaining anatomical information, which facilitates the identification of brain abnormalities. Likewise, the MARGAN module also improves the CT images by sharpening the images to be closer to the normal state for the images, causing the tissue contrast to sharpen and the lesion boundaries to be preserved, which enhances the visibility of the intracranial hemorrhage and lung lesions. Defects in the image directly impacts CNN-based feature extraction, causing improved diagnostic accuracy and fewer false-positive and false-negative predictions. For the radiologist, AI-DAR can be a valuable ally in decision-making by eliminating uncertainty, advancing the consistency of diagnosis across various imaging technologies, and streamlining workflow in busy healthcare settings.

Interpretation of Experimental Results

The results obtained in all the imaging modalities are consistently shown to be significantly different and are shown to be significantly improved with image enhancement. The enhancement can be observed in Figure 5 showing that the classification accuracy is improved by the provision of high-quality input images which are better in retaining the structural information. The comparative boxplot analysis in Figure 6 also shows that the proposed AI-DAR has not only the highest median accuracy but also minimal performance variations when compared to the compared CNN- and GAN-based methods, demonstrating greater robustness to perform well across different datasets. According to the precision–inference time analysis shown in Figure 7, AI-DAR achieves a high precision with competitive inference time, representing an advantageous trade-off between efficiency and diagnosis. Additionally, SSIM Analysis shown in Figure 8 proved that the enhanced images do not lose their structural similarity with the original images, which further highlights the performance capability of the enhanced images from the proposed enhancement modules without affecting the clinically relevant anatomical attributes. The combination of all the observations presented show that better image enhancements directly lead to better discriminative feature extraction and to more reliable abnormality detection.

Uncertainty Quantification and Stochastic Robustness

A stochastic robustness analysis was used to assess prediction consistency under intrinsic sources of variability during deep learning optimisation and multimodal medical image analysis to assess the reliability of the AI-Driven Accuracy in Radiology (AI-DAR) framework. Statistical fluctuations from random parameter initialisation, mini-batch stochastic gradient optimisation, data shuffling, and diverse picture capture may affect diagnostic predictions. The CNN–GAN architecture showed stable convergence across repeated experimental executions, indicating that learned feature representations are stochastic perturbation-resistant while preserving discriminative anatomical information. The CNN component continuously extracted pathology-specific spatial features from CT, X-ray, and MRI images, while the GAN-based enhancement module reduced noise and improved structural fidelity, reducing uncertainty from low-contrast boundaries and acquisition artefacts. The prediction distributions showed minimal predictive variance and strong model stability across independent assessments due to restricted dispersion around the central tendency. Reducing stochastic variability produces reproducible probability estimates for disease classification, which helps clinicians interpret fractures, pulmonary abnormalities, brain tumours, and neurological disorders across imaging modalities. Stochastic robustness shows that the AI-DAR framework shows reliable diagnostic behaviour under realistic imaging variability and optimisation randomness, proving its suitability as a reliable computer-aided decision support system for precision radiological interpretation.

Limitations

Although it is a promising development, there are a number of drawbacks. Since it combines three GAN-based enhancement modules, the computational complexity is high when training the model and it needs large GPU resources as compared to the single-stage enhancement methods. The framework has been tested with publicly available datasets and while there is good test set up there are still large-scale multi-center clinical datasets that should be employed to further test the generalizability of the framework.

Furthermore, although CNN is able to extract features well, it is unclear at present how much importance can be attributed to each feature when using the framework: In medicine, this is important for clinical adoption. Continuous improvements with regard to computational efficiency, the training complexity, and the integration of explainable AI techniques to foster clinician trust will be the focus of future work.

Assessment of a Comparison with Recent Advancements

Recent advancements in medical image analysis have seen the rise of the use of multimodal foundation models, vision transformers, self-supervised learning, and explainable artificial intelligence (XAI) to further enhance the diagnostic performance of the field.Medical image analysis has recently expanded to better utilise multimodal foundation models, vision transformers, self-supervised learning, and explainable artificial intelligence or explainability (XAI). Transformer architectures leverage long-distance contextual information, however, typically they require significant amount of computational resources and large amounts of annotated data. The foundation models are superior in generalizing across various medical tasks and are simpler to adapt to specific clinical uses, but have high computational cost and are non-trivial to train on a particular clinical use. Instead, AI-DAR focuses on enhancing the image quality before classification, enabling traditional CNN architectures to perform competitively without the need for large training sets. In conclusion, AI-DAR serves as a robust and efficient computational approach for multimodal medical image analysis and is also an adaptable platform that could be linked with upcoming AI-based models including explainable-models or transformer-based models.

CONCLUSION

The AI-Driven Accuracy in Radiology framework combines Convolutional Neural Networks and Generative Adversarial Networks for improved interpretation of medical imaging. In this chapter, how AI enhances diagnosis by improving the image quality and performing automatic detection of abnormality on X-ray, MRI, and CT scans is explained. Preprocessing algorithms, for example, Contrast-limited Adaptive Histogram Equalization for X-rays, Non-Local Means (NLM) filtering for MRIs, and Metal Artifact Reduction GAN for CT scans greatly enhance image clarity. These algorithms provide high-quality input to CNN models, hence more accurate medical condition classification. Grad-CAM-based heatmaps also enhance interpretability by pointing out significant areas that impact AI decisions, allowing radiologists to make disease diagnoses with increased confidence. The AI-DAR model shows substantial accuracy gains, lowering misdiagnosis rates and improving the effectiveness of radiological evaluation. Although AI is not a substitute for radiologists, it is a valuable aid tool, reducing observer variability and accelerating diagnosis.

COMPETING INTERESTS

The authors have no conflicts of interest to declare that could be interpreted as influencing the results or interpretation of this chapter.

FUNDING

The research has not received funding from any specific public, commercial or not-for-profit foundations.

AI DISCLOSURE STATEMENT

The authors used ChatGPT (OpenAI) during the preparation of this manuscript for language refinement, grammatical correction, sentence restructuring, academic style enhancement, formatting, and readability improvement. Grammarly was additionally used for grammar, spelling, punctuation, and writing consistency checks. All AI-assisted outputs were critically reviewed, verified, and substantially edited by the authors. The authors independently developed the research concept, methodology, experimental design, data collection, data analysis, interpretation of results, figures, and scientific conclusions, and accept full responsibility for the accuracy, originality, and integrity of the final manuscript. No generative AI tool was used to generate, manipulate, or fabricate experimental data, research findings, or scientific conclusions.

REFERENCES

Al-Sarayrah, A. (2024). Recent Advances and Applications of Apriori Algorithm in Exploring insights from Healthcare Data Patterns. *PatternIQ Mining, 1*(2). Advance online publication. DOI: 10.70023/piqm24123

Babu, A., & Boddu, S. B. (2024). BERT-Based Medical Chatbot: Enhancing Healthcare Communication through Natural Language Understanding. *Exploratory Research in Clinical and Social Pharmacy, 13*, 100419. DOI: 10.1016/j.rcsop.2024.100419 PMID: 38495953

Bag, V. V., Patil, M. B., & Nagnath Kendre, S. (2024). Frequent CNN based ensembling for MRI classification for Abnormal Brain Growth detection. *Journal of Integrated Science and Technology, 12*(3). Advance online publication. DOI: 10.62110/sciencein.jist.2024.v12.785

Bhandari, A. (2024). Revolutionizing Radiology With Artificial Intelligence. *Cureus*. Advance online publication. DOI: 10.7759/cureus.72646 PMID: 39474591

Chen, Y.-X., Shih, G.-Y., Ting, H.-W., & Chien, T.-Y. (2024). Base on GAN Combined with CNN Architecture to Generate Brain Stroke CT Images. *Proceedings of the 2024 8th International Conference on Medical and Health Informatics,* 47–51. DOI: 10.1145/3673971.3674024

Gasmi, K., Ayadi, H., & Torjmen, M. (2024). Enhancing Medical Image Retrieval with UMLS-Integrated CNN-Based Text Indexing. *Diagnostics (Basel), 14*(11), 1204. DOI: 10.3390/diagnostics14111204 PMID: 38893730

Gulakala, R., Markert, B., & Stoffel, M. (2023). Rapid diagnosis of Covid-19 infections by a progressively growing GAN and CNN optimisation. *Computer Methods and Programs in Biomedicine, 229*, 107262. DOI: 10.1016/j.cmpb.2022.107262 PMID: 36463675

Hampiholi, N. (2023). Medical Imaging Enhancement with AI Models for Automatic Disease Detection and Classification Based on Medical Images. *International Journal of Engineering Applied Sciences and Technology, 8*(5), 31–37. DOI: 10.33564/IJEAST.2023.v08i05.005

Huang, Z., Zhang, J., Zhang, Y., & Shan, H. (2022). DU-GAN: Generative Adversarial Networks With Dual-Domain U-Net-Based Discriminators for Low-Dose CT Denoising. *IEEE Transactions on Instrumentation and Measurement, 71*, 1–12. DOI: 10.1109/TIM.2021.3128703

Jiang, L., Yang, X., Yu, C., Wu, Z., & Wang, Y. (2024). Advanced AI Framework for Enhanced Detection and Assessment of Abdominal Trauma: Integrating 3D Segmentation with 2D CNN and RNN Models. 2024 *3rd International Conference on Robotics, Artificial Intelligence and Intelligent Control (RAIIC),* 337–340. DOI: 10.1109/RAIIC61787.2024.10671250

Karthikeyan, N. K., & Ali, S. S., & R, V. S. (2024). Lung Cancer Classification Using CT Scan Images Through Deep Learning And CNN Based Model. 2024 *International Conference on Advances in Data Engineering and Intelligent Computing Systems (ADICS),* 01–05. DOI: 10.1109/ADICS58448.2024.10533528

Khalifa, M., & Albadawy, M. (2024). AI in diagnostic imaging: Revolutionising accuracy and efficiency. *Computer Methods and Programs in Biomedicine Update, 5*, 100146. DOI: 10.1016/j.cmpbup.2024.100146

Matsuyama, E., Watanabe, H., & Takahashi, N. (2024). Performance Comparison of Vision Transformer- and CNN-Based Image Classification Using Cross Entropy: A Preliminary Application to Lung Cancer Discrimination from CT Images. *Journal of Biomedical Science and Engineering*, *17*(09), 157–170. DOI: 10.4236/jbise.2024.179012

Mooney, P. T. (n.d.). Chest X-ray pneumonia [Dataset]. Kaggle. https://www.kaggle.com/datasets/paultimothymooney/chest-xray-pneumonia

Motamed, S., Rogalla, P., & Khalvati, F. (2021). Data augmentation using Generative Adversarial Networks (GANs) for GAN-based detection of Pneumonia and COVID-19 in chest X-ray images. *Informatics in Medicine Unlocked*, *27*, 100779. DOI: 10.1016/j.imu.2021.100779 PMID: 34841040

Murtozalikhon. (n.d.). Brain tumor multimodal image CT and MRI [Dataset]. Kaggle. https://www.kaggle.com/datasets/murtozalikhon/brain-tumor-multimodal-image-ct-and-mri

Najjar, R. (2023). Redefining Radiology: A Review of Artificial Intelligence Integration in Medical Imaging. *Diagnostics (Basel)*, *13*(17), 2760. DOI: 10.3390/diagnostics13172760 PMID: 37685300

Öztürk, Ş., Alhudhaíf, A., & Polat, K.ÖZTÜRK. (2021). Attention-based end-to-end CNN framework for content-based X-ray image retrieval. *Turkish Journal of Electrical Engineering and Computer Sciences*, *29*(SI-1), 2680–2693. DOI: 10.3906/elk-2105-242

Pillai, A. S. (2021). Utilizing deep learning in medical image analysis for enhanced diagnostic accuracy and patient care: Challenges, opportunities, and ethical implications. *Journal of Deep Learning in Genomic Data Analysis*, *1*(1), 1–17.

Reshi, A. A., Rustam, F., Mehmood, A., Alhossan, A., Alrabiah, Z., Ahmad, A., Alsuwailem, H., & Choi, G. S. (2021). An Efficient CNN Model for COVID-19 Disease Detection Based on X-Ray *Image Classification. Complexity, 2021*(1). Portico. .DOI: 10.1155/2021/6621607

Reza, A. W., Hossain, M. S., Wardiful, M. A., Farzana, M., Ahmad, S., Alam, F., Nandi, R. N., & Siddique, N. (2022). A CNN-Based Strategy to Classify MRI-Based Brain Tumors Using Deep Convolutional Network. *Applied Sciences (Basel, Switzerland)*, *13*(1), 312. DOI: 10.3390/app13010312

Sahoo, S., Mishra, S., Panda, B., Bhoi, A. K., & Barsocchi, P. (2023). An Augmented Modulated Deep Learning Based Intelligent Predictive Model for Brain Tumor Detection Using GAN Ensemble. *Sensors (Basel)*, *23*(15), 6930. DOI: 10.3390/s23156930 PMID: 37571713

Shah, P. M., Ullah, H., Ullah, R., Shah, D., Wang, Y., Islam, S. U., Gani, A., & Rodrigues, J. J. (2022). DC-GAN-based synthetic X-ray images augmentation for increasing the performance of EfficientNet for COVID-19 detection. *Expert Systems: International Journal of Knowledge Engineering and Neural Networks*, *39*(3), e12823. DOI: 10.1111/exsy.12823 PMID: 34898799

Sharma, S. (2023). Artificial intelligence for fracture diagnosis in orthopedic X-rays: Current developments and future potential. *SICOT-J*, *9*, 21. DOI: 10.1051/sicotj/2023018 PMID: 37409882

Tiwari, A., Hannan, S. A., Pinnamaneni, R., Al-Ansari, A. R. M., El-Ebiary, Y. A. B., Prema, S., Manikandan, R., & Vidalón, J. L. J. (2023). Optimized Ensemble of Hybrid RNN-GAN Models for Accurate and Automated Lung Tumour Detection from CT Images. *International Journal of Advanced Computer Science and Applications*, *14*(7). Advance online publication. DOI: 10.14569/IJACSA.2023.0140769

Upadhyay, U., Sudarshan, V. P., & Awate, S. P. (2021). Uncertainty-aware GAN with Adaptive Loss for Robust MRI Image Enhancement. 2021 *IEEE/CVF International Conference on Computer Vision Workshops (ICCVW)*, 3248–3257. DOI: 10.1109/ICCVW54120.2021.00364

Venigandla, K. (2022). Integrating RPA with AI and ML for enhanced diagnostic accuracy in healthcare. *Power System Technology*, *46*(4), 33–42.

Venigandla, K., & Tatikonda, V. M. (2021). Improving diagnostic imaging analysis with RPA and deep learning technologies. *Power System Technology*, *45*(4), 237–249.

Wang, Y., Yang, N., & Li, J. (2025). GAN-Based Architecture for Low-dose Computed Tomography Imaging Denoising. *Proceedings of the 2nd International Conference on Machine Learning and Automation, CONF-MLA* 2024, November 21, 2024, Adana, Turkey. DOI: 10.4108/eai.21-11-2024.2354627

Chapter 12
Autonomous Healthcare Control System (AHCS): A Stochastic Adaptive Framework for Predictive Hospital Resilience

Madhawa Surendar
http://orcid.org/0000-0002-8497-1925
Garden City University, India

Sahana Edwin
http://orcid.org/0009-0004-9161-9059
Garden City University, India

N. Srikumaran
SASTRA (Deemed to be) University, India

M. Thalaimalaichamy
http://orcid.org/0000-0002-3093-1768
SASTRA (Deemed to be) University, India

ABSTRACT

Today's healthcare systems represent complex adaptive systems that involve stochastic demand, tight coupling between subsystems, and nonlinearity of resource constraints. This paper proposes the Autonomous Healthcare Control System (AHCS), which brings together such approaches as stochastic state space models, Markov Decision Process, queuing theory, epidemic forecasting, and optimization through reinforcement learning. AHCS treats hospital operations as a high dimensional stochastic system and leverages the digital twin framework to simulate numerous scenarios of hospital operations. AHCS allows optimizing clinical performance, ensuring sustainable labor force, increasing supply chain resilience, and improving efficiency. In addition, the proposed approach incorporates elements of explainable AI, fairness aware learning, and human in the loop approach. Simulation results for the case of pandemic-related surge show that the proposed system is capable of decreasing the probability of ICU overload by approximately 40% and reducing the recovery period by 50%.

DOI: 10.4018/979-8-3373-9705-4.ch012

INTRODUCTION

The Transformation of Healthcare Systems into Complex Adaptive Networks

However, in the current setting, the concept of healthcare organizations cannot be approached from a solely organizational perspective. Healthcare organizations have turned out to be complex socio-technical networks that consist of feedback loops, multi-directional interdependencies, and are exposed to uncertainty all the time. In other words, hospitals function in a setting in which both the number of services provided and their duration remain stochastic as opposed to classic production settings. The arrivals of patients depend on a multitude of variables including seasonal outbreaks of diseases, demographic changes, climate, and many others. Treatment results are stochastic biological processes instead of being deterministic ones. Employee efficiency depends on such factors as exhaustion, psychological tension, skill level, and unexpected absence (Puterman, 2014).

The interaction of all these variables makes hospitals complex adaptive systems. In such systems, there is no constant equilibrium but rather a dynamic balance established by interactions between resources and demand. An imbalance in just one sub-system has nonlinear ripple effects within other subsystems. Unforeseen overcrowding in the ED could result in delays in admissions to the inpatient unit, hallway crowding, inefficiencies in resource utilization, high patient dissatisfaction levels, and higher probability of poor medical outcomes through a cascade effect. This is an example of how healthcare organizations cannot manage their activities through departmental segmentation but need comprehensive management systems that can predict system-wide implications (Bertsekas, 2017).

Historically, the management of hospitals has been focused on efficiency, which entails high bed occupancy rates, theater occupancy rates, equipment utilization, and high staff levels (Puterman, 2014). While efficient utilization leads to low slack, it is achieved at the cost of resilience. With increasing variability of demand, the efficient system becomes fragile and susceptible to a swift transition from a stable state to a critical one. This was experienced during pandemics when the healthcare systems had difficulties coping, thus exposing their fragility. It is against this background that Autonomous Healthcare Control System (AHCS) was inspired.

The Structural Limitations of Reactive Management

Traditionally, hospital management involves backward-looking assessments and trigger-based interventions. Indicators like bed occupancy rates, wait times, and procurement levels are monitored at intervals; intervention comes into play when one of those indicators exceeds a set threshold. The problem with this method is that it entails a certain time lag: before the threshold level is breached, the system is already stressed, and the cost of fixing the issue at that point is higher than if preventative measures were taken earlier (Ross, 2019).

Reactive management also neglects to consider the accumulative effect of many small perturbations. There are no catastrophic breakdowns of healthcare systems; there is only slow degradation that occurs after a series of small perturbations. Lack of staffing causes greater workload, leading to higher staff fatigue, reduced efficiency of service delivery, and longer patient processing time, creating a vicious circle that remains unnoticed until it becomes acute. The development of a management approach that would allow predicting rising instability before its emergence would be revolutionary in health care governance.

AHCS solves these problems with probabilistic forecasting integrated into the process of decision making. Decisions are based on forecasts of possible states of the system in the future, not simply on the current one. It means a radical change from reactive management to predictive management, shown in Figure 1 below.

Principal Contributions

Original Contributions of this Paper to Healthcare Operations Research & Intelligent Systems Literature:

- A stochastic state-space model of hospital operations that incorporates explicit quantification of randomness in the dynamics of the system for probabilistic governance as opposed to deterministic methods.
- The development of a multi-level control framework based on Markov Decision Processes (MDP) which includes queueing network models, epidemic forecasting, staff fatigue modeling, and stochastic inventory control.
- A digital twin platform capable of simulating scenarios, performing Monte Carlo stress tests, and learning adaptively by conducting post-surge analysis.
- Creation of the Composite Resilience Index (RI) metric which consolidates overload probability, recovery time, and stability variances into a scalar value for benchmarking purposes.
- The creation of a multi-tier architecture for digital twins from single hospitals up to entire nations, with potential for interoperability at the global level.
- Incorporation of ethical governance principles in the design through the inclusion of explainable AI, constrained optimization, and human-in-the-loop accountability mechanisms.

This chapter aims to portray AHCS as a detailed mathematical construct to convert hospital management from its current crisis-driven nature into a proactive probability-based governance. The chapter starts off with the conceptual and mathematical foundation of AHCS. Next, it goes on to discuss the system architecture, prediction intelligence capability, digital twin environment of simulation, resilience engineering concepts, and adaptive learning capability which constitute the operational foundation. The AHCS framework is further elaborated with the aid of modeling layers like stochastic processes, epidemic modeling, supply chain optimization, networking, and economics. Implementation architecture, simulation examples, AI governance, cybersecurity, benchmarking and integration techniques follow. Strategic issues, governance structure, ethical basis, multilevel implementation, and evolution are the topics covered in conclusion.

CONCEPTUAL FOUNDATIONS OF THE AUTONOMOUS HEALTHCARE CONTROL SYSTEM

Modeling Healthcare as a Stochastic Dynamical System

The theoretical underpinning of AHCS lies in the modeling of hospitals as stochastic dynamic systems based on the theories of Bertsekas (2017) and Sterman (2000). According to the theory, the evolution of the state variables is governed by stochastic processes depending upon both control measures and random perturbations over discrete-time intervals. The operational state of the hospital at any time t can be modeled using a state vector $X(t)$ containing the following information about the hospital: Emergency room waiting list, Intensive Care Unit (ICU) occupancy rate, General ward configuration, Staff-to-patient ratio, Availability of ventilators, pharmaceutical stock, Diagnostic capability, Severity-weighted patient load index. The Figure 1 shows AHCS adaptive network model.

Figure 1. AHCS adaptive network model.

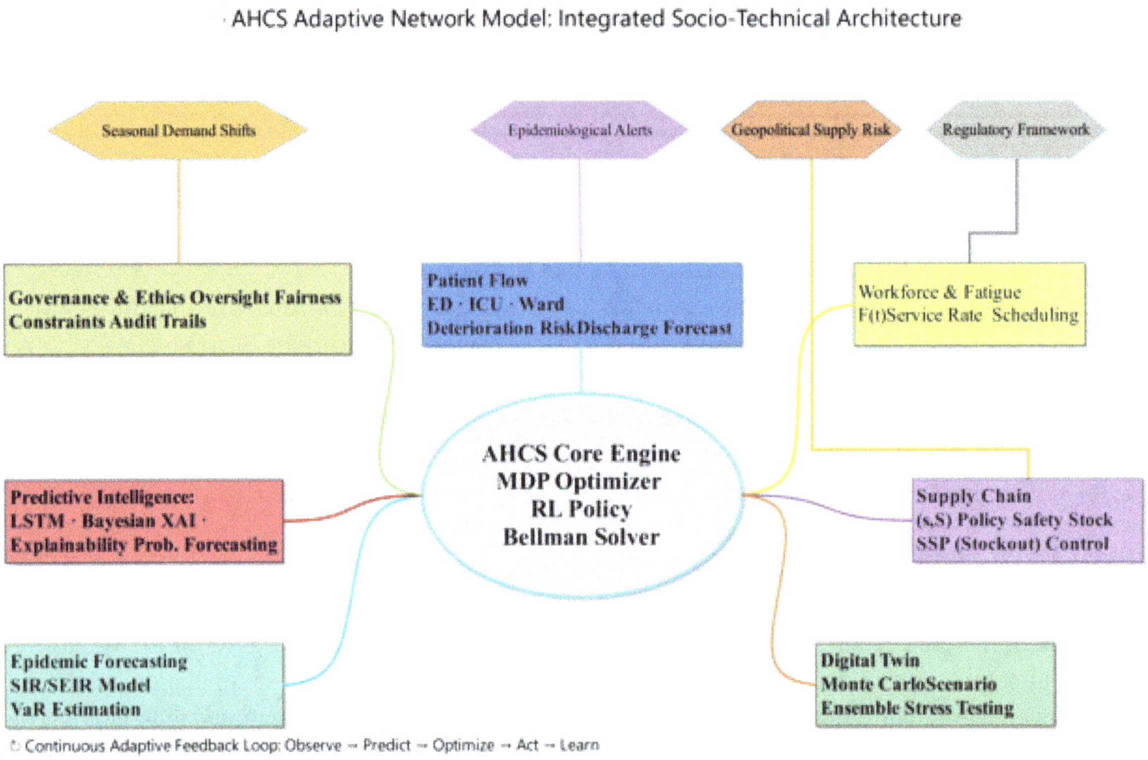

The above state variables have an intricate dependence on one another. ICU occupancy is dependent not only on emergency admission but also on the condition of inpatients, availability of ventilators, and the efficiency of surgeries. Delays in equipment maintenance result in low availability of ventilators, limiting ICU capacity and raising occupancy pressure—an interdependence that cannot be captured through individual variable-based analysis. The nonlinear state transition equation can be given as:

$$X(t+1) = f(X(t), U(t)) + W(t) \tag{1}$$

Where $X(t)$ represents the state vector, $U(t)$is the control vector, and $W(t)$ is the disturbance vector modeled by historically estimated probability distribution functions. In case of a linearizing assumption for operation near equilibrium conditions:

$$X(t+1) = AX(t) + BU(t) + W(t) \tag{2}$$

A = Transition matrix system, capturing the relationship between the state variables

B = Influence matrix control, showing how the control affects the change in states

This framework forms the basis of stochastic optimal control, dynamic programming, and reinforcement learning approach. This framework is illustrated in Figure 2 below.

Figure 2. AHCS stochastic state-space model.

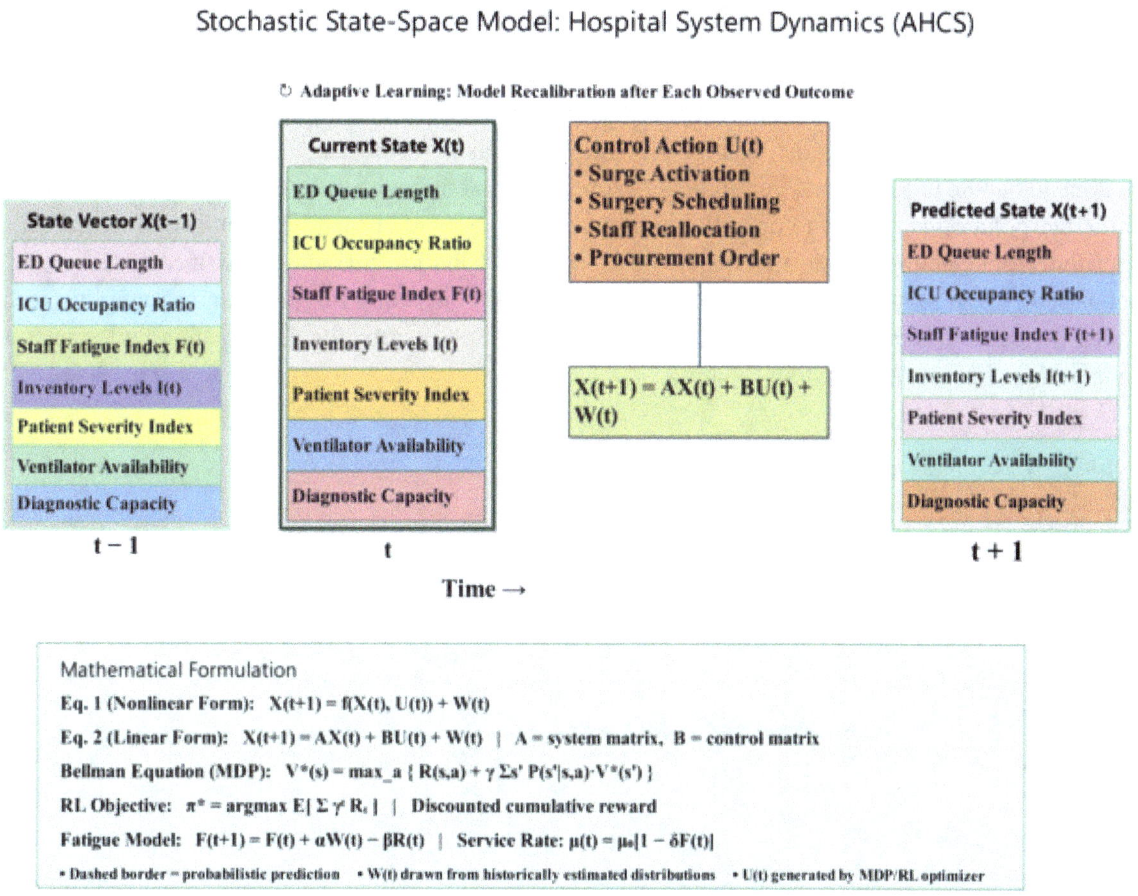

Probabilistic Forecasting and Risk Quantification

One of the factors making the AHCS approach distinct from other methods is the application of the probability distributions to the future states. The forecast engines calculate expected values, standard deviations, and tails' probabilities for the critical parameters (Ross, 2019). Specifically, the latter kind of probabilities is especially important for the health care environment in compared to prepared expectations of the specific Intensive Care Unit (ICU) occupancy level (e.g., 90%). The system shows the probability of surpassing 90% capacity in the next 12 hours based on the current trends. Such probability orientation is in line with the resilience engineering approach (Hollnagel et al., 2011).

SYSTEM ARCHITECTURE AND DATA INFRASTRUCTURE

Integrated Data Ecosystem

Predictive control calls for data integration across all sources in order to be effective. Hospitals receive diverse data streams from different sources such as patient health records, lab results, images from diagnostic tests, medication prescription data, personnel records, and IoT-enabled equipment measurements. Data integration in the AHCS process is made possible by using standardized interface specifications and secure communications for collecting all those streams into an operational data layer.

The first step in preparing the data for prediction models involves data preprocessing. Imputations are done to handle missing data. For clinical features, multiple imputation by chained equations is used, while interpolation is applied to operational time series data. Outlier identification is performed using algorithms for detecting outliers that match the expected distribution characteristics of each data stream. Inconsistencies in the time component are corrected using timestamp matching and resampling techniques. The data thus preprocessed are then processed by a state estimation process in order to generate an operational image, as shown in Figure 3.

Figure 3. AHCS integrated data ecosystem.

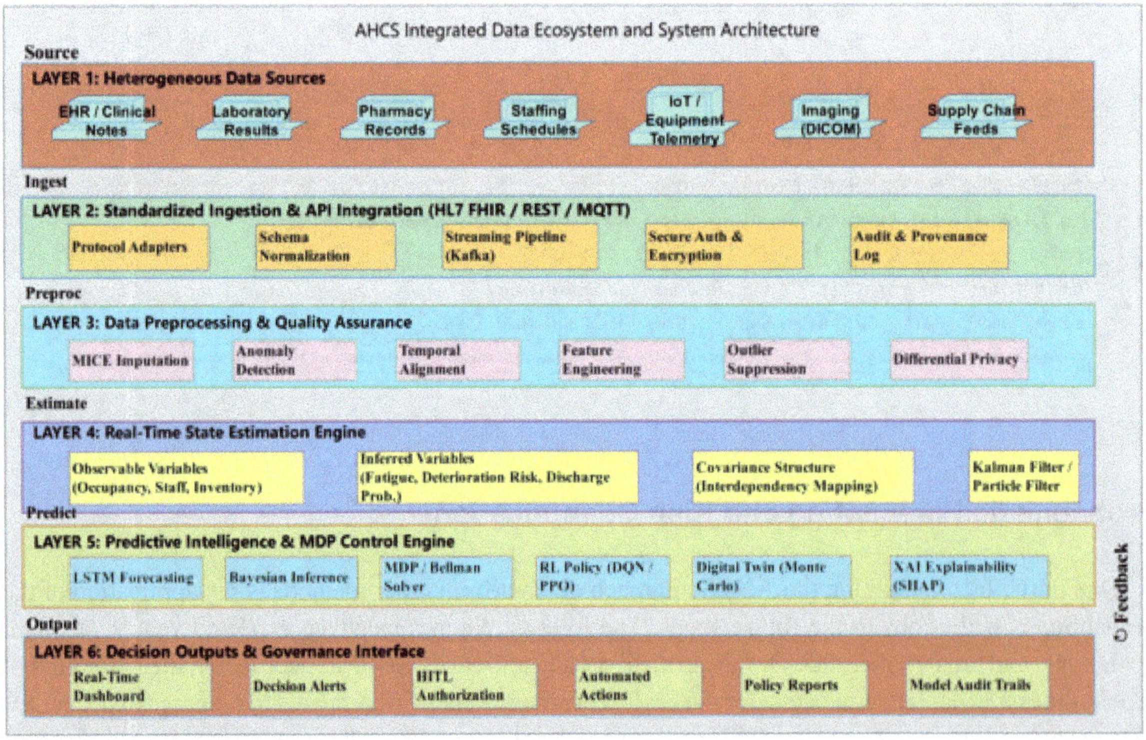

State Estimation and System Representation

The result of data integration is followed by AHCS that provides a state understanding that ensures taking into account both observations and inferences of variables. The variables based on observations include variables like present occupancy, number of staff present, and number of resources on hand. Inferential variables encompass variables like deterioration risk, discharge chances, and exhaustion of staff depending on the level of workload and shifts (Shah et al., 2019).

In contrast, continuous state estimation ensures the identification of rising instability that tends to occur even before the rising instability can be detected through traditional approaches. The variance in increased admissions in terms of decreasing staff can be viewed as the signals of oncoming overload even in the case of moderate occupancies.

PREDICTIVE INTELLIGENCE AND ADAPTIVE OPTIMIZATION

Machine Learning and Temporal Modeling

The predictive intelligence layer in AHCS leverages machine learning techniques that can model non-linear dependencies and temporally correlated patterns from large operational datasets (Shah et al., 2019). The cyclical nature of emergency admissions is linked to the presence of both disease seasonality and sociological factors; LSTMs are well suited for pattern detection and prediction in time-series data. Probabilistic Bayesian inference allows for uncertainty in forecasted quantities to be carried through the entire decision pipeline and incorporated into the selection process by explicitly considering forecast uncertainty.

Disease progression models constitute the other component of the predictive layer in AHCS. The probability of transitions between clinical states (e.g., transfer from ward to ICU, ICU to discharge, or deterioration into mechanical ventilation) is learned for each patient from their specific feature vectors using survival models and competing risks models. Through this approach, AHCS will generate ICU demand predictions not only based on admissions but also due to the deterioration of current patients.

Multi-Objective Decision Optimization

Based on forecasted future operational scenarios, AHCS uses optimization techniques to analyze candidate intervention plans. Decisions made for healthcare always have competing goals since maximizing surge capacity makes hospitals more resilient while increasing their operational cost, whereas delaying elective surgeries helps keep the ICU space occupied but lowers revenues. It is critical to apply multi-objective optimization, not a single-objective technique.

Using reinforcement learning, the AHCS can train itself by interacting with the simulated environment, the digital twin (Sutton & Barto, 2018; Silver et al., 2016). This is achieved through the discounted cumulative reward optimization goal:

$$\pi * = argmax\pi\, E[\Sigma t = 0\, \infty\, \gamma\, t\, Rt] \quad (3)$$

$\pi*$ = Optimal intervention policy

Rt = Composite reward at time t (clinical, operational, and financial components)
γ = Discount factor governing the trade-off between immediate and long-term outcomes

DIGITAL TWIN SIMULATION AND SCENARIO ANALYSIS

The digital twin part of AHCS ensures that there is an ongoing real-time replication of the hospital environment based on actual operational data collected (Batty, 2018; Tao et al., 2019). Instead of only replicating the current status, the twin generates a probability distribution of thousands of potential operational trajectories using the stochastic simulation method. Sampling of probability distributions for arrival rates, service times, and the likelihood of equipment failure through Monte Carlo Simulation enables this process.

In this setting, interventions in response to extreme events can be evaluated without risking the real-life operational system (Brailsford et al., 2009). It becomes a risk-free experimental platform to prepare the health system for future extreme scenarios. Probabilistic approaches become a basis for building a solid strategy as uncertainty is considered explicitly. A three-level hierarchy of baseline, stress, and worst-case scenarios enables proportionate risk planning, as shown in Figure 4.

Figure 4. AHCS digital twin simulation architecture.

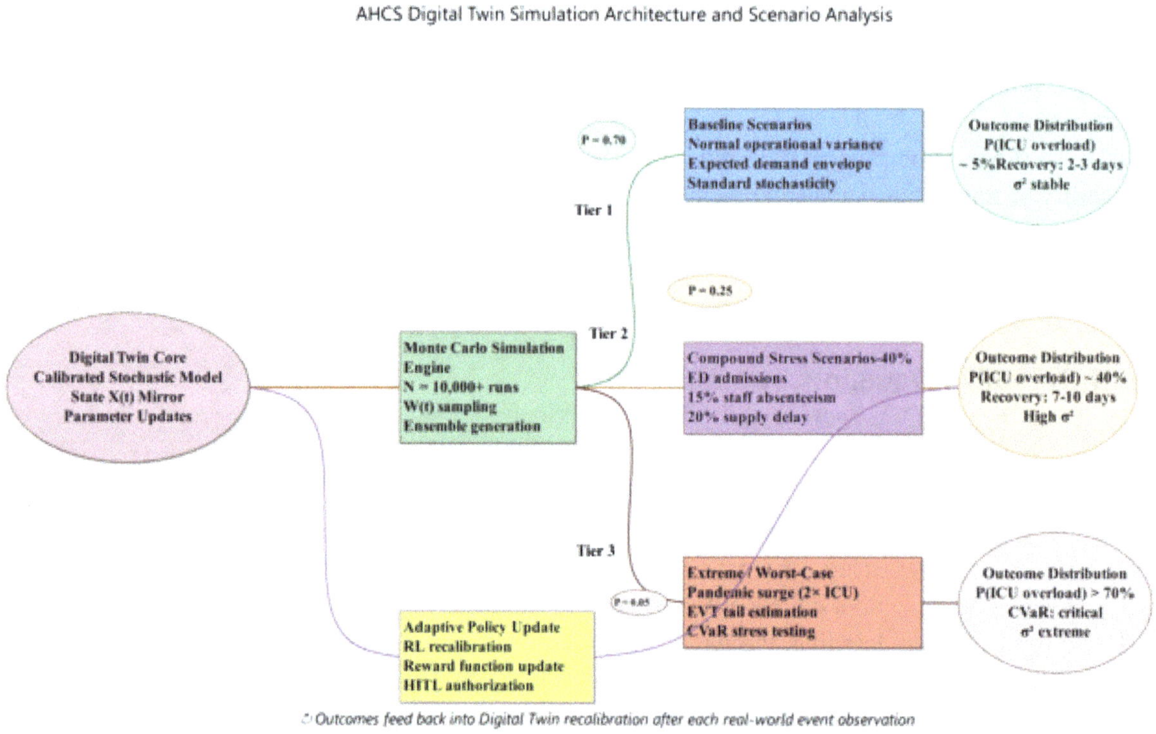

RESILIENCE ENGINEERING AND SYSTEM STABILITY

Resilience concept is interpreted in the context of healthcare through the capacity to accommodate perturbations and maintain necessary services, as well as quickly revert back to the basis level of operation (Hollnagel et al., 2011). Resilience metrics in AHCS consist of: probability of overload (po); recovery time index (tr); and stability variance (σ^2). Recovery time refers to the duration between the surge incident and the attainment of equilibrated performance back from the level prior to the surge.

The implementation of adaptive buffer management conceives transforming measures of resilience into operational management actions. The fact of the matter is that the staying power-utilization goal does not change within the AHCS framework. However, the staying power-utilization goal changes as it is modified by the amount of risk. If the risk is low, the staying power takes advantage of the efficiencies in full with very few bullets. However, with the increase of the risk, the bullets are built by the time criticality sets in.

CONTINUOUS LEARNING AND INSTITUTIONAL TRANSFORMATION

Institutions are continuously improved through the closed-loop adaptive learning process performed by AHCS: data acquisition, state estimation, probabilistic forecasting, multi-objective optimization, intervention delivery, and impact assessment. Differences between actual and expected results are leveraged to refine parameters, state transition probabilities, and rewards in the model. This cyclical process allows for adaptation to changing operating environment, demographics, diseases, and incorporates institutional experience into the control algorithm.

At a strategic level, AHCS revolutionizes the way healthcare organizations operate. Management of crises shifts towards proactive risk management based on probability theory. Decisions made by stakeholders become informed, justified, and predictable. Budget planning is optimized through pre-planned resource allocation, resulting in reduced emergency costs. Workforce is satisfied as overworking is prevented by schedule optimization. Patients benefit from reduced waiting times due to alleviated congestion in the system. The governance shift made possible by the application of AHCS can be summarized in Figure 5.

Figure 5. AHCS closed-loop adaptive learning cycle illustrating the six-stage process.

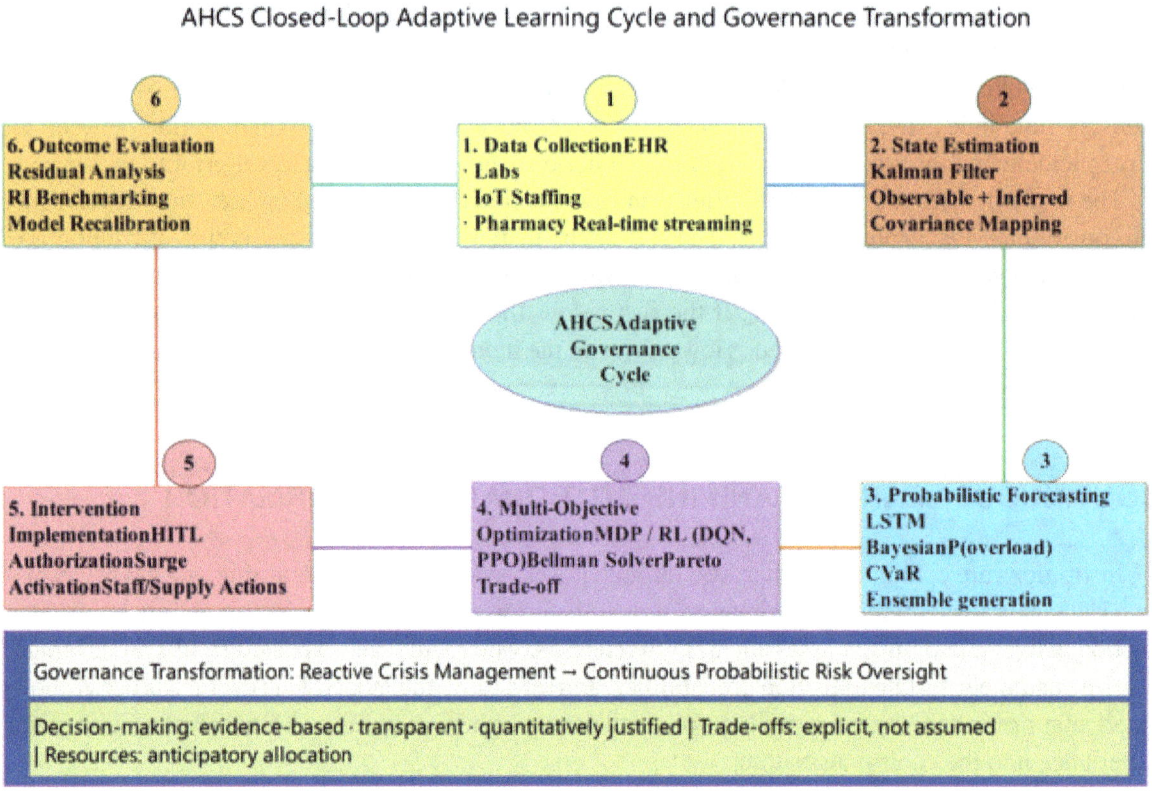

ADVANCED STOCHASTIC MODELING FRAMEWORK

Formal State-Space Representation of Hospital Dynamics

The advanced modeling level leverages the fundamental system representations from the conceptual foundations to develop a formal stochastic state-space model for the functioning of hospitals (Bertsekas, 2017; Sterman, 2000). At any point in time t, the state vector contains all the parameters related to the hospital operation, which were introduced in the conceptual foundations section. Changes in states follow stochastic difference equations of the type expressed in Equations (1) and (2). With such a model, one can employ stochastic optimal control theory, Markov decision processes, and dynamic programming approaches. Most importantly, however, one can optimize according to criteria sensitive to risks, including those based on the variance of outcomes and CVaR restrictions (Puterman, 2014; Bertsekas, 2017).

Markov Decision Process Formulation

The control problem for AHCS is mathematically modeled using Markov Decision Processes (Puterman, 2014). Here, the MDP states represent the operating state vector X(t), and actions include any possible management decisions such as changes in the surgical scheduling, opening of surge units, resource relocation, etc. Justification for the use of the Markov property is given by consideration of the state variables that include queue length, utilization, fatigue rates, and inventory levels, which make future behavior independent of past behavior conditional on the current state.

Multi-criteria objective function considers weighted criteria of clinical efficiency, employee well-being, resource utilization, and profitability. Extensions of Markov decision processes to risk-aware policies involve the addition of CVaR conditions that help to penalize rare and extreme catastrophic events (Puterman, 2014). The Bellman optimality equation for selecting the policy is:

$$V^*(s) = max_a R(s,a) + \gamma \Sigma s'' P(s''s,a) \cdot V^*(s'') \tag{4}$$

$V^*(s)$ = Value function at state s
$R(s,a)$ = Reward for action a in state s
γ = Discount factor ($0 < \gamma < 1$)
$P(s'|s,a)$ = Probability of transitioning to state s'', given (s, a)

For problems having large state spaces that cannot be solved analytically, approximation through dynamic programming and Deep Reinforcement Learning become feasible solutions. DQN was proposed by Mnih et al. (2015) in the context of high-dimensional state spaces, whereas PPO was proposed by Schulman et al. (2017) as a policy gradient algorithm for continuous actions space.

Queueing Network Modeling of Departmental Interdependencies

The different departments in a hospital represent a network of coupled nodes, the effectiveness of which depends on the flow of patients routed from one node to another (Gross et al., 2018). The queueing network model helps in studying the issues related to congestion, delay, and efficiency of the process when arrival and service processes follow random behavior. In AHCS, each individual department is represented by a service node along with estimates of its arrival rate, service time distribution, and capacity.

M/M/1 represents a simple queueing model that helps understand the utilization factor that is:

$$\rho = \frac{\lambda}{\mu} \tag{5}$$

λ = Mean arrival rate
μ = Mean service rate
ρ = Utilization factor

The stability condition requires $\rho < 1$ (mean capacity must exceed mean demand):

$$\rho < 1 \tag{6}$$

The expected waiting time in queue is:

$$Wq = \frac{\lambda}{[\mu(\mu - \lambda)]} \tag{7}$$

Queue simulation for all nodes of the network under different demand situations highlights key capacity limits as well as nodes that are most crucial in terms of the infrastructure to be invested in. Figure 6 demonstrates the modeling approach in a single framework.

Figure 6. AHCS advanced stochastic modeling framework.

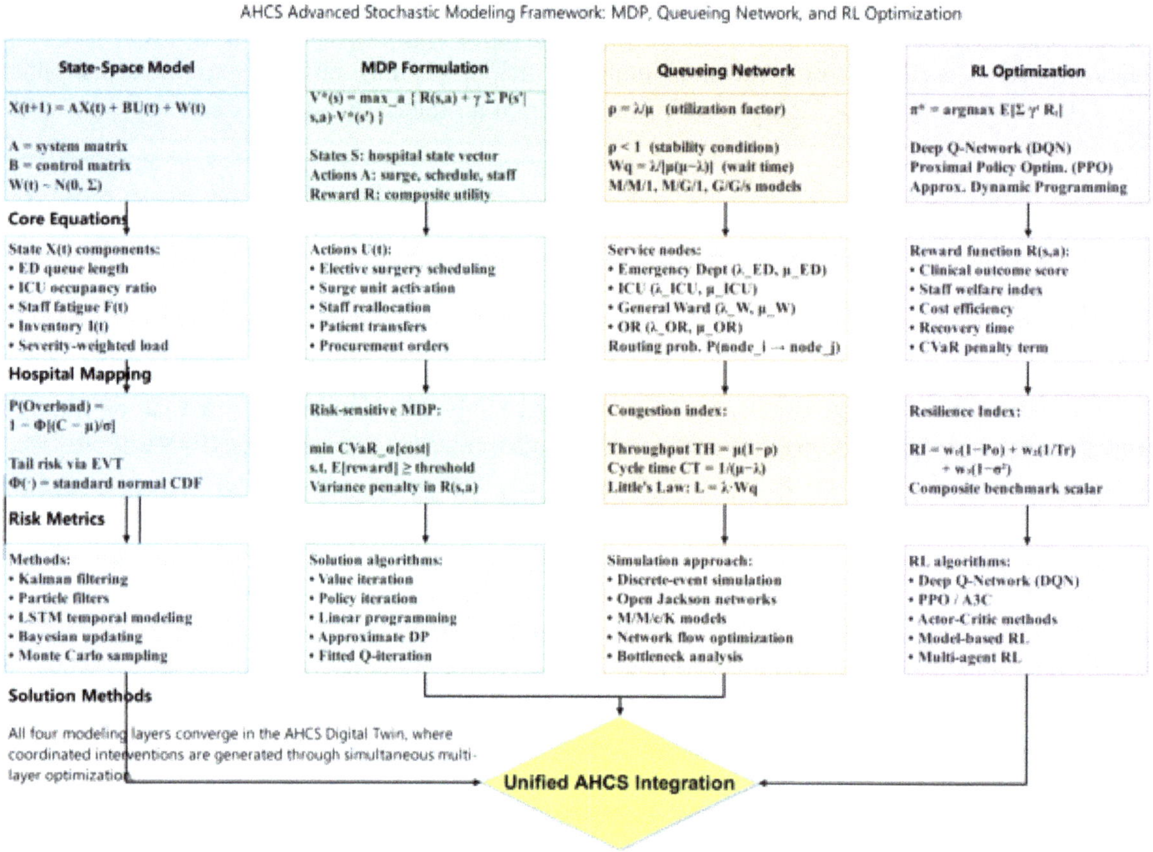

EPIDEMIC AND SURGE MODELING

Compartmental Disease Modeling Integrated with Hospital Capacity

For predicting mass-scale health disasters, AHCS combines the application of compartment models of infectious diseases with hospital capacity management models (Kermack & McKendrick, 1927). The SIR model involves dividing the population into three different compartments: Susceptible (S),

Infected (I), and Recovered (R). The complete system of ordinary differential equations governing the SIR dynamics is given below (Eqs. 8–10):

$$dS/dt = -\beta SI \tag{8}$$

$$dI/dt = \beta SI - \gamma I \tag{9}$$

$$dR/dt = \gamma I \tag{10}$$

β = Transmission rate
γ = Recovery rate
The basic reproduction number characterizing epidemic growth potential is:

$$R^0 = \beta\frac{N}{\gamma} \tag{11}$$

N = Total population size (normalization factor ensuring mass-action consistency)

Stochastic formulations consider both β and γ as stochastic variables with their probability distribution being fitted to actual outbreaks data, thus allowing for ensemble forecasting of hospital admission demands. The digital twin system explores the effects of various measures—medicinal and behavioral interventions and isolation strategies—on hospital needs. This is illustrated by the epidemic surge modeling methodology shown in Figure 7.

Figure 7. AHCS epidemic and surge modeling framework.

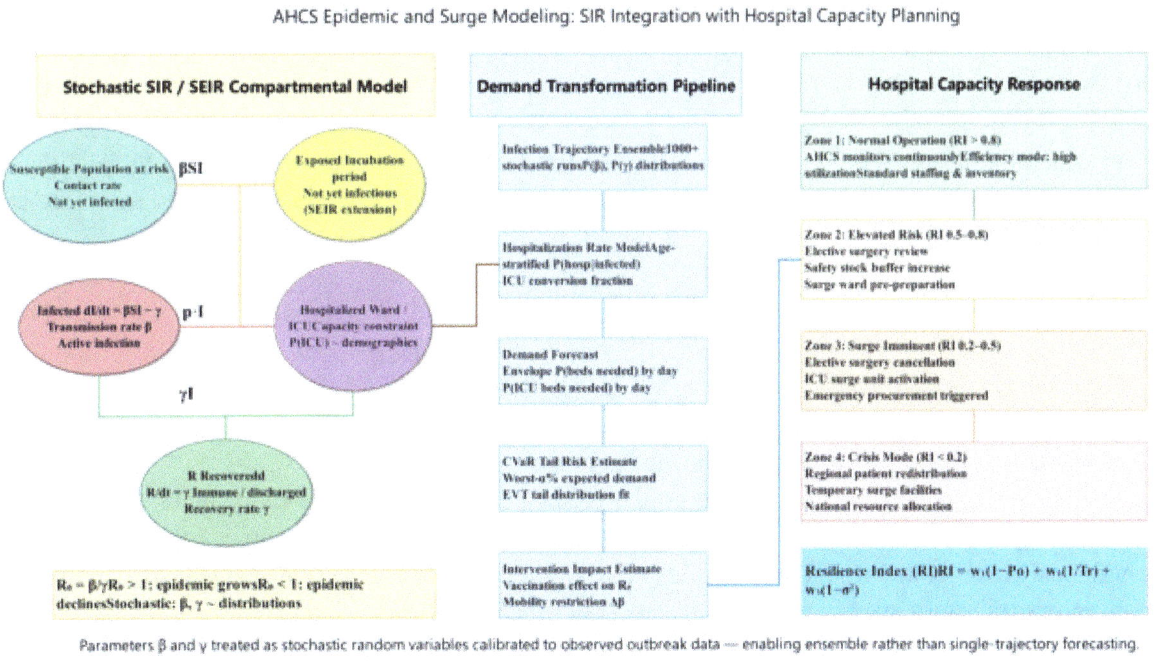

Extreme Event Simulation and Tail Risk Estimation

The most disruptive risks to the stability of the healthcare system are presented in cases which fall outside the bounds of historical experience and cannot be forecasted usually using the conventional methods. The main shortcoming of the conventional risk prediction lies in the fact that the extremes of the risks occur very seldom in the history. This can be remedied by AHCS by means of the use of the approach of extreme value theory and adversarial stress testing. In the framework of the extreme value theory the parametric distribution for the tails (Gumbel, Fréchet, or Weibull) is estimated on the exceedance data set, what allows the statistical estimation of the occurrence of the event above historical maxima. In the context of adversarial stress testing, the artificial compound cases such as double increase of ICU admissions and 20% illness absenteeism among the staff.

SUPPLY CHAIN AND RESOURCE OPTIMIZATION

Operational robustness of AHCS is not limited to its throughput performance but encompasses its logistics for material and human resources. The engineering view of the system considers the supply chains and the work force as subsystems whose performance influences service delivery and recovery ability.

Stochastic Inventory Modeling

Healthcare logistics systems run amidst conditions of uncertainty regarding demand and lead time. This makes deterministic methods of determining reorder policies inadequate. AHCS uses stochastic models of inventory management that take into account the random distribution of demands and uncertain lead times. Demand function D(t) is defined as:

$$D(t) \sim Poisson(\lambda_t) or D(t) \sim N(\mu_t, \sigma_t^2) \tag{12}$$

in which the parameters λt, μt, and σt are calculated based on predictions of future clinical load, ensuring that procurement actions are proactive in nature. Safety stock will be determined from service level requirements:

$$SS = z \cdot \sigma_L \tag{13}$$

SS = Safety stock amount

z = Service level factor (normal quantile corresponding to the required service level probability)

σL = Standard deviation of demand during lead time L

In AHCS, z is recalibrated depending on the predicted surge status. The dynamic (s, S) replenishment strategy will place an order whenever $I(t) \leq s$ and restock inventory to target level S, where s is continuously recalibrated from the epidemic and ICU forecasts. By conducting Monte Carlo simulation of inventory trajectory, we can calculate the stockout probability::

$$P(Stockout) = P(D_L > I(t)) \tag{14}$$

Where, D_L is the cumulative demand during lead time

Workforce Dynamics and Fatigue Modeling

The greatest constraint on the resources in healthcare management is that of human capital. As opposed to physical inventory, human capital deteriorates under continued stress. The AHCS includes a model of fatigue dynamics:

$$F(t+1) = F(t) + \alpha W(t) - \beta R(t) \tag{15}$$

$F(t)$ = Cumulative fatigue level at time t
$W(t)$ = Workload intensity at time t
$R(t)$ = Rest and recovery duration at time t
α = Workload sensitivity coefficient
β = Recovery efficiency coefficient
Fatigue affects operational throughput through a performance degradation function:

$$\mu(t) = \mu^0[1 - \delta F(t)] \tag{16}$$

$\mu(t)$ = Effective service rate at time t
μ^0 = Baseline productivity at zero fatigue
δ = Performance degradation factor
Constraint: the fatigue parameter $F(t)$ has an upper bound $F_m ax = 1/\delta$, implying that $\delta F(t) \leq 1$and hence $\mu(t) \geq 0$ for all t. Operationally, this constraint is ensured by the optimization process in Eq. (17), preventing fatigue accumulation beyond a safe limit. The two-process mathematical model of fatigue (Folkard & Akerstedt, 2004) provides experimental justification for this linear recovery/accumulation framework.

AHCS uses RL and constrained optimization to determine roster schedules minimizing the weighted-sum cost function:

$$min \{ \alpha c \cdot C\_overtime + \beta c \cdot C\_fatigue + \gamma c \cdot C\_understaffing \} \tag{17}$$

with $\alpha c, \beta c, \gamma c$ being institutional priority weights, subject to minimum staffing requirements, maximum fatigue levels, and policy restrictions. This weighted-sum formulation is the right multi-objective model; the model also compares various policies, such as rotational ICU teams, surge staffing pools, and cross-training programs.

The supply and workforce subsystems are interconnected; insufficient supplies increase infections, resulting in more staff absenteeism; staff fatigue decreases productivity, making demand more volatile. The AHCS captures this connectivity through the state space model to avoid cascades.

MULTI-HOSPITAL NETWORK INTEGRATION

Regional Capacity Coordination

Healthcare resilience is not confined to individual organizations (Sutton & Barto, 2018). Networked regions facilitate the redistribution and sharing of resources. Under the AHCS multiple hospitals system, each hospital system in the region is modeled through a node in a regional network of healthcare systems. The model takes into account the possibility of patients being transferred and the delay times associated with this process and limitations on communication among institutions. Regional optimization seeks to find the best redistribution strategy such that the probability of simultaneous overload within the system is minimized.

National-Level Digital Twin Architecture

The scaling up of the AHCS digital twin into a nationwide scope involves the use of a hierarchical modeling approach. The local hospital twins are rolled up regionally and then nationally into a combined digital twin of the national health care system (Silver et al., 2016). The national digital twin facilitates decision-making based on a real representation of the complete national health care system by evaluating options such as resource allocation during emergencies, travel restrictions, or vaccination programs. Figure 8 shows how the regional digital twin can be used to simulate an outbreak in the region along with 10% staff infection, conducted via thousands of Monte Carlo simulations.

Figure 8. AHCS multi-hospital network integration architecture.

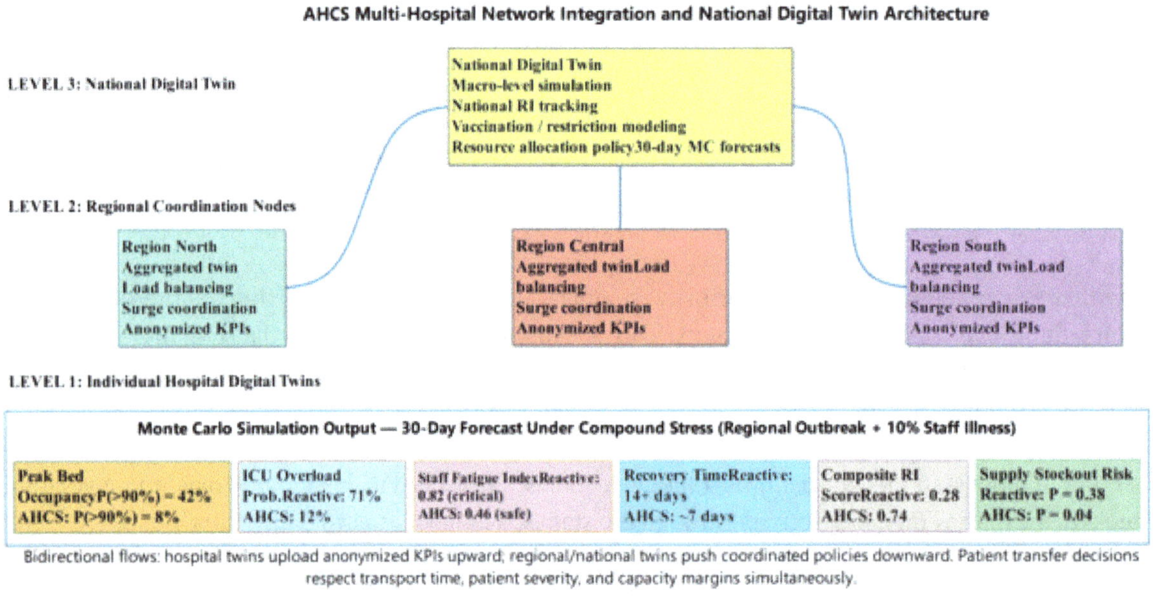

ECONOMIC AND COST-BENEFIT MODELING

Cost of Overload Versus Cost of Preparedness

The costs associated with building resilience involve preparedness costs like maintaining surge capacity, building up safety stock, and investing in predictive infrastructure, balanced against the potential disaster costs of being unprepared. The AHCS model uses a cost analysis tool to measure both types of costs. Overload costs include additional procurement costs due to an emergency, costs related to paying overtime and hiring temporary workers, lost revenues from canceling elective procedures, risks associated with deaths, reputational risks, and fines. Costs related to preparedness include:

$$E[C] = Cp + Po \cdot Cf \tag{18}$$

Cp = Preparedness cost
Po = Overload probability
Cf = Expected cost conditional on overload occurring

Assuming overload probability decreases with preparedness investment, we model Po as a decreasing function $Po(Cp)$, capturing the intuition that greater preparedness reduces overload risk. Under this specification, the expected cost $E[C] = Cp + Po(Cp) \cdot Cf$ is minimized at the optimal preparedness level satisfying the first-order condition:

$$\frac{dE[C]}{dCp} = 0 \Rightarrow 1 + \left(\frac{dPo}{dCp}\right) \cdot Cf = 0 \tag{19}$$

Cost analysis using simulation repeatedly shows that spending on predictive infrastructure pays off economically over a period of several years. The fact that operations become less volatile also reduces insurance costs.

Value of Information and Predictive Intelligence

The economic value of predictive modeling could be determined by the use of value of information (VOI). An increase in predictive accuracy helps in decreasing the uncertainty in decisions made, thus leading to accurate allocation of resources. The AHCS model determines the marginal benefit in reducing the variability of cost due to an improvement in predictive accuracy. This analysis shows that it is economically sensible to invest in the development of a predictive capacity because the saving of expected overload cost makes up for implementation costs despite the existence of costs in maintaining the system. For near-capacity operating regimes where the normal approximation is reasonable, the overload probability at occupancy threshold C is approximated as:

$$P(Overload) = 1 - \Phi\,[\,(C - \mu)\,/\,\sigma\,] \tag{20}$$

C = Institutional capacity threshold (e.g., 90% bed occupancy)
μ = Mean occupancy under current operational state
σ = Standard deviation of occupancy

$\Phi(\cdot)$ = Standard normal cumulative distribution function

Note: For tail-risk estimation beyond this near-capacity regime, extreme value theory (EVT) methods—as employed in the stress-testing subsection—should be used in place of the Gaussian approximation, since occupancy distributions are bounded and right-skewed under surge conditions.

LARGE-SCALE IMPLEMENTATION ARCHITECTURE

Phased Deployment Strategy in Complex Healthcare Environments

Rollout of AHCS in an active hospital would require careful phase-out to avoid disruptions to the patient treatment process. The implementation approach consists of four separate phases, each building upon the previous phase.

Phase 1 — Data Infrastructure Integration: The first phase sets up the basic data infrastructure. In most hospitals, there are disparate data systems that operate independently from one another in the realms of radiology, pharmacy management, ward management, and staff management. Phase 1 sets up the communication channels that standardize the process; establishes the data schema; and builds the pipelines for ingest and pre-processing of the data for processing in the state estimation layer. Ensuring data completeness is the main success metric for this phase.

Phase 2 — Read-Only Predictive Intelligence: This involves switching on the predictive algorithms and digital twin system, which operates separately from the current managerial processes in what amounts to a shadow mode. This phase sees the output of various predictions made by the models and digital twin (occupancy, overload likelihood, supply depletion prediction). These are recorded in a separate system but not considered for decision-making purposes. This helps ensure model accuracy and predictability.

Phase 3 – Decision Support under Human Authorization: In this phase, decision-making workflows are updated to include AHCS recommendations as advice that must receive specific human authorization prior to execution. Clinicians and administrators consider risk and scenarios analysis and intervention suggestions before accepting or overriding them. Every decision, whether from algorithmic recommendations or from human override, is recorded with complete audit trails. This phase builds experience with probabilistic governance while defining boundary limits where autonomous operations can be expanded.

Phase 4 – Adaptive Autonomous Governance within Policy Limits: After successful piloting of Phase 1 to 3, AHCS shifts to adaptive autonomous governance using a limited number of decision areas pre-authorized by the institution (such as dynamic bed allocation, safety stock ordering, and routine scheduling changes). Autonomous decisions are constrained by institutional policy parameters. Unauthorized decision types remain under human authorization. Performance tracking, model audits, and governance reviews continue during this phase.

Infrastructure Requirements and Computational Architecture

The computer platform of the AHCS has to be sufficiently powerful, scalable, and robust. The real-time prediction and stochastic simulation using a digital twin model demand computer performance that is able to process a massive amount of information and perform thousands of iterations of simulation.

The choice between distributed cloud-based architecture and on-premises solutions depends on the need for data sovereignty of some organizations.

The pipeline should allow the analytics to be performed in real-time mode with minimal latency from the moment when the data is produced until a result is predicted. Real-time dashboards display the results of computations such as probabilistic risk indicators, probability of an overload, and proposed actions in operational terms.

The model governance constructs form an integral part of the computational infrastructure and allow for versioning of the predictive models, datasets used for training purposes, and updates to the parameters. This enables documentation and ensures transparency and accountability in algorithmic decision making. Predictive models can be updated incrementally to ensure their continued predictive performance under changing operational conditions. The architecture is illustrated in Figure 9.

Figure 9. AHCS large-scale implementation architecture.

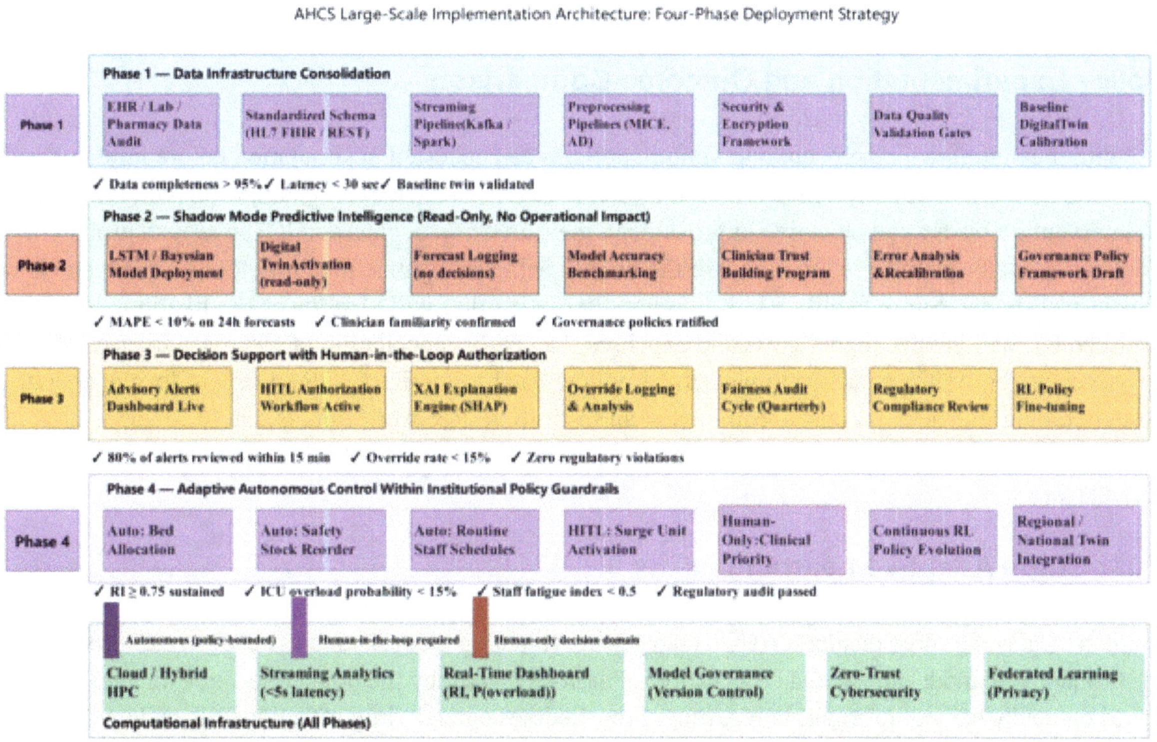

PANDEMIC SURGE CASE SIMULATION

Scenario Design and Parameterization

For example, if we wish to demonstrate the functionality of the AHCS under such a surge condition where the virus transmission is escalating and there is a significant uncertainty regarding the probability of hospitalization, then the digital twin will factor in the existing capacity limits and model a surge profile up to 30 days into the future. Here, β and γ transmission parameters will be modeled as probability distributions that are reflective of the uncertainty associated with estimating R_0 and compliance with measures. The probability of hospitalization and conversion rate of cases to ICU wards will be provided in the form of demographic-specific distributions.

Through stochastic modeling, a large number of outbreak scenarios are run through the simulation in order to derive the distribution of outcomes in the form of maximum use of ICU beds, need for ventilators, probability of absenteeism on account of staff infections, and mortality risks based on current capacity limits.

Policy Experimentation and Outcome Comparison

With the digital twin approach, intervention policies can be tested in simulation before implementation. The simulation of early cancellation of elective surgeries provides an example showing how such an intervention leads to an objective improvement, measured as a decrease in ICU overload probability. The administrator would need to compare the benefit achieved against potential losses in revenue and patient well-being. Surge facility use is another alternative that will also lower the likelihood of ICU overload but will involve higher costs and expenses than early cancellation of elective surgeries.

Accordingly, AHCS selects optimal sets of policies that minimize CVaR of failure for the hospital system, taking into account cost constraints at an institution. Recovery time is one of the comparative metrics used by AHCS. The latter measures the period from the peak ICU surge to reaching its pre-surge level.

Post-Surge Adaptive Learning

In the wake of a surge incident, AHCS engages in evaluating inconsistencies between the forecasts of the probabilistic model and actual observations. Parameters used by the predictive algorithm are refined based on newly gained information regarding how diseases spread, drug effectiveness, and operational patterns. Thus, each occurrence of an epidemic enhances the accuracy of forecasting and control measures within the framework of AHCS. While traditional contingency plans are left unchanged until the next disaster strikes, AHCS constantly updates its database, adding operational knowledge to its algorithms and thereby creating an institutional legacy of sorts. The relative efficiency of alternative approaches in the simulation experiment is presented in Table 1.

Table 1. Comparative performance of pandemic surge intervention strategies across three key operational dimensions under the 30-day AHCS simulation scenario.

Strategy	ICU Overload Risk	Operational Cost Impact	System Recovery Time
Status Quo (Reactive)	High (>70% within 5 days)	Baseline (elevated crisis costs)	Extended (>2 weeks)
Early Elective Cancellation	Moderate (~40% reduction)	Moderate (elective revenue loss)	Rapid (<1 week)
Temporary Surge Wards	Low (~60% reduction)	High (capital + staffing)	Moderate (~10 days)
AHCS Adaptive Control	Minimal (<10% probability)	Optimized (pre-emptive)	Shortest (~3–4 days)

ARTIFICIAL INTELLIGENCE GOVERNANCE AND ETHICAL OVERSIGHT

Transparency and Explainability in Clinical Decision Support

The use of AI-driven controllers in the domain of health creates important ethical and organizational issues that should be considered and addressed in advance (Topol, 2019). The decisions about patient care, resource management, and clinical priorities should be understandable, auditable, and explainable to clinicians and administrators using this knowledge. Explainable AI algorithms are incorporated into AHCS: SHAP (SHapley Additive exPlanations) value attribution (Lundberg & Lee, 2017) and LIME (Local Interpretable Model-agnostic Explanations) (Ribeiro et al., 2016), thus allowing clinicians to understand why the system makes its decisions. For instance, when recommending delay in non-emergency procedures, AHCS provides probabilistic overload projections, surgical schedule sensitivity, and confidence intervals.

This framework guarantees the ability of the physician to exercise his or her own judgment and makes ethically acceptable decisions based on clinical reasoning rather than unreflective obedience. Uncertainty estimation is performed alongside any probabilistic estimate to ensure no overconfidence.

Bias Mitigation and Fair Resource Allocation

Disparities found within healthcare data have been inherited from past inequities caused by social stratification, discrimination, and lack of access. Models built without fairness considerations have the potential to reinforce these inequalities by predicting systematic biases in resource allocation. This is mitigated by AHCS through the explicit inclusion of fairness constraints within the optimization framework. Fairness constraints act as penalties against demographic bias within predictions, while fairness-based learning algorithms adapt model training to lower differences in prediction error rates between subpopulations (Topol, 2019). Bias auditing checks ensure that forecast errors do not unfairly burden disadvantaged groups, and if necessary, models are retrained with re-weighting.

Accountability and Human-in-the-Loop Governance

Although AHCS allows more automation in making decisions, human beings are still responsible for making decisions on quality of healthcare. It is clear from the governance model that there are certain types of decisions that are permitted to be automated using algorithms, while there are certain types of decisions that have to be automated after human approval, and there are certain types of decisions that only clinical judgments can make. In short, the priority decision of a patient's care is solely the clinician's.

Decision making process is well-audited through maintenance of complete documentation in terms of algorithm results, consideration of confidence intervals, decisions taken by humans from algorithms, decision override as well as reason of override. There exists a hierarchy of decision overrides whereby, decision taken by algorithms can be overridden by clinicians. Analysis of override patterns helps in learning the systematic cases where there exist differences between human and algorithmic decisions.

CYBERSECURITY AND DATA PROTECTION FRAMEWORK

Threat Landscape and Risk Mitigation

Healthcare delivery systems represent significant targets of cyber-attacks owing to the sensitive nature of information contained within healthcare systems, critical importance of the systems supported by such information, and vulnerabilities that may be exploited through aging information technology infrastructure. Incorporation of autonomous prediction control systems increases the risks associated with cyber-attacks in terms of the capacity to manipulate the data stream, which may result in distortion of the estimation of state and the triggering of interventions not based on sound predictions. The AHCS uses several measures to ensure the safety of its systems, including end-to-end data stream encryption, multi-factor authentication to access the systems, user-controlled access to data, and anomaly detection.

Privacy-Preserving Analytics

Big data analysis requires that vast amounts of clinical and operational data be used. This causes the privacy problem, which needs to be addressed with regard to the current legal regulations. In AHCS, federated learning (McMahan et al., 2017) is used as the primary technology for collaborative training of models; rather than collecting patient data in one place, all participants learn their own updates of the model, which are then sent to other organizations with encrypted gradient updates. This way, it is possible to improve the collaborative model and at the same time protect the sensitive patient data from any leakages from the organizations participating in the learning process. The privacy preserving technology provides a very strict mathematical bound on the privacy loss caused by inclusion of any individual record to the training data set. Data governance committees' activities help with ensuring the compliance with nationally and internationally applicable laws on data privacy.

LONG-TERM ADAPTIVE EVOLUTION OF AHCS

Self-Improving Predictive Ecosystems

The long-term goal of the AHCS goes well beyond mere implementation and into continuous improvement of the predictive environment. As more data becomes available, predictive algorithms will be updated to incorporate changes to the epidemiological context, population characteristics, and operating procedures. Predictive feedback based on outcome data will allow for better calibration of transition probabilities and rewards functions, enhancing the system's knowledge of local operating conditions. The incorporation of novel data sources, such as biosensor signals from wearable devices, risk stratification at the genomic level, and environmental sensor data, further enhances the predictive capability of the system.

Scaling Toward National and Global Networks

In the last stage of complete implementation, the AHCS systems are implanted over the regions' health care network systems and are connected through secure digital twin technologies to provide demand forecasting at a macro level as well as epidemic monitoring. The collected information is used for monitoring the national resilience index and evidence-based policy making. The global systems interoperability framework will help to respond to any health crisis at an international level in distribution of vaccines, drugs, and other emergency services.

COMPREHENSIVE INTEGRATED CASE STUDY: SYSTEM-WIDE STRESS EVALUATION

Baseline Operational Profile

In order to evaluate the overall performance of AHCS, think of a theoretical large tertiary hospital whose operational dynamics reflect those of a top-performing facility (Obermeyer & Emanuel, 2016). Such an organization has an average bed utilization rate of over 85%. There is a maximum possible number of electives surgeries carried out in order to ensure profitability. In addition, emergency admissions have moderate variation with respect to their long-term mean. This is how a typical healthcare facility performs under traditional management. From the perspective of resilience engineering, however, such an organization is extremely fragile in relation to external disturbances.

AHCS Digital Twin produces the corresponding baseline model, taking into account all the above-mentioned characteristics. Thus, expected waiting times, distributions of ICU beds, staff workloads, functions of discharge rates, and supply turnovers can be predicted. Moreover, variance and covariance of the corresponding random variables determine their dependence.

Multi-Dimensional Stress Scenario Design

The stress test uses the model of compound disturbance involving a combination of three stress elements, including a 40% rise in the number of patients seeking medical services owing to the outbreak within the community, a 15% decrease in nurse availability caused by their illness and quarantine, and finally, a 20% delay in delivery of vital supplies owing to logistical disturbances. Compound stress is fundamentally different from the use of sensitivity analysis using a single element since there are inherent non-linear interactions in real-world situations.

Stress Propagation Analysis

Analysis of the digital twin model for compound stress through conventional reactive management shows the typical cascading effect associated with the scenario. Over the first 48 hours, higher emergency admission rates deplete ED capacity, leading to increased boarding times and diverting nurses from attending to their ward patients. The decreased number of staff members lowers service output per shift and increases patient handling times, further exacerbating queue formation. An increasing number of ICU patients results as patients boarded in the ED need more care due to their condition.

The simulation results show that the ICU overload level is reached after five days when the probability exceeds 70%. System recovery in terms of restoring pre-stress occupancy takes more than two weeks in a reactive approach, where elective procedures pile up in the process. The results from the CVaR measure demonstrate high mortality risk from adverse scenarios. This is due not only to the patient's conditions, but also due to congestion-related resource shortages.

Outcome Analysis Under AHCS Adaptive Control

If AHCS is also involved at the same time in the compounded stress situation, then the application of probabilistic forecasting makes clear that there is the development of an increased chance of overload in the first 24 hours after the start of the surge event. The best combination of strategies suggested by the digital twin could include such strategies as the temporary suspension of elective surgeries, proactive migration of the medical staff from low acuity units, activation of the surge unit before the level of critical occupancy, and rapid inventory restocking.

The ICUs' occupancies will never cross the collapse points within most simulation situations. The recovery time is reduced by nearly halfway more than the reactive approach. There are no fatigue problems for the staff because dynamic staff allocation with the assistance of workloads is utilized. Statistical analysis performed on the simulations concludes that the cvar and mortality rates are statistically significantly lower than the reactive approach. In addition to that, the digital twin gives information concerning the weakness in the infrastructure, which is the lack of ventilator system equipment redundancy.

ECONOMIC IMPACT AND COST-BENEFIT ANALYSIS

Direct Operational Cost Modeling

The AHCS measures both direct and indirect costs associated with instabilities in the system (Kaplan et al., 2002). Direct costs include overtime and emergency staffing costs, expedited procurement charges, revenue loss because of canceled electives, and costs incurred in activating a temporary facility. Indirect costs include damages to reputation and a long-term reduction of patients' confidence. In the case of reactive strategy, response to an incident means emergency procurement at a premium rate and revenue loss during the whole recovery period. With an application of AHCS, the costs will be spread across time via pre-emptive measures and extreme financial costs are avoided. Early canceling of electives leads to revenue loss, but significantly reduces the duration of recovery process and total financial effects over time.

Quantifying the Value of Resilience

The economic value of resiliency may be defined as the expected loss saving due to lower probability of overload that is created by the AHCS in comparison with reactive approaches. The saving estimates are calculated as the expected loss during stress scenarios with and without AHCS taken from the probability of each event. Such savings consist of the loss of life, elimination of legal concerns, and reputation savings, which was not accounted in the operational efficiency earlier.

Sensitivity analysis for various frequencies and intensities of the stresses shows that the predictive infrastructure has positive roi even under conditions of high environmental variability, therefore the argument for AHCS implementation is validated. The probability of overload considering occupancy, the normal distribution, is calculated by means of equation (19).

QUANTITATIVE RESILIENCE BENCHMARKING

Development of a Composite Resilience Index

Resilience is measured as an RI by AHCS, which consists of a composite index from all individual metrics of the institution's resilience. The RI is calculated using a formula involving Po, Tr, and σ^2, weighted depending on the institutional priorities (Kermack & McKendrick, 1927):

$$RI = w\left(1 - Po\right) + w\left(\frac{(1)}{Tr}\right) + w\left(1 - \sigma^2\right) \tag{21}$$

Po = Overload probability

Tr = Recovery time (normalized)

σ^2 = Stability variance (normalized)

w , w , w = Institutional priority weights (summing to 1)

The monitoring of RI evolution longitudinally on a quarterly basis gives the institution a window for identifying deteriorations in trends before they become critical, as well as for benchmarking on a regional and national scale.

Comparative Analysis Across System Configurations

A number of simulations are carried out to compare these three approaches. (1) traditional reactive management. (2) predictive alarms based on rules without the optimization module. (3) predictive alarms with adaptive control. The first approach demonstrates the high variability and long recovery time. The second approach displays the superior performance in the first stage of detecting deteriorations, but it does not have the optimization module to apply the predictions into actions and get the undesired balance between costs and resilience. The third approach outperforms most other criteria.

INTEGRATION OF ADVANCED MODELING LAYERS

Unified Stochastic-Control Architecture

The integrated case study illustrates how stochastic modeling, queueing networks, epidemic prediction, worker dynamics, and supply chains optimization combine into a common AHCS framework (Glasserman, 2004). Each of the modeling layers adds its unique perspective: stochastic state-space models describe system dynamics, queueing models consider congestion/throughput aspects, the epidemic model predicts external demands, the fatigue model controls worker dynamics, while the inventory models assure material supply. The digital twin represents a common ground where the modeling layers interact and are evaluated together.

The control layer combines all the outputs produced by different modeling layers to develop an intervention plan. An example of such an intervention would be the decision whether to activate surges. In the proposed framework, this kind of decision would be made taking into account predictions produced not only by the epidemic model but also queue length predictions, fatigue models, and material supplies.

Adaptive Policy Evolution Through Reinforcement Learning

Each time the RL optimization tool is implemented, it becomes further competent at identifying the appropriate time for an intervention to be executed as well as the size of that intervention. It has already realized that an intervention that is implemented earlier and within a moderate scale is always better and more cost-efficient than an intensive intervention done later. This is one of the several principles of resilience engineering; which is that it is always faster and cheaper to anticipate a problem than to react to it. Policy is formulated based on past experience; this is almost like the organization's own memorization system. Any change in the environment will affect the policy as well.

STRATEGIC IMPLICATIONS FOR HEALTHCARE GOVERNANCE

Institutional Transformation

As illustrated in this paper, through modeling and benchmarking, AHCS is not only an enhancement of technology but a shift in the philosophy of governance as well (Chaudhry et al., 2006). In the decision-making model, there is a move from a process marked by reactive crisis management towards a system of ongoing probabilistic risk management. Decision-making is based on factual information and the compromises that result from it are explicitly made. Leadership involves a move towards transparent and collaborative management among doctors, managers, data analysts, and engineers.

Implications for Policy and Regulation

Benchmarking of resilience through the use of quantitative metrics enables the setting of benchmarks for resilience on the basis of quantitative metrics rather than qualitative metrics. Resilience indexes can be incorporated into insurance risk models and provide a financial incentive to invest in resilience. National digital twins from the public health authorities can be used for the planning of regional reservoir capacities. The regulators' implementation of a framework that is conformant with the AHCS formalism extends the field of application for the predictive resilience from institutional to ecosystem levels of healthcare management.

GOVERNANCE ARCHITECTURE FOR AUTONOMOUS HEALTHCARE SYSTEMS

Institutional Governance Transformation

The evolution of AHCS reflects a structural change in governance within an institution and not merely a technological innovation (Dekker, 2011). Traditional governance in hospitals is conducted using vertical reportage structures, backward-looking performance reviews, and crisis management escalation procedures. In the context of AHCS, the approach involves real-time updates to risk probabilities and proactive anticipation of intervention opportunities using the digital twin's predictive power. Such a shift creates a new dynamic at the intersection of executive management, clinical units, and decision algorithms.

AHCS governance takes place on three layers, which are all nested together. Operational governance consists of short-term decision-making that includes bed distribution decisions, scheduling changes for staffing, and scheduling elective procedures. Tactical governance consists of medium-term decisions regarding capacity expansion planning, safety stock planning, and cross training efforts. Strategic governance involves long-term decisions concerning technology purchases, infrastructural capital investment, and organizational resiliency.

Decision Rights and Accountability Structures

Among other critical decisions that need to be made in the realm of autonomous systems is the decision-making authority distribution. In the case of AHCS, this is clearly outlined where some decisions can be taken algorithmically within certain policy parameters, others must be authorized by humans and yet others are reserved exclusively for the human domain. Algorithmic execution of dynamic bed allocations and predictive inventory reorders falls into the former category where they can be algorithmically executed within the constraints provided by policy rules, while the latter category will include the prioritizing of patients' care.

In order to ensure accountability, all decisions are logged. Each algorithmic decision recommendation includes its associated probabilities, input variables and confidence intervals which allows retrospective analysis in case of any issues. Clinicians have the authority to override the recommendations made by the algorithms in their areas and provide reasoning in doing so. Override data is reviewed regularly and serves as a feedback mechanism into the models to enhance the decision-making.

Dynamic Policy Updating and Institutional Learning

The environment of healthcare organizations is continuously changing, as it depends on various parameters like dynamics of the diseases, changes in demographic situation and technological developments. Governance frameworks must also be dynamic in response to this. At the AHCS, for example, the system of regular reviews of already existing policies takes place when there are statistical abnormalities in the errors in model predictions or at predetermined time periods. Whenever the model predicts poorly, it starts the procedure of an alarm that initiates the session for discussion of the nature of abnormality by the data analysts, doctors and managers as the issue of abnormality may represent a problem with data, environmental changes or concept drift of the model.

ETHICAL FOUNDATIONS OF PREDICTIVE HEALTHCARE CONTROL

Human-Centered AI Integration

Predictive control systems in medicine should retain the priority of human dignity and ethical judgment. Integration from an ethical perspective requires starting with recognizing the drawbacks of optimizing through probabilities, namely, the difficulty of capturing human experiences, subtleties in particular clinical cases, and ethical considerations into a reward function. For this reason, AHCS is built to support but not substitute for decision-making, as explainability modules describe prediction results in narratives, scenario analysis enables counterfactual reasoning, and uncertainty helps prevent overconfidence.

Fairness and Bias Mitigation

Systemic disparities emerge within healthcare data due to socioeconomic issues, access problems, and discrimination. The issue of disparity in the context of AHCS is addressed by incorporating fairness algorithms into model training in order to mitigate the likelihood of such disparities. Disparity is measured by examining performance metrics for each demographic variable (including age, geographical locations, and socioeconomic status). Algorithmic auditing is carried out to determine if there is a bias in the prediction errors against certain communities. These techniques include reweighting, adversarial fairness, and counterfactual approaches. Fairness constraints are incorporated in the optimization framework.

Privacy Preservation and Data Governance

The success of the AHCS is based on the precision of clinical data. It requires that access to the data must be as qualified as possible. This fact brings about certain data privacy issues, resolution of which is possible with help of various methods. The use of federated learning provides an opportunity to learn a model without gathering any data centrally (McMahan et al., 2017). Also, differential privacy ensures that the levels of individual data vulnerability will stay within specified limits. In addition to that, end-to-end encryption can provide secure conditions for the data transfer. Lastly, data privacy governance can be provided with the help of the creation of boards that include representatives of the clinical field, lawyers, and data scientists.

MULTI-LEVEL DEPLOYMENT ARCHITECTURE

Hospital-Level Implementation

Hospital-scale deployment begins by constructing a digital twin based on historical data, calibrated by stochastic models for state transitions with considerations of patient throughput, personnel behavior, and the logistics chain. Hospital-scale deployment is carried out in the phased deployment manner described earlier, with four phases: consolidation of the data environment, testing in shadow mode, human-in-the-loop decision support, and autonomous operation within policy constraints.

Regional Network Coordination

The association of hospital twins is made at the regional level by way of a coordination layer where all situational information is shared while respecting organizational independence. Hospitals feed data from performance indicators anonymously to a regional layer of aggregation that predicts risks in terms of a system-wide outlook as well as detects weaknesses in the process. Load balancing methods analyze potential patient transfer scenarios under a variety of stresses, taking into account not only the transportation time, but also patient acuity and capacity availability. The focus is on reducing the risk of regional overload in the system rather than maximizing the performance of hospitals individually.

National Strategic Integration

Deployment at national scale incorporates epidemic modeling and hospital capacity analysis via a hierarchy of digital twin that includes regional twins. National scale simulation involves the simulation of the spread of disease considering the constraints of the existing health facilities infrastructure, which allows for the assessment of the prioritization of vaccination campaigns, mobility controls, and emergency resource allocation. Resilience indices at national level can be developed using the aggregated hospital performance data to guide fair allocation of resources.

Global Interoperability Framework

Global health crises require cross-border cooperation at a level that can't be achieved by national digital twin strategies alone. The AHCS helps achieve global interoperability through consistent data models and federation of analytics infrastructures (McMahan et al., 2017), allowing international agencies to assess overall readiness metrics without getting access to personal health records. Interdependencies of global supply chains have been modeled in order to detect potential bottlenecks in the cross-border transport of essential equipment, which, consequently, helps implement cooperative procurement strategies that help avoid shortages due to conflicting interests. Achieving full interoperability on a global scale will require consistent data standards, common privacy regulations, and cooperation between international health agencies—issues for which the AHCS system has been designed.

CYBER-PHYSICAL RESILIENCE AND INFRASTRUCTURE INTEGRITY

Cybersecurity Architecture

The implementation of an autonomous control system results in the emergence of unique cybersecurity risks that need to be countered. AHCS uses zero-trust networks, intrusion detection systems that use both signatures and behavior analysis, encryption for all data flows, and multifactor authentication for any form of administration. There is also the provision for predictive anomaly detection that monitors any anomalies in the operational data that can imply cybersecurity risk – for instance, biases in sensors that might alter state estimations and lead to unnecessary interventions. Cybersecurity becomes a fundamental part of AHCS resilience.

Physical Infrastructure Redundancy

Reliable performance of AHCS requires proper functionality of its power sources, communication networks, and environmental control facilities. The system is able to forecast energy consumption needs and can foresee peak demand scenarios, allowing the system to place backup sources of energy in advance, ensuring non-stop operation. In cases where central servers fail, the local nodes are capable of performing their functions of prediction and control of processes within the system.

Environmental Sustainability Integration

Healthcare is highly resource-intensive. The implementation of the AHCS leads to more sustainable practices with regard to the fact that procurement takes place in accordance with the demand calculated, so there is no waste due to excessive procurement. Energy usage models illustrate the spots where waste is observed in the systems like HVAC, equipment scheduling, and facilities management. Adaptive scheduling is helping to conserve more energy since the system works only when it is really necessary based on the number of patients calculated.

LONG-TERM EVOLUTION AND TECHNOLOGICAL EXPANSION

Integration with Precision Medicine

The future AHCS design will integrate genomics analysis and risk stratification to allocate resources according to the biological risks unique to each patient, thus allowing for better prediction of demands. This will be accomplished by utilizing wearable biosensors for continuous monitoring of patients' physiological parameters, which in turn would allow for dynamic updates in their deterioration scores and trigger interventions before a critical state is reached. This will enhance the accuracy of demand forecasting and avoid unnecessary ICU admissions.

Artificial General Intelligence and Advanced Simulation

AI advancements will one day allow the creation of a holistic model for the numerous biological and social relationships affecting demand for health care. Multi-agent simulation systems could even create complete models of the health care ecosystem, taking into consideration reactions to policy initiatives, economic incentives, and even demographic changes over a long period of time. The result would be much further strategic planning out than just days ahead.

Continuous Cultural Adaptation

There should also be cultural change in conjunction with technological change. Literacy in probabilistic reasoning should play a key role in the training done by healthcare organizations on various levels of organizational hierarchies so that clinicians, managers, and policymakers are aware of the nature, strengths, and weaknesses of the predictions made through the probabilistic reasoning. The fact that data scientists and healthcare professionals work in an interdisciplinary manner when building and implementing the system leads to the generation of tools with analytic and clinical validity. Cultural dimension of AHCS implementation is very important as the system is fully operating only if it is properly.

CONCLUSION

The Autonomous Healthcare Control System (AHCS) embodies a scientifically sound paradigm change in healthcare management from an efficiency-driven reaction mode of management to a resilience-focused mode of anticipatory control. In its consideration of hospitals as multidimensional stochastic dynamic systems, AHCS transforms uncertainty in healthcare management into a measurable factor of governance. AHCS is built on the foundation of stochastic state space models, adaptive optimization using MDPs, queueing network models, compartment models for predicting epidemics, dynamics of fatigue in workers, and stochastic control of inventory in a digitally simulated environment. Each of the models adds a different dimension of operational intelligence, collectively defining a multidimensional description of hospital operation.

The resulting Resilience Index offers a composite scalar metric for the system's robustness that allows institutional benchmarking as well as trends analysis over time. Through simulations, it can be shown that the proposed AHCS system leads to a significantly lower ICU overload risk, cuts down on the recovery time by roughly 50% when compared to reactive benchmarks, and keeps staff fatigue at operationally acceptable levels while also increasing patient care, ensuring work safety, and stabilizing finances. The ethical governance framework guarantees that these results are attained through processes aligning with medical ethics: human agency is maintained through explain ability, unfairness is avoided in optimization, and accountability mechanisms are provided.

Scalability from the individual hospitals to regional cooperation to digital twin hierarchies at the nation state level renders AHCS an ideal foundation for the development of a whole new era of healthcare governance infrastructure. The eventual horizon towards which the AHCS framework would have to grow and evolve, based on its current architectural design, would be a world of interoperability in terms of predictive resilience in which the world's nations coordinate their efforts through digital twins against global health threats.

AI DISCLOSURE STATEMENT

The authors wish to state that the use of artificial intelligence (AI) writing assistance software was utilized while working on this chapter. In particular, large language model-based writing assistance software was used to help enhance grammatical accuracy and formatting. All intellectual material, research methodology, mathematical calculations, and scholarly conclusions are solely the work of the authors. The manuscript has been seen, revised, and approved by all authors.

REFERENCES

Batty, M. (2018). *Digital twins*. MIT Press.

Bertsekas, D. P. (2017). *Dynamic programming and optimal control* (4th ed.). Athena Scientific.

Brailsford, S. C., Harper, P. R., Patel, B., & Pitt, M. (2009). An analysis of the academic literature on simulation and modelling in health care. *Journal of Simulation*, *3*(3), 130–140. DOI: 10.1057/jos.2009.10

Chaudhry, B., Wang, J., Wu, S., Maglione, M., Mojica, W., Roth, E., Morton, S. C., & Shekelle, P. G. (2006). Systematic review: Impact of health information technology on quality, efficiency, and costs. *Annals of Internal Medicine*, *144*(10), 742–752. DOI: 10.7326/0003-4819-144-10-200605160-00125 PMID: 16702590

Dekker, S. (2011). *Drift into failure: From hunting broken components to understanding complex systems*. CRC Press.

Folkard, S., & Akerstedt, T. (2004). Trends in the risk of accidents and injuries and their implications for models of fatigue and performance. *Aviation, Space, and Environmental Medicine*, *75*(3), A161–A167. PMID: 15018280

Glasserman, P. (2004). *Monte Carlo methods in financial engineering*. Springer.

Gross, D., Shortle, J. F., Thompson, J. M., & Harris, C. M. (2018). *Fundamentals of queueing theory* (5th ed.). Wiley.

Hollnagel, E., Paries, J., Woods, D. D., & Wreathall, J. (2011). *Resilience engineering in practice: A guidebook*. Ashgate.

Kaplan, E. H., Craft, D. L., & Wein, L. M. (2002). Emergency response to a smallpox attack: The case for mass vaccination. *Proceedings of the National Academy of Sciences of the United States of America*, *99*(16), 10935–10940. DOI: 10.1073/pnas.162282799 PMID: 12118122

Kermack, W. O., & McKendrick, A. G. (1927). A contribution to the mathematical theory of epidemics. *Proceedings of the Royal Society of London. Series A, Containing Papers of a Mathematical and Physical Character*, *115*(772), 700–721. DOI: 10.1098/rspa.1927.0118

Lundberg, S. M., & Lee, S.-I. (2017). A unified approach to interpreting model predictions. In *Advances in Neural Information Processing Systems* (pp. 4765–4774).

McMahan, B., Moore, E., Ramage, D., Hampson, S., & Arcas, B. A. y. (2017). Communication-efficient learning of deep networks from decentralized data. In *Proceedings of the International Conference on Artificial Intelligence and Statistics* (pp. 1273–1282).

Mnih, V., Kavukcuoglu, K., Silver, D., Rusu, A. A., Veness, J., Bellemare, M. G., Graves, A., Riedmiller, M., Fidjeland, A. K., Ostrovski, G., Petersen, S., Beattie, C., Sadik, A., Antonoglou, I., King, H., Kumaran, D., Wierstra, D., Legg, S., & Hassabis, D. (2015). Human-level control through deep reinforcement learning. *Nature*, *518*(7540), 529–533. DOI: 10.1038/nature14236 PMID: 25719670

Obermeyer, Z., & Emanuel, E. J. (2016). Predicting the future—Big data, machine learning, and clinical medicine. *The New England Journal of Medicine*, *375*(13), 1216–1219. DOI: 10.1056/NEJMp1606181 PMID: 27682033

Puterman, M. L. (2014). *Markov decision processes: Discrete stochastic dynamic programming*. Wiley.

Ribeiro, M. T., Singh, S., & Guestrin, C. (2016). Why should I trust you?: Explaining the predictions of any classifier. In *Proceedings of the ACM SIGKDD International Conference on Knowledge Discovery and Data Mining* (pp. 1135–1144). DOI: 10.1145/2939672.2939778

Ross, S. M. (2019). *Introduction to probability models* (12th ed.). Academic Press.

Schulman, J., Wolski, F., Dhariwal, P., Radford, A., & Klimov, O. (2017). Proximal policy optimization algorithms. *arXiv:1707.06347.*

Shah, N. H., Milstein, A., & Bagley, S. C. (2019). Making machine learning models clinically useful. *Journal of the American Medical Association*, *322*(14), 1351–1352. DOI: 10.1001/jama.2019.10306 PMID: 31393527

Silver, D., Huang, A., Maddison, C. J., Guez, A., Sifre, L., van den Driessche, G., Schrittwieser, J., Antonoglou, I., Panneershelvam, V., Lanctot, M., Dieleman, S., Grewe, D., Nham, J., Kalchbrenner, N., Sutskever, I., Lillicrap, T., Leach, M., Kavukcuoglu, K., Graepel, T., & Hassabis, D. (2016). Mastering the game of Go with deep neural networks and tree search. *Nature*, *529*(7587), 484–489. DOI: 10.1038/nature16961 PMID: 26819042

Sterman, J. D. (2000). *Business dynamics: Systems thinking and modeling for a complex world.* McGraw-Hill.

Sutton, R. S., & Barto, A. G. (2018). *Reinforcement learning: An introduction* (2nd ed.). MIT Press.

Tao, F., Zhang, H., Liu, A., & Nee, A. Y. C. (2019). Digital twin in industry: State-of-the-art. *IEEE Transactions on Industrial Informatics*, *15*(4), 2405–2415. DOI: 10.1109/TII.2018.2873186

Topol, E. J. (2019). *Deep medicine: How artificial intelligence can make healthcare human again.* Basic Books.

Chapter 13
Implications of Stochastic AI and Adaptive Systems for Cloud-Driven Digital Healthcare:
Ethical, Legal, and Societal Concerns

Prantosh Kumar Paul
http://orcid.org/0000-0003-1140-3369
Raiganj University, India

Suchismita Das
http://orcid.org/0009-0000-5006-3331
Raiganj University, India

Tanusree Chakraborty
http://orcid.org/0000-0003-0322-3990
Great Lakes Institute of Management, India

Gangotri Ganguly
Eastern Institute for Integrated Learning in Management (EIILM), Kolkata, India

Saibabu Neyyila
http://orcid.org/0000-0001-6054-2053
Skyline University Nigeria, Nigeria

Manoj Deva Yeddu
Adikavi Nannaya University, India

Rohit Kumar Pal
http://orcid.org/0000-0002-7525-0771
Lincoln University College, Malaysia

ABSTRACT

Digital healthcare increasingly uses artificial intelligence (AI), cloud computing, and adaptive systems for predictive, personalized, continuous care. These systems face uncertainty from incomplete observations, heterogeneous data, changing patient states, and variable treatment responses. This chapter synthesizes literature on stochastic adaptive healthcare and cloud-enabled AI from technological, ethical, legal, and regulatory perspectives. It examines Bayesian updating, MDPs/POMDPs, uncertainty quantification, and queueing networks as foundations for adaptive clinical decision-making. It distinguishes aleatory and epistemic uncertainty and shows how probabilistic outputs affect trust, accountability, bias, consent, and regulation. The chapter proposes the Cloud-Based Adaptive Healthcare Governance and

DOI: 10.4018/979-8-3373-9705-4.ch013

Implementation Framework (CAHGIF 2.0–Stochastic), integrating stochastic reasoning, organizational readiness, governance, and health outcomes. Responsible adaptive healthcare requires AI and measurement, communication, monitoring, and governance of uncertainty across AI lifecycle.

INTRODUCTION

The healthcare management industry is undergoing a transformation brought about by artificial intelligence (AI), adaptive systems, and cloud computing (Fahim et al., 2025). Patient data can be noisy or incomplete, disease progression can differ between patients, and treatment response can vary even among patients receiving the same therapies (Bica et al., 2021). This means an adaptive healthcare system should account not only for predictions but also for the probabilities and uncertainties associated with them. Consequently, this necessitates examining adaptive AI from the standpoint of stochastic and probabilistic perspectives in which states, transitions, observations, and decisions in healthcare are seen as uncertain processes and not as deterministic results.

This perspective is grounded in stochastic reasoning. Bayesian analysis allows adaptive systems to update prior information when new patient data enter the system (Irie et al., 2025). Markov processes allow modeling of transitions between changing health states and make it possible to view treatment selection as a series of decisions under uncertain transitions (Chen et al., 2026a). Furthermore, probabilistic models enable quantification of uncertainty. When the patient's physiological state is incompletely observed (de Jong et al.,2026), Partially Observable Markov Decision Processes (POMDPs) provide a decision-making framework.

In addition, AI solutions can be combined with cloud computing technologies. Cloud computing supplies an extensive array of computational and storage resources (Aunugu & Vathsavai,2025) allowing for fast processing of heterogeneous healthcare data that require numerous inferences, simulations, model updates, and real-time analytical work (Nawaz, 2025). However, technology does not guarantee clinical success. Adaptive and probabilistic systems raise the question of how to measure, describe, and verify uncertainty. A predictive model may be very good but may not be usable in clinical contexts due to poor characterization of its uncertainty, while the accuracy of another model may not look impressive, but it can be considered useful if its confidence level is high enough (Campagner et al., 2025).

The challenges of using adaptive AI technologies become even more serious because algorithms must adapt to incoming data. The iterative process of updating makes it harder to manage accountability, reproducibility, and oversight of the algorithms (Paul, P. et al., 2024). Algorithmic bias, data privacy, cybersecurity, explainability, human oversight, and accountability for computer-powered decisions are major issues highlighted in this chapter.

This chapter discusses AI-based stochastic adaptive healthcare in the cloud with respect to technology, probability, organization, ethics, and regulation. Special emphasis is placed on the role of Bayesian updating, Markovian decision processes, stochastic modeling, uncertainty quantification, and queueing networks in making adaptive healthcare better without undermining trust. The chapter also explains how probabilistic reasoning connects to governance and regulation.

Overall, this chapter aims to:

- Examine the role of adaptive systems and AI in improving digital health.
- Assess the use of AI and related technologies in building adaptive, patient-oriented systems.

- Review previous academic work on AI and digital systems in healthcare.
- Evaluate ethical, legal, governance, and regulatory issues associated with AI in adaptive healthcare.
- Identify emerging trends in methodologies for implementing AI in adaptive healthcare.
- Integrate stochastic reasoning and uncertainty quantification into governance and implementation.

BACKGROUND

Digital healthcare has progressed from electronic records and telemedicine to intelligent systems that perform predictive analytics, support personalized treatment, and maintain continuous patient observation. The combination of AI, cloud technologies, the Internet of Medical Things (IoMT), big data analytics, and wearables has allowed healthcare organizations to work with diverse data and make more responsive clinical management decisions (Bhatia et al., 2025; Brahman & Pandey, 2026). AI contributes through machine learning, predictive analytics, computer vision, and natural language processing, facilitating diagnostics, clinical decision-making, patient monitoring, and healthcare management.

At the same time, healthcare environments are characterized by changing patient conditions, noisy measurements, incomplete observations, and heterogeneous data. Therefore, adaptive healthcare systems must not only achieve predictive accuracy but also account for uncertainty when making clinical recommendations. Stochastic and probabilistic approaches give adaptive healthcare systems this additional capability. Through Bayesian inference, clinical beliefs can be corrected when new evidence about patients becomes available (Ali, H., 2022). Models based on Markov processes can be used for modeling patient health changes and making sequential treatment decisions. Gaussian and other probabilistic models allow predictions with uncertainty distributions, so doctors can assess prediction reliability.

Cloud computing has emerged as a critical enabler of these adaptive capabilities. The scalability, flexibility, and computational power of cloud platforms allow healthcare organizations to process large volumes of heterogeneous data in real time, supporting the iterative model updates that adaptive AI requires (Nawaz, 2025). Cloud-based architectures facilitate the integration of diverse data sources, including electronic health records, medical imaging, wearable devices, and IoMT sensors, creating a comprehensive data ecosystem for adaptive healthcare systems.

However, integrating cloud computing with adaptive AI introduces new challenges. Data privacy and security concerns become more complex when sensitive health information is processed across distributed cloud environments. Regulatory compliance must address jurisdictional differences in data protection laws. Interoperability between different cloud platforms and healthcare systems remains a significant technical and organizational challenge. These issues are particularly relevant for stochastic adaptive systems, which require continuous data flows and frequent model updates.

Table 1 presents definitions of adaptive AI and related concepts. Table 2 summarizes stochastic modeling and decision-making approaches in healthcare.

Table 1. Definitions of Adaptive AI and Related Concepts

AI Type	Core Characteristic	Learning After Deployment	Typical Healthcare Example	StochasticCore Mechanism
Static AI	Uses a fixed model trained before deployment	No	Disease prediction model requiring periodic retraining	Fixed model; no post-deployment stochastic updating
Adaptive AI	Continuously updates predictions or recommendations using new validated data while operating	Yes	Personalized treatment recommendations that adjust to patient responses	Online Bayesian updating / stochastic gradient descent
Generative AI	Creates new content such as text, images, reports, or code	Not necessarily	Automated clinical documentation, medical report generation, patient communication	Probabilistic diffusion models / variational autoencoder encoding
Agentic AI	Autonomously plans, coordinates, and executes multi-step tasks to achieve defined goals	Yes, with autonomous decision-making	AI coordinating appointments, diagnostics, follow-up, and clinical workflows	Partially observable Markov decision processes
ContinuouslyLearning AI	Continuously improves predictive performance from incoming data	Yes, primarily through model optimization	Predictive models refined using new patient outcomes	Sequential stochastic optimization and model updating under uncertainty

Source: Compiled by the authors.

Table 2. Stochastic Modelling and Decision-Making Approaches in Healthcare

Stochastic / Decision Concept	Approach	Example in Healthcare
Markov Chains	Models how a system moves between different states over time, where the next state depends mainly on the current state.	Tracking a chronic disease patient moving between stable → worsening → hospitalized → recovered/stable health states.
PoissonProcesses	Models the number or frequency of random events occurring over a period of time.	Estimating how many patients arrive at an emergency department per hour or how frequently adverse events occur.
GaussianProcesses	Models uncertain continuous variables and helps predict values while providing uncertainty/error ranges.	Forecasting a patient's blood glucose, blood pressure, or temperature while estimating uncertainty around the prediction.
Brownian / WienerProcesses	Models continuous random fluctuations over time.	Representing unpredictable short-term changes in a patient's disease progression or physiological measurements.
BayesianInference	Updates beliefs about a patient's condition when new evidence becomes available.	A doctor initially estimates a patient's probability of having a disease; after receiving a new test result, the probability is updated.
MarkovDecisionProcesses (MDPs)	Helps make sequential decisions when different actions lead to different possible future states and outcomes.	Choosing whether to continue medication, change treatment, or hospitalize a patient based on current condition and expected future outcomes.

continued on following page

Table 2. Continued

Stochastic / Decision Concept	Approach	Example in Healthcare
Partially Observable Markov Decision Processes (POMDPs)	Supports sequential decision-making when the patient's true health state cannot be directly observed.	Selecting treatment when clinicians do not have complete information and must combine symptoms, test results, and previous observations.
QueueingNetworks	Models flow, waiting, congestion, and service capacity in systems with random arrivals and service times.	Managing emergency department waits, intensive care unit bed allocation, telemedicine triage queues, and cloud-based inference workloads.

Source: Compiled by the authors.

STOCHASTIC FOUNDATIONS FOR ADAPTIVE HEALTHCARE GOVERNANCE

Adaptive healthcare exists in a scenario where patients' conditions change, observations might be incomplete, data remains heterogeneous, measurements are noisy, and treatment responses are uncertain. Therefore, adaptive AI must do more than continuously learn. It must also account for uncertainty. Stochastically speaking, healthcare states, observations, transitions, and outcomes are probabilistic rather than deterministic.

Bayesian Inference and Online Updating

Bayesian inference allows an adaptive healthcare system to update its beliefs based on new evidence (Kim et al., 2025). Before new patient data emerge, there is a prior probability. This prior is combined with new data to produce a posterior belief. For example, an adaptive treatment-support system can predict the efficacy of treatment based on previously acquired data and patient indications. As more information on treatment outcomes, laboratory results, and possible side effects becomes available, the system may alter the predicted probability of success.

This differs from traditional batch learning, where a model is trained on a fixed dataset and recalibrated only when enough new data are gathered. Sequential Bayesian updating is naturally suitable for adaptive medicine because knowledge can be integrated gradually. Bayesian updating allows individualized treatment while explicitly taking uncertainty into consideration (Berry, 2025). Techniques range from conjugate priors to more advanced Markov Chain Monte Carlo methods for complex posterior distributions. Cloud computing can support such computationally intensive probabilistic inference (Revathy et al., 2026).

The mathematical foundation of Bayesian updating can be expressed through Bayes' theorem, which relates the posterior probability of a hypothesis given observed data to the likelihood of the data given the hypothesis, multiplied by the prior probability of the hypothesis. In healthcare contexts, this means that a clinician's or system's belief about a patient's condition is continuously refined as new test results, symptoms, or treatment responses are observed. This approach is particularly valuable in chronic disease management, where patient states evolve over time and treatment effectiveness may change.

However, continuous Bayesian updating may change how a model functions after deployment. Therefore, adaptive Bayesian systems require constant monitoring, checking, documentation, and regulatory oversight. The challenge for governance is to ensure that these updates remain within acceptable bounds and that any significant changes in model behavior are detected and addressed promptly.

Markov Decision Processes, POMDPs, and Reinforcement Learning

In healthcare, the state signifies indicators of patient health; the action signifies an intervention; the transition depicts the probabilistic movement of health state; and the reward describes a sought-after outcome, such as improved health or reduced adverse consequences. Reinforcement learning (RL) uses this idea to identify actions that lead to desirable long-term consequences. This is relevant to dynamic treatment strategies because the outcome of an intervention can affect future patient states and future decisions (Shin et al., 2026).

The MDP framework provides a formal structure for sequential decision-making under uncertainty. At each decision point, the system observes the current state, selects an action, receives a reward, and transitions to a new state according to probabilistic transition dynamics. The goal is to find a policy that maximizes expected cumulative reward over time. In healthcare, this translates to finding treatment strategies that optimize long-term patient outcomes while accounting for the uncertainty inherent in disease progression and treatment response.

Clinical situations are rarely fully observable. Laboratory results, vital signs, and imaging findings may be incomplete or delayed (Sadanandan, 2026). This means that clinicians have access only to partial information about the physiological state of the patient. POMDPs address this problem by allowing the system to hold probabilistic beliefs regarding an unobservable state and to use new measurements to update those beliefs. MDPs and POMDPs therefore provide a basis for adaptive clinical decision-making and indicate the need for human intervention in highly uncertain situations (Cleynen et al., 2026).

For governance, the key issue is accountability. When a system recommends a treatment pathway based on an MDP or POMDP, who bears responsibility if a probabilistic recommendation leads to an adverse outcome? The answer cannot be purely technical. It must involve human oversight, documentation, and clear allocation of responsibility among clinicians, healthcare organizations, developers, and regulators. This requires new governance mechanisms that account for the probabilistic nature of AI recommendations and the distributed nature of decision-making in adaptive healthcare systems.

Uncertainty Quantification for Clinical Trust

Uncertainty quantification (UQ) means that an AI system should provide not only a prediction but also information about how reliable that prediction is (He et al., 2026). Two types of uncertainty are important.

Aleatoric uncertainty is inherent to variability in healthcare data and biological processes, such as fluctuations in physiology and noise during measurement (Hall, 2026). This type of uncertainty cannot be reduced by collecting more data because it reflects genuine randomness in the underlying processes. For example, even with perfect knowledge of a patient's condition, there may be inherent variability in how they respond to a treatment.

Epistemic uncertainty results from shortcomings in available data, knowledge, or model specification, for example, when an AI system works with a rare disease or a patient group not regularly represented in training data (Srivatsa, 2026). Unlike aleatoric uncertainty, epistemic uncertainty can potentially be reduced by acquiring more data or improving the model.

This distinction has practical implications. Aleatoric uncertainty may be present everywhere. Epistemic uncertainty may signal that more work, testing, or human review is needed. Probabilistic systems can provide credible intervals, prediction intervals, posterior distributions, and confidence measures (Martin, 2026). As a result, uncertainty can serve as a safety signal in decision-making.

For ethics and law, uncertainty affects informed consent, liability, and fairness. If an AI system says a patient has an 85% probability of a condition rather than a definitive "yes" or "no," clinicians and patients must interpret that information. When probabilistic predictions lead to different treatment decisions, questions arise about bias, transparency, accountability, and the standard of care. The governance challenge is to establish norms and standards for how probabilistic information should be communicated and acted upon in clinical settings.

Queueing Networks and Real-Time Adaptive Care

Queueing networks model flow, waiting, congestion, and service capacity in systems with random arrivals and service times. In healthcare, queueing networks are relevant to emergency department waits, intensive care unit bed allocation, telemedicine triage queues, operating room scheduling, and cloud-based inference workloads.

This is directly relevant to the chapter's stochastic framework. Adaptive healthcare systems do not operate in isolation (NIST, 2023;OECD., 2021; Martin, 2026). . They depend on cloud resources, clinical workflows, and human attention, all of which can become congested. If an AI system continuously updates predictions in real time, it may generate additional alerts, recommendations, or requests for human review. This can create new queues and new forms of uncertainty.

For example, an adaptive triage system may prioritize patients probabilistically. If the model's uncertainty is high, it may refer more cases to clinicians. This can increase waiting times for other patients. Queueing networks help explain these trade-offs. They also connect stochastic reasoning to organizational readiness, resource allocation, and health equity.

The integration of queueing theory with adaptive AI governance is particularly important in cloud environments, where computational resources are shared among multiple applications and users. If an adaptive healthcare system requires frequent model updates or extensive probabilistic computations, it may compete for cloud resources with other critical applications. This creates a need for resource-aware governance that considers both computational and clinical queues.

Ethical, Legal, and Societal Implications of Probabilistic Outputs

The uncertainties inherent in stochastic models amplify ethical concerns such as bias, fairness, and accountability. If a model's probabilistic outputs are systematically less reliable for certain populations, then adaptive learning may reproduce or worsen disparities. Epistemic uncertainty can reveal where a model lacks knowledge. Governance systems should therefore require uncertainty reporting by population group, clinical context, and data source.

Legal and regulatory frameworks are needed to govern stochastic decision-making systems where outcomes are probabilistic rather than deterministic. Current regulatory approaches often focus on safety and efficacy at a point in time. Adaptive systems change over time. Regulators need mechanisms for post-market monitoring, model change documentation, uncertainty thresholds, and human override requirements.

Transparency and explainability are also challenging when clinical decisions are informed by complex stochastic processes. It is not enough to explain a model's architecture. Stakeholders need to understand what a probabilistic output means, how uncertain it is, and what action is appropriate. This requires probabilistic literacy among clinicians, administrators, patients, and policymakers.

Societal implications include trust, equity, and the distribution of responsibility. If adaptive systems continuously update their behavior based on real-time probabilistic inference, then patients and clinicians may find it difficult to know why a decision was made. Governance must therefore ensure that adaptive systems remain transparent, accountable, and trustworthy.

The ethical framework for stochastic adaptive healthcare must also address the question of consent. Traditional informed consent models assume that patients can understand the risks and benefits of a proposed treatment. When those risks are expressed as probabilities that may change over time, new approaches to consent may be needed. This could include dynamic consent mechanisms that are updated as the system's recommendations evolve, or tiered consent that allows patients to specify their preferences for different levels of uncertainty.

REVIEW OF LITERATURE AND RESEARCH GAP

AI-drivenCloud Technologies for Predictive and Diagnostic Healthcare

The first stream of research considers the use of AI and cloud computing for predictive analytics, diagnostics, and clinical decision-making. Cloud-based AI systems support computation and storage of large, heterogeneous health data. Narla et al., (2020) illustrate how machine learning and deep learning can support disease prediction and diagnosis in cloud environments. Koppolu et al., (2022) show how cloud-based health system frameworks create opportunities for integration and interoperability, while Nayak (2025) introduces cloud-based solutions for improved design.

The literature demonstrates significant progress in developing cloud-based AI systems for healthcare. These systems leverage the scalability and computational power of cloud platforms to process large volumes of data and support complex machine learning models. Applications range from medical imaging analysis to predictive analytics for patient outcomes. However, most studies focus on technical performance metrics such as accuracy, sensitivity, and specificity, with limited attention to uncertainty quantification or prediction reliability in real-world conditions (Paul, P. K., 2026). In stochastic terms, this is a major limitation. It is not enough to know whether a predictive system can predict an outcome. It is also necessary to evaluate prediction reliability under changing conditions. This gap is particularly important for adaptive systems, which are designed to operate in dynamic environments where data distributions may shift over time.

The healthcare industry is undergoing a revolutionary transformation by Cloud computing and AI. The research identified how a secure cloud-based healthcare analytics framework implementation happens with the help of AI for the betterment of healthcare outcomes and securing data(Chen et al, 2026b). This study highlights the use of Machine learning in the healthcare system. The researcher also analyses the cloud ecosystems, which also assist integration between healthcare providers, collaboration and smooth data sharing. The researcher also mentioned some challenges in this study, such as data breaches, algorithmic bias, and infrastructure complexity, among others. To overcome these challenges, the author proposed the analytical framework. The researcher also suggests that future work of this study can be health care institution needs to improve the data standardization framework, etc. The potential of these technologies are dedicated to convert the healthcare delivery service and improve process optimizationindependently (Koppolu, H. K. R., et al, 2022). In generally cloud computing is advancing healthcare systems as depicted in Figure-1. Integration of advanced AI and Cloud Computing played a crucial role in the healthcare industry. With the assistance of AI and Cloud computing along with Big data enhancing healthcare services are easy to deliver, manage, and effective with best for nutritional solutions (Paul, et al., 2025). An adaptive healthcare system is an intelligent and versatile architecture that uses patients' clinical data, Treatment outcomes, and ambient conditions to improve healthcare services and decision-making.

Figure 1. Cloud Infrastructure in Smart Healthcare for the Healthcare Transformation

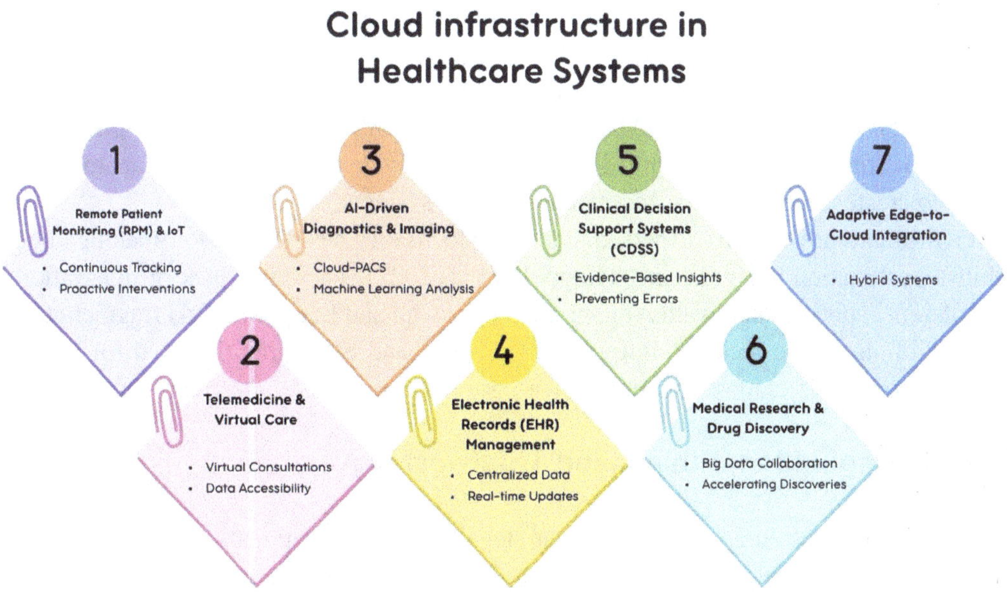

An adaptive Healthcare system in a cloud environment offers Data processing power, Scalable data storage, live accessibility, budget friendly medical treatments (Narla, et al., 2020). The combination of AI and cloud computing transforms manual healthcare services into a modern, tech-driven healthcare system and this new-edge tech-friendly medical system is focused on personalized patient care, data-driven and reactive.

The integration of AI into the healthcare system assist to analyse large volumes of medical data sets to find patterns, disease assessment, course of treatment, critical treatment evaluation, etc. These skills of AI are responsible for the betterment of precision diagnostics, reduced oversight and boosting the delivery of healthcare services. On the other hand, integration of Cloud computing into the healthcare system serves as a digital foundation of the adaptive healthcare system (Amutha, M., 2026). Cloud computing offers an adaptive healthcare system with all the computing resources, a huge storage capacity, and rapid data processing (Chen et al, 2026b). In the healthcare industry, the Electronic Health Record, patients' imaging documents, smart healthcare gadgets, and lab results generate a huge amount of medical datasets, which require a scalable storage to store, manage, and process all the data.

Stochastic and Probabilistic AI in Adaptive Healthcare

A growing body of research addresses the applicability of stochastic approaches in making health services adaptive to uncertainty. Rather than focusing only on prediction accuracy, stochastic methods consider state dynamics, imprecise observations, and the probabilities of different outcomes. Ali (2022) shows that reinforcement learning can change treatment planning, including chemotherapy scheduling, insulin dosing, and rehabilitation organization, based on patient responses. This method is based on MDPs, with patient health as the state, treatment as the action, health transitions as transition probabilities, and healing as the goal. (Ilic et al., 2026) show the significance of adaptation by tracking changes in patient data distributions and adjusting predictive models as needed.

Other stochastic methods offer additional advantages. Kalman filters can estimate changing health states from noisy observations. Bayesian networks can display relationships among symptoms, risk factors, and diagnoses (Junior et al., 2025). Markov models can provide information on transitions between health states and estimates of uncertainty. These methods provide complementary capabilities that can be combined to create comprehensive adaptive healthcare systems.

However, the literature remains dispersed. It tends to focus on adaptive decision-making, model drift, or probabilistic estimation independently (Koppolu et al, 2022). There is a lack of integration among stochastic inference, uncertainty evaluation, clinical approval, and licensing. This fragmentation limits the translation of stochastic methods into clinical practice and highlights the need for an integrated framework that connects technical capabilities with governance and organizational readiness.

Governance, Regulation, Ethics, and Trustworthy AI

Another stream focuses on governance, ethical, legal, and social implications of AI-enabled healthcare. Alowais et al., (2023) highlight ethical ambiguity, workforce preparedness, and legal uncertainty as main obstacles to AI adoption. Singh (2023) examines algorithmic ambiguity and accountability in cloud-based healthcare systems. Amutha (2026) states that privacy, cybersecurity, and compliance issues remain serious.

Stakeholder perspectives vary. Junior et al., (2025) note that government officials often discuss fairness and transparency, while technology developers are more interested in system efficiency. Although algorithmic bias and privacy remain central, solutions differ among stakeholders. An important observation is that internationally recognized governance models are not well represented in academic literature. Despite guidelines from organizations such as WHO and FDA, studies on AI implementation in healthcare often do not compare their findings with these frameworks (WHO, 2021).

The governance literature also reveals a gap in addressing the specific challenges posed by adaptive and stochastic systems. Most governance frameworks assume static AI systems that do not change after deployment. Adaptive systems require continuous monitoring and governance mechanisms that can respond to changes in model behavior over time. This includes mechanisms for detecting and responding to model drift, ensuring that updates maintain safety and fairness, and maintaining accountability across multiple versions of a model.

Implementation and Organizational Readiness

The implementation literature explains that effective application of AI-enhanced healthcare does not depend only on technology. Organizational preparedness, funding, managerial support, technical infrastructure, skilled human resources, and information sharing among systems are main prerequisites (Kee et al., 2024; Junior et al., 2025). These requirements are higher for systems employing stochastic and probabilistic methods because users must deal with uncertainty when acting on AI recommendations.

The matter is more acute in developing countries, which may experience lack of facilities, insufficient finances, limited qualifications, and unequal access to digital technologies (Rabiee, 2026). Therefore, it is necessary to combine technology with organizational capacity, data management, and law. From a stochastic perspective, inadequate probabilistic knowledge is a key implementation barrier. Healthcare workers should be able to understand uncertainty estimates and recognize when it is necessary to confirm or check AI decisions.

Organizational readiness also involves developing appropriate workflows and decision-making processes that integrate AI recommendations with clinical judgment. This requires not only technical training but also changes in organizational culture and professional norms. The introduction of probabilistic AI systems may challenge traditional notions of clinical expertise and decision-making authority, requiring careful change management and stakeholder engagement.

Research Gap

Three linked gaps emerge from the synthesis. First, most AI-cloud studies evaluate predictive accuracy but include few uncertainty estimates or systematic probabilistic validation. This limits understanding of how reliable AI systems are in real-world conditions and undermines clinical trust.

Second, stochastic tools such as Bayesian updating, MDPs, and probabilistic estimation are rarely used alongside governance and clinical responsibility. The literature on stochastic methods and the literature on AI governance remain largely separate, with limited integration between technical capabilities and governance mechanisms.

Third, governance and regulatory procedures stress rational use of AI, but there are few recommendations regarding uncertainty measures and probabilistic credibility in validation and approval. Current regulatory frameworks do not adequately address the specific challenges of adaptive systems, including how to validate systems that change over time and how to ensure ongoing safety and effectiveness.

An integrated framework is therefore necessary. Such a framework should connect stochastic methods with governance, address uncertainty at multiple levels, and provide practical guidance for implementation in healthcare organizations.

METHODS

This chapter uses a systematic integrative literature review that synthesizes different knowledge domains, including AI, adaptive medical systems, cloud computing, digital healthcare transformation, ethics, and regulation. The integrative review was chosen because the work touches on healthcare management, computer science, information systems, medical informatics, and public policy.

Sources were drawn from Scopus, Web of Science, PubMed/MEDLINE, IEEE Xplore, ACM Digital Library, ScienceDirect, SpringerLink, Wiley Online Library, Taylor & Francis Online, Emerald Insight, and Google Scholar. Studies and guidance documents from the FDA, NIST, OECD, and the European Commission were also included. Boolean operators connected keyword groups such as "artificial intelligence," "machine learning," "deep learning," "adaptive AI," "healthcare," "cloud computing," "ethics," "governance," "privacy," "security," "responsible AI," "stochastic modeling," "probabilistic modeling," "Bayesian inference," "Markov decision processes," "uncertainty quantification," and "Monte Carlo simulation."

The review included sources published between 2018 and 2026, with older significant publications included where necessary for theoretical background. Eligible publications were peer-reviewed articles, reviews, conference proceedings, books and chapters, and reports from internationally recognized organizations. Editorials, news items, blogs, duplicates, and low-relevance studies were excluded.

The integrative approach allowed for synthesis of diverse perspectives and identification of common themes across disciplines. This was particularly important for addressing the research gaps identified in the literature, which require integration of technical, organizational, ethical, and regulatory perspectives.

RESULTS AND DISCUSSION

Digital Healthcare Systems and AI: Context for Stochastic Adaptation

Digital healthcare has progressed from electronic records and telemedicine to intelligent systems that can perform predictive analytics, ensure personalized treatment, and maintain continuous patient observation. The combination of AI, cloud technologies, IoMT, big data analytics, and wearables allows healthcare organizations to work with diverse data and make more responsive clinical management decisions (Bhatia et al., 2025; Brahman & Pandey, 2026).

AI acts as a factor in this process through machine learning, predictive analytics, computer vision, and natural language processing. At the same time, healthcare environments are characterized by changing patient conditions, noisy measurements, insufficient observations, and heterogeneous data. Therefore, adaptive healthcare systems involve not only predictive accuracy but also accounting for uncertainty while making clinical recommendations.

Stochastic and probabilistic approaches give this additional capability. Bayesian inference helps correct clinical beliefs when new evidence about patients becomes available. Markov process models can be used for modeling patient health changes and making sequential treatment decisions. Gaussian and other probabilistic models allow predictions with uncertainty distributions, helping doctors understand whether predictions are reliable. The collaboration among AI, stochastic modeling, and cloud computing creates premises for adaptive healthcare systems capable of processing new information continuously and managing evidence-based decision-making.

The evolution toward stochastic adaptive systems represents a fundamental shift in how healthcare AI is conceptualized. Rather than treating AI as a static tool that provides definitive answers, the stochastic approach recognizes that healthcare decisions are inherently probabilistic and that effective AI systems must embrace and communicate uncertainty (Bhatia et al., 2025). This shift has implications for system design, clinical workflows, governance, and professional education.

AI in Healthcare Management and Sustainable Healthcare

Healthcare systems face challenges caused by increasing costs, staff shortages, an ageing population, advancing diseases, and unequal access to healthcare. AI may help manage healthcare through its capability to analyze large amounts of clinical, administrative, and patient data (Kaul et al., 2023; Aceto et al., 2024). In adaptive healthcare, the value of AI goes beyond automation and prediction. It may help make necessary adjustments as the patient's health condition changes along with operational needs.

This capability is enhanced by stochastic and probabilistic models that help healthcare systems capture and measure variability and uncertainty. For instance, probabilistic forecasting may assist in predicting uncertainty in demand for services and resources. Bayesian approaches may aid in updating treatment or risk estimates in light of new patient data. Uncertainty-aware predictive models may help healthcare workers distinguish between trustworthy and less reliable recommendations. Therefore, AI may contribute to sustainable healthcare not only through efficiency but also through more efficient and evidence-based allocation of resources. As depicted in Table.3 regarding emerging AI & allied technologies in Adaptive Healthcare Applications.

Sustainability in healthcare also encompasses environmental considerations. Cloud-based AI systems consume significant computational resources, and the energy consumption of large-scale machine learning models is a growing concern. Adaptive systems that continuously update their models may require even more computational resources than static systems. This creates a tension between the benefits of adaptive AI and the environmental costs of computation. Governance frameworks should consider these trade-offs and promote energy-efficient approaches to stochastic inference.

Table 3. Core AI Technologies and Their Adaptive Healthcare Applications

AI Technology	Adaptive Healthcare Application	Stochastic / Probabilistic Link
Machine Learning	Risk prediction, diagnosis support, patient stratification	Probabilistic classifiers, Bayesian updating
Deep Learning	Medical imaging, early deterioration detection	Predictive uncertainty, Monte Carlo dropout
ReinforcementLearning	Dynamic treatment regimes, resource allocation	MDPs, POMDPs
Natural Language Processing	Clinical documentation, patient communication	Probabilistic language models
Cloud AI	Scalable inference, model updating, simulation	Distributed Bayesian inference, MCMC
Digital Twins	Simulation of patient scenarios and treatment outcomes	Gaussian processes, uncertainty propagation

Source: Compiled by the authors.

Stochastic-Driven Adaptive Healthcare Systems

Stochastic techniques assist adaptive healthcare through effective use of AI. With AI technologies, stochastic processes can be applied to produce predictions based on adaptable variables in the healthcare system. Algorithms can keep modifying predictions based on updated information from various sources.

The integration of stochastic methods with AI creates new possibilities for personalized medicine and adaptive care. By explicitly modeling uncertainty and incorporating probabilistic reasoning, these systems can provide more nuanced and reliable recommendations that account for the inherent variability in healthcare.

Probabilistic Clinical Diagnosis and Decision-Making

AI in medicine uses information from imaging, laboratory results, previous treatments, and prior experiments. Bayesian updating makes it possible to change results based on new information (Kaul et al., 2023). Probabilistic models of diagnosis can provide information about alternative diseases along with the probability of each.

This approach contrasts with traditional diagnostic systems that provide binary outputs (disease present or absent). Probabilistic diagnosis acknowledges that clinical evidence is often ambiguous and that multiple conditions may be possible. By providing probability estimates for different diagnoses, AI systems can help clinicians make more informed decisions and communicate uncertainty to patients.

The governance implications of probabilistic diagnosis include the need for clear standards on how probability estimates should be interpreted and acted upon. What probability threshold should trigger further testing? How should patients be informed about uncertain diagnoses? These questions require both technical and ethical consideration.

Adaptive Treatment and Personalized Healthcare

MDPs and reinforcement learning enable successful decisions during treatment. A patient's current health condition can be modelled as the current state, actions as interventions, and treatment outcomes as factors that influence subsequent decisions. Patient response during treatment is taken into account to enhance personalized treatment. POMDPs can support diagnosis and treatment because the patient's full physical condition cannot always be observed directly.

Adaptive treatment systems represent a significant advance over static treatment protocols. By continuously updating recommendations based on patient response, these systems can optimize outcomes and reduce adverse effects. However, they also raise questions about accountability and transparency. If a treatment recommendation changes over time, how should clinicians and patients understand the rationale for different recommendations at different points?

Continuous Monitoring and Predictive Management

Stochastic filtering and probabilistic forecasting enable continuous monitoring of physiological indicators and health conditions. Kalman filters, Gaussian processes, and similar techniques can distinguish meaningful changes from measurement noise. This information allows specialists to intervene earlier or manage chronic disease effectively.

Continuous monitoring systems generate large volumes of data and require sophisticated algorithms to extract meaningful signals. The challenge is not only technical but also organizational. Healthcare systems must develop workflows and protocols for responding to alerts and recommendations generated by continuous monitoring systems. This includes defining action thresholds, ensuring appropriate human oversight, and managing clinicians' cognitive load.

Queueing and Resource-Aware Adaptation

Queueing networks add a further dimension. Adaptive AI systems consume computational resources and generate outputs that require human review. If uncertainty is high, the system may request more clinician attention. This can create queues, delays, and resource competition. A governance framework for stochastic adaptive healthcare should therefore include queue-aware monitoring. It should track not only model accuracy but also waiting times, referral volumes, and the distribution of human oversight.

Queue-aware adaptation highlights the importance of considering the broader system in which AI operates. An AI system that performs well in isolation may create problems when integrated into a healthcare system with limited human and computational resources. Governance must therefore take a systems perspective that considers the interactions between AI, clinical workflows, and resource constraints.

Stochastic Adaptive Systems in Cloud Environments

Cloud computing contains the scalable infrastructure necessary for computationally intensive stochastic and adaptive applications in healthcare (Chen et al., 2026b). Cloud mechanisms can process large, varied data from electronic health records, medical imaging, wearables, and IoMT systems, enabling continuous analysis through probabilistic calculations. The integration of cloud computing and stochastic AI is especially applicable to Bayesian inference, Monte Carlo simulations, MCMC techniques, and uncertainty estimation.

Cloud computing also allows development of systems that continuously monitor models. At the same time, reliance on the cloud requires stronger security, interoperability, and access control because cloud environments hold sensitive health information. Thus, the significance of the cloud environment extends beyond data storage and computational capacity. It also includes governance of probabilistic computation, auditability, and jurisdictional compliance.

The distributed nature of cloud computing creates both opportunities and governance challenges. On one hand, cloud platforms can provide centralized monitoring and logging of model behavior, making it easier to track changes and detect problems (Rabiee, 2026). On the other hand, distributing data and computation across multiple jurisdictions creates complex regulatory challenges. Healthcare organizations must navigate different data protection laws, professional standards, and liability regimes depending on where data is processed and where decisions are made.

Ethical, Legal, and Governance Implications of Stochastic Adaptive Healthcare

Stochastic adaptive AI creates governance challenges different from those of traditional AI. Privacy, cybersecurity, algorithmic bias, transparency, explainability, and accountability remain central (Alowais et al., 2023; Amutha, 2026). However, adaptive systems produce varying probabilistic results, so it is necessary to follow not only model performance but also changes in uncertainty and model behavior over time.

Uncertainty is especially important for clinical accountability. A probabilistic recommendation should express the confidence or uncertainty accompanying the prediction so the clinician can decide whether to accept, consult, or reject it. High epistemic uncertainty might indicate that the patient and clinical case are poorly covered by the model's knowledge. Responsible implementation requires continuous validation, transparent documentation of model changes, human control, data governance, and proper regulation.

The WHO stresses fairness, transparency, human control, privacy, and sustainability. The FDA and NIST provide bases for monitoring AI-related risks. Therefore, managing stochastic adaptive healthcare must go beyond understanding whether an AI system is correct. It should provide details of how uncertainty is measured, communicated, monitored, and included in clinical and regulatory decisions.

The legal framework for stochastic adaptive healthcare must address several novel issues. First, liability allocation becomes more complex when decisions are based on probabilistic recommendations from adaptive systems that change over time. Second, regulatory approval processes designed for static systems may not be appropriate for systems that continuously update. Third, privacy protections must account for the continuous data flows required by adaptive systems. These issues require new legal and regulatory approaches that are specifically designed for stochastic adaptive healthcare.

PROPOSED CLOUD-BASED ADAPTIVE HEALTHCARE GOVERNANCE AND IMPLEMENTATION FRAMEWORK (CAHGIF 2.0–STOCHASTIC)

This chapter proposes the Cloud-Based Adaptive Healthcare Governance and Implementation Framework (CAHGIF 2.0–Stochastic). The framework extends the original CAHGIF by integrating stochastic reasoning and uncertainty quantification into the process of transforming technology into better healthcare outcomes. It addresses the gap between AI effectiveness and governance.

The framework consists of six interconnected layers. Figure 2 presents the framework.

Figure 2. CAHGIF 2.0–Stochastic Framework

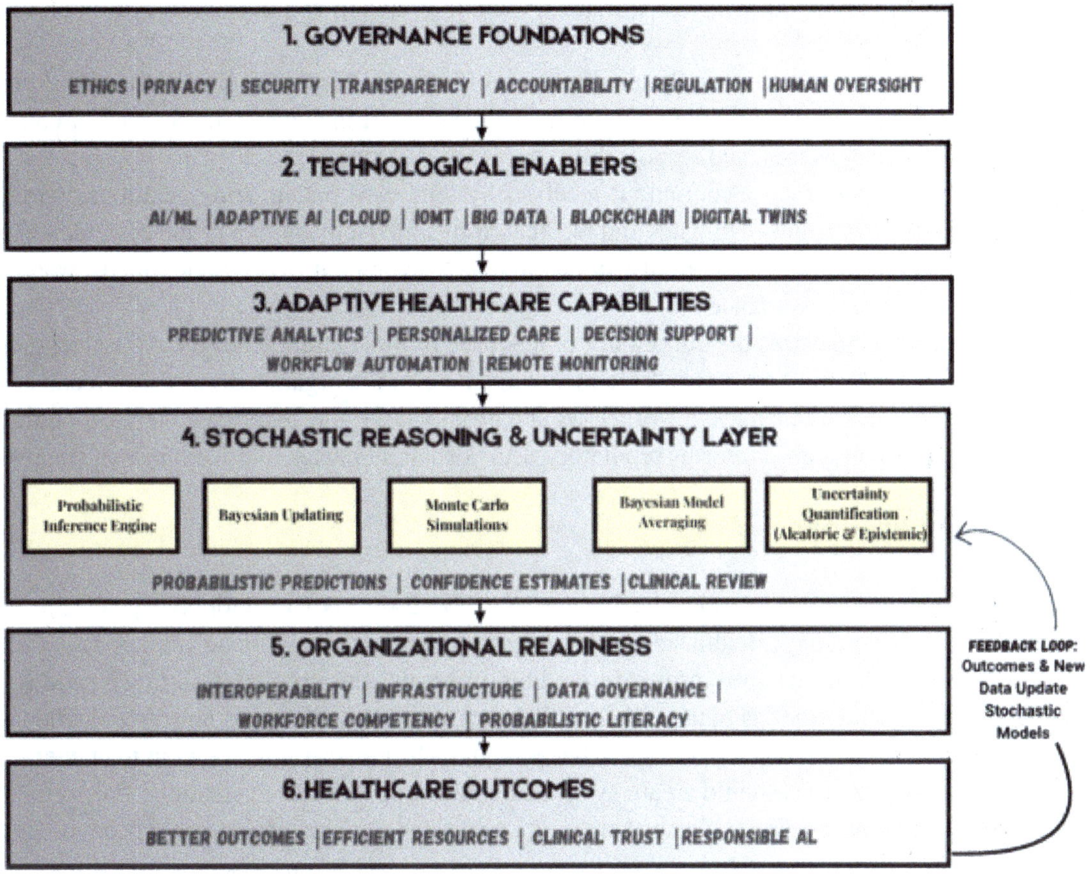

Layer 1: Governance Foundations. Ethics, privacy, security, transparency, accountability, regulation, and human oversight. This foundational layer establishes the normative and regulatory context for adaptive healthcare systems. It includes principles for responsible AI, data protection requirements, and mechanisms for accountability.

Layer 2: Technological Enablers. AI/machine learning, adaptive AI, cloud computing, IoMT, big data, blockchain, and digital twins. This layer encompasses the technical infrastructure and capabilities required for stochastic adaptive healthcare. It includes both the computational resources provided by cloud platforms and the algorithms that enable adaptive behavior.

Layer 3: Adaptive Healthcare Capabilities. Predictive analytics, personalized care, decision support, workflow automation, and remote monitoring. This layer represents the clinical applications that stochastic adaptive AI enables. It connects technical capabilities to healthcare outcomes.

Layer 4: Stochastic Reasoning and Uncertainty. Probabilistic inference engine, Bayesian updating, Monte Carlo simulation, Bayesian model averaging, uncertainty quantification, and queue-aware monitoring. This layer connects aleatoric and epistemic uncertainty. It represents the core innovation of CAHGIF 2.0–Stochastic, integrating probabilistic reasoning into every aspect of the adaptive healthcare system.

Layer 5: Organizational Readiness. Interoperability, infrastructure, data governance, workforce competency, and probabilistic literacy. This layer recognizes that technology alone is not sufficient for successful implementation. Organizations must develop the capacity to understand and act on probabilistic information.

Layer 6: Healthcare Outcomes. Better outcomes, efficient resources, clinical trust, and responsible AI. This layer represents the ultimate goals of the framework. It includes both clinical outcomes and process outcomes such as trust and responsibility.

The framework operates as a continuous feedback system. New patient and operational data update stochastic models. Uncertainty estimates and medical results feed into another round of model updating. Adaptation is therefore governed not only by continuous learning but also by continuous probabilistic assessment and human governance.

The framework emphasizes the importance of feedback loops at multiple levels. At the technical level, new data and uncertainty estimates drive model updates. At the organizational level, feedback from clinical outcomes informs changes in workflows and protocols. At the governance level, monitoring of model behavior and outcomes informs regulatory decisions and updates to governance mechanisms.

Practical Implications

To implement stochastic adaptive healthcare, organizations must develop competencies beyond conventional AI technology. Healthcare practitioners must learn probabilistic literacy to understand probability estimates, uncertainty measures, credible intervals, and prediction intervals, and to avoid treating AI recommendations as binary choices. This training helps clinicians understand when an AI-generated answer is sufficiently reliable and when it requires further examination or human intervention.

Healthcare organizations should create systems that allow continuous evaluation of adaptive model performance, predictive accuracy, changes in data distributions, and post-deployment behavior(Alowais et al., 2023). An efficient override strategy is especially important when epistemic uncertainty is high, and the AI recommendation contradicts clinicians' conclusions.

From a managerial standpoint, implementation should combine data governance, cybersecurity, interoperable infrastructure, regulatory compliance, and workforce competencies. Cloud platforms must provide robust, scalable probabilistic computing while ensuring the safety of sensitive health information. Responsible implementation therefore requires organizations to develop not only AI capabilities but also capabilities for managing uncertainty.

The practical implications extend to clinical workflow design. Adaptive AI systems require new workflows that accommodate probabilistic recommendations and uncertainty information (Bhatia et al., 2025). This includes protocols for when to accept AI recommendations, when to seek additional information, and when to override the system. Clinical decision support systems must be designed to present uncertainty information in ways that are actionable and understandable.

Education and training are also critical. Healthcare professionals need to develop probabilistic literacy, understanding concepts such as confidence intervals, posterior distributions, and uncertainty decomposition. This requires changes in medical education and continuing professional development. Interdisciplinary collaboration among clinicians, data scientists, ethicists, and regulators is essential to develop and implement effective governance mechanisms.

Future Research Directions

Several areas require further research to advance stochastic adaptive healthcare. First, researchers need to develop methods for validating adaptive systems that change over time. Traditional validation approaches assume static models, but adaptive systems require ongoing validation that accounts for model evolution.

Second, research is needed on how to communicate uncertainty effectively to different stakeholders. How should probabilistic information be presented to clinicians, patients, and policymakers? What formats and visualizations are most effective for different audiences?

Third, the ethical and legal frameworks for adaptive healthcare need further development. Questions of liability, consent, and fairness in probabilistic adaptive systems require interdisciplinary research that bridges technical, legal, and ethical perspectives.

Fourth, research on the organizational and workforce implications of stochastic adaptive healthcare is needed. How should healthcare organizations restructure to accommodate adaptive AI systems? What new roles and competencies are required?

Fifth, the environmental sustainability of large-scale stochastic adaptive systems requires attention. Methods for reducing the computational footprint of adaptive AI while maintaining performance and reliability should be explored.

CONCLUSION

Artificial intelligence, cloud computing, and adaptive technologies are changing healthcare. A key challenge in healthcare development is the uncertainty in processes such as healthcare adaptation due to changing patient states or surges. This chapter presents a deeper analysis of adaptive healthcare through the lens of stochastic and probabilistic reasoning. Bayesian updating, Markovian decision processes, and probabilistic modeling allow changes in medical beliefs, consideration of current health statuses, recognition of decision possibilities, and understanding of prediction reliability.

The CAHGIF 2.0–Stochastic framework shows how these approaches can be combined with technical issues, governance, and healthcare system efficiency. Responsible adaptive healthcare must go beyond AI accuracy. It requires adaptive systems that can function under uncertainty and communicate the reliability of the information they provide.

The chapter has argued that stochastic reasoning is not merely a technical enhancement but a fundamental requirement for trustworthy adaptive healthcare. By explicitly modeling and communicating uncertainty, adaptive systems can support more informed clinical decision-making, enable appropriate human oversight, and maintain accountability over time. However, this requires new approaches to governance, education, and organizational design that are attuned to the challenges of probabilistic adaptive systems.

Integrating stochastic methods with AI governance represents a significant advance in the field. By connecting technical capabilities with governance mechanisms, the CAHGIF 2.0–Stochastic framework provides a roadmap for responsible implementation of adaptive healthcare systems. As healthcare continues to evolve toward greater personalization and adaptivity, such integrated approaches will become increasingly essential.

AI DISCLOSURE STATEMENT

The authors used AI-assisted writing tool during the preparation of this chapter. It was used primarily for language refinement, grammar correction, restructuring of sentences, and improving clarity and readability. The authors reviewed, verified, and edited all AI-assisted content and retain full responsibility for the accuracy, originality, and final content of the chapter.

REFERENCES

Aceto, G., Persico, V., & Pescapé, A. (2024). Artificial intelligence for healthcare sustainability: Challenges, opportunities, and future directions. *Journal of Healthcare Engineering*, *2024*, 1–18.

Ali, H. (2022). Reinforcement learning in healthcare: Optimizing treatment strategies, dynamic resource allocation, and adaptive clinical decision-making. *International Journal of Computer Applications Technology and Research*, *11*(3), 88–104.

Alowais, S. A., Alghamdi, S. S., Alsuhebany, N., Alqahtani, T., Alshaya, A. I., Almohareb, S. N., Aldairem, A., Alrashed, M., Bin Saleh, K., Badreddin, H. A., Al Yami, M. S., Al Harbi, S., & Albekairy, A. M. (2023). Revolutionizing healthcare: The role of artificial intelligence in clinical practice. *BMC Medical Education*, *23*(1), 689. Advance online publication. DOI: 10.1186/s12909-023-04698-z PMID: 37740191

Amutha, M. (2026). Cloud-powered intelligent ecosystems for secure healthcare analytics with artificial intelligence-driven innovation. *International Journal of Technology. Management and Humanities*, *12*(1), 108–115.

Aunugu, D. R., & Vathsavai, V. G. (2025). Cloud-based AI solutions for scalable and intelligent enterprise modernization. *ICCK Transactions on Emerging Topics in Artificial Intelligence*, *2*(2), 81–89. DOI: 10.62762/TETAI.2025.100106

Berry, D. A. (2025). Adaptive Bayesian clinical trials: The past, present, and future of clinical research. *Journal of Clinical Medicine*, *14*(15), 5267. Advance online publication. DOI: 10.3390/jcm14155267 PMID: 40806890

Bhatia, M., Nagpal, M., & Jaswal, A. (2025). Adaptive therapeutics through AI-enhanced nanoscale sensors: Innovations in real-time health monitoring. In *3rd International Conference on Disruptive Technologies (ICDT)* (pp. 845–850). IEEE. DOI: 10.1109/ICDT63985.2025.10986393

Bica, I., Alaa, A. M., Lambert, C., & Van Der Schaar, M. (2021). From real-world patient data to individualized treatment effects using machine learning: Current and future methods to address underlying challenges. *Clinical Pharmacology and Therapeutics*, *109*(1), 87–100. DOI: 10.1002/cpt.1907 PMID: 32449163

Brahman, K. S., & Pandey, A. (2026). AI-driven adaptive patient care framework for personalized medicine and optimized health outcomes. In *Recent advances in technology & management* (pp. 170–174). CRC Press., DOI: 10.1201/9781003768630-33

Campagner, A., Biganzoli, E. M., Balsano, C., Cereda, C., & Cabitza, F. (2025). Modeling unknowns: A vision for uncertainty-aware machine learning in healthcare. *International Journal of Medical Informatics*, *203*, 106014. Advance online publication. DOI: 10.1016/j.ijmedinf.2025.106014 PMID: 40603232

Chen, S., Liu, T., Sun, Z., Jia, J., Hang, D., & Zhang, W. (2026a). Markov Decision Process–Based Personalized Follow-Up Planning for Type 2 Diabetes: Retrospective Cohort Study. *JMIR Medical Informatics*, *14*(1), e88206. DOI: 10.2196/88206 PMID: 42686193

Chen, S., Zhang, X., Liu, E., Xiong, Y., Wang, L., Gu, X., Wang, Z., Guo, J., & Luo, T. (2026b). Privacy-preserving cloud-based dermatological image processing for medical applications: A review. *Journal of Cloud Computing (Heidelberg, Germany)*, *15*(1), 46. Advance online publication. DOI: 10.1186/s13677-026-00886-6

Cleynen, A., de Saporta, B., Rossini, O., Sabbadin, R., & Vernay, A. (2026). *Bridging impulse control of piecewise deterministic Markov processes and Markov decision processes: Review and open challenges.*

de Jong, I. P., Sburlea, A. I., & Valdenegro-Toro, M. (2026). Uncertainty quantification in machine learning for biosignal applications-a review. *Journal of Healthcare Informatics Research*, ●●●, 1–55. DOI: 10.1007/s41666-026-00249-5

European Commission. (2021). *Proposal for a regulation laying down harmonised rules on artificial intelligence.* AI Act.

Fahim, Y. A., Hasani, I. W., Kabba, S., & Ragab, W. M. (2025). Artificial intelligence in healthcare and medicine: Clinical applications, therapeutic advances, and future perspectives. *European Journal of Medical Research*, *30*(1), 848. Advance online publication. DOI: 10.1186/s40001-025-03196-w PMID: 40988064

FDA. (2021). *Artificial intelligence/machine learning (AI/ML)-based software as a medical device (SaMD) action plan.* U.S. Food and Drug Administration.

Hall, J. (2026). Personalized treatment response modeling from multimodal patient profiles across heterogeneous diseases, clinical interventions, and longitudinal outcomes with calibrated predictive uncertainty estimation. *International Journal of Machine Learning and Engineering*, *2*(1), 1–13.

He, W., Jiang, Z., Xiao, T., Xu, Z., & Li, Y. (2026). A survey on uncertainty quantification methods for deep learning. *ACM Computing Surveys*, *58*(7), 1–35. DOI: 10.1145/3786319

Ilic, A. S., Ilic, M., Stojanovic, N., & Stojanovic, D. (2026). Adaptive healthcare monitoring through drift-aware edge-cloud intelligence. *Future Internet*, *18*(3), 156. Advance online publication. DOI: 10.3390/fi18030156

Irie, K., Minar, P., Reifenberg, J., Boyle, B. M., Noe, J. D., Hyams, J. S., & Mizuno, T. (2025). Hybrid Population Pharmacokinetic–Machine Learning Modeling to Predict Infliximab Pharmacokinetics in Pediatric and Young Adult Patients with Crohn's Disease. *Clinical Pharmacokinetics*, *64*(11), 1669–1679. DOI: 10.1007/s40262-025-01564-7 PMID: 40885855

Junior, A. A., Ndayizigamiye, P., Bokaba, T., & Idemudia, E. C. (2025). Resilient healthcare systems through AI-powered cloud computing: Perspectives on resource allocation. In *Proceedings of the 58th Hawaii International Conference on System Sciences* (pp. 3310–3319).

Kaul, V., Enslin, S., & Gross, S. A. (2023). History of artificial intelligence in medicine. *Gastrointestinal Endoscopy*, *97*(5), 807–812. PMID: 32565184

Kee, K. A. L., Hashim, J. H., & Tan, S. S. L. (2024). The adoption of advanced healthcare technologies in the private healthcare industry: Case of IHH Healthcare Berhad, Malaysia. *Jesselton Journal of Educators and Scholars*, *1*(1), 46–67. DOI: 10.68440/3009-0881.1005

Kim, M. J., Prieto-Merino, D., Nicholas, J., Allen, L., Burton, M. J., Bastawrous, A., & Macleod, D. (2025). Evidence-based approaches to quality improvement: A narrative review of integrating Bayesian adaptive trials into health services. *Journal of Evaluation in Clinical Practice*, *31*(5), e70197. Advance online publication. DOI: 10.1111/jep.70197 PMID: 40618403

Koppolu, H. K. R., Recharla, M., & Chakilam, C. (2022). Revolutionising patient care with AI and cloud computing: A framework for scalable and predictive healthcare solutions. *International Journal of Scientific and Engineering Research*, *11*(12), 1457–1472.

Martin, R. (2026). Possibilistic inferential models: A review. *Journal of the American Statistical Association*, *121*(553), 807–826. DOI: 10.1080/01621459.2025.2606127

Narla, S., Valivarthi, D. T., & Peddi, S. (2020). Cloud computing with artificial intelligence techniques: GWO-DBN hybrid algorithms for enhanced disease prediction in healthcare systems. *Journal of Current Science & Humanities*, *8*(1), 14–30.

Nawaz, A.Dr. Ali Nawaz. (2025). Cloud computing and edge computing: Converging technologies for real-time data processing. *Multidisciplinary Research in Computing Information Systems*, *5*(3), 157–179. DOI: 10.71465/mrcis93

Nayak, K. (2025). Adaptive multi-cloud AI architectures for predictive healthcare analytics and cybersecurity automation. *International Journal of Science. Resources and Technology*, *8*(6), 15359–15368.

NIST. (2023). *Artificial intelligence risk management framework (AI RMF 1.0)*. National Institute of Standards and Technology.

OECD. (2021). *Recommendation of the Council on artificial intelligence*. OECD.

Paul, P. K. (2026). Demystifying Digital Healthcare Systems: Aspects of Emerging Technologies, Initiatives, Opportunities and Issues—The Indian Context. *International Journal of Information Science and Computing*, *12*(2), 259–265.

Paul, P. K., Bandyopadhyay, A., Kayyali, M., Das, N., Chatterjee, R., & Sharma, S. K. (2025). Integrating Big Data and AI in nutrition: Current trends and future directions. [IJRQEH]. *International Journal of Reliable and Quality E-Healthcare*, *14*(1), 1–22. DOI: 10.4018/IJRQEH.372690

Paul, P. K., Pradhan, U., Jena, S. K., Bommali, T., Kayyali, M., & Saavedra, R. (2024). Emerging Healthcare Systems with AI based Medicine, EHRs, VHAs, & Precision Healthcare: A Scientific Study. *International Journal of Applied Science and Engineering*, *12*(2), 133–151. DOI: 10.30954/2322-0465.2.2024.3

Rabiee, P. (2026). Artificial intelligence in healthcare systems of low- and middle-income countries: Opportunities, challenges, and pathways to ethical integration. In Malawana, J., Arjomandi Rad, A., Vardanyan, R., & Miller, G. (Eds.), *Artificial intelligence in healthcare and biomedical visualization* (pp. 157–170). Springer Nature Switzerland., DOI: 10.1007/978-3-032-06520-9_9

Revathy, G., Dinesh, L., Sathish, P., & Selvan, S. T. (2026). Support systems: Revolutionizing patient care in Industry 6.0: Integrating cloud computing and IoT for enhanced patient care. In *Generative AI revolution: Transforming healthcare and life sciences towards sustainable development in Industry 6.0* (p. 73).

Sadanandan, B. (2026). Multimodal deep learning for early prediction of patient deterioration in the ICU: Integrating time-series EHR data with clinical notes. arXiv. https://arxiv.org/abs/2603.14719

Shin, D.-H., Lee, D.-J., Son, Y.-H., & Kam, T.-E. (2026). Treatment stitching with Schrödinger bridge for enhancing offline reinforcement learning in adaptive treatment strategies. *Proceedings of the AAAI Conference on Artificial Intelligence*, *40*(21), 17697–17705. DOI: 10.1609/aaai.v40i21.38826

Singh, K. (2023). Artificial intelligence & cloud in healthcare: Analysing challenges and solutions within regulatory boundaries. *SSRG International Journal of Computer Science and Engineering*, *10*(9), 1–9.

Srivatsa, S. S. (2026). Epistemic uncertainty in clinical machine learning: Sources, detection, and mitigation. *JVS-Vascular Insights*. Advance online publication. DOI: 10.1016/j.jvsvi.2026.100492

WHO. (2021). *Ethics and governance of artificial intelligence for health*. World Health Organization.

ADDITIONAL READING

Rajkomar, A., Dean, J., & Kohane, I. (2019). Machine learning in medicine. *The New England Journal of Medicine*, *380*(14), 1347–1358. DOI: 10.1056/NEJMra1814259 PMID: 30943338

Sutton, R. S., & Barto, A. G. (2018). *Reinforcement learning: An introduction* (2nd ed.). MIT Press.

Topol, E. J. (2019). High-performance medicine: The convergence of human and artificial intelligence. *Nature Medicine*, *25*(1), 44–56. DOI: 10.1038/s41591-018-0300-7 PMID: 30617339

Chapter 14

Equity-Aware Agentic AI Architectures and Governance With SDG-Aligned Healthcare Innovation

Dhanshri Parihar
http://orcid.org/0009-0005-4249-9051
Department of CSE (AI & ML), Krishna Institute of Engineering and Technology (KIET), Ghaziabad, India

Sachin Jain
http://orcid.org/0000-0002-2948-7858
Department of Computer Science and Engineering, Ajay Kumar Garg Engineering College, Ghaziabad, India

Aastha Sharma
http://orcid.org/0009-0000-5511-3131
Department of Computer Science and Engineering, Ajay Kumar Garg Engineering College, Ghaziabad, India

Divya Sharma
http://orcid.org/0000-0002-3787-5017
Department of Electronics and Communication Engineering, Ajay Kumar Garg Engineering College, Ghaziabad, India

ABSTRACT

Agentic AI marks a shift from static forecasting to autonomous, goal-oriented systems for healthcare workflows. Unlike conventional AI models, agentic AI integrates adaptive learning with planning, execution, monitoring, and coordination within multi-agent architectures. This chapter explores how these systems collaborate with UN SDGs 3, 9, 10, and 17—directly related to health equity. The chapter formally models the proposed system as a Partially Observable Markov Decision Process (POMDP), introducing stochastic foundations including transition dynamics, belief updating, and Bellman optimality for policy learning under uncertainty. Probabilistic fairness metrics evaluate disparities using confidence intervals.

DOI: 10.4018/979-8-3373-9705-4.ch014

Uncertainty quantification addresses aleatoric and epistemic uncertainty via risk-aware optimization. The suggested Equity-Aware Agent Architecture integrates governance, federated learning, fairness constraints, and human oversight. Combining subgroup equity data with clinical metrics enables agentic AI to reduce inequities while maintaining efficiency.

INTRODUCTION

Public health developments do not benefit all individuals, regardless of the amount of money invested in healthcare systems and state-of-the-art medical technology. This is true both nationally and internationally. Health outcomes vary for many systemic reasons, including poverty, social isolation, a shortage of trained medical personnel, and remoteness from urban centers. To close these gaps, the SDGs and other global frameworks lay forth moral standards; nevertheless, in order to achieve these lofty goals on a large scale, we require innovative technologies that are both smart and ethical. Recent advances in artificial intelligence (AI) systems that integrate goal-driven planning, autonomy, multi-agent collaboration, and adaptive learning are bringing complex health systems one step closer to making situationally aware decisions (Borkowski, 2025).

Traditional AI systems, particularly those dominant between 2000 and 2022, were primarily designed as task-specific predictive tools. These systems operated within a static input-output framework, where data were fed into a trained model to generate a prediction or classification. Mathematically, such systems can be represented as $y=f(x)$, where input data x are mapped to output y through a learned function f. The machine's job was done once it made the output. Individuals who made standard choices were still in charge of how to understand predictions and what to do about them. This represented a moment when AI was a tool to help people make decisions, not an independent agent.

Traditional AI designs lacked long-term planning capabilities, permanent memory, and extensive contextual awareness. In the medical field, for instance, a more conventional AI model would make an educated guess as to the likelihood that a patient will fall ill or require a return visit to the hospital. The onus for patients to notify their doctors of any changes, arrange for follow-up appointments, or alter their care routes remained on them. Even in the financial sector, alarms from fraud detection systems were relayed to humans, who then had to conduct follow-up investigations and make decisions. That is why the scope of classical AI was narrow, and its influence was limited to a subset of decision-making.

Conversely, a major shift in the operation of creative systems is brought about by the advent of agentic AI. Agentic AI systems can act on their own and have long-term goals. Instead of making predictions on their own, those systems get or set high-level goals and then break them down into smaller goals on their own. They can plan, carry out, watch the results, and make changes all at once. Agentic AI systems are mathematically analogous to reinforcement learning frameworks where a policy π seeks to optimize cumulative reward over time, as indicated by $\max_{\pi} \sum_{t=0}^{T} R(s_t a_t)$, where s_t represents the system state at time t, a_t represents actions, and R represents reward. This formulation records the sequential, adaptive, and objective-oriented features of agentic systems.

There are different parts that make up agentic AI that function together. These parts include planning components, execution agents, monitoring systems, memory subsystems, and maybe even governance or oversight systems. Agentic systems are distinct from standard models in that they are more endogenous and have memory that lasts. This implies they may remember the context from one session to the next and alter to match new conditions. They can also work with other AI agents to create multi-agent ecosystems that are spread out. One essential thing about these systems is the fact that they can work ahead of time. An agentic AI system in healthcare, for example, would not only be able to predict a patient's risk of readmission, but it would also be able to automatically schedule follow-up visits, send reminders to take medications as needed, change remote monitoring activities as needed, change the care plan if compliance is low, or let clinicians know about any unusual events. In this case, AI is not a fixed predictor; instead, it is a manager of processes (Borkowski, 2025).

Classical AI and agentic AI are not only different in how they think about things, but they are also different in how they affect how we split up work between computers and people. Agentic AI will show us the way and help us solve problems. Over time, more and more people will be able to take part in government and watching. We establish boundaries, moral guidelines, and objectives. A lot of people call this new way of connecting "Hybrid Intelligence." People set broad goals and moral limits, while agentic systems handle rollout and making things run more smoothly.

However, just a subset of options were often affected by these concerns. The opposite is true with agentic AI systems, which operate throughout complex workflows and interconnected systems. This makes them more likely to make changes and puts the whole system at danger. Investigating agentic deployment—cases of unforeseen damage caused by an autonomous AI system exercising authority—reveals specific categories of threats, including chain reaction decision errors and excessive autonomy. Because these systems have an independent effect on how resources are used, services are delivered, and policies are carried out, governance systems need to grow as the level of autonomy grows. Over the years, AI went through three main phases of expansion. We worked on rule-based and statistical models that could be employed as working computational tools from 2000 to 2015. From 2015 to 2022, algorithms using deep learning improved AI's ability to execute predictions, making it more like a smart assistant. The age of Assistant AI started before 2023. These were straightforward workers who could only work on modest social and technical systems. The change entails moving from static prediction to dynamic control systems and from separate outputs to continuous decision orchestration.

In line with the SDGs, this chapter walks through the design and governance of agentic AI to help achieve health fairness. The following topics span all areas of focus: equity, openness, data governance, human supervision, and strengthening local capacities (Borkowski, 2025). The subsequent sections provide a comprehensive treatment of the stochastic foundations, SDG alignment, architectural design, evaluation frameworks, and governance mechanisms required for responsible deployment of equity-aware agentic AI in healthcare.

FORMAL STOCHASTIC FOUNDATIONS

Mdp/Pomdp Formulation of the Equity-Aware Agentic System

The proposed equity-aware agentic healthcare system is formally modeled as a Partially Observable Markov Decision Process (POMDP) defined by the tuple $\langle S, A, \Omega, T, O, R, \gamma \rangle$, where each component captures a distinct aspect of the healthcare decision-making environment under uncertainty.

The **state space** S encompasses all relevant clinical and contextual information. This includes patient health conditions such as disease progression stage, vital signs, laboratory results, and medication adherence history. Demographic characteristics such as age, socioeconomic status, geographic location, and social determinants of health are also incorporated to enable equity-aware decision-making. Additionally, healthcare resource availability—including bed capacity, staff availability, medication stock, and equipment functionality—is represented within the state space to enable realistic resource-constrained planning.

The **action space** A comprises the full range of interventions available to the healthcare system. These actions include diagnostic procedures, treatment recommendations, medication adjustments, resource allocation decisions, patient outreach interventions, follow-up scheduling, and care coordination activities. Each action represents a discrete or continuous choice that the agentic system can execute to influence patient outcomes and system efficiency.

The **observation space** Ω represents the incomplete information available to the agent. In healthcare settings, observations are inherently partial and noisy. These may include self-reported symptoms from patients, incomplete medical histories, delayed laboratory results, imaging reports with varying quality, and fragmented data from different healthcare providers. The observation function captures the probabilistic relationship between true states and the observations received.

The **transition probability function** $T(s',|sa) = P(s_{t+1}= s' \mid s_t = sa_t = a)$ captures the stochastic dynamics of patient health evolution and resource utilization under a given action. This function models the inherent randomness in disease progression, treatment response variability, and the unpredictable nature of healthcare resource consumption. For example, a patient with congestive heart failure may improve, remain stable, or deteriorate following medication adjustment, with probabilities influenced by individual characteristics and environmental factors.

The **observation probability function** $O(o,|s'a) = P(o_t= o \mid s_t = s'a_{t-1} = a)$ models the likelihood of receiving observation o given the true state and previous action. This function accounts for the measurement error, reporting delays, and data incompleteness that characterize healthcare information systems. A patient may fail to report symptoms accurately, laboratory results may be lost or delayed, and socioeconomic data may be missing or outdated.

The **reward function** $R(s,a)$ encodes both clinical and equity objectives in a unified framework. The reward can be expressed as $R(s,a) = \alpha \cdot \text{ClinicalBenefit}(s,a) - \beta \cdot \text{Cost}(s,a) - \gamma \cdot \text{InequityPenalty}(s,a)$, where α, β, and γ are weighting coefficients that balance competing objectives. The clinical benefit term captures improvements in patient health outcomes such as reduced mortality, avoided hospitalizations, and enhanced quality of life. The cost term accounts for resource consumption and financial expenditure. The inequity penalty is a novel addition that penalizes actions that disproportionately benefit privileged demographic groups, thereby encoding equity as an explicit optimization objective. For instance, if an action leads to a 10% improvement in survival for urban patients but only 2% for rural patients, the inequity penalty would be substantial, incentivizing the agent to select actions that provide more balanced benefits across groups.

The **discount factor** $\gamma \in [0,a)$ determines the relative importance of immediate versus future rewards. A higher discount factor encourages long-term planning and sustained investments in patient health, while a lower discount factor prioritizes immediate interventions.

The agent maintains a **belief state** $b(s)$—a probability distribution over possible states given the history of actions and observations. The belief state serves as the sufficient statistic for decision-making under partial observability, capturing all relevant information from past interactions. Upon taking action a and receiving observation o, the belief is updated via Bayes' rule:

$$b'(s') = \eta \cdot O(o,|s'a) \sum_{s\in S} T(s',|sa) b(s)$$

where $\eta = \left[\sum_{s'' \in S} O(o, |s''a) \sum_{s \in S} T(s'', |sa) b(s)\right]^{-1}$ is the normalization constant ensuring that the updated belief sums to unity. This belief update equation captures the core learning mechanism of the agentic system, allowing it to refine its understanding of patient states and system conditions as new information arrives.

The agent's objective is to learn an optimal policy $\pi^*: b \mapsto a$ that maximizes the expected discounted cumulative reward over the planning horizon. The optimal value function for a belief state satisfies the Bellman optimality equation:

$$V^*(b) = \max_{a \in A} \left[\sum_{s \in S} R(s, a) b(s) + \gamma \sum_{o \in \Omega} P(o, |\ ba) V^*(b')\right]$$

where $P(o, |ba) = \sum_{s' \in S} O(o, |s'a) \sum_{s \in S} T(s', |sa) b(s)$ is the probability of observing o given belief b and action a. This equation decomposes the value of a belief state into immediate expected reward plus the expected future value after taking action and receiving an observation.

Probabilistic Fairness Metrics

To ensure equitable decision-making, the framework employs probabilistic fairness metrics rather than deterministic constraints. Traditional fairness approaches impose hard equality constraints, such as requiring that true positive rates be exactly equal across groups. However, such deterministic requirements are often unrealistic in healthcare settings characterized by heterogeneous populations, limited data, and inherent statistical variability. A probabilistic approach recognizes that observed performance disparities may arise from sampling variability, measurement error, or limited sample sizes, and it provides a principled framework for distinguishing between systematic bias and benign statistical fluctuation.

Let G denote the set of demographic or socioeconomic groups relevant to the healthcare context. For each group $g \in G$, define the group-specific performance metrics of interest. The true positive rate (TPR) for group g is defined as:

$$TPR_g = \frac{TP_g}{TP_g + FN_g}$$

where TP_g is the number of true positive predictions and FN_g is the number of false negative predictions for individuals in group g. Similarly, the false positive rate (FPR) is:

$$FPR_g = \frac{FP_g}{FP_g + TN_g}$$

where FP_g is the number of false positive predictions and TN_g is the number of true negative predictions for group g. Additional metrics such as precision, recall, positive predictive value, and negative predictive value can be defined analogously.

The disparity metric between groups g_1 and g_2 for a given performance measure μ is defined as:

$$D_{g_1, g_2} = |\ \mu_{g_1} - \mu_{g_2}\ |$$

where μ_g represents the estimated performance metric for group g. To account for sampling uncertainty, the disparity metric is accompanied by a confidence interval:

$$D_{g_1,g_2} \pm z \cdot SE\left(D_{g_1,g_2}\right)$$

where z is the critical value corresponding to the desired confidence level (e.g., $z = 1.96$ for 95% confidence) and $SE\left(D_{g_1,g_2}\right)$ is the standard error of the disparity estimate.

The standard error can be computed using various statistical methods. Bootstrapping is a non-parametric approach that resamples the data with replacement to generate an empirical distribution of the disparity metric, from which confidence intervals can be directly computed. Bayesian credible intervals can be obtained by placing prior distributions on the group-specific performance metrics and computing the posterior distribution of the disparity. Hoeffding's inequality provides a distribution-free concentration bound:

$$P\left(|\ \hat{\mu}_g - \mu_g\ | \geq \epsilon\right) \leq 2\exp\left(-\frac{2n_g\epsilon^2}{(b-a)^2}\right)$$

where $\hat{\mu}_g$ is the empirical estimate, μ_g is the true value, n_g is the sample size for group g, and $[ab]$ is the range of the performance metric. This inequality can be inverted to obtain confidence bounds that hold with high probability regardless of the underlying data distribution.

The probabilistic fairness criterion is operationalized as follows: the system is considered fair with respect to a given disparity metric if the confidence interval for D_{g_1,g_2} falls entirely below a pre-specified threshold δ_{g_1,g_2}, or if the probability that the true disparity exceeds the threshold is sufficiently small:

$$P\left(D_{g_1,g_2} > \delta_{g_1,g_2}\right) < \alpha$$

where α is a pre-specified significance level. This probabilistic formulation provides more realistic and robust fairness guarantees in healthcare settings where data are limited and populations are heterogeneous. It acknowledges that perfect equality is an unrealistic ideal and instead focuses on ensuring that any observed disparities are consistent with statistical variability rather than systematic discrimination.

The framework also supports differential fairness, where different thresholds may be applied to different disparity metrics or different group comparisons.

Uncertainty Quantification in Resource Allocation and Patient Outcomes

The proposed framework explicitly quantifies uncertainty in both healthcare resource allocation and patient outcome prediction. Healthcare environments are characterized by multiple sources of uncertainty: resource availability fluctuates unpredictably, patient demand varies seasonally and epidemically, and treatment effectiveness depends on individual patient characteristics that are only partially observed.

Resource availability is modeled as a probabilistic variable. For example, the number of available hospital beds B on a given day can be represented as:

$$B \sim \mathcal{N}\left(\mu_B, \sigma_B^2\right)$$

where μ_B is the expected number of available beds and σ_B^2 captures day-to-day variability. Similarly, medication stock levels, staff availability, and equipment functionality can be modeled using appropriate probability distributions depending on the nature of the variable (e.g., Poisson distributions for count data, beta distributions for proportions, or gamma distributions for positively-skewed continuous variables). Patient demand for healthcare services can be modeled as a stochastic process, with emergency admissions following a Poisson process and scheduled appointments following time-varying arrival patterns.

The framework distinguishes between two fundamental types of uncertainty: aleatoric uncertainty and epistemic uncertainty. Aleatoric uncertainty, also known as statistical uncertainty, arises from inherent randomness in the data-generating process. This type of uncertainty is irreducible; it captures the natural variability in patient outcomes, treatment responses, and disease progression that cannot be eliminated even with perfect models. Epistemic uncertainty, also known as model uncertainty, arises from limited knowledge about the true underlying relationships. This type of uncertainty is reducible through additional data collection, improved model specifications, and better understanding of the causal mechanisms.

Predictive uncertainty is estimated through statistical and machine learning techniques that explicitly model the distribution of outcomes rather than just point estimates. Bayesian neural networks place prior distributions on network weights and compute posterior distributions conditioned on the observed data, yielding predictive distributions that capture both aleatoric and epistemic uncertainty. Monte Carlo dropout provides an approximation to Bayesian inference by applying dropout at test time and collecting multiple stochastic forward passes, generating an empirical distribution of predictions. Ensemble methods train multiple independent models and aggregate their predictions, with the variance across ensemble members serving as an estimate of epistemic uncertainty. Conformal prediction provides distribution-free prediction intervals that are guaranteed to contain the true outcome with a specified probability.

The integration of uncertainty quantification enables risk-aware decision-making through chance-constrained optimization. Rather than optimizing expected outcomes under the assumption that all variables are known with certainty, the agentic system optimizes subject to probabilistic constraints. A general chance-constrained optimization formulation is:

$$\max_{\pi} \mathbb{E}[R(\pi)] \text{ subject to } P(g(x,\xi) \leq 0) \geq 1-\epsilon$$

where $g(x,\xi) \leq 0$ represents a constraint on resource consumption or patient outcomes, ξ captures the random variables in the system, and ϵ is a small tolerance parameter specifying the acceptable probability of constraint violation. This formulation ensures that the system maintains high reliability even in the face of uncertainty.

The practical implementation of risk-aware decision-making in the agentic healthcare system involves several mechanisms. First, the system identifies high-risk cases where predictive uncertainty is large, either because the patient is unusual or because data are sparse. In such cases, the system prioritizes human oversight, escalating decisions to clinicians rather than taking autonomous actions. Second, the system adapts its confidence thresholds dynamically, being more conservative when resources are scarce or when the consequences of errors are severe. Third, the system provides clinicians with uncertainty estimates alongside its recommendations, enabling informed judgment about when to accept or override AI suggestions. Finally, the system continuously monitors its predictive performance, detecting when uncertainty metrics diverge from expected patterns and triggering model updates or human review. These mechanisms collectively improve the reliability, transparency, and safety of AI-driven healthcare interventions while ensuring that uncertainty is explicitly managed rather than ignored.

HEALTH EQUITY AND THE SDG FRAMEWORK

Health equity states that everyone should have a fair chance to be as healthy as they can be. The SDGs are a mechanism to make sure that modern technology breakthroughs are made and used in a way that aids society fulfil its goals. SDG 3 (good health and well-being), SDG 9 (industry, innovation, and infrastructure), SDG 10 (reducing disparities), and SDG 17 (partnerships for the goals) are among the targets most directly relevant to health equity. However, health equity cannot be accomplished only through healthcare services; there is a need to deal with wider societal variables, indicators, and organizations that determine how easy it is to get care, how good the care is, and how healthy people are (Lampropoulos et al., 2024). The United Nations established the Sustainable Development Goals as a global framework that has both direct and indirect effects on health equity. The following analysis demonstrates that all of the SDGs reduce inequalities in distinct ways, and the subsequent discussion connects each SDG to specific agentic AI capabilities.

SDG 1: No Poverty

One of the most major things that causes bad health is being deficient. People that are deprived do not have sufficient food, a safe place to live, or medical attention. Poverty is both a cause and a consequence of poor health: illness can push families into poverty through medical expenses and lost income, while poverty limits access to preventive care, nutritious food, and healthy living conditions. Health equity requires ways to keep people safe from money problems and assist them get out of poverty, such as insurance, social protection programs, and affordable healthcare services. When health care expenses are reduced, fewer families have to choose between health care and their fundamental needs, allowing them to invest in education, housing, and other determinants of health.

Agentic AI can contribute to SDG 1 by optimizing the allocation of financial protection programs, identifying households at highest risk of catastrophic health spending, and automating enrollment in social protection schemes. The system can analyze patient data alongside socioeconomic indicators to predict which families are most vulnerable to medical impoverishment and proactively connect them with financial assistance. By reducing administrative barriers and ensuring that resources reach those who need them most, agentic AI supports poverty reduction while also improving health outcomes.

SDG 3: Health and Well-Being

SDG 3's goal is the one that has the most to do with health. It aims to ensure healthy lives and promote well-being for all at all ages. The specific targets include universal health coverage (UHC), maternal and child health, disease prevention, mental health care, access to essential medicines, and reduction of non-communicable diseases. The divide between affluent and poor people grows less when everyone can access and pay for health care. More immunization programs, better care for pregnant women, and more screenings for people who are at risk make sure that no one is left behind. Lower death rates are linked to better access to early detection and treatment for everyone, not only people who live in cities or have a lot of money.

Agentic AI directly supports SDG 3 by enabling proactive and preventive care, as discussed in subsequent sections. The system can detect early warning signs of disease, automate follow-up care, optimize treatment pathways, and ensure that patients in underserved areas receive timely interventions.

By incorporating equity-aware planning, the system specifically targets populations that have historically been left behind, ensuring that UHC becomes a reality rather than merely an aspiration. The integration of clinical decision support with resource allocation ensures that even in resource-constrained settings, the most vulnerable patients receive appropriate care.

SDG 4: Quality Education

A higher level of education is linked to better health literacy, which means being able to understand health facts, know your rights when it comes to health care, and take precautions. Research has found that people with more education are more likely to get preventative care, stick with their treatments, and make smart decisions about their health (Berdahl et al., 2023). For example, people are more likely to get vaccinated when they know more about the benefits and risks. Education also empowers individuals to navigate complex healthcare systems, advocate for their own health, and engage in shared decision-making with clinicians.

Agentic AI can support SDG 4 by delivering personalized health education and literacy interventions. The system can identify patients with low health literacy through proxy indicators such as educational attainment, language barriers, or prior engagement with health information. It can then generate tailored educational materials in appropriate languages and formats, deliver reminders and explanations through accessible channels, and assess comprehension through interactive dialogue. By integrating education into the care pathway, agentic AI ensures that patients are informed participants in their own care rather than passive recipients.

SDG 5: Gender Equality

High rates of maternal death prove that reproductive health is insufficient. The main reason is that men and women access reproductive health services differently. Inequities in freedom and opportunities for women: women residing in low-income environments lack sufficient freedom, educational opportunities, and health care resources (Borkowski, 2025). If we could achieve gender equality and give all women more power, it would have a major impact on health equity. Women with equal rights and decision-making power receive better reproductive health care, quicker postpartum recovery care, and are less likely to be victims of violence against women. Consequently, equitable access to both obstetric and prenatal care has been shown to result in health outcomes for mothers that are at least as good, while significantly reducing mortality.

Agentic AI can address gender-based health disparities by ensuring that reproductive health services are equitably distributed, that maternal health risks are identified early, and that postpartum care is automated and accessible. The system can detect patterns of gender-based discrimination in care delivery, flag disparities in access to reproductive services, and recommend interventions to address identified gaps. Additionally, by ensuring that women's health concerns are not dismissed or minimized in clinical decision-making, the system promotes more equitable care.

SDG 9: Industry, Innovation, and Infrastructure

For accessible and efficient services, strong healthcare systems need stable infrastructure, effective digital tools, and continual innovation. Good care is still difficult in many distant and low-resource communities due to poor infrastructure and limited medical facilities. Telemedicine, electronic health records (EHRs), and remote monitoring might improve healthcare infrastructure by plugging care gaps and enabling care beyond hospital walls (Berdahl et al., 2023). These technologies can make doctor-patient communication easier, saving time and money while making healthcare accessible to previously underserved populations.

Agentic AI is itself an innovation that enhances healthcare infrastructure. The system integrates with existing EHRs, telemedicine platforms, and remote monitoring devices to create a coordinated digital infrastructure that spans primary, secondary, and tertiary care. Investment in infrastructure and new ideas creates more open, effective, and flexible healthcare systems that satisfy the needs of many people. By enabling decentralized, intelligent care coordination, agentic AI strengthens healthcare systems in both high-resource and low-resource settings.

SDG 10: Reduced Inequalities

SDG 10 aims to end global and national inequality. Because geography, social position, and health are strongly linked, systemic issues like income inequality and racism typically cause health inequities. Health disparities might worsen due to a lack of qualified medical staff, infrastructure, or poor or distant residents. Health equality requires more access to basic medical care and social safety nets. These plans provide cheap health care to all. Some groups will receive assistance, and low-income facilities and services will improve. When these programs uncover unjust treatment, some groups may receive fair treatment. The difference in health care between cities and rural areas is getting smaller, as more healthcare facilities, digital healthcare solutions, outreach programs, and transportation providers have made it possible for people in rural areas to get the same level of care as people in big towns. The result of efforts to lower inequality is health outcomes that are more evenly spread, fairer, and easier to get.

Agentic AI is explicitly designed with SDG 10 in mind, as the equity-aware framework ensures that inequality reduction is a primary optimization objective rather than an afterthought. The system continuously monitors for disparities in access, quality, and outcomes across demographic and socioeconomic groups, adjusting its recommendations to close identified gaps. By actively countering the systemic biases that perpetuate health inequalities, agentic AI serves as a tool for structural change in healthcare delivery.

SDG 17: Partnerships for the Goals

SDG 17 emphasizes global cooperation, financing, and knowledge sharing. Health challenges such as pandemics require cross-border coordination and resource mobilization. Partnerships enable equitable distribution of vaccines, medicines, and funding during health crises, protecting vulnerable nations and ensuring that global health security benefits all countries rather than just the wealthiest. Agentic AI can facilitate such partnerships by enabling secure data sharing across institutions through federated learning, coordinating multinational responses to health emergencies, and distributing resources based on equity principles rather than political or economic power. Cross-border disease response improves global resilience and protects vulnerable nations during health crises.

RELATIONSHIP BETWEEN AGENTIC COMPONENTS AND SDGS

The agentic architecture presented in this chapter aligns with the SDGs through its constituent components. Perception agents collect data from diverse sources, enabling monitoring of health and inequality (SDG 3 and SDG 10). Planner agents develop strategic care plans that bridge health objectives with innovation infrastructure (SDG 3 and SDG 9). Federated learning modules enable collaborative model training across institutions without sharing sensitive data (SDG 9 and SDG 17). Simulation agents model disease transmission and resource needs, facilitating partnerships and global health coordination (SDG 17). Governance agents ensure institutional accountability and equity oversight (SDG 10). This multi-SDG alignment demonstrates how agentic AI can serve as an integrated platform for achieving multiple global development objectives simultaneously.

MOTIVATION AND OPPORTUNITIES

Bridging the Gap between Detection and Intervention

The "prediction-action gap" is an important issue with conventional AI in healthcare. Most systems accurately categorize patients by risk, but they do not take action to ensure fair health outcomes. A conventional risk prediction model might identify a patient as high-risk for hospital readmission, but the responsibility for acting on that prediction falls on overburdened clinicians who may not have the time or resources to follow up appropriately. This creates a dangerous disconnect between knowledge and action, where AI identifies problems but fails to solve them.

Agentic AI bridges this gap by integrating planning modules, execution agents, monitoring systems, and re-planning mechanisms into a unified framework. The system does not merely identify high-risk patients; it automatically schedules follow-up visits, sends medication reminders, adjusts care plans based on real-time data, and escalates concerning cases to clinicians. For example, when the system detects a pregnant patient with signs of pre-eclampsia, it autonomously schedules additional prenatal visits, tracks compliance with blood pressure monitoring, provides educational materials about warning signs, and alerts the care team if readings exceed thresholds. By closing the loop between detection and intervention, agentic AI ensures that predictive insights translate into tangible improvements in patient care.

Alignment with the Sustainable Development Goals

The SDGs provide a normative framework for ensuring that everyone can get health care, reducing inequality, building infrastructure, and encouraging countries to work together (Jain & Jain, 2024). Agentic AI offers the opportunity to build SDG priorities into the design of systems from the ground up. When people make decisions, they may not only look for efficiency, but also fairness. As an example, they might try to close the performance gaps between ethnic groups or focus on groups of people who are not getting enough help. This equity-aware optimization is explicitly encoded through the constrained optimization framework presented earlier, where the objective function includes both clinical performance and equity metrics. The result is a system that actively works to reduce disparities rather than perpetuating existing inequalities.

Proactive and Preventive Care Systems

A lot of the change in healthcare is due to agentic AI. Care is moving from being reactive to being proactive and protective. Agents of intelligence can spot early signs of disease up to six months in advance by keeping an eye on patient data, environmental signals, and patterns of behaviour. So, treatment can start before things get worse. This feature can be very helpful when it comes to long-term, non-communicable diseases like diabetes, heart disease, and lung disease. Agentic systems also make it easier for the community to keep an eye on public health by finding new risks and making it easier to respond quickly (Jain et al., 2025).

Proactive care systems contribute to long-term cost savings by reducing the need for costly hospital stays and intensive treatments. Through the provision of earlier, more widespread, and more personalized therapies for previously overlooked or underrepresented populations, agentic AI contributes to the advancement of health equity. By eliminating issues like delayed diagnosis and inadequate access to care, these systems aim to reduce disparities. At the same time, they encourage healthcare delivery models that are more inclusive, accessible, and long-lasting. The integration of predictive analytics with autonomous intervention ensures that patients receive appropriate care at the right time, regardless of their background or circumstances.

Resource Optimization in Low-Resource Settings

There is a severe lack of doctors, hospital beds, and other medical supplies in many middle- and low-income nations. Agentic AI has the ability to dynamically optimize the distribution of resources by prioritizing high-need cases, scheduling staff efficiently, predicting supply demand, and allocating mobile clinics strategically. This promotes fairness since it targets those most in need, rather than those with the most extensive networks, with scarce resources. In rural areas with limited healthcare infrastructure, agentic AI can triage patients based on severity, direct them to appropriate care facilities, and ensure that essential medications are available when needed. By making the most of limited resources, agentic AI enables high-quality care even in settings where conventional systems would struggle.

Hybrid Intelligence and Human-AI Collaboration

Instead of doing away with human intervention altogether, agentic AI only reimagines it. Agents of artificial intelligence carry out and enhance operational procedures in Hybrid Intelligence systems, with humans defining objectives, ethical limits, and supervision thresholds. Scalability is assured without sacrificing responsibility in this well-rounded paradigm. Working together in this way improves institutional efficiency without sacrificing the use of human judgment in delicate or potentially dangerous matters (Jaidka & Jain, 2023). Clinicians remain in control of overarching care goals, ethical boundaries, and complex medical decisions, while the agentic system handles routine coordination, monitoring, and optimization. This partnership leverages the strengths of both humans and machines, ensuring that AI serves as a powerful tool rather than a replacement for human expertise.

Scalable Public Health Governance

Pandemics and other public health emergencies demonstrate the critical importance of well-coordinated, flexible systems. By connecting monitoring data, simulating the transmission of disease, distributing testing resources, and easing cross-regional collaboration, agentic AI can serve as a digital coordinating layer. During the COVID-19 pandemic, for example, an agentic system could have automated contact tracing, coordinated vaccine distribution based on equity principles, monitored hospital capacity in real time, and dynamically adjusted public health recommendations. Aligning with public health objectives led by the SDGs, this skill fosters global resilience and ensures that health emergencies are managed with both efficiency and fairness.

TECHNICAL FOUNDATIONS: ARCHITECTURES AND EVALUATION

Equity-Aware Agent Architecture

We present the Equity-Aware Agent Architecture (EAA), which divides an agentic healthcare system into five coordinated components that facilitate scalable, fair, and coordinated decision-making across all healthcare processes.

Perception Agents: The Intake Layer

The first step is the introduction of Perception Agents, which act as the sensory input for the system. These agents use "heterogeneous data," which does not come from clinical records alone like standard models do. The data sources include therapeutic information from electronic health records, real-time data from medical sensors and self-reports from mobile devices, and background information from geographical markers and Social Determinants of Health (SDoH). These agents make sure the system can identify outside obstacles, including geographical isolation or a lack of transportation, by collecting data outside of the hospital (Gupta et al., 2025). By incorporating these diverse data streams, perception agents ensure that the system has a comprehensive view of each patient's circumstances and can tailor interventions accordingly.

Interpretation Agents: The Diagnostic Layer

Interpretation Agents carry out the normalization and annotation processes after data has been ingested. They primarily serve the purpose of computing clinical risk scores in the context of identifying "access risks" and checking for inherent biases to rule out the possibility of biased results caused by historical biases in the incoming data. This layer provides a morally sound basis for decisions by transforming raw data into something usable. For example, if historical data underrepresents certain ethnic groups, interpretation agents can flag this issue and adjust the interpretation accordingly. By detecting and mitigating bias at the point of data ingestion, interpretation agents prevent biases from propagating through the system.

Planner Agents: The Strategic Layer

Agents that act as planners are like the "brain" of an agentic network. The multi-horizon planning process is their responsibility; it entails dividing broad health objectives into more manageable, multi-stage processes. Most importantly, equity restrictions are a part of this strategy. If the plan calls for a follow-up meeting, it is the planner's job to make sure the patient can make it. If they cannot, they can try something different (like telemedicine) to help the patient. The planner agents operationalize the constrained optimization framework described earlier, balancing clinical effectiveness against equity considerations to generate care plans that are both effective and fair.

Actuator Agents: The Execution Layer

The Actuator Agents make the system get stuff done as soon as it knows something. These bots actually do something to reduce the risk, while most AI only sends a warning. They are responsible for beginning to request referrals and telephone consultations, performing automated resource movement, and communicating with third-party workflow applications (APIs for transport, appointments, or messaging). This independence frees doctors and patients from administrative worries and ensures that interventions are implemented promptly and reliably.

The Governance Agent: The Supervisory Oversight

The Governance Agent checks things. A group monitors the procedure to ensure honesty and fairness. Its key roles include ensuring that the policy meets everyone's privacy and fairness needs, being accountable for all decisions through comprehensive audit trails, and building hospital trust by creating models of what needs to be done. That means managing "escalation logic," which ensures that the technology delivers difficult cases to real people if confidence is low or if fairness constraints are at risk of being violated.

Deployment Lifecycle for Equity-Aware Agentic AI

Two critical decision gates ensure safety, justice, and equity before the framework is widely employed. The first decision, "Pass Fairness Checks?" ensures game fairness. We evaluate the model using established fairness indicators. If it does not pass, deployment development is halted and the team returns to model design with fairness constraints. After that, the system goes through Federated Training and Local Validation steps whereas only model parameters are shared and data remains at the local sites. For the sake of generalizability and equity, each location verifies performance within its particular context. Redesigning the model is the next step in the process if problems arise. Clinicians can examine and veto AI recommendations in Pilot Deployment with Human-in-the-Loop (HITL) oversight, revealing usability, safety, or fairness issues in actual workflows. All of these things—performance, equity measurements, safety problems, and model drift—are monitored in an ongoing Monitoring and Governance Loop (Anderson & Visweswaran, 2025). Reaching equity and performance goals is the focus of the second decision gate, which assesses whether scaling is feasible. The system is sent back for redesign if the targets are not met. After these checks are passed, Scale Deployment can commence, and in the event that any harm or inequities occur, options to rollback or redesign are available (Dychiao et al., 2024).

Mathematical Formalization

We formalize the equity-aware planning objective as a constrained optimization. Let $R(\pi)$ denote expected cumulative reward over horizon H when following policy π, and $D_g(\pi)$ denote an equity metric (disparity) across demographic groups $g \in G$. The equity-aware optimization becomes:

$$\max_{\pi} R(\pi) \text{ subject to } D_g(\pi) \leq \delta_g, \ \forall g \in G$$

Equivalently, using Lagrangian relaxation with multiplier λ:

$$\max_{\pi} \mathscr{L}(\pi) = R(\pi) - \lambda \sum_{g \in G} \max\left(0, D_g(\pi) - \delta_g\right)$$

where δ_g are acceptable disparity thresholds per group. The fairness penalty term can be instantiated as difference in service coverage rates, difference in true positive rates, or a more domain-specific utility gap. These equations connect high-level policy objectives to implementable optimization algorithms in planner agents.

Evaluation Metrics (Equity-Aware Suite)

Standard machine learning metrics such as accuracy, area under the receiver operating characteristic curve (AUC-ROC), and area under the precision-recall curve (PR-AUC) are insufficient for equity evaluation. We adopt a mixed suite that captures performance, equity, system efficiency, and human oversight.

Performance Metrics: The system is evaluated using standard metrics including AUC-ROC, which measures the ability to distinguish between positive and negative outcomes across all thresholds; PR-AUC, which is particularly important in imbalanced healthcare datasets; and Brier score, which measures calibration of predicted probabilities.

Equity Metrics: The core equity metrics include group true positive rate (TPR) and false positive rate (FPR) gaps, defined as:

$$\Delta TPR_{g_1, g_2} = | \ TPR_{g_1} - TPR_{g_2} \ |$$

$$\Delta FPR_{g_1, g_2} = | \ FPR_{g_1} - FPR_{g_2} \ |$$

The coverage difference metric captures disparities in the proportion of each group that receives a particular intervention. The HEAL (Health Equity Assessment of ML) metric provides a composite measure that combines multiple equity dimensions.

System Metrics: Resource utilization fairness is measured through per-capita resource allocation variance across groups. Timeliness is measured as median time to treatment across groups, with disparities flagged if some groups systematically experience longer delays.

Human Oversight Metrics: The system tracks frequency of human escalations, explanation fidelity, and clinician acceptance rates. High escalation rates may indicate that clinicians do not trust the system, while low acceptance rates may suggest that recommendations are not clinically appropriate. These metrics provide continuous feedback on the human-AI collaboration quality.

The evaluation framework employs subgroup reporting as a minimum standard. Such reporting is being more and more anticipated by regulators in healthcare AI submissions. The equity-aware suite tests for biases across multiple demographic dimensions, including but not limited to age, gender, race, ethnicity, socioeconomic status, geographic location, and insurance type. A balanced evaluation reports both absolute performance and equity measures, recognizing that high overall performance may conceal significant subgroup disparities. Trade-offs between performance and equity are explicitly acknowledged and discussed, with acceptable trade-offs determined by clinical context and stakeholder values.

ETHICS, GOVERNANCE, AND REGULATION

WHO Guidance and Rights-Based Grounding

In order to ensure fairness, accountability, and human well-being, a rights-based framework must be needed to use AI in healthcare. The World Health Organization states that human rights, fairness, and equity should be at the forefront of minds when developing and implementing health programs (Weldon et al., 2024). According to the WHO guidelines, some of the key principles are openness, explainability, data privacy, and good human oversight. These rules are particularly critical when dealing with Agentic AI, in which systems have greater autonomy and capacity to act. The WHO identifies six core principles for AI in healthcare: (1) protecting human autonomy, (2) promoting human well-being and safety, (3) ensuring transparency and explainability, (4) fostering responsibility and accountability, (5) ensuring inclusiveness and equity, and (6) promoting AI that is responsive and sustainable.

These recommendations can be achieved by ensuring that agentic AI systems incorporate governance tools such as audit trails, explanation modules, and policy-enforcing governance agents. Biases and unintended harm can develop in systems, or technical problems can occur, and the governance agent ensures that such issues are detected and addressed promptly. Second, new guidance from the World Health Organization highlights the need to have ongoing governance loops in place, especially when working with systems where humans are practically no longer in charge because of large multimodal models or systems that learn on their own. These loops ensure that AI systems do not cross the boundaries of ethics over time. Community engagement is also an ingredient, enabling stakeholders, including patients and healthcare providers, to engage in the development of socially acceptable norms and thresholds for decisions from AI-driven systems.

Algorithmic Fairness and Clinical Risk

For using AI in healthcare, algorithmic justice is a bigger challenge (Xu et al., 2022; Jaidka & Jain, 2023). Earlier work describes different manifestations of bias, such as under-representation of some demographic groups in training datasets, roundabout indicators of socioeconomic disadvantage via proxy variables, or miscalibration between demographic groups. These issues might worsen health inequities and require specialised care. For example, if a model is trained primarily on data from urban, affluent patients, its predictions may be systematically inaccurate for rural, low-income patients, leading to inappropriate care recommendations.

Agentic AI requires several justice methods. Model training can utilize reweighting, bias mitigation strategies, and subgroup-specific calibration to be fair (Eggleton, 2023). Reweighting assigns higher importance to underrepresented groups during training to ensure that the model performs well across all groups. Bias mitigation strategies include preprocessing techniques that remove or adjust biased features, in-processing techniques that incorporate fairness constraints during training, and post-processing techniques that adjust predictions to achieve fairness goals. Subgroup-specific calibration ensures that predicted probabilities are well-calibrated for each group, preventing systematic overconfidence or underconfidence.

Fairness tests must go beyond overall performance numbers. Subgroup analyses, domain-level fairness indicators, and stakeholder criteria should also be included. We must prospectively validate across numerous cohorts to ensure our models work in real life. "Agentic AI justice" requires ongoing review and improvement. The system must be continuously monitored for emerging biases, and governance mechanisms must be in place to trigger corrective actions when disparities are detected.

Explainability, Trust, and Human Oversight

Explainable AI (XAI) is needed to build trust in AI systems used in healthcare (Dychiao et al., 2024). Patients and doctors must understand AI discoveries. Because AI does so much, its intentions are both rigid and fluid, making it tougher to describe. That is why good explanations should explain processes rather than individual predictions. According to Weldon et al. (2024), an agentic system should be able to explain why a certain action was taken, how the patient and his or her surroundings affected the decision-making process, and how resources were distributed among different needs. For example, when the system recommends a particular treatment plan, it should explain the clinical rationale, the expected outcomes, the evidence supporting the recommendation, and any equity considerations that influenced the decision.

For security and responsibility, HITL tools are needed. These technologies allow doctors to approve or amend AI judgments, keeping everything in check. Explainable AI researchers emphasise testing interfaces with users, getting feedback iteratively, and designing with humans in mind while creating new interfaces. These methods reduce automated bias, improve system reliability, and make clinician acceptance easier. The governance agent also plays a crucial role in ensuring that explanations are provided at the appropriate level of detail for different audiences, from patients who need simple explanations to clinicians who require comprehensive technical justifications.

Data Governance, Privacy, and Federated Models

Healthcare data is confidential and must be secured according to all laws and morals. Agentic systems need various data governance levels, such as encrypted storage, access rules, and clear permissions. The General Data Protection Regulation (GDPR) in the European Union and the Health Insurance Portability and Accountability Act (HIPAA) in the United States establish strict requirements for handling healthcare data, including requirements for consent, purpose limitation, data minimization, and individual rights of access and erasure. Agentic systems must comply with these regulations, which may require specific architectural choices such as storing data in the jurisdiction where it was collected and ensuring that data use is transparent and auditable.

Federated learning lets students from different schools collaborate without sacrificing data privacy. This works by letting models be trained on datasets that are spread out, without having to share raw data (Prayitno et al., 2021). Instead, each institution trains the model on its own data and only shares model updates with a central server. This approach preserves patient privacy while still enabling the system to learn from diverse populations, improving generalizability and reducing bias.

However, different data from different institutions might worsen bias if not managed correctly. To fix this, federated frameworks should include methods for regularization and fairness-aware aggregating. It is important to keep an eye on and review the model all the time to make sure that techniques that protect privacy do not hurt its performance or make it less fair. The governance agent plays a critical role in this process, ensuring that data governance policies are enforced consistently across all participating institutions.

FUTURE RESEARCH DIRECTIONS

We suggest the following areas of focus for future study in order to ethically develop Agentic AI for health equity:

Equity-Aware Multi-Agent Learning: Create algorithms that ensure there is limited difference in planner results between groups. These algorithms should incorporate equity-aware multi-agent learning techniques that coordinate the behavior of multiple agents to achieve collective fairness. Research is needed on how to design reward structures, communication protocols, and coordination mechanisms that incentivize equitable outcomes across all agents.

Robust Federated Fairness Systems: Develop federated fairness systems with comprehensive fairness diagnostics and solutions for aggregating corrections. This includes developing methods for detecting bias in federated settings where data distributions vary significantly across institutions, and for aggregating model updates in ways that preserve fairness guarantees. Privacy-preserving techniques that maintain both privacy and fairness simultaneously are a particularly important research direction.

Explainability for Plans: Conduct research in XAI that provides an explanation of multi-step plans and the projected equality consequences. This goes beyond explaining individual predictions to explaining whole care pathways, including how different decisions interact over time and how equity considerations influence each step. User interface research is needed to present these complex explanations in ways that are understandable and actionable for clinicians and patients.

Regulatory Evaluation Systems: Develop systems for evaluating regulations, such as audits and standards for self-driving healthcare agents. According to the World Health Organization, there should be controlled trials done in places with few resources to find out how well programmes work and how well they are accepted by society (Bouderhem, 2026). Research is needed on how to design regulatory frameworks that are both rigorous and flexible enough to accommodate the rapid evolution of agentic AI technologies.

Longitudinal Equity Monitoring: Develop methods for monitoring equity impacts over time, recognizing that biases can emerge or change as populations evolve and as the system learns from new data. This includes developing early warning systems that detect emerging disparities and automated response mechanisms that trigger corrective actions.

Community-Centered Design: Research participatory design approaches that involve communities in the development and governance of agentic AI systems. This includes understanding community concerns, incorporating diverse perspectives into system design, and building trust through transparency and accountability.

CONCLUSION

Agentic AI is a paradigm shift in healthcare because it allows us to transition from antiquated, fixed prediction instruments to new, goal-oriented systems that can autonomously orchestrate complex tasks. Agentic AI can unify planning, execution, monitoring, and governance under one framework. This will finally enable health care workers to learn the missing link between identifying a problem and solving it. This implies that we can systematically accelerate health equity if, and only if, the UN's Sustainable Development Goals for health, inequality, infrastructure, and relationships align with these systems.

The proposed Equity-Aware Agent Architecture is a system that enables fairness constraints, federated learning, and human oversight. It can be used to measure success and it can be used to close the gap in terms of clinical performance between demographic groups. All of this requires ongoing monitoring, governance checkpoints, and feedback loops that can scale to ensure that they are safe and fair to use. The formal stochastic foundations developed in this chapter provide the mathematical rigor necessary for rigorous evaluation and regulatory approval.

Agentic AI, like all technology, is a moving target: there is endemic potential for bad things to happen from its use and misuse. The big open question on whether one of its emerging promises comes true will depend on how it gets used and regulated and also how much money goes into building an equitable structure. By making sure that fairness is the main thing that is thought about during design and not just an afterthought, agentic AI could have a direct effect on healthcare systems all over the world. How this will make systems stronger and more open in line with the SDGs depends on continued research, careful governance, and sustained commitment to equity.

AI DISCLOSURE STATEMENT

The author(s) confirm that artificial intelligence (AI) assisted technologies were used solely for language refinement, structural editing, and formatting to improve readability and ensure compliance with IGI Global Scientific Publishing guidelines. No AI tools were used for the generation of original research content, scientific analysis, or intellectual contributions. The core concepts, theoretical framework, mathematical formulations, and substantive arguments presented in this chapter are the original work of the author(s).

REFERENCES

Anderson, J. W., & Visweswaran, S. (2025). Algorithmic individual fairness and healthcare: A scoping review. *JAMIA Open*, *8*(1), ooae149. DOI: 10.1093/jamiaopen/ooae149 PMID: 39737346

Berdahl, C. T., Baker, L., Mann, S., Osoba, O., & Girosi, F. (2023). Strategies to improve the impact of artificial intelligence on health equity: Scoping review. *JMIR AI*, *2*, e42936. DOI: 10.2196/42936 PMID: 38875587

Borkowski, A. (2025). Multiagent AI systems in health care: Envisioning next-generation intelligence. *Federal Practitioner : for the Health Care Professionals of the VA, DoD, and PHS*, *42*(5), 188–195. DOI: 10.12788/fp.0589 PMID: 40831649

Bouderhem, R. (2026). Artificial intelligence in healthcare: Ethical challenges and promoting clinical equity and transparency. In *Handbook of Tissue Reconstruction and Regeneration* (pp. 1–29). Springer Nature Singapore. DOI: 10.1007/978-981-96-7448-0_29-1

Dychiao, R. G., Nazer, L., Mlombwa, D., & Celi, L. A. (2024). Artificial intelligence and global health equity: Regulation and monitoring are needed to prevent harmful bias in AI tools. *BMJ (Clinical Research Ed.)*, *387*, e079845.

Eggleton, A. (2023). Dr Robot: Robotics and AI in healthcare. In *Research Handbook on Patient Safety and the Law* (pp. 336–368). Edward Elgar Publishing.

Gupta, S., Gupta, P., Goel, L., & Jain, S. (2025). Enabling decentralized clinical insights: Federated learning in smart healthcare systems. In *Enabling Collaborative Health Intelligence with Federated Learning* (pp. 149–180). IGI Global. DOI: 10.4018/979-8-3373-3306-9.ch006

Jaidka, P., & Jain, S. (2023). Performance analysis of various deep learning techniques for brain tumor classification. *2023 International Conference on Power, Instrumentation, Energy and Control (PIECON)*, 1–6. DOI: 10.1109/PIECON56912.2023.10085796

Jain, S., & Jain, V. (2024). MRI based brain tumor segmentation with ensemble deep learning. *2024 1st International Conference on Advanced Computing and Emerging Technologies (ACET)*, 1–5.

Jain, S., Jain, V., & Chatterjee, J. M. (2025). Ensemble based brain tumor classification technique from MRI based on K fold validation approach. *Journal of Integrated Science and Technology*, *13*(5), 1114. DOI: 10.62110/sciencein.jist.2025.v13.1114

Lampropoulos, G., Garzón, J., Misra, S., & Siakas, K. (2024). The role of artificial intelligence of things in achieving sustainable development goals: State of the art. *Sensors (Basel)*, *24*(4), 1091. DOI: 10.3390/s24041091 PMID: 38400249

Prayitno, S., Shyu, C.-R., Putra, K. T., Chen, H.-C., Tsai, Y.-Y., Hossain, K. S. M. T., Jiang, W., & Shae, Z.-Y. (2021). A systematic review of federated learning in the healthcare area: From the perspective of data properties and applications. *Applied Sciences (Basel, Switzerland)*, *11*(23), 11191. DOI: 10.3390/app112311191

Weldon, M. N., Thomas, G., & Skidmore, L. (2024). Establishing a future-proof framework for AI regulation: Balancing ethics, transparency, and innovation. *Tennessee Journal of Business Law*, *25*(2), 2–24.

Xu, J., Xiao, Y., Wang, W. H., Ning, Y., Shenkman, E. A., Bian, J., & Wang, F. (2022). Algorithmic fairness in computational medicine. *EBioMedicine*, *84*, 104250. DOI: 10.1016/j.ebiom.2022.104250 PMID: 36084616

Chapter 15

Constitutional Governance of Stochastic Healthcare Decisions:
From Probability to Accountability

Rajiv Gurugopinath
http://orcid.org/0000-0003-3845-6778
Ramaiah College of Law, India

Ramya Krishnappa
http://orcid.org/0000-0001-8900-454X
Christ University, India

ABSTRACT

Healthcare systems increasingly rely on probabilistic tools—risk scores, predictive models, and adaptive algorithms—to allocate resources, prioritise patients, and guide public health interventions. These tools transform uncertainty into institutional power, raising constitutional and administrative law questions that deterministic frameworks cannot resolve. Drawing primarily on Indian constitutional law, with comparative reference to international human rights instruments and regulatory approaches in the EU, UK, US, Canada, and Australia, this chapter argues that learning health systems require "stochastic-compatible regulation." Such regulation governs not merely algorithms but the production and operationalisation of probability: who sets decision thresholds, how uncertainty is disclosed, whether models are calibrated, how predictive errors are distributed, when reassessment is triggered, and who bears legal responsibility. It develops an operational framework for probabilistic decision standards, risk-based classification, lifecycle governance, and institutional accountability.

INTRODUCTION

Uncertainty has always shaped healthcare decision-making. Disease trajectories cannot be forecast with precision, patient demand varies, treatment responses differ, and medical institutions routinely confront shortages of facilities, staff, medicines, and diagnostic capacity. What has changed is how uncertainty is modelled and how that modelling affects institutional action. Predictive analytics, risk-scoring tools, probabilistic forecasting, queueing models, and AI-powered systems are now used to anticipate future

DOI: 10.4018/979-8-3373-9705-4.ch015

events and inform clinical and administrative decisions. Together, these developments are producing learning health systems, in which information generated during care delivery is continuously applied to subsequent decisions, policies, and resource allocation (Koppolu, 2025; Lyu, 2025).

This transformation is not merely a question of AI regulation. A stochastic healthcare system must make decisions under conditions in which outcomes are unknown and therefore represented as probabilities, distributions, estimated risks, and updated predictions (Allen et al., 2026). A patient may be modelled as having a specific probability of deterioration; a community as having an elevated probability of infection; intensive care capacity as likely to be overwhelmed. Crucially, the legal consequence does not follow from the estimate itself. It follows when an institution converts probability into action by establishing an intervention threshold, assigning priority, imposing monitoring, or allocating resources (Jellema, 2025).

This separation is the chapter's central concern. A statement that a patient has a seventy per cent probability of deterioration is informational. That information becomes institutional power when a policy provides that patients with a calculated risk above seventy per cent receive priority access to an intervention. Who receives attention and who does not depends on the threshold selected. That selection embodies judgments about tolerable risk, resource scarcity, the relative weight of false positives and false negatives, and the consequences of each. Stochastic healthcare governance therefore poses legal challenges that conventional automated decision-making frameworks cannot adequately address (Geßler, 2026).

Traditional legal oversight assumes reasonably stable rules, identifiable decision-makers, and ascertainable criteria. Learning health systems unsettle these assumptions. Predictions change as new information arrives. Thresholds, error rates, and variables may vary across populations or institutional contexts, and models are recalibrated (Spanos et al., 2024). A system that was reliable when introduced may later degrade because of demographic change, shifting clinical practice, new disease patterns, or data drift (Duan et al., 2026). Regulatory responsibility must therefore extend beyond deployment to ongoing performance and modification.

These developments also raise distinctive rights concerns. Probabilistic systems can deliver population-level efficiency while producing serious individual effects. A model may optimise allocation of scarce resources overall while misclassifying a particular patient, or may achieve higher aggregate accuracy at the cost of elevated false-negative rates for rural communities or groups historically underrepresented in healthcare data (Yang et al., 2024). Statistical rationality and legal fairness are not equivalent at the individual or group level.

India's constitutional framework provides a particularly apt setting for examining these questions. Articles 14 and 21, the constitutional protection of informational privacy, administrative-law review, and the emerging digital data protection regime together supply normative resources for regulating probabilistic healthcare decisions. The principles of equality, non-arbitrariness, dignity, medical treatment, reasonableness, and proportionality can be extended to cases in which governmental or institutional action rests on probabilities rather than certainties (Kushwaha, 2026; Mukherjee, 2025).

The chapter's scope is not confined to India. Healthcare governance is both transnational and probabilistic. International human rights instruments recognise health, dignity, privacy, and non-discrimination as constraints on healthcare governance, and jurisdictions including the European Union, the United Kingdom, the United States, Canada, and Australia are developing varied approaches to adaptive decision systems, health data, medical technologies, and artificial intelligence (Skaletska, 2026). Across all of them, systems that learn, adapt, and generate uncertain outputs cannot be governed adequately by one-off approval or conventional technology safeguards (Pang & Szlitzer, 2026).

The chapter argues that learning health systems require stochastic-compatible regulation. Such regulation addresses not only algorithms but the production and operationalisation of probability. Relevant questions include: who sets the threshold for a probabilistic decision; how uncertainty is reported; whether a model is properly calibrated; how false-positive and false-negative errors are distributed; when performance change triggers regulatory re-evaluation; and who is legally accountable when an adaptive model contributes to a harmful decision.

The chapter develops a legal structure in which probability levels, uncertainty estimates, calibration, error distribution, and dynamic model updating become questions of constitutional and administrative responsibility. It does not argue that healthcare decisions should never rest on probability. Well-designed stochastic systems can improve responsiveness, resource utilisation, and patient outcomes (Saleh et al., 2025). The legal objective is to ensure that their capacity to learn and adapt remains subject to legality, equality, dignity, transparency, proportionality, and reviewability.

Three questions organise the analysis. First, how should thresholds, uncertainty, error, and adaptive updating in high-impact healthcare systems be understood from a constitutional and administrative law perspective? Second, what are the procedural and substantive limits on the institutional consequences that follow? Third, how can technological adaptation be reconciled with persistent legal responsibility? The chapter thus shifts the legal debate from the general regulation of AI in healthcare to regulating stochastic decision-making itself.

India's lack of a dedicated AI regulatory framework creates enforcement challenges compared with more concentrated approaches such as the European Union's. The EU operates a mandatory risk-based classification system with clearly defined supplier obligations, whereas India's framework is fragmented across sectoral laws and the Information Technology Act, 2000 (Kaur & Kaur, 2025). This decentralisation is often not matched by robust mechanisms to address algorithmic bias and transparency in autonomous diagnostic support. Uncertainty about liability for diagnostic error makes it difficult to allocate fault among developers, healthcare providers, and clinical institutions. Judicial precedents such as *Jacob Mathew v. State of Punjab* reflect traditional conceptions of medical negligence centred on human conduct and do not directly address systems in which AI-recommended practices shape outcomes.

The black-box character of many algorithms compounds the difficulty. Without explainability, it is hard to determine whether a harmful recommendation resulted from a technical fault, poor training data, or inadequate clinician oversight. The lack of specific requirements for periodic algorithmic assessment leaves institutions without adequate tools to govern autonomous decision support (Pal, 2025). Moreover, the Digital Personal Data Protection Act, 2023, though foundational, contains broad exemptions for public health data that may undermine robust data governance. Addressing these gaps requires both technical infrastructure and clear clinical research procedures for anonymisation and informed consent.

BACKGROUND

Evolution of Healthcare Decision-Making

Healthcare regulation historically developed around clear professional responsibilities, institutional norms, and relatively stable administrative rules. Clinical decisions turned on professional judgment, while health administration rested on defined procedures, epidemiological data, budgetary planning, and retrospective demand analysis. Uncertainty has always been present in medicine; the legal approach generally identified the authority or professional who made the decision in accordance with the applicable standard at the time (Domargard, 2026).

Digitalisation has transformed this structure. Electronic health records, digital diagnostic systems, hospital information platforms, disease surveillance systems, and increasingly interoperable datasets now permit analysis of health information at a scale and speed unavailable to traditional administration (Hawsawi et al., 2024). Data has evolved from recording past activity to forecasting future events. It is now used to predict patient deterioration, anticipate admissions, identify susceptible populations, schedule procedures, allocate staff, and prioritise scarce resources (Ali, 2026).

The distinction between retrospective and predictive information is legally significant. A record describes what occurred; a predictive model projects what may occur and can influence future intervention (Tamba, 2026). Legal systems must therefore address decisions grounded in estimated possibilities rather than established facts.

Artificial intelligence and machine learning have accelerated this shift, but "stochastic healthcare governance" is not synonymous with AI. Probabilistic decision-making predates AI and encompasses risk scores, statistical forecasting, survival analysis, queueing processes, epidemiological modelling, and transition models. What these share is that decisions are made under the assumption that the future may take multiple states, and that estimating probable outcomes is the appropriate basis for action.

Emergence of Learning Health Systems

A learning health system is one in which healthcare institutions systematically leverage information generated during routine care to improve future practice. Care delivery and institutional evaluation are not separated; information about outcomes, errors, patient pathways, resource use, and evolving disease patterns continuously informs subsequent decisions and organisational policy (Curcin et al., 2025; Foley & Horwitz, 2025).

Institutional feedback is the defining feature. A conventional system implements a protocol and maintains it until formally amended. A learning system adjusts recommendations in real time as patterns change. A hospital may revise admission forecasts as new patients arrive, and a public health official may adjust outbreak risk assessments as case numbers evolve. This flexibility can improve safety and efficiency.

Continuous learning also challenges traditional regulatory assumptions. If the model, data, or operating thresholds change substantially after approval, the approved system may no longer govern the system actually in use. The regulatory object is no longer static, which explains the growing emphasis on lifecycle approaches in healthcare AI and adaptive systems discourse (Haakman et al., 2021).

For law, the central issue is not learning as such but the possibility that learning alters the basis for institutional power. A change in prediction can affect a person's treatment, the speed of treatment, whether a population is monitored, or how limited resources are allocated. Adaptive capacity therefore requires adaptive accountability.

Stochastic Processes and Probabilistic Decision-Making in Healthcare

A stochastic process is one in which future states are not known exactly but are modelled using probabilities. Healthcare offers numerous examples. Emergency department arrivals fluctuate over time, patients move through phases of illness and recovery, outbreaks evolve according to transmission factors, and treatment outcomes vary even among patients presenting with similar disease.

Stochastic methods describe different aspects of uncertainty. Queueing models may be used to model patient arrivals, waiting times, and service capacity. Transition models describe the probability of moving between health states. Risk models estimate the likelihood of treatment failure, rehospitalisation, deterioration, or death. Epidemiological models estimate the occurrence and spread of infection or other health events within populations.

Table 1. Key Stochastic Concepts and Their Legal Significance in Learning Health Systems

Concept / Method	Meaning in a Stochastic Health System	Potential Legal Significance
Queueing models	Estimate patient arrivals, waiting times, service demand and available capacity	May influence allocation of beds, staff, emergency services and treatment priority; legal scrutiny arises where allocation adversely affects access to care
Transition models	Estimate probability of moving between health states (recovery, deterioration, progression)	Decisions based on predicted transitions may affect treatment, monitoring and eligibility, requiring transparency and clinical oversight
Risk models	Calculate likelihood of treatment failure, rehospitalisation, deterioration or death	Risk scores may influence consequential clinical and administrative decisions; a probabilistic prediction should not be treated as a certain determination about an individual
Epidemiological models	Estimate occurrence, spread or likelihood of infection and other health events within populations	May inform public health interventions, resource deployment and preventive measures; where measures restrict rights, proportionality and evidentiary justification become relevant
Probability estimate	Expresses likelihood rather than certainty; an 80% predicted risk does not mean the event will occur for a particular patient	Institutions should avoid treating probabilities as established facts; decisions affecting treatment or rights should recognise inherent uncertainty
Decision threshold	Specifies the predicted probability at which clinical or administrative action is triggered	Thresholds transform statistical predictions into consequential institutional decisions; their selection should be clinically justified, transparent and periodically reviewed
Calibration	Measures how closely predicted probabilities correspond with actual outcomes	Poor calibration makes apparently precise predictions unreliable; continued reliance may raise questions of negligence, accountability and reasonableness
Uncertainty estimates	Confidence or predictive intervals indicating the degree of uncertainty surrounding a prediction	Presenting only a point estimate may create unjustified impressions of precision; material uncertainty should be communicated where predictions influence significant decisions
False positive	Model predicts a risk or event that does not occur	May result in unnecessary treatment, surveillance, testing or diversion of scarce resources; legal significance depends on frequency and severity
False negative	Model fails to identify a risk or event that subsequently occurs	May result in delayed diagnosis, denial of intervention or failure to provide necessary treatment, potentially engaging questions of negligence and rights

Table 1 identifies the principal stochastic concepts underpinning learning health systems and explains their legal relevance. Queueing, transition, risk, and epidemiological models assist in predicting patient flows, health outcomes, and population-level events, but their outputs remain probabilistic rather than certain. Decision thresholds, calibration, uncertainty estimates, false positives, false negatives, and model drift become legally significant because they determine how statistical predictions translate into clinical or administrative action. The legal concern is not with mathematical formulae but with whether institutions understand the limits of prediction, justify the thresholds at which action is triggered, communicate uncertainty appropriately, account for the consequences of error, and periodically reassess models whose reliability may change.

From Probability to Legal Consequence

When an institution establishes a rule connecting a predicted level of risk with a consequential choice, probability acquires legal significance. The model's output is only one component of the governance structure; equally important is the institutional rule governing what follows once that output is produced (Akarkach, 2026).

Consider a system predicting the probability that patients will require intensive care. The model may prioritise patients by risk estimate. The hospital must then determine whether the prediction is advisory or determinative, whether a minimum threshold triggers priority treatment, and whether clinicians may depart from it. Each of these choices is normative.

Threshold selection necessarily involves error. Raising a threshold reduces unnecessary interventions but increases the risk that someone who needs help falls below it. Lowering a threshold reduces missed cases but increases false positives and strains scarce resources (Miche et al., 2024). No technically defined threshold exists. Determining acceptable error is a function of the interest at stake, available resources, and the consequences of an incorrect determination.

From an administrative-law perspective, model design cannot be divorced from policy design. The department or hospital adopting a threshold must be able to explain why that threshold was considered appropriate. Stronger justification is required where the interference with rights is substantial, such as restrictive surveillance or denial of emergency treatment (Widlas-Klimsiak, 2025).

Temporality is also legally relevant. A decision made during scarcity may become disproportionate once capacity increases. Calibration established in one population may not hold in another. Legality therefore cannot rest on prior technical validation alone; it must be continuously addressed.

Regulatory Responses and Working Concepts

Existing law addresses some of these issues, but not within a coherent field of stochastic healthcare regulation. International human rights instruments provide broad protection for health, dignity, privacy, and equality. Constitutional systems impose obligations of non-discrimination, lawful administration, and procedural fairness. Data protection regimes govern personal data, and medical device and healthcare regulators increasingly address software and AI-based technologies (Papadopoulou et al., 2025).

European regulation has moved toward risk-based governance, data protection, and accountability for high-impact automated systems. The United Kingdom has established governance frameworks and standards specifically for healthcare data technologies. The United States has focused regulatory attention on software in medical devices and on the challenges posed by systems that can be updated after initial review. Canada and Australia have launched comparable initiatives addressing automated decision-making, responsible AI, digital health, and medical technologies (Holdbrook et al., 2026; Reddy, 2024).

These are significant but fragmented approaches. Medical device regulation may address safety and clinical performance without engaging constitutional or public-law questions about governmental allocation. Data protection law may protect personal data without adequately addressing the distribution of probabilistic error. AI governance may require transparency or risk management without asking what probability is sufficient to justify denial or delay of healthcare.

This fragmentation justifies a stochastic-compatible approach. Such an approach does not replace constitutional, administrative, health, or data protection law; it connects them through legal norms tailored to decisions made under conditions of probability and uncertainty.

For the purposes of this chapter, the following working concepts apply. A learning health system is a healthcare system in which information generated through care delivery is systematically integrated into subsequent clinical, administrative, or policy decisions. Stochastic healthcare governance is governance exercised through systems substantially dependent on probability, uncertainty, predictive modelling, or distributions of possible outcomes. Probabilistic decision-making is the use of probabilities, rather than settled facts, to inform or determine consequential healthcare decisions. A probabilistic decision threshold is a predetermined operational level of estimated probability at which classification, prioritisation, restriction, or intervention is triggered. Adaptive regulation is regulation responsive to a system's lifecycle, adjusting to changing data, model performance, operational environments, and material system changes. Finally, stochastic-compatible regulation accepts the necessity of probabilistic reasoning in healthcare while subjecting thresholds, uncertainty, calibration, error distribution, model updating, and institutional responsibility to standards of legality, equality, transparency, proportionality, and reviewability.

These definitions frame the central thesis: law should not remove uncertainty from healthcare decision-making, but it should specify the conditions under which uncertainty may legitimately be translated into institutional action.

RIGHTS-BASED FOUNDATIONS OF STOCHASTIC HEALTHCARE GOVERNANCE

Article 21: Right to Health Under Probabilistic Allocation

Article 21 requires that State action affecting fundamental interests of life be just, fair, and reasonable. In *Parmanand Katara v. Union of India*, the Supreme Court confirmed that preservation of human life is paramount and that injured persons must receive immediate medical assistance without avoidable procedural delay. In *Paschim Banga Khet Mazdoor Samity v. State of West Bengal*, the Court held that failure by a government hospital to provide timely treatment violates Article 21 and that the State must establish an adequate system of medical care (Gurugopinath & Venugopal, 2024; Kaur & Kaur, 2025; Nale, 2025). These determinations establish that resource scarcity or administrative inconvenience does not license the State to abandon its constitutional obligation to provide meaningful access to essential treatment.

Stochastic allocation complicates this framework, since treatment may be prioritised according to predicted survival, anticipated benefit, urgency, or projected need. Probability-based decisions are not inherently unconstitutional. Difficult choices must be made under scarcity, and evidence-based prioritisation may be more rational than unstructured discretion. However, a probabilistic recommendation is not a conclusive reason for refusing care. A model may underestimate benefit if records are incomplete, if it relies on population-level assumptions, or if it fails to represent particular communities accurately (Ennis et al., 2023; Meier, 2022).

Denial or postponement of treatment may breach Article 21 where it rests solely on an opaque risk score, disregards relevant individual circumstances, or forecloses clinical reconsideration (Arora et al., 2023; Molbæk-Steensig & Scheinin, 2025). "Reasonable access" must encompass more than aggregate efficiency. It requires minimum guarantees of emergency treatment, disclosure of the material grounds of prioritisation, verification of relevant data, and an accessible process for urgent appeal. *Maneka Gandhi v. Union of India* established that any procedure bearing on life or liberty must be fair rather than arbitrary.

Article 21 thus requires a further distinction between the accuracy of a model and the validity of the institutional rule attached to its prediction. The constitutional question is not confined to technical accuracy. It also concerns the level of probability at which a consequence attaches. Where a scarce treatment is allocated by criteria, the criterion is a question of law. Authorities must be able to justify the threshold, the consequences of falling above or below it, and the alternatives considered.

Procedural rights should be commensurate with the gravity of the consequences. Limited safeguards may suffice for a model projecting hospital inventory. A model affecting emergency treatment, intensive care allocation, or access to essential medicines requires considerably stronger protection, since misclassification may directly affect life or bodily integrity. In such cases, Article 21 should require disclosure not merely of the model's output but of the material uncertainty underlying it, an opportunity for clinical reconsideration, and a rapid mechanism for correcting inaccurate information.

This does not mean that all healthcare predictions must attain certainty before being used. Managing healthcare probabilistically would otherwise be impossible. The constitutional question is whether the uncertainty surrounding a prediction is proportionate to the gravity of the proposed intervention. The more serious the potential false negative or false positive, the stronger the justification required.

Article 21 may therefore be read as imposing a probabilistic due process that is impact-sensitive. Where probability materially affects access to care, the State or responsible institution must demonstrate that the prediction is sufficiently reliable for its purpose, that the decision threshold is clinically and administratively justified, that material uncertainty is not concealed, and that meaningful human reconsideration is available. Probabilistic optimisation may assist the State in meeting its healthcare obligations, but it cannot be used to deny access to vital health services without adequate justification.

Article 14: Equality and the Distribution of Probabilistic Error

Article 14 prohibits unequal treatment and unwarranted State action. In *E.P. Royappa v. State of Tamil Nadu*, the Supreme Court defined arbitrariness as fundamentally incongruent with equality (Joshi & Wamankar, 2025; Pandey & Singh, 2025). A healthcare model that does not expressly classify patients by prohibited attributes may still offend Article 14 if its variables, data sources, thresholds, and operational effects lack a rational connection to a legitimate healthcare purpose.

Historical healthcare data may reflect disparities in access rather than disparities in need. A model trained on prior hospital utilisation may assign lower priority to those already socially disadvantaged—rural, poor, or disabled patients—because they previously encountered difficulty accessing treatment (Abràmoff et al., 2023; Chen et al., 2023). This constitutes indirect discrimination, in which ostensibly neutral criteria perpetuate structural disadvantage.

Algorithmic classification must therefore rest on an intelligible basis and bear a rational connection to the goal pursued (Cossette-Lefebvre & Maclure, 2022; Voeneky et al., 2022). This requires regular review for disparate impact, reasoned prioritisation criteria, and a prohibition on treating statistical averages as definitive statements about individuals. Individual constitutional protection cannot be displaced by population-level optimisation. Stochastic allocation is constitutionally defensible only where design is evidence-based, use is transparent, and results are subject to open review and correction.

Equality and the Distribution of Probabilistic Error

Equality analysis must extend beyond the model's variables to the distribution of its errors. Any forecasting system will produce error. The constitutional question is not whether all predictions are accurate but whether errors are distributed equally and non-arbitrarily.

Substantial disparities in subgroup accuracy may be masked by aggregate measures. A model may achieve high overall accuracy while performing poorly for specific groups. It may be less reliable for rural patients if developed in a different setting. Outcome probabilities for persons with disabilities may be systematically distorted by historical data reflecting discriminatory assumptions about quality of life. Socio-economic variables may function as proxies for unequal access to care.

Article 14 scrutiny should therefore distinguish overall model performance from subgroup performance. Regulators and institutions should examine differences in false-positive rates, false-negative rates, and calibration across relevant populations. A model well calibrated for the population as a whole may be constitutionally problematic if identical predicted risk scores correspond to materially different actual risks for particular groups.

Treating people equally is not the same as treating risk equally. Applying a uniform threshold may appear formally equal, but where a model systematically underestimates the needs of one population, uniform thresholds can reinforce inequality. Formal uniformity cannot substitute for substantive analysis of the conditions generating the data.

Article 14 should therefore require authorities deploying high-impact stochastic allocation systems to determine whether materially significant differences in predictive performance exist across materially affected groups, to investigate such differences, and to correct them where they cannot be reasonably justified. Remedies may include recalibration, variable modification, improved datasets, additional clinical review, or withdrawal of the model from specific applications.

This does not mean that every statistical difference constitutes discrimination. The question is whether there is a rational connection between a material imbalance of error and a legitimate healthcare goal, supported by reliable evidence and proportionate to the consequences imposed. Where harmful error rates are materially higher for a vulnerable population and the institution continues to rely on the model without modification, justification by reference to the constitutional prohibition on arbitrariness becomes increasingly difficult.

Equality in stochastic healthcare governance therefore requires attention not only to how individuals are classified but also to the risk that the model is wrong.

International Human Rights Foundations

The constitutional analysis developed in the Indian context forms part of a broader global framework of human rights obligations concerning healthcare access, dignity, equality, and State accountability. Article 25 of the Universal Declaration of Human Rights recognises medical care as part of the standard of living adequate for health and well-being. Article 12 of the International Covenant on Economic,

Social and Cultural Rights affirms the right of everyone to "the highest attainable standard of physical and mental health."

The Committee on Economic, Social and Cultural Rights has elaborated the content of Article 12 in General Comment No. 14. The right to health does not guarantee that everyone will remain healthy. It requires States to establish conditions, facilities, and services enabling meaningful enjoyment of the right. The criteria of availability, accessibility, acceptability, and quality provide a useful framework for assessing stochastic healthcare systems.

Availability is engaged where predictive tools determine the distribution of beds, medicines, or personnel. Accessibility is engaged where risk models prioritise certain patients or where digital systems create barriers for particular populations. Acceptability concerns dignity, autonomy, and how patients are informed about consequential probabilistic assessments. Quality requires that clinical validity, data quality, calibration, and ongoing reliability of stochastic models be adequate.

International human rights law thus distinguishes probabilistic optimisation from rights-compatible allocation. A model may improve overall system efficiency while reducing access for a particular population. Aggregate improvement alone does not demonstrate compliance with the right to health, because it may predictably exclude or disadvantage those already facing barriers to care.

Non-discrimination is likewise central. Beyond technical bias, the legal concern arises where differential error rates or systematically different risk assessments affect particular populations because of historically unequal datasets. Whether data-driven governance reproduces unequal access to healthcare becomes a question of rights compliance.

Regional rights systems offer comparable protections. Although the European Convention on Human Rights contains no explicit general right to health, health-related interests may be engaged through Article 2 (right to life), Article 8 (respect for private life), and Article 14 (prohibition of discrimination). These provisions illustrate how rights may be implicated in technologically mediated healthcare decisions—including probabilistic assessments affecting life and death, informational autonomy, and unequal treatment. The Charter of Fundamental Rights of the European Union is more explicit, recognising access to preventive healthcare and medical treatment in Article 35 and prohibiting discrimination on extensive grounds in Article 21.

The chapter's general argument—that stochastic healthcare governance must be assessed not only by predictive accuracy or efficiency—is therefore consistent with international human rights standards. The legality of such systems depends on their capacity to preserve meaningful access to healthcare, distribute error fairly, maintain dignity and privacy, and remain justifiable and reviewable.

Comparative Rights Perspectives

Healthcare rights differ across legal systems. India relies principally on Article 21 read with Article 14. The European Union expressly provides for access to preventive healthcare and medical treatment under Article 35 of the Charter, alongside privacy, data protection, and non-discrimination guarantees. The European Convention system addresses health-related harms indirectly through rights to life, private life, and non-discrimination. Other jurisdictions rely more heavily on statutory health entitlements, administrative-law obligations, anti-discrimination legislation, and sectoral regulation than on a constitutional right to health.

These institutional differences do not preclude common legal principles for stochastic healthcare systems. Across regulatory traditions, healthcare decisions should have a lawful basis, serve a legitimate aim, rest on adequate evidence, and be subject to procedures commensurate with their impact. Probabilistic decision-making compounds each requirement, because the evidence supporting intervention is itself expressed in probabilistic terms.

Comparative analysis should therefore focus less on whether jurisdictions share constitutional language and more on the functional protections they provide. These include review of the evidence supporting predictions, justification of decision thresholds, protection against discriminatory error, transparency regarding material uncertainty, ongoing validation of adaptive systems, and opportunities for meaningful human reconsideration.

India thus serves not as the exclusive jurisdictional frame but as a primary constitutional case study. Its principles of non-arbitrariness, dignity, fair procedure, proportionality, and positive duties to provide healthcare illustrate how established public law principles may be applied to probabilistic governance. The framework developed below builds on these principles and identifies standards capable of application across legal systems.

Table 2. Rights-Based Legal Scrutiny of Stochastic Healthcare Decisions

Stochastic Feature	Rights Concern	Legal Safeguard
Probability of treatment benefit	Right to health and life	Individual clinical reconsideration
Decision threshold	Fair procedure	Reasoned threshold justification
Calibration error	Equality and non-discrimination	Periodic calibration audit and recalibration
Subgroup error distribution	Equality	Disaggregated error analysis and corrective action
Uncertainty estimate	Transparency and dignity	Material uncertainty disclosure
Model drift	Continuing legality	Pre-defined reassessment triggers
Automated recommendation	Non-abdication of discretion	Meaningful human override
Inferred classification	Privacy	Notice, explanation, correction and reconsideration

Table 2 addresses the movement from statistical output to legal consequence. A stochastic prediction becomes legally significant when it is used to trigger, deny, prioritise, or modify healthcare action. The legality of such use depends not merely on predictive accuracy but on transparency, proportionality, equality, contestability, and continuing review. In learning health systems, safeguards must address both the uncertainty inherent in probabilistic models and the real-world consequences of error, bias, poor calibration, and model drift.

ADMINISTRATIVE LAW AND ADAPTIVE REGULATION OF PROBABILISTIC HEALTH SYSTEMS

Healthcare governance in India is largely administrative. Resource allocation and public health interventions typically result from government schemes, clinical guidelines, standard operating procedures, digital dashboards, technical advisories, and executive directions (Bocean & Vărzaru, 2024; Mahendra et al., 2025). Reliance on algorithmic systems adds a further administrative dimension, since their logic shifts with new data.

An authority does not lose discretion by using an algorithm; it shares discretion with officials, software developers, data analysts, hospital administrators, and clinical staff. Selecting data, risk variables, prediction thresholds, and acceptable error rates involves subjective judgment (Parycek et al., 2023; Tracey, 2025). A model prioritising patients by survival likelihood reflects administrative decisions about urgency, benefit, and resource efficiency. These choices must be traceable to a legally accountable public body.

The principle that the authority entrusted with statutory discretion must exercise it constrains delegation to technical systems. Technical assistance may be used, but authority may not be abdicated to an automated recommendation or private vendor (Langer, 2024; Miller, 2023). Mechanical application of a risk score without regard to individual factors may constitute abdication of discretion. Human oversight must therefore be substantive, not symbolic.

Administrative Legality of Probabilistic Decision Thresholds

The legal significance of stochastic healthcare systems becomes clearest when probability translates into administrative consequence. Predictive models typically produce scores, rankings, or likelihood estimates. These outputs have no inherent consequences. An administrative authority, healthcare institution, or clinical governance body must determine the probability at which intervention, priority, surveillance, or exclusion is triggered. Threshold selection is therefore not merely technical; it is an exercise of administrative discretion.

Consider a system predicting patient deterioration. A hospital may determine that patients with a predicted risk above a specified level require immediate specialist review. The model produces the probability; the institution determines when that probability alters the individual's legal or practical position. Thresholds produce markedly different distributions of healthcare resources and differing rates of false-positive and false-negative outcomes.

Administrative law should impose a threshold justification standard. At minimum, where a probabilistic threshold materially affects access to healthcare, the responsible authority should record: the clinical or administrative purpose for which the threshold was established; the evidence supporting its selection; the consequences of false-positive and false-negative classification at that threshold; reasonably considered alternatives; and the circumstances in which clinical or administrative departure from the threshold is permitted.

This follows established principles requiring administrative power to be exercised lawfully, for a lawful purpose, on relevant considerations, and without arbitrariness. A further principle is that a statutory body cannot abdicate its discretion. In *Purtabpore Co. Ltd. v. Cane Commissioner of Bihar*, the Supreme Court reiterated that an authority vested with statutory discretion cannot delegate it or act on another's instructions. The concern in stochastic healthcare governance is analogous: where an institution treats a vendor-supplied rating or software recommendation as given, similar difficulties arise.

Human review alone cannot resolve this problem if the reviewing officer accepts the output mechanically. The nature and limits of the prediction, the individual circumstances requiring consideration, and the decision-maker's authority to depart from the model in legally and clinically legitimate ways are all essential.

Thresholds should therefore be treated as a subject of administrative policy. Characterising a determining factor as a technical parameter in software cannot obscure the fact that the hospital or public authority bears responsibility for it. Where that parameter conditions access to treatment or priority access to a significant benefit, it is subject to the same requirements of legality, relevance, reasonableness, and accountability as conventional administrative parameters.

Adaptive policies complicate judicial review. Conventional review focuses on a specific time and the legality of a rule or decision. A stochastic system may alter its classifications or recommendations through model updates (Lopes, 2026). Courts and regulators must therefore consider not only initial implementation but also the processes for revising, validating, and ongoing use of the system.

Review should rest on reasonableness and proportionality. A model-assisted measure should pursue a legitimate healthcare purpose, rest on relevant and reliable data, bear a rational relation to that purpose, and avoid unnecessary burdens on patients (Farah et al., 2024; Welzel et al., 2023). Where reasonable alternatives exist with fewer restrictions on rights, exclusive reliance on automated prioritisation may be inappropriate.

Reasonableness, Proportionality and Probabilistic Evidence

Reasonableness and proportionality take on distinct meanings where administrative action rests on probabilistic evidence. Indian administrative law already permits judicial review of whether government action serves a legitimate purpose, rests on relevant considerations, and imposes burdens proportionate to the aim pursued. In *Om Kumar v. Union of India*, the Supreme Court treated proportionality as a significant principle in reviewing administrative action; in *Tata Cellular v. Union of India*, the Court affirmed that judicial review is confined to the legality of the decision-making process and does not substitute judicial preference for administrative expertise.

A court evaluating a stochastic healthcare decision need not identify the mathematically optimal prediction or replace an expert model with its own assessment. Judicial review may instead examine the institutional pathway by which probabilistic evidence became administrative action. Relevant questions include whether the model was validated for the population to which it was applied, whether the authority considered material uncertainty, whether the selected threshold had a rational evidentiary basis, and whether the authority understood the consequences of different forms of predictive error.

The seriousness of error is also relevant to proportionality. A false positive in an inventory-forecasting system may have limited legal consequences. A false positive resulting in restrictive surveillance, or a false negative resulting in denial of life-saving treatment, raises far greater concern. The degree of predictive uncertainty that is tolerable should therefore correspond to the nature and reversibility of the administrative consequence.

This approach may be described as "stochastic proportionality." A reviewing authority should ask whether the probabilistic measure serves a legitimate healthcare purpose; whether the model is sufficiently reliable and calibrated for that use; whether the threshold is rationally connected to the purpose; whether less rights-restrictive or less error-prone alternatives exist; and whether the expected public benefit justifies the nature and distribution of the risks imposed.

Reasoned decision-making is also required. The Supreme Court's emphasis on the importance of reasons in administrative decision-making, as in *Kranti Associates Pvt. Ltd. v. Masood Ahmed Khan*, is particularly relevant where the operative logic is technically complex. A stochastic decision need not disclose all mathematical detail, but it should identify the fundamental basis of the prediction, the applicable threshold, the material factors influencing the outcome, and the rationale in the circumstances.

Administrative review should therefore adapt rather than retreat in the face of technical complexity. Courts should remain attentive to clinical and scientific expertise while holding authorities accountable for evidence-based, lawful, and proportionate exercises of probabilistic power.

Material Model Changes and the Continuing Duty of Reassessment

Administrative legality is not determined solely by initial implementation. Adaptive models may change over time through new training data, recalibration, altered variables, or changing operating environments. A system that was accurate, non-discriminatory, and proportionate when introduced may become inaccurate, discriminatory, or disproportionate without any formal amendment of the legal instrument authorising its use.

This creates a continuing administrative duty to reassess. High-impact stochastic systems should be documented with a description of purpose, data sources, variables, assumptions, thresholds, known error rates, known limitations, validation population, and permitted fields of use. This documentation should serve as an administrative record demonstrating that continued reliance remains reasonable.

Not every technical change requires a full regulatory process. The law should distinguish operational adjustments from material model changes. A change is material if it could reasonably be expected to materially affect the affected population, the distribution of error, the probability assigned to patients, the decision threshold, the nature of the consequence attached to the output, or the model's clinical field of application.

Where a material change occurs, assessment should be repeated. This may involve recalibration, subgroup analysis, clinical validation, re-evaluation of the decision threshold, and approval by the relevant healthcare body commensurate with the risk. A hospital should not be permitted to rely on prior validation where the model is subsequently used in materially different circumstances.

Ongoing monitoring is particularly important because model performance may deteriorate through data or population drift. The relationship between historical data and future outcomes changes with prevalence, treatment, demographics, and access to care. A probability that was well calibrated when a model was introduced may not remain accurate over time.

The administrative duty should therefore include pre-established review triggers. These may include high rates of false negatives or false positives, substantial subgroup disparities, significant deterioration in calibration, introduction of new variables, changes to decision thresholds, deployment in a new population, or serious adverse incidents connected to model-assisted decision-making.

An audit trail should be maintained for regulatory and judicial review of such changes and evaluations. The general rule that an authority must be able to account for the exercise of its power applies with particular force here. Conventional administration may enjoy long-term stability; an adaptive system must periodically demonstrate continuing legality.

Stochastic governance of healthcare therefore requires a shift in the conception of legality from approval to lifecycle. The legal question is not only whether deployment was reasonable when the model was developed, but whether it remains reasonable given changing probabilities, populations, and institutional conditions.

Judicial Review of Changing Probabilistic Policies

Judicial review of adaptive healthcare systems should recognise that the object of review may evolve. Courts typically review material available at the time a decision was made. In a learning health system, however, subsequent model changes may produce different classifications, thresholds, or performance without the creation of a new formal administrative instrument.

Authorities should therefore maintain version histories identifying the model, dataset, and threshold in use at the time of a consequential decision. Such records are essential for affected patients and for courts seeking to understand the basis of a decision and assess the administrative process.

Judicial review should distinguish the current model from the decision-time model. Subsequent improvement cannot establish that an earlier decision was wrongful, nor does subsequent deterioration necessarily establish that an earlier decision was unreasonable. Meaningful review must be version-specific and therefore requires auditability.

Courts should also be empowered to require production of validation records, calibration reports, and adverse incident documentation where relevant to legality. Commercial confidentiality may justify proportionate protection against unrestricted disclosure, but it should not bar courts or regulators from examining the basis of public healthcare decisions.

Table 3. Administrative-Law Standards for Probabilistic Healthcare Decisions

Administrative Issue	Required Standard	Evidence to Be Maintained
Model adoption	Lawful purpose and clinical necessity	Approval record and intended use
Probability threshold	Reasoned threshold justification	Threshold rationale and alternatives
Model reliability	Fitness for intended use	Validation and calibration record
Error trade-off	Proportionate allocation of error	False-positive and false-negative analysis
Subgroup performance	Non-arbitrary operation	Disaggregated error analysis
Human discretion	No mechanical abdication	Override and review protocol
Model modification	Reassessment of material changes	Version and change log
Model drift	Continuing reasonableness	Periodic performance reports
Adverse incident	Corrective administrative action	Incident report and response
Judicial review	Reconstruction of decision-time logic	Archived model version and decision record

Table 3 addresses administrative accountability and the evidentiary record. Lawful use of stochastic models in healthcare requires institutions to maintain an auditable record of how and why they adopt, configure, modify, and rely on algorithmic tools. Administrative accountability extends beyond initial model approval to justifying probability thresholds, validation and calibration, assessment of error trade-offs, subgroup performance, human override mechanisms, and ongoing monitoring for model drift. When an adverse incident occurs, the institution should be able to identify the model version used, reconstruct the decision-making process, and demonstrate the corrective steps taken. Such documentation is particularly important for judicial or regulatory review, because a decision's legality may depend on whether the model was reasonable, fit for its intended purpose, and appropriately supervised when the decision was made.

DATA PROTECTION, CONSENT AND PROBABILISTIC INFERENCE

Stochastic healthcare systems depend on continuous and extensive digital health data. Electronic health records, diagnostic history, demographics, genomic data, treatment outcomes, insurance data, and behavioural data may be combined to predict disease, classify patients, and allocate resources, alongside data from wearable devices, telemedicine systems, mobile applications, and public health surveillance (Chigboh et al., 2024; Mohammed et al., 2024). Such processing can benefit diagnosis, prevention, and institutional planning, but it raises legal challenges that consent alone cannot resolve.

The constitutional right to privacy underpins regulation of such processing. Privacy encompasses individual control over the collection, use, and dissemination of personal information. Personal health information is particularly sensitive and may reveal illness, disability, reproductive history, mental health, genetic susceptibility, and future medical risk (Beyan et al., 2019; Velmovitsky et al., 2021). The constitutionality of health data processing requires legality, legitimate purpose, necessity, proportionality, and procedural safeguards.

The Digital Personal Data Protection Act, 2023 establishes the general statutory framework in India. It addresses lawful purpose, notice, consent, specified legitimate uses, security protection, accuracy requirements, grievance redressal, and accountability of data fiduciaries. The Digital Personal Data Protection Rules, 2025 provide for phased commencement and impose enhanced obligations on significant data fiduciaries, including data protection impact assessments, regular audits, and due diligence on technical measures such as algorithms that can affect data principals' rights.

These provisions are important for learning health systems but should not displace healthcare-specific legal analysis. The DPDP framework governs digital personal data generally and does not create a distinct category of sensitive health data with heightened protection. The sensitivity of health information must be addressed through the nature of the processing, its consequences for the individual, constitutional privacy principles, and the specific risks arising from clinical and probabilistic uses—all of which require sectoral governance.

A further limitation is that information generated by a stochastic health system may be legally relevant even if the data principal did not provide it directly. Where a dataset contains accurate age, diagnosis history, treatment, and location data, it may support a prediction about future deterioration, treatment adherence, or healthcare costs. The underlying data may be accurate, yet the inference is probabilistic and may misrepresent reality. Data protection law must therefore distinguish input accuracy from the validity of the conclusions drawn from it.

In such systems, consent is fragile. Health data is collected repeatedly and reused for purposes unanticipated at the time of consent. Consenting to the use of information for immediate diagnosis does not imply awareness that the information will be used for commercial research, automated eligibility determinations, population surveillance, or risk prediction. Consent fatigue resulting from repeated requests and lengthy technical notices may reduce consent to a formality rather than an expression of genuine informational autonomy (Vedder & Spajić, 2023).

Consent in a Continuously Learning Data Environment

India's digital health architecture illustrates both the value and the limits of consent. The Ayushman Bharat Digital Mission's Health Data Management Policy is built on federated, consent-based health data exchange. This offers important protection against uncontrolled centralisation and unauthorised sharing. However, consent to exchange or use existing health information does not necessarily constitute meaningful consent to all probabilistic inferences that may subsequently be drawn from it.

This distinction matters in a learning health system. A patient may understand that a hospital must retain a diagnosis for current treatment but may not reasonably expect the same information to be used in a model continuously analysing treatment adherence, readmission, future healthcare costs, or clinical deterioration risk. The further a secondary use is removed from the context in which information was provided, the less likely it is that the original consent provides a valid basis for that use.

Regulation should therefore distinguish consent to data processing from accountability for consequential inferences. Predictive uses may have a lawful basis, but institutions should ensure that predictive tools remain consistent with the purpose of collection, that materially different secondary purposes are adequately justified, and that high-impact inferences are sufficiently reliable for their intended use. Consent should function as one component of a health data governance framework rather than as an absolute barrier to subsequent privacy risks. Consent to processing does not entail agreement to inaccurate classification, unjustified risk profiling, or denial of treatment on that basis.

A further difficulty arises from probabilistic inference. A model may draw conclusions about a person's potential illness or disability, likely treatment, life expectancy, or future healthcare costs, even where those matters were never made explicit to the individual. Inferred information can affect triage, insurance, employment health assessment, and public health surveillance (Hummel et al., 2024; Mittelstadt, 2022). Privacy protection must therefore extend beyond data to the consequential profiles, predictions, and classifications it generates. The law should not be defeated by the fact that sensitive information has been statistically deduced rather than directly collected.

From Data Accuracy to Inference Validity

Traditional data protection analysis focuses on the accuracy of personal data. Stochastic healthcare systems require an additional question: whether the inference drawn from accurate information is a valid basis for the decision in which it is used. These are distinct regulatory inquiries.

Consider a patient record accurately documenting age, previous admissions, diagnosis, and location. Those accurate facts may be used in a model to predict a sixty-five per cent likelihood of readmission. Correcting the underlying data will not resolve the legal issue if the model is poorly calibrated, was validated in a different population, or produces materially higher error rates for that population.

High-impact health systems should therefore be subject to a duty regarding inferences. Before an inferred health profile forms the basis for treatment, prioritisation, surveillance, or another consequential decision, the responsible institution should demonstrate its reliability for that specific decision and population.

At least four considerations govern inference validity. First, the model must have demonstrated predictive validity for the healthcare context in which it is used. Second, probability estimates must be properly calibrated. Third, the model must convey prediction uncertainty to the human decision-maker. Fourth, error rates must be measured at the level of relevant subgroups rather than only for the population as a whole.

The temporal validity of an inference also matters. Dynamic health information can quickly render predictions outdated. A risk classification should not acquire perpetual legal force merely because it was lawfully generated. Where a prediction materially affects subsequent action, the system should indicate when further information, recalculation, or reassessment is required.

This supports a functional interpretation of correction rights in learning health systems. Correcting factual data may be insufficient. Individuals should also be able to challenge consequential classifications derived from that data and to seek human reconsideration where a prediction materially affects access to healthcare.

Group-level harms may also arise from stochastic modelling. A model may designate a geographic, occupational, ethnic, or socio-economic community as higher risk. Even without disclosure of individual records, stigma, heightened surveillance, denial of services, or discriminatory treatment may follow. Historical datasets may carry unequal healthcare access (Cho et al., 2024; Rucinski et al., 2024). A system trained on past utilisation may misinterpret low hospital attendance as low medical need when it in fact reflects poor infrastructure, discrimination, distance, or poverty.

Individualised data protection models are poorly suited to group-level probabilistic harm. A person may be disadvantaged without any wrongful conduct by the information provider, simply because they have been assigned the statistical characteristics of a group. A locality with higher disease prevalence may serve as a proxy for individual risk even where the individual does not share that risk. Legal analysis should therefore address not only individual informational control but also the validity and proportionality of group-based inferences. Where such inferences affect access to essential services, privacy, equality, and administrative reasonableness are all engaged.

Regulatory intensity should increase where an inference affects emergency treatment, eligibility, or surveillance, or where it concerns significant interests such as scarce resources. Relevant safeguards include purpose limitation, data minimisation, security measures, documented provenance, retention limits, validation of inferred attributes, and restrictions on incompatible secondary use. Integrated privacy, equality, clinical, and algorithmic impact assessments should be conducted for high-impact stochastic systems before deployment. Such assessment should determine the data used, the inference drawn, the affected population, calibration, expected error rates, subgroup performance, proposed decision thresholds, and the means by which human reconsideration will occur.

The enhanced obligations applicable to significant data fiduciaries provide a useful statutory basis for lifecycle oversight. The notified DPDP Rules contemplate periodic data protection impact assessments and audits, together with appropriate care regarding algorithmic software capable of harming data principals. In the health sector, these obligations could be operationalised through guidance requiring stochastic health models to incorporate inference validity, calibration, subgroup error, and threshold justification into the impact-assessment process. This would not create a new data protection regime but would apply existing requirements to the specific circumstances of probabilistic healthcare processing.

Where an inferred profile materially affects a healthcare decision, the individual should receive intelligible notice that a probabilistic assessment has been made, the factors underlying the classification, and, where applicable, the degree of uncertainty in the prediction. The purpose is not to provide a technical statistical document but to prevent probabilistic estimates from being treated as established facts.

Individuals should also have a meaningful way to challenge consequential inferences. This should permit correction of inaccurate input data, reconsideration of outdated or inappropriate inferences, and review by a competent human decision-maker. Where urgent decisions are required—such as triage or allocation of a life-saving resource—reconsideration should occur within a timeframe that preserves the underlying healthcare interest.

Data fiduciaries and healthcare institutions remain accountable when they contract data processing to vendors or integrate third-party models into clinical systems. Contracting out technical development does not transfer constitutional or administrative responsibility for consequential healthcare decisions.

Constitutional privacy in a learning health system is therefore not confined to secrecy and control over disclosure. It requires governance across the inferential chain: collection, combination, prediction, classification, decision, updating, and consequence. The health record is no longer the sole legal object; the probabilities generated from it, and the institutional power exercised on the basis of those probabilities, are equally relevant (Crowson et al., 2026; Hurley et al., 2024).

EMERGENCY POWERS AND STOCHASTIC DECISION-MAKING IN PUBLIC HEALTH CRISES

The legal significance of probabilistic inference becomes particularly evident during public health emergencies. In ordinary healthcare administration, misprediction may affect a single patient or an institutional allocation decision. In an epidemic or system-wide crisis, predictive architecture may underpin restrictions affecting entire populations. Infection rates, projected hospitalisation requirements, and estimated mortality may drive surveillance, movement restrictions, and emergency allocation. The governance problem shifts from individual probabilistic profiles to collective action under rapidly evolving uncertainty.

Public health emergencies increase governmental reliance on prediction. During COVID-19, decisions on lockdowns, containment zones, surveillance, and allocation of limited medical resources rested on epidemiological forecasts, infection rates, mobility data, hospital capacity estimates, and projected oxygen requirements. These models were necessarily stochastic, since they had to operate with incomplete and rapidly changing information.

In India, the Disaster Management Act, 2005, the Epidemic Diseases Act, 1897, State public health legislation, and public health directions provided the principal legal basis for pandemic measures (Anand, 2025; Mishra et al., 2022; Pal, 2025). The Disaster Management Act establishes a general institutional structure for disaster prevention, mitigation, and response, while the Epidemic Diseases Act empowers the government to take special measures where ordinary law is inadequate to address a dangerous epidemic disease. These powers are broad but not unlimited.

Emergency Probability Bounds and Intervention Thresholds

When predictive models are used in public health emergencies, an unresolved question is how high a predicted risk must be to justify government intervention. Epidemiological models do not establish that harm will occur. They rest on assumptions about transmission, behaviour, treatment capacity, and other variables, and estimate ranges of possible outcomes. Where such predictions support state coercion—restricting movement, intensifying surveillance, or diverting limited healthcare resources—they function as evidence.

Emergency regulation should therefore incorporate an "Emergency Probability Bounds" standard. The responsible authority should establish the indicators, predicted risks, or capacity conditions that justify escalation of an emergency measure, and those that would warrant relaxation or withdrawal.

At minimum, an emergency decision should identify five elements. The authority should state the public health harm it seeks to anticipate. It should identify the principal evidence or predictive model on which the intervention rests. It should explain the threshold or combination of indicators deemed sufficient to trigger the measure. It should state the degree of uncertainty in the prediction where that uncertainty is material to the decision. It should specify a review period or de-escalation condition.

Requiring an activation threshold does not oblige public authorities to await confirmed harm. Preventive public health action must often be taken before full knowledge is available. But precaution should not justify unfettered discretion. The greater the interference with fundamental rights, the stronger the evidentiary and procedural support required for reliance on uncertain forecasts.

De-escalation thresholds are equally important. Emergency governance frequently specifies conditions for imposing restrictions without defining conditions for their withdrawal. Where restrictions are imposed because hospital occupancy, infection rates, or another relevant measure crosses a threshold, they should ordinarily be reconsidered once risk falls materially below that threshold.

Probability bounds should also prevent point estimates from acquiring artificial certainty. Decision-makers should not reflexively adopt the worst-case scenario where forecast scenarios diverge materially, without explaining why the worst case warrants intervention. Nor should they rely exclusively on the most optimistic projection where life and health are at stake. The administrative task is to demonstrate a reasoned connection between the expected level of consequences, the severity of potential harm, and the degree of action taken.

Emergency legality should therefore be understood as a continuing state rather than a single event. An exceptional measure remains justified only while the evidence, predicted risk, and institutional circumstances supporting it persist.

Model-driven executive action must be backed by legislation, pursue a legitimate public health purpose, and satisfy constitutional requirements of necessity, reasonableness, and proportionality. A predictive model may justify pre-emptive action, but it is not equivalent to legal reasoning. Restrictions on movement, livelihood, privacy, and access to healthcare should rest on relevant evidence and be re-evaluated as circumstances change. In *Anuradha Bhasin v. Union of India*, the Supreme Court held that restrictions on fundamental rights must be proportionate and should not be maintained without review for an unlimited period (Bijjargi, 2026; Mukherjee, 2025). Although decided outside the public health context, its requirements of publication, necessity, and periodic review apply directly to model-based restrictions in emergencies.

Temporal Validity, Conflicting Forecasts and Dynamic Proportionality

Periodic review is especially important where the factual basis for governmental action is probabilistic and dynamic. The justifications for intervention at one stage of an epidemic may not hold weeks later. Disease prevalence, healthcare capacity, treatment availability, population behaviour, and model performance all change. The evidentiary basis for emergency action is therefore temporal.

This requires "dynamic proportionality." Proportionality should not be assessed solely at the time of the initial measure. Authorities must reassess the relationship between anticipated harm and restrictive intervention periodically. A measure considered necessary when hospital capacity was expected to be insufficient may cease to be necessary once capacity has been expanded or demand is projected to fall materially.

Authorities should therefore specify a maximum period during which an emergency decision may rest on a model without re-evaluation. Review should consider new evidence rather than restating the reasons for the original decision. Automatic renewal based on a prior forecast would defeat the requirement that exceptional action reflect current need.

A further challenge arises where credible models produce divergent predictions. Stochastic uncertainty may generate conflicting estimates of infection spread, mortality, or healthcare need. Government action need not eliminate disagreement, but it should acknowledge material model disagreement and explain the preference for particular evidence. Relevant considerations include model validation, assumptions, population relevance, prior performance, and the consequences of under- or over-estimating risk.

Public authorities should not present a particular forecast as scientific fact where uncertainty is substantial. Acknowledging uncertainty should not be treated as governmental inaction. The law should require action in light of uncertainty, not certainty.

Dynamic proportionality thus ties emergency power to evolving probability. The more intrusive and prolonged the restriction, the greater the State's burden to demonstrate that the anticipated public health threat persists.

Similar considerations arise in resource allocation. During the second wave of COVID-19, the Supreme Court in *In re: Distribution of Essential Supplies and Services During Pandemic* examined the availability of oxygen, supply of essential medicines, hospital infrastructure, and vaccination policy (Bhardwaj & Johari, 2022; Lind, 2023; Srinivasan, 2022). The proceedings illustrate that allocation policies, however technical, are reviewable where they affect equality, access to medical care, and life. Courts may rely on expert evaluation rather than perform calculations, but they must ensure that information, formulae, assumptions, and reasons are shared.

These proceedings matter because they concern legal architecture rather than technical expertise. Courts need not determine the optimal epidemiological model or calculate precise institutional oxygen requirements. They may ask about the basis of the allocation formula, whether current and relevant evidence was considered, whether assumptions were disclosed, whether changes in demand were accounted for, and whether particular States, hospitals, or populations were systematically disadvantaged. Probabilistic allocation is thus subject to institutional limits on judicial review while remaining required to be reasoned, auditable, and open to correction.

Sunset Clauses, Post-Emergency Stochastic Audit and Accountability

The temporary character of emergency authority should be reflected in the design of model-based interventions. Restrictions premised on the likelihood of harm should include sunset clauses, fixed reconsideration periods, or objectively identifiable sunset conditions. Continuation should not be automatic; it should require fresh justification. This is particularly important where the initial measure rested on incomplete information and worst-case forecasting.

In stochastic governance, a sunset clause serves two purposes. It constrains the intensity of extraordinary power and requires the authority to revisit the assumptions about the probabilities that originally justified intervention. The expiry of an order need not end the governmental response where serious risk persists, but renewal should rest on new evidence and fresh proportionality assessment.

Transparency obligations should accompany this. In high-impact emergencies, authorities should maintain and, subject to legitimate confidentiality interests, disclose the principal indicators, assumptions, thresholds, and evidentiary sources supporting action. Not every technical aspect of an epidemiological model needs to be published. What is required is sufficient disclosure to enable affected persons, legislatures, auditors, and courts to understand the reasons for intervention and its continuation.

Accountability should not end when the emergency subsides. After stabilisation, significant model-based interventions should undergo a thorough stochastic audit. Such an audit should examine how closely predictions corresponded with actual experience, whether material uncertainty was adequately identified, how frequently predictions changed, whether assumptions were revised when contrary evidence emerged, and whether particular groups were disproportionately burdened (Bjørnskov & Voigt, 2021; Norheim et al., 2020).

Audits should also compare the effects of over-prediction and under-prediction. Excessive pessimism may produce unnecessary restrictions, economic disruption, or misallocation of healthcare resources. Excessive optimism may produce inadequate hospital capacity, delayed intervention, or preventable deaths. Both forms of error should be evaluated, not merely whether the predicted adverse event occurred.

Critically, a forecast should not be judged retrospectively solely on the ground that the predicted outcome did not materialise. Measures taken to prevent harm may alter the course being forecast. Post-emergency review should instead consider whether the model and governmental response were reasonable given the evidence available at the time, and whether the authority took a reasonable stance as evidence evolved (Lock et al., 2023).

Records of the model version used, key data, prediction ranges, decision thresholds, reassessment dates, and reasons for continuing or relaxing measures should therefore be retained for significant emergency decisions. This supports legislative review, independent audit, judicial review, and institutional emergency preparedness.

In a crisis, the rule of law does not require governments to possess certainty. It requires that uncertainty be temporary, reviewable, and structured. Alertness to stochastic evidence is not sufficient to authorise rapid preventive action, nor may it conceal assumptions or normalise measures taken during exceptional circumstances.

STOCHASTIC-COMPATIBLE HEALTH REGULATION: AN OPERATIONAL LEGAL FRAMEWORK

The preceding analysis identifies legal issues arising at multiple levels from stochastic healthcare governance. Constitutional rights constrain the impact of probabilistic error on individuals and groups. Administrative law governs thresholds, discretion, and continuing regulation of model use. Data protection law regulates the inferential chain linking data to predictions. Emergency law sets conditions for extraordinary measures based on uncertain forecasts. These doctrines provide necessary protections but remain fragmented. This section integrates them into a unified regulatory structure for stochastic healthcare systems (Gevorkova, 2025; Madej et al., 2021).

The framework rests on three propositions. First, regulatory intensity should correspond to the potential impact of the stochastic decision rather than merely the technical complexity of the model. Second, the probabilistic features of the system must be subject to legal examination. Third, accountability must persist throughout the system's lifecycle, since initial validation does not guarantee continuing legality.

Core Principles of Stochastic-Compatible Regulation

Five principles underpin the use of stochastic healthcare systems.

Procedural constitutionalism. Consequential probabilistic decisions must be fair, reasonable, and contestable. When treatment, triage, surveillance, or allocation of essential resources is materially affected by a model, the responsible institution must determine and record the model's lawful purpose, document its decision criteria, and establish adequate means of reconsideration. The constitutionality of the system must be assessed both when uncertainty is translated into institutional action and at the level of final outcomes.

Impact-sensitive explainability. The depth of explanation should correspond to the impact of the decision. Disclosure of source code is not ordinarily required. Where an individual has been denied treatment, assigned lower priority, or subjected to restrictive health measures, the institution should provide an intelligible explanation of the principal considerations, the decision threshold, and, where relevant, the uncertainty associated with the prediction.

Stochastic equality. The distribution of predictive error must be examined. Where population groups differ significantly in false-positive or false-negative rates, aggregate accuracy is insufficient. High-impact systems should therefore be assessed for subgroup performance, calibration, and differential error before and during deployment.

Adaptive legality. Legality is continuing rather than one-off. A model that was lawful at deployment may become unreliable as demographics, clinical practice, disease patterns, training data, or model behaviour change. Assessment is therefore not merely technical quality control but part of an ongoing legal obligation.

Human accountability. Every consequential stochastic system must be linked to an identifiable, publicly accountable authority, healthcare institution, or designated officer. Although technical development may be outsourced, legal responsibility for using predictive outputs cannot be transferred to a vendor or software.

If stochastic-compatible regulation is to become binding law, these principles must be translated into specific standards.

Probabilistic Decision Standards for Stochastic Healthcare Systems

Threshold justification standard. Every clinically and administratively significant probability threshold must be explicitly justified. The record should identify the threshold's purpose, the evidence supporting it, the alternative thresholds considered, and the likely consequences of each. Scrutiny should intensify where the threshold results in denial or delay of healthcare, priority access to scarce resources, mandatory surveillance, or another significant consequence. Changing a consequential threshold should be treated as a material model change even if the prediction model itself is unaltered.

Uncertainty disclosure standard. Probability should not be presented as certainty. Where uncertainty is material to a consequential decision, the institution should provide adequate information to the clinician or administrator responsible for the decision. The form of disclosure should be context-sensitive. A clinician may require detailed information about predictive reliability; a patient should ordinarily receive a brief, intelligible explanation that the decision rested on probabilistic assessment rather than established fact.

Calibration standard. High-impact stochastic systems should undergo regular calibration assessment. A model assigning numerical probabilities should demonstrate reasonable correspondence between predicted probabilities and actual outcomes for the population to which it is applied. Calibration should be examined overall and within clinically and legally meaningful subgroups. Persistent miscalibration should be investigated, recalibrated, and, where it cannot be shown to be harmless, result in restricted use or withdrawal.

Error distribution standard. Errors produced by high-impact systems should be documented and assessed for both false positives and false negatives. Assessment should not rely solely on aggregate accuracy. The legal significance of an error depends on its consequences: a false negative that denies prompt treatment raises more serious rights concerns than an incorrect administrative prediction with no clinical effect. Regulators should therefore consider both the number and severity of errors. Subgroup analysis should identify whether adverse outcomes are more likely for groups defined by disability, location, gender, economic status, or other relevant characteristics.

Dynamic reassessment standard. Stochastic systems should be subject to pre-planned reassessment triggers. Reassessment should occur on significant model drift, deterioration in calibration, substantial changes in error rates, introduction of new variables, deployment in a new population, modification of decision thresholds, or serious adverse incident. Institutions should not be permitted to treat initial validation as permanently sufficient.

Probability communication standard. Where a probabilistic classification materially affects a person, communication should distinguish prediction from fact. Statements such as "the patient will not benefit" should not substitute for a probabilistic formulation indicating that, on the available evidence, the probability of benefit is low. Communication should be sufficiently clear to permit meaningful discussion, challenge, and human reconsideration, balancing technical precision against communicative accessibility.

Emergency probability bounds standard. Where action affects a population, the responsible authority should specify the predicted risk or indicator triggering activation, the evidence supporting it, the duration of the measure, and the conditions for review or de-escalation. Emergency probability should thus remain bounded in time and evidence rather than serving as an open-ended licence for exceptional authority.

Risk-Based Regulatory Classification

Healthcare systems should not be regulated uniformly. The intensity of scrutiny should depend primarily on the severity of consequences flowing from probabilistic outputs, the vulnerability of the affected population, the degree of automation, and the reversibility of an incorrect decision. Three classifications provide a starting point.

Tier I: Low-risk stochastic systems. These are systems whose predictions are used principally for internal administration and do not ordinarily determine individual access to healthcare. Examples include inventory forecasting, scheduling, and non-consequential service demand estimation, as well as workforce planning. Basic requirements of documented purpose, data quality, security, validation, and periodic performance review should apply. Where predictions do not create a substantial patient interest, formal individual explanation and appeal mechanisms may not be necessary.

Tier II: Moderate-risk stochastic systems. These are systems used for clinical decision support, non-emergency risk stratification, preventive prioritisation, or resource planning that may materially affect individual care but does not directly determine access to life-saving treatment. Such systems should be documented, validated, subject to impact assessment and periodic review, calibrated, assessed for subgroup performance, and clinically supervised. Material model modifications should be recorded. Where a prediction materially affects an individual decision, the affected person should receive an appropriate explanation and an opportunity for reconsideration.

Tier III: High-risk stochastic systems. These are systems that determine or substantially shape emergency triage, intensive care prioritisation, access to scarce life-saving medicines or procedures, denial or delay of treatment, compulsory public health surveillance, restrictive emergency measures, or other decisions with significant impact on life, health, equality, privacy, or liberty. Such systems should be subject to the most stringent requirements. Before deployment, they should undergo integrated clinical, privacy, equality, and stochastic impact assessment covering purpose, validation population, calibration, error distribution, relevant subgroups, threshold justification, expected false-positive and false-negative rates, alternatives considered, and human review arrangements. High-risk systems should also have an accountable officer, documented override procedures, regular independent audit, adverse incident reporting, and mandatory review following material change. Consequential decisions should remain open to meaningful and timely human reconsideration.

Risk classification should not be static. Where a system initially used for administrative forecasting is subsequently used to deny or prioritise patient care, it becomes high-risk. Classification should therefore attach to use and consequence rather than to technology alone.

Lifecycle Governance of Stochastic Systems

Stochastic-compatible regulation should operate throughout the system's life.

Pre-deployment. Before adoption, the responsible institution should determine the lawful purpose and clinical necessity of the system, assess whether a probabilistic model is appropriate for the function, and document reasonable alternatives. Moderate- and high-risk systems should undergo impact assessment covering data quality, intended population, validation, calibration, error rates, subgroup performance, decision thresholds, privacy implications, and anticipated patient consequences.

Validation and pilot. High-risk systems should initially be deployed through limited validation or pilot arrangements. Evaluation should occur under conditions and in environments closely resembling intended use. Pilot assessment should examine not only model accuracy but also the calibration of generated probabilities, the clinical significance of tolerable error, and differences in model performance across relevant factors.

Deployment. The institution should identify the model version, threshold, and responsible decision-maker. High-impact recommendations should receive meaningful clinical and administrative review. An adverse probability generated by an automated system should not justify denial of vital care where the system lacks a mechanism for considering individual circumstances.

Monitoring. Institutions should monitor model performance during deployment. Indicators may include calibration, false-positive and false-negative rates, subgroup error rates, override rates, adverse incidents, and evidence of model drift. Review frequency should correspond to system risk and the rate of change in the operating environment.

Modification. Material changes should trigger reassessment. These may include substantial changes in training data, predictive variables, decision thresholds, target population, or clinical application. Version histories should record when changes occurred and which model version was used for particular consequential decisions.

Incident and corrective action. Serious adverse incidents connected to model-assisted decisions should be documented and investigated formally. Where necessary, institutions should suspend use, adjust thresholds, recalibrate the system, add clinician safeguards, or withdraw the model.

Retirement. A stochastic healthcare system should be withdrawn where it can no longer be shown to be reliable, where it produces a material discriminatory effect that cannot reasonably be remedied, or where it is demonstrably no longer proportionate in light of safer and more appropriate alternatives. Retirement should not entail loss of adequate records for audit, investigation, and judicial review.

Institutional Responsibility, Compliance Evidence and Enforcement

Responsibility must be clearly allocated for the framework to operate. Stochastic healthcare governance should distinguish the obligations of healthcare institutions, public health authorities, developers, and individual clinical decision-makers.

Healthcare institutions. An institution operating a moderate- or high-risk stochastic system should maintain a register of stochastic decision systems in use; identify their intended use and risk classification; maintain current validation and calibration records; document consequential thresholds; designate a responsible medical or administrative officer for high-risk systems; establish human review and override procedures; maintain adverse incident and model change records; and provide adequate grievance and reconsideration processes.

Health authorities and regulators. Relevant health authorities should establish minimum technical and procedural standards for high-risk systems. They should have authority to require validation documentation, audit calibration and subgroup performance records, direct corrective action, and restrict further use where significant risk cannot be adequately controlled. High-risk stochastic systems implemented in public healthcare programmes may warrant independent pilot evaluation or assessment before wider adoption.

Developers and vendors. Developers should provide deploying institutions with sufficient information about intended use, training and validation populations, known limitations, calibration, performance, and material modifications. Information required for regulatory supervision or judicial review should not be withheld on grounds of contractual confidentiality. Developers should also notify institutions of changes or updates to underlying architecture or software that could materially affect probabilities, thresholds, or error distributions.

Medical and administrative decision-makers. Individual clinicians should not be expected to audit technical models. Their responsibility should focus on reasonable operation of the system within its designated purpose, attention to individual circumstances, and use of available human override where a probabilistic recommendation materially diverges from clinical judgment. Responsibility should not be allocated in a way that leaves clinicians legally liable for technical matters they could not reasonably discover, nor that allows healthcare institutions to attribute all harm caused by software to an external vendor.

Compliance evidence. The responsible institution should be able to demonstrate continuing legal compliance. Relevant records include lawful purpose and clinical necessity assessment; validation and calibration reports; false-positive and false-negative analysis; subgroup performance assessment; threshold justification; impact assessment; version and change management documentation; human override policy; incident reports; periodic reassessment records; and evidence of remedial action. Together, these constitute an administrative evidence trail of stochastic governance, enabling regulators and courts to understand why a probabilistic system was considered appropriate at the relevant time.

Enforcement responses. Regulatory action should be proportionate to the extent of non-compliance. Available measures include corrective directions, required recalibration, threshold modification, increased human oversight, temporary suspension, restriction of population or use, and withdrawal from use.

Where systemic failure results in unlawful denial of treatment, ordinary administrative, constitutional, contractual, professional, or tort remedies should remain available under applicable law.

Enforcement should not mean punishment for every inaccurate prediction, since some error is unavoidable in stochastic systems. The regulatory role is to address unjustified error, failure to monitor known risks, concealed limitations, thresholds set too high or too low, discriminatory performance, non-compliance with reassessment requirements, and continued use of systems no longer shown to be suitable.

Practicality of Implementation

The proposed framework does not necessarily require a new independent regulatory body. It may be implemented incrementally through existing healthcare regulation, hospital accreditation, public health governance, data protection compliance, medical device regulation, and hospital governance.

Initial priority should be given to Tier III systems affecting emergency treatment, triage, allocation of life-saving resources, or restrictive public health interventions. Deployment of such systems should begin with limited implementation, integrated impact assessment, and enhanced monitoring before wider adoption.

An accountable medical or administrative officer should be designated for each institution employing a high-risk stochastic system. This officer should be responsible for institutional compliance, review of model changes and adverse incidents, and coordination of remediation. The role should not require personal responsibility for all clinical decisions but should provide a clearly specified institutional accountability point.

Periodic review can be integrated into existing hospital accreditation and quality assurance processes. Calibration reports, subgroup error assessments, cybersecurity controls, and incident records could be incorporated into existing compliance and accreditation mechanisms rather than requiring an entirely new regulatory structure.

Implementation should remain risk-sensitive and proportionate. The objective is not to impose so many procedural steps that clinically useful technology becomes impractical. Minimum requirements should address matters central to lawful stochastic governance: a stated purpose; reliable and representative data; validation appropriate to intended use; justified thresholds; ongoing performance monitoring; meaningful human oversight; and effective means of correcting consequential error.

The framework thus combines technological flexibility with institutional responsibility. A stochastic healthcare system must be able to learn, and the institution implementing it must also learn—from miscalibration, adverse incidents, differential error, patient grievances, and regulatory scrutiny. Adaptation should occur within, not outside, the rule of law.

Table 4. Lifecycle Compliance Framework for Stochastic Healthcare Systems

Lifecycle Stage	Required Measure	Stochastic Metric or Evidence	Responsible Actor	Regulatory Consequence
Pre-deployment	Establish lawful purpose and clinical necessity	Intended use and alternatives assessment	Health institution or authority	Do not deploy if necessity cannot be demonstrated
Pre-deployment	Conduct integrated impact assessment	Calibration, baseline error, subgroup error, privacy risk	Institution with independent experts	Modify or reject system
Pilot	Conduct limited real-world validation	Prospective performance and calibration	Health authority or institution	Expand, modify, or terminate pilot
Threshold approval	Justify consequential cut-off	Threshold rationale and error trade-off	Clinical governance body	Revise unjustified threshold
Deployment	Assign accountable officer	Responsibility and override protocol	Healthcare institution	Correct governance deficiency
Decision	Require meaningful human review for high-risk outputs	Review and override record	Clinician or review committee	Reconsider affected decision
Monitoring	Assess ongoing performance	Calibration, false positives, false negatives, subgroup performance	Institution or auditor	Recalibrate or restrict use
Drift detection	Identify declining reliability	Performance change from baseline	Institution or developer	Mandatory reassessment
Model modification	Review material changes	Version log, new validation and threshold analysis	Institution and developer	Approval required before continued high-risk use
Adverse incident	Investigate serious harm	Incident record and causal analysis	Institution or regulator	Corrective action or suspension
System failure	Maintain alternative pathway	Availability of clinician-led or non-digital route	Healthcare institution	Restore alternative access
Retirement	Withdraw unsuitable system	Continuing risk assessment	Health authority or institution	Terminate deployment
Judicial review	Preserve decision-time evidence	Archived model version, threshold and decision record	Institution	Enables effective legal review

Table 4 presents lifecycle compliance as a continuing legal commitment rather than a one-off approval. Compliance begins with establishing a lawful and clinically justified purpose, followed by data governance, model validation, calibration, threshold justification, and error evaluation. During deployment, institutions should ensure meaningful human oversight, acknowledge material uncertainty, monitor subgroup performance, and maintain review and contestation processes. After implementation, the model should be monitored for drift, changing clinical conditions, discriminatory outcomes, and adverse incidents. Version histories, audit records, and decision logs should be maintained, with revalidation following material change. Where performance is no longer acceptable as regards safety, fairness, or reliability, the model should be modified, suspended, or withdrawn. The lifecycle approach thus connects directly with legal notions of reasonableness, proportionality, equal treatment, transparency, and continuing institutional accountability.

Future Directions for Research and Regulatory Development

Legal scholarship on stochastic healthcare systems remains nascent and requires substantially more empirical and doctrinal work. Existing research has largely addressed AI, data security, clinical bias, and automated decision-making as discrete concerns, with limited attention to the stochastic properties—probability thresholds, calibration, uncertainty estimates, and distributions of predictive error—as they occur in actual healthcare settings.

Empirical research on the use of probabilistic decision systems in hospitals, public health programmes, insurance schemes, and emergency resource allocation is a first priority. Such research should determine not only whether predictive models are used but how institutional rules convert predictions into decisions. Specific questions include who sets decision thresholds, whether they are documented, how frequently models are recalibrated, and what procedures exist when clinicians disagree with probabilistic recommendations.

A second priority concerns the distribution of error. Future studies should examine whether false-positive and false-negative rates differ systematically across populations defined by geography, disability, gender, socio-economic position, and other legally relevant characteristics. Such research is important because substantial inequities in the allocation of predictive error may be concealed by aggregate accuracy. Comparative empirical research across public and private healthcare institutions may also reveal whether differences in data quality, institutional capacity, and accountability regimes produce differing legal risks.

Third, further work is needed on the relationship between model calibration and legal standards of reasonableness. The question of what degree of predictive reliability is sufficient to justify denial, prioritisation, or restrictive intervention is rarely addressed in legal scholarship. Future research could develop standards for different categories of healthcare risk and identify the evidence required to satisfy them.

Fourth, comparative regulatory research on adaptive and probabilistic healthcare systems is needed. Useful points of comparison include the European Union's risk-based regulatory architecture, the United Kingdom's approach to health technology governance, United States approaches permitting adaptive medical software, and emerging Canadian and Australian frameworks. Particular attention should be given to healthcare systems in the Global South, where infrastructure limitations, incomplete information systems, and unequal access to care may generate distinctive patterns of stochastic risk.

Fifth, institutional capacity for regulating stochastic systems should be assessed to determine whether existing regulatory bodies can perform these functions without undue administrative duplication. Hospital accreditation, medical device regulation, public health administration, and data protection compliance may offer routes for incorporating calibration audits, threshold documentation, incident reporting, and lifecycle reassessment into existing governance processes.

Finally, standardised regulatory instruments should be developed, including stochastic impact assessment templates, model registers, threshold justification forms, calibration reporting formats, and procedures for challenging consequential probabilistic decisions. Longitudinal studies should then test the effectiveness of these mechanisms for patient safety, equality, and accountability without imposing disproportionate regulatory burden.

The future research agenda should therefore shift from asking whether healthcare institutions are using AI to asking how they are implementing it. The more legally relevant questions concern the production of probability, the point at which it may be acted upon, the consequences of predictive error, and the institutional mechanisms ensuring continuing legal review as probabilities change.

CONCLUSION

Uncertainty has become a defining feature of contemporary healthcare governance. Decisions that were once made in the face of uncertainty are now increasingly made through predictions of risk, probability distributions, dynamic forecasts, and continuously updated models. The resulting legal question is not merely one of AI governance but of governing decisions in which probability itself determines treatment allocation, risk classification, restrictions on conduct, and the distribution of scarce healthcare resources.

This chapter has argued that probabilistic decision-making has a legitimate place within constitutional and public law frameworks. Stochastic systems can improve patient flow, detect risks earlier, and enhance planning and resource utilisation. The law need not demand absolute certainty in order to permit innovation. What it must do is identify the conditions under which uncertainty may legitimately be translated into institutional power.

The Indian constitutional framework is particularly instructive. Article 21 mediates between probabilistic allocation and the requirements of dignity, meaningful access to healthcare, fair procedure, and protection of life. Article 14 requires equality analysis to extend beyond facially neutral classification to the distribution of predictive error. A model may be generally accurate yet constitutionally problematic because of false negatives, miscalibration, or thresholds that disadvantage historically underserved populations.

Administrative law provides a further layer of accountability. Predictive outputs carry no inherent legal consequence. Institutions select models, variables, thresholds, and error tolerances, and decide whether to depart from automated recommendations. These are exercises of institutional judgment and must be justified. Reliance on technical expertise does not relieve public decision-making of responsibility or exempt consequential decisions from scrutiny.

The same applies to health data governance. Inaccurate personal data may generate erroneous inferences, and poor calibration may produce systematic over- or under-estimation. Privacy regulation must therefore extend beyond the accuracy of input data to the validity, purpose, and consequences of probabilistic classifications. Similarly, governments acting during emergencies must recognise that forecasts have a temporal horizon. A prediction reasonably relied upon today may cease to be reasonable tomorrow as conditions change.

Thresholds, uncertainty, calibration, error distribution, model drift, and model updating are therefore legally relevant characteristics, as the framework developed in this chapter demonstrates. That framework integrates probabilistic standards with risk-based classification, lifecycle supervision, identifiable institutional responsibility, meaningful human reconsideration, and proportionate enforcement. Systems affecting emergency treatment, scarce resources, or fundamental rights should be subject to substantially greater requirements than administrative forecasting systems.

Although developed primarily from Indian constitutional and administrative law, the framework yields broader insights for adaptive healthcare governance. Its requirements can be incorporated through constitutional rights, human rights instruments, medical device regulation, data protection law, health service regulation, or administrative review in different jurisdictions. While institutional pathways may differ, five principles are transferable: consequential thresholds must be justified; material uncertainty must not be concealed; calibration must be continuously verified; the distribution of predictive error must be examined for equality; and adaptive systems require adaptive legal oversight.

The central claim is therefore straightforward. The distinctive task of stochastic-compatible regulation is to make probability legally accountable. A model need not predict the future perfectly, but it must be demonstrated to predict it adequately. Law must determine who may act on a prediction, how much uncertainty is acceptable, who bears the risk when a prediction is wrong, and when changed evidence requires reconsideration of a decision.

A legitimate learning health system must learn from more than clinical outcomes and operational data. It must also learn from miscalibration, exclusions, adverse incidents, unequal error distributions, patient challenges, and regulatory scrutiny. Accountability can evolve alongside adaptive healthcare without sacrificing innovation. The objective is neither to prescribe clinical judgment nor to demand mathematical certainty, but to ensure that where probability shapes life, health, and access to care, it remains bounded by dignity, equality, reasoned administration, transparency, and the rule of law.

AI DISCLOSURE STATEMENT

This chapter was prepared and revised with the assistance of AI tool ChatGPT (OpenAI) to assist in structuring and reorganizing sections, developing and refining preliminary draft formulations, clarifying and synthesizing interdisciplinary concepts, and improving the language and content coherence and readability. The authors were fully involved in every aspect of the outputs generated by AI, including their critical review, significant revision, and incorporation. The authors have confirmed and verified the legal analysis, authorities, citations, and substance of the chapter as well as the conclusions drawn, and assume sole responsibility for the accuracy, originality, integrity and scholarly nature of the chapter. The AI tool was not seen as an author, and did not make research interpretation decisions or decisions to publish.

REFERENCES

Abràmoff, M. D., Tarver, M. E., Loyo-Berríos, N., Trujillo, S., Char, D., Obermeyer, Z., Eydelman, M., & Maisel, W. H. (2023). Considerations for addressing bias in artificial intelligence for health equity. *NPJ Digital Medicine, 6*(1), 170. DOI: 10.1038/s41746-023-00913-9 PMID: 37700029

Akarkach, M. (2026). *Inference as the exposure event: Implications for legal discovery, audit, and institutional governance. Zenodo.* DOI: 10.5281/zenodo.18993386

Ali, M. A. (2026). A broad review of AI and machine learning in healthcare informatics for predictive analytics, data analytics, and healthcare supply chain systems. *Global Trends in Science and Technology, 43*, 43. Advance online publication. DOI: 10.70445/gtst.2.2.2026.43-63

Allen, T., Manjunatha, I. G., Khoni, N. S., & Allen, A. (2026). *Noise-aware mathematical frameworks for artificial intelligence in predictive clinical decision-making: From stochastic dynamics to regulatory compliance. Zenodo.* DOI: 10.5281/zenodo.18501207

Anand, A. (2025). Beyond the Epidemic Diseases Act, 1897: Rethinking India's public health laws for pandemic preparedness—Lessons from Singapore. *The Journal of Communicable Diseases, 57*(1), 33–43. DOI: 10.24321/0019.5138.202504

Arora, A., Alderman, J., Palmer, J., Ganapathi, S., Laws, E., McCradden, M. D., Oakden-Rayner, L., Pfohl, S., Ghassemi, M., McKay, F., Treanor, D., Rostamzadeh, N., Mateen, B. A., Gath, J., Adebajo, A. O., Kuku, S., Matin, R., Heller, K., Sapey, E., & Liu, X. (2023). The value of standards for health datasets in artificial intelligence-based applications. *Nature Medicine, 29*(11), 2929–2938. DOI: 10.1038/s41591-023-02608-w PMID: 37884627

Beyan, O., Choudhury, A., van Soest, J., Kohlbacher, O., Zimmermann, L., Stenzhorn, H., Karim, M. R., Dumontier, M., Decker, S., da Silva Santos, L. O. B., & Dekker, A. (2019). Distributed analytics on sensitive medical data: The Personal Health Train. *Data Intelligence, 2*(1-2), 96–107. DOI: 10.1162/dint_a_00032

Bhardwaj, K., & Johari, V. (2022). COVID-19 vaccines in India: Judicial blind spots in upholding the right to health. *Socio-Legal Review, 18*(1), 119. DOI: 10.55496/EONP8082

Bijjargi, P. (2026). Digital human rights under the Indian Constitution: Emerging jurisprudence and policy challenges. *International Journal for Multidisciplinary Research, 8*(1), 69665. Advance online publication. DOI: 10.36948/ijfmr.2026.v08i01.69665

Bjørnskov, C., & Voigt, S. (2021). This time is different?—On the use of emergency measures during the corona pandemic. *European Journal of Law and Economics, 54*(1), 63–81. DOI: 10.1007/s10657-021-09706-5 PMID: 35924085

Bocean, C. G., & Vărzaru, A. A. (2024). Assessing social protection influence on health status in the European Union. *Frontiers in Public Health, 12*, 1287608. DOI: 10.3389/fpubh.2024.1287608 PMID: 38528863

Chen, Y., Clayton, E. W., Novak, L. L., Anders, S., & Malin, B. (2023). Human-centered design to address biases in artificial intelligence. *Journal of Medical Internet Research*, *25*, e43251. DOI: 10.2196/43251 PMID: 36961506

Chigboh, V. M., Zouo, S. J. C., & Olamijuwon, J. (2024). Health data analytics for precision medicine: A review of current practices and future directions. *International Medical Science Research Journal*, *4*(11), 973–984. DOI: 10.51594/imsrj.v4i11.1732

Cho, H., Froelicher, D., Dokmai, N., Nandi, A., Sadhuka, S., Hong, M. M., & Berger, B. (2024). Privacy-enhancing technologies in biomedical data science. *Annual Review of Biomedical Data Science*, *7*(1), 317–343. DOI: 10.1146/annurev-biodatasci-120423-120107 PMID: 39178425

Cossette-Lefebvre, H., & Maclure, J. (2022). AI's fairness problem: Understanding wrongful discrimination in the context of automated decision-making. *AI and Ethics*, *3*(4), 1255–1269. DOI: 10.1007/s43681-022-00233-w

Crowson, M. G., Tan, J. Z. H., Dunn, J., Bhatt, J., Schneider, Z., Forger, D. B., Celi, L. A., Dorotić, M., & Malin, B. (2026). The need to develop health data transaction disclosure requirements to balance transparency, privacy, and progressive use. *The Lancet. Digital Health*, *8*(2), 100947. DOI: 10.1016/j.landig.2025.100947 PMID: 41792017

Curcin, V., Delaney, B., Alkhatib, A., Cockburn, N., Dann, O., Kostopoulou, O., Leightley, D., Maddocks, M., Modgil, S., Nirantharakumar, K., Scott, P., Wolfe, I., Zhang, K., & Friedman, C. (2025). Learning health systems provide a glide path to safe landing for AI in health. *Artificial Intelligence in Medicine*, *173*, 103346. DOI: 10.1016/j.artmed.2025.103346 PMID: 41506062

Domargard, A. (2026). *Standing on shifting ground: Clinical decision-making in a non-linear world. Zenodo*. DOI: 10.5281/zenodo.18221943

Duan, M., Liu, X., Yeung, W., Hao, S., Raffa, J. D., Hu, P., Liu, C., Chen, L., Li, Z., Gao, Z., Li, T., Cao, D., Zhou, F., Zhang, Z., Zhang, Z., & Celi, L. A. (2026). Multicenter validation and updating of the ELDER-ICU model for severity assessment in elderly critical illness. *NPJ Digital Medicine*, *9*(1), 498. Advance online publication. DOI: 10.1038/s41746-026-02472-1 PMID: 41957287

Ennis, J. S., Riggan, K. A., Nguyen, N. V., Kramer, D. B., Smith, A. K., Sulmasy, D. P., Tilburt, J. C., Wolf, S. M., & DeMartino, E. S. (2023). Triage procedures for critical care resource allocation during scarcity. *JAMA Network Open*, *6*(8), e2329688. DOI: 10.1001/jamanetworkopen.2023.29688 PMID: 37642967

Farah, L., Borget, I., Martelli, N., & Vallée, A. (2024). Suitability of the current health technology assessment of innovative artificial intelligence-based medical devices: Scoping literature review. *Journal of Medical Internet Research*, *26*, e51514. DOI: 10.2196/51514 PMID: 38739911

Foley, T., & Horwitz, L. I. (2025). Learning health systems. In *Cambridge University Press eBooks*. Cambridge University Press., DOI: 10.1017/9781009325912

Geßler, T. (2026). *Why probabilistic AI resists auditability: From explainability to verifiable responsibility in high-risk AI systems. Zenodo*. DOI: 10.2139/ssrn.6103587

Gevorkova, E. (2025). The concept and essence of human genetic information as an object of constitutional law regulation. *Bulletin of the South Ural State University Series Law, 25*(2), 66–73. DOI: 10.14529/law250211

Gurugopinath, R., & Venugopal, B. (2024). Judicial interventions in environmental health and the right to health: A critical analysis of landmark endosulfan case in India and similar cases in USA, UK, Canada, and Australia. *Revista de Gestão Social e Ambiental, 18*(9), e07577. Advance online publication. DOI: 10.24857/rgsa.v18n9-110

Haakman, M., Cruz, L., Huijgens, H., & van Deursen, A. (2021). AI lifecycle models need to be revised. *Empirical Software Engineering, 26*(5), 95. Advance online publication. DOI: 10.1007/s10664-021-09993-1

Hawsawi, H. M. A., Al-Rashidi, S. A., Alghamdi, W. A. E., Alghamdi, M. A. M., Althagafi, M. E., Alsalmy, B. O., Alharthi, M. A., Alharthi, A. A., Alshawqab, A. S., Alshehri, M. M., Dosar, A. M. A., & Alhuzali, H. S. (2024). The role of health administration, social services, health informatics, and public health in driving digital transformation in healthcare systems: An integrative review. *Journal of Posthumanism, 4*(2), 2189–2195. DOI: 10.63332/joph.v4i2.3713

Holdbrook, R. O., Obanla, A. K., Ani, C. P., Eboh, N. A., & Oboh, R. (2026). A comparative study of regulatory guidelines, digital pharmacovigilance, and software as a medical device across high- and low-to-middle-income countries. *Journal of Pharma Insights and Research, 4*(2), 304–319. DOI: 10.69613/mdb50d20

Hummel, P., Braun, M., Bischoff, S., Samhammer, D., Seitz, K., Fasching, P. A., & Dabrock, P. (2024). Perspectives of patients and clinicians on big data and AI in health: A comparative empirical investigation. *AI & Society, 39*(6), 2973–2987. DOI: 10.1007/s00146-023-01825-8

Hurley, M. E., Lang, B., Kostick, K. M., Smith, J. N., & Blumenthal-Barby, J. (2024). Patient consent and the right to notice and explanation of AI systems used in health care. *The American Journal of Bioethics, 25*(3), 102–114. DOI: 10.1080/15265161.2024.2399828 PMID: 39288291

Jellema, H. (2025). Standards of proof for future crimes and decision theory. *Quaestio facti: Revista internacional sobre razonamiento probatorio, 10*. DOI: 10.33115/udg_bib/qf.i10.23144

Joshi, P. B., & Wamankar, Y. (2025). Algorithmic policing and due process in cybercrime investigations: A constitutional analysis under Articles 14, 19 and 21 of the Indian Constitution. *ShodhSamajik Journal of Social Studies, 2*(2), 153–167. DOI: 10.29121/ShodhSamajik.v2.i2.2025.57

Kaur, S., & Kaur, S.Ms. Navjot KaurMrs. Rajinder Kaur. (2025). Article 21: A lifeline to new rights in a progressive society. *International Journal on Science and Technology, 16*(2), 4692. Advance online publication. DOI: 10.71097/IJSAT.v16.i2.4692

Koppolu, H. K. R. (2025). *The intersection of data, artificial intelligence, and healthcare: Creating predictive and personalized care models* (pp. 128–143). DOI: 10.70593/978-93-49910-67-6_8

Kushwaha, G. (2026). *From Gian Kaur to living wills: The changing landscape of euthanasia law in India. Zenodo.* DOI: 10.5281/zenodo.19152320

Langer, C. (2024). Decision-making power and responsibility in an automated administration. *Discover Artificial Intelligence*, *4*(1), 59. Advance online publication. DOI: 10.1007/s44163-024-00152-1

Lind, Y. (2023). Pandemocracy in Europe: Power, parliaments and people in times of COVID-19. *The American Journal of Comparative Law*, *71*(2), 491–494. DOI: 10.1093/ajcl/avad025

Lock, D., de Londras, F., & Hidalgo, P. G. (2023). Delegated legislation in the pandemic: Further limits of a constitutional bargain revealed. *Legal Studies*, *43*(4), 695–733. DOI: 10.1017/lst.2023.25

Lopes, F. P. (2026). *From human-in-the-loop to institutional oversight of judicial decision support systems*. Tilburg University Research Portal. https://research.tilburguniversity.edu/en/publications/e1f1c14a-464b-473b-b7fb-e517ea3cc100

Lyu, G. (2025). Data-driven decision making in patient management: A systematic review. *BMC Medical Informatics and Decision Making*, *25*(1), 239. DOI: 10.1186/s12911-025-03072-x PMID: 40598137

Madej, M., Sąsiadek, M., & Witt, M. (2021). Genetic testing—Whether to allow complete freedom? Direct to consumer tests versus genetic tests for medical purposes. *Journal of Applied Genetics*, *63*(1), 119–126. DOI: 10.1007/s13353-021-00670-z PMID: 34826052

Mahendra, R. R., Cahya, D. A., Ningsih, N., Kurniawan, L. S., & Judijanto, L. (2025). Critique of the concept of efficiency in public health management: A qualitative review of social justice-based health policy. *Health Leadership and Quality of Life*, *4*, 762. DOI: 10.56294/hl2025762

Meier, L. J. (2022). Systemising triage: COVID-19 guidelines and their underlying theories of distributive justice. *Medicine, Health Care, and Philosophy*, *25*(4), 703–714. DOI: 10.1007/s11019-022-10101-3 PMID: 35796935

Miche, M., Strippoli, M. F., Preisig, M., & Lieb, R. (2024). Evaluating the clinical utility of an easily applicable prediction model of suicide attempts, newly developed and validated with a general community sample of adults. *BMC Psychiatry*, *24*(1), 217. DOI: 10.1186/s12888-024-05647-w PMID: 38509477

Miller, P. L. (2023). A new 'machinery of government. In *Cambridge University Press eBooks* (pp. 116–135). Cambridge University Press., DOI: 10.1017/9781009334297.010

Mishra, A., Naik, B. N., Kumar, S., & Agarwal, N. (2022). Covid-19: Catalyst for a comprehensive law to combat potential pandemics in India. *Indian Journal of Medical Ethics*, *7*(3), 231–236. DOI: 10.20529/IJME.2022.039 PMID: 35699302

Mittelstadt, B. (2022). Protecting health privacy through reasonable inferences. *The American Journal of Bioethics*, *22*(7), 65–68. DOI: 10.1080/15265161.2022.2075980 PMID: 35737503

Mohammed, S. Y., Jumaah, N. S., Abbas, E. H., Ali, H. M., & Aljanabi, M. (2024). Healthcare intelligence and decision making: Big data's role in predictive analytics for clinical decision-making. *Mesopotamian Journal of Big Data*, *2024*, 223–229. DOI: 10.58496/MJBD/2024/016

Molbæk-Steensig, H., & Scheinin, M. (2025). Human rights and artificial intelligence in healthcare-related settings: A grammar of human rights approach. *European Journal of Health Law*, *32*(2), 139–164. DOI: 10.1163/15718093-bja10146 PMID: 40368349

Mukherjee, S. P. (2025). Balancing liberty and legality: The expanding horizon of the doctrine of proportionality in Indian administrative law after Puttaswamy. *International Journal on Science and Technology*, *16*(4), 9423. Advance online publication. DOI: 10.71097/IJSAT.v16.i4.9423

Nale, G. S. (2025). Right to speedy trial: A critical study. *Indian Journal of Legal Review*, *5*(13), 678. DOI: 10.65393/OWJF3694

Norheim, O. F., Abi-Rached, J. M., Bright, L. K., Bærøe, K., Ferraz, O. L. M., Gloppen, S., & Voorhoeve, A. (2020). Difficult trade-offs in response to COVID-19: The case for open and inclusive decision making. *Nature Medicine*, *27*(1), 10–13. DOI: 10.1038/s41591-020-01204-6 PMID: 33340033

Pal, J. (2025). Assessing India's readiness for public health emergencies: Governance, policy, and executive powers. *International Journal for Multidisciplinary Research*, *7*(6), 61769. Advance online publication. DOI: 10.36948/ijfmr.2025.v07i06.61769

Pandey, A., & Singh, R. (2025). Article 14 and social justice: A constitutional mandate for an egalitarian society. *International Journal of Research Publication and Reviews*, *6*(8), 3723–3729. DOI: 10.55248/gengpi.6.0825.3087

Pang, G., & Szlitzer, M. (2026). Governing AI in operations: Ethical risks, accountability mechanisms, and responsible digital operations. *AI and Ethics*, *6*(4), 338. Advance online publication. DOI: 10.1007/s43681-026-01191-3

Papadopoulou, E., Exarchos, T. P., Jenko, S., Krepelkova, K., & Namorado, J. (2025). Artificial intelligence (AI) in health systems: Introducing a 'Do Good' approach. *AI and Ethics*, *5*(6), 6339–6357. DOI: 10.1007/s43681-025-00757-x

Parycek, P., Schmid, V., & Novak, A.-S. (2023). Artificial intelligence (AI) and automation in administrative procedures: Potentials, limitations, and framework conditions. *Journal of the Knowledge Economy*, *15*(2), 8390–8415. DOI: 10.1007/s13132-023-01433-3

Reddy, S. (2024). Global harmonization of artificial intelligence-enabled software as a medical device regulation: Addressing challenges and unifying standards. *Mayo Clinic Proceedings. Digital Health*, *3*(1), 100191. DOI: 10.1016/j.mcpdig.2024.100191 PMID: 40207007

Rucinski, K. B., Knight, J., Willis, K., Wang, L., Rao, A., Roach, M. A., Phaswana-Mafuya, N., Bao, L., Thiam, S., Arimi, P., Mishra, S., & Baral, S. (2024). Challenges and opportunities in big data science to address health inequities and focus the HIV response. *Current HIV/AIDS Reports*, *21*(4), 208–219. DOI: 10.1007/s11904-024-00702-3 PMID: 38916675

Saleh, M., Awad, O. R. D., Bizun, H. K. M., & Oufi, M. R. H. (2025). Advanced statistical techniques in healthcare: Innovations in data analysis and decision making. In *Bright Sky Publications eBooks*. DOI: 10.62906/bs.book.293

Skaletska, Z. S. (2026). International legal regulation of medical algorithms: Challenges and prospects for control of artificial intelligence in healthcare. *Uzhhorod National University Herald Series Law*, *5*(92), 250–257. DOI: 10.24144/2307-3322.2025.92.5.34

Spanos, S., Dammery, G., Pagano, L., Ellis, L. A., Fisher, G., Smith, C. L., Foo, D., & Braithwaite, J. (2024). Learning health systems on the front lines to strengthen care against future pandemics and climate change: A rapid review. *BMC Health Services Research*, *24*(1), 829. Advance online publication. DOI: 10.1186/s12913-024-11295-3 PMID: 39039551

Srinivasan, S. (2022). The vaccine mandates judgment: Some reflections. *Indian Journal of Medical Ethics*, *8*(2), 134–140. DOI: 10.20529/IJME.2022.056 PMID: 36880474

Tamba, H. (2026). *The institutional production of causation: Predictive classification and the governance of human behaviour. Zenodo*. DOI: 10.2139/ssrn.6412758

Tracey, P. (2025). *The atomization of vulnerability: An ethnographic investigation of quantification and automation in Philadelphia's homeless services coordinated entry system*. Deep Blue. DOI: 10.7302/27071

Vedder, A., & Spajić, D. (2023). Moral autonomy of patients and legal barriers to a possible duty of health related data sharing. *Ethics and Information Technology*, *25*(1), 23. Advance online publication. DOI: 10.1007/s10676-023-09697-8

Velmovitsky, P. E., Bevilacqua, T., Alencar, P., Cowan, D., & Morita, P. P. (2021). Convergence of precision medicine and public health into precision public health: Toward a big data perspective. *Frontiers in Public Health*, *9*, 561873. DOI: 10.3389/fpubh.2021.561873 PMID: 33889555

Voeneky, S., Burgard, W., Tallinn, J., Misselhorn, C., Thoma, J., Durt, C., Risse, M., Burri, T., Schmidt, T., Shen, W., Metzinger, T., Zittrain, J., Wendehorst, C., von Hein, J., Hinsch, W., von Ungern-Sternberg, A., Poscher, R., & Paal, B. P. (2022). *The Cambridge handbook of responsible artificial intelligence*. Cambridge University Press., DOI: 10.1017/9781009207898

Welzel, C., Cotte, F., Wekenborg, M., Vasey, B., McCulloch, P., & Gilbert, S. (2023). Holistic human-serving digitization of health care needs integrated automated system-level assessment tools. *Journal of Medical Internet Research*, *25*, e50158. DOI: 10.2196/50158 PMID: 38117545

Widlas-Klimsiak, K. (2025). The ECtHR and mental health jurisprudence: Progressive interpretation or doctrinal stagnation? *Prawo i Więź*, *59*(6), 8. Advance online publication. DOI: 10.36128/w78k2k58

Yang, Y., Zhang, H., Gichoya, J. W., Katabi, D., & Ghassemi, M. (2024). The limits of fair medical imaging AI in real-world generalization. *Nature Medicine*, *30*(10), 2838–2848. DOI: 10.1038/s41591-024-03113-4 PMID: 38942996

Chapter 16
Governing Uncertainty in Adaptive Healthcare:
Ethical and Legal Frameworks for Probabilistic Systems

Abba Amsami Elgujja
http://orcid.org/0000-0003-0476-8810
King Saud University Medical City, Nigeria

Hayam Alrasheed
http://orcid.org/0009-0002-6186-848X
College of Pharmacy, Princess Nourah bint Abdulrahman University, Riyadh, Saudi Arabia

ABSTRACT

Healthcare systems increasingly rely on probabilistic models, such as Markov processes, to manage uncertainty and allocate resources in dynamic clinical settings. While these models improve efficiency and predictive capacity, they also introduce ethical and legal challenges inherent in the traditional governance systems. In probabilistic systems, outcomes emerge from system-level trajectories rather than isolated decisions, creating risks of structural bias and collective harm. This chapter develops a framework for the ethical governance of probabilistic healthcare systems by integrating stochastic modelling with comparative regulatory analysis and Islamic bioethical principles. Drawing on regulatory perspectives from different jurisdictions, the chapter examines how governance systems address uncertainty and algorithmic decision-making. A Markov-based outbreak response case study shows how non-ergodic system dynamics may produce unintended disparities. The chapter proposes design principles to guide relevant stakeholders in governing probabilistic healthcare systems ethically.

INTRODUCTION

Healthcare systems operate in environments characterized by pervasive uncertainty. Patient demand fluctuates unpredictably, disease trajectories evolve dynamically, resources remain constrained, and information is frequently incomplete or delayed. Historically, healthcare governance frameworks have attempted to manage this uncertainty through deterministic protocols, standardized clinical pathways,

DOI: 10.4018/979-8-3373-9705-4.ch016

and retrospective quality assurance mechanisms. While these approaches have been effective in relatively stable environments, they struggle to address the complexity and variability inherent in modern healthcare systems.

In response, healthcare organizations increasingly rely on probabilistic modelling approaches drawn from stochastic processes and operations research. Methods such as Markov decision processes, queueing theory, stochastic optimization, and simulation modelling allow healthcare systems to represent uncertainty explicitly and optimize decisions under conditions of incomplete information (Ross, 2014; Gross et al., 2018; Green, 2006; Hulshof et al., 2012). These models enable adaptive resource allocation, improved patient flow management, and enhanced outbreak response capabilities. When integrated with artificial intelligence and real-time data streams, probabilistic models can support continuously learning healthcare systems capable of responding dynamically to changing conditions.

Despite these advantages, probabilistic decision systems raise significant ethical and legal concerns. Traditional governance frameworks assume that decisions can be traced to identifiable actors and evaluated at discrete points in time. Probabilistic systems, however, operate differently. Outcomes emerge from sequences of probabilistic transitions across system states, rather than from individual choices. A decision that appears reasonable at a particular moment may contribute to inequitable outcomes when repeated over time across populations.

This shift from discrete decisions to system trajectories introduces new forms of ethical risk. For example, probabilistic scheduling systems designed to optimize operating room utilization may systematically delay certain categories of patients. Similarly, predictive models used in outbreak response may allocate resources in ways that inadvertently concentrate risk in particular communities. These patterns often emerge gradually through repeated interactions between system rules and population characteristics, making them difficult to detect through conventional oversight mechanisms.

Scholars of algorithmic governance have increasingly recognized that many harms associated with automated decision systems arise not from explicit bias but from structural dynamics embedded within optimization processes (Bertsimas & Dunn, 2017). In stochastic healthcare systems, these dynamics may manifest as persistent occupancy of high-risk states, unequal recovery probabilities across patient groups, or long-run distributional inequities. These patterns may remain invisible when systems are evaluated solely through point-in-time performance metrics.

The chapter therefore advances trajectory-level accountability as its central governance principle. Instead of assessing isolated outputs alone, oversight should examine transition probabilities, cumulative exposure to high-risk states, recovery pathways, and long-run outcome distributions across patient groups. This consolidated shift from discrete decisions to system trajectories aligns ethical and legal review with the mathematical structure of adaptive stochastic systems.

Legal frameworks are also beginning to grapple with these challenges. In the European Union, emerging regulatory approaches to artificial intelligence emphasize risk-based classification and continuous monitoring of high-impact systems (European Union, 2024). In the United States, oversight remains more fragmented, relying on sector-specific regulators and outcome-based liability frameworks. Meanwhile, countries such as Saudi Arabia are developing hybrid governance models that combine centralized digital health oversight with ethical principles rooted in Islamic jurisprudence and public interest considerations (SDAIA, 2023; Albar, 2018).

These diverse approaches reflect broader debates about how societies should govern algorithmic decision-making under uncertainty. In healthcare, the stakes are particularly high because decisions directly affect human health, access to care, and allocation of scarce resources. Ethical governance must therefore balance efficiency and innovation with commitments to justice, transparency, and public trust.

This chapter develops a framework for governing probabilistic healthcare systems by treating uncertainty as a governable feature rather than a technical nuisance. Integrating stochastic modelling, regulatory governance, and bioethics, it proposes design principles that embed ethical oversight within system architecture.

The chapter first explains the stochastic foundations needed for the governance analysis, then examines ethical risk and comparative regulatory approaches. A worked outbreak-response case study illustrates how non-ergodic dynamics can generate structural harm. The chapter then develops design principles and practical implementation guidance for regulators, healthcare organizations, and system designers before concluding with the broader implications of governing uncertainty.

This chapter contributes to the literature in three ways. First, it develops a conceptual framework for governing probabilistic healthcare systems that shifts ethical analysis from discrete decisions to long-run system trajectories. Second, it integrates stochastic modelling concepts such as ergodicity and transition dynamics into the evaluation of healthcare fairness and accountability. Third, it translates these theoretical insights into practical governance mechanisms—including dynamic equity thresholds, automated ethical tripwires, and institutional responsibility matrices—capable of guiding real-world implementation.

STOCHASTIC PROCESSES IN ADAPTIVE HEALTHCARE SYSTEMS

Healthcare systems operate within environments characterized by inherent uncertainty. Patient arrivals fluctuate unpredictably, disease trajectories evolve differently across individuals, treatment durations vary, and resource availability may shift rapidly in response to demand. Traditional deterministic models attempt to simplify these complexities by assuming fixed relationships between inputs and outputs. While such models may provide useful approximations in stable settings, they often fail to capture the dynamic variability that characterizes real healthcare systems.

Stochastic processes provide a more appropriate mathematical framework for modelling these dynamics. Unlike deterministic models, stochastic models explicitly incorporate randomness and probabilistic transitions between system states. By representing uncertainty as an integral component of system behaviour, stochastic models enable healthcare administrators, clinicians, and policymakers to analyse how complex systems evolve over time under conditions of incomplete information (Ross, 2014). These models allow decision-makers to evaluate expected outcomes, assess risk distributions, and design policies that perform robustly across a range of possible scenarios.

Stochastic modeling has become increasingly important in healthcare operations research, epidemiology, and health systems engineering. Hospitals and public health institutions use stochastic models to optimize patient flow, manage resource allocation, predict disease progression, and design adaptive response strategies for public health emergencies. By capturing the probabilistic nature of healthcare processes, these models provide decision-makers with tools for managing uncertainty in ways that deterministic frameworks cannot.

Markov Models and State Transitions

A Markov model represents movement among defined health or operational states through a transition matrix P, where P is the probability of moving from state i to state j during the next time interval. When a policy or action influences those transitions, the model becomes a Markov decision process. In healthcare, these models support analyses of disease progression, patient flow, treatment pathways, and outbreak response (Ross, 2014).

For governance, the important question is not merely whether the next prediction is accurate, but whether transition patterns produce persistent disadvantage. Relevant metrics include subgroup-specific transition probabilities, expected time in adverse states, probability of recovery, and long-run state distributions.

Queueing Theory and Patient Flow

Queueing theory models systems in which entities, such as patients, arrive according to a stochastic process and wait for service from limited resources, such as clinicians, beds, or equipment. Arrival rates, service rates, queue lengths, waiting times, and utilization are used to assess congestion and capacity (Green, 2006; Gross et al., 2018).

In governance terms, average waiting time is insufficient. Organizations should also measure the upper tail of waiting times, repeated delay, abandonment, and subgroup disparities, because an apparently efficient queue may still impose concentrated burdens on complex or vulnerable patients.

Stochastic Optimization and Simulation

Stochastic optimization selects policies under uncertain demand, clinical progression, and resource availability. Simulation complements optimization by testing how policies behave across many plausible scenarios before clinical deployment (Hulshof et al., 2012).

Governance metrics should translate ethical commitments into measurable constraints—for example, maximum waiting-time disparities, minimum admission or recovery probabilities for high-risk groups, and alert thresholds for material shifts in transition probabilities. Sensitivity analysis should show whether these safeguards remain effective when assumptions about demand, capacity, or disease severity change.

Implications for Adaptive Healthcare Governance

The increasing use of stochastic models reflects a broader transformation in healthcare systems toward adaptive decision-making. Rather than relying solely on fixed protocols, modern healthcare systems increasingly incorporate data-driven models that update predictions and policies in response to changing conditions.

Real-world adaptive systems include radiology worklists that reprioritize examinations by predicted urgency, deterioration alerts that update as new clinical observations enter the electronic health record, and outbreak dashboards that revise forecasts as surveillance data change. These applications demonstrate why governance must extend beyond initial validation to longitudinal monitoring of performance, equity, and model drift (Rajkomar et al., 2019; World Health Organization, 2021).

While these tools enhance system efficiency and resilience, they also introduce governance challenges. Because stochastic systems generate outcomes through probabilistic trajectories rather than deterministic decisions, their ethical and legal implications must be evaluated at the system level rather than at individual decision points.

Understanding the mathematical foundations of stochastic modelling is therefore essential for effective governance. Policymakers, healthcare administrators, and regulators must recognize how probabilistic models shape system behaviour over time, including how they distribute risk, allocate resources, and influence patient outcomes.

The discussion that follows builds on this foundation by examining the ethical risks associated with probabilistic decision-making in healthcare systems.

PROBABILISTIC DECISION-MAKING AND ETHICAL RISK

The increasing integration of probabilistic models into healthcare decision-making represents a fundamental shift in how healthcare systems manage uncertainty. Rather than relying solely on deterministic rules or static protocols, healthcare organizations now employ stochastic models that explicitly incorporate randomness, variability, and incomplete information. These models enable decision-makers to anticipate future states of complex systems and allocate resources accordingly. However, the same probabilistic mechanisms that improve efficiency and adaptability also introduce new ethical risks that traditional governance frameworks struggle to detect or regulate.

Probabilistic decision-making in healthcare commonly relies on mathematical frameworks such as Markov decision processes, queueing networks, and stochastic optimization models. These approaches treat healthcare systems as dynamic state-based processes, in which transitions between states occur with certain probabilities (Ross, 2014). For example, a patient may move from a low-risk clinical state to a higher-risk state depending on treatment decisions, disease progression, and system capacity. Similarly, hospital resources such as intensive care beds, diagnostic equipment, or surgical slots can be modelled as queues with stochastic arrival and service rates (Gross et al., 2018).

Such models allow healthcare administrators and policymakers to optimize decision-making under uncertainty. For instance, queueing theory can be used to minimize waiting times in emergency departments, while stochastic optimization models can guide allocation of scarce resources during infectious disease outbreaks. When integrated with machine learning and real-time monitoring systems, probabilistic models can support adaptive decision policies that continuously update as new information becomes available.

Despite these advantages, probabilistic decision systems present distinctive ethical challenges. Unlike deterministic systems, where decisions and outcomes can be clearly attributed to specific actions, stochastic systems generate outcomes through probabilistic transitions across multiple system states. This means that harm may emerge not from a single decision but from repeated interactions between system rules, patient characteristics, and environmental conditions.

A key ethical concern is the emergence of trajectory-dependent harm. In stochastic systems, individuals may follow different pathways through the system depending on probabilistic transitions. Over time, certain groups may become disproportionately represented in unfavourable system states. Consequently, algorithmic decision systems may generate structural inequities even when explicit discrimination is absent (Barocas & Selbst, 2016; Obermeyer et al., 2019). For example, predictive triage systems may assign lower priority scores to patients whose clinical indicators historically correlate with lower survival rates. While such decisions may appear statistically justified, repeated application of these rules can lead to structural disadvantage for particular patient populations.

These dynamics are closely related to the concept of non-ergodicity, which refers to systems in which long-run outcomes differ systematically across individuals or groups depending on their initial conditions or trajectories. In ergodic systems, long-term averages converge across individuals, meaning that no group remains permanently disadvantaged. Non-ergodic systems, by contrast, may produce persistent inequalities because certain states are difficult to escape once entered. In healthcare contexts, this may manifest as prolonged waiting times, reduced access to specialized care, or repeated exposure to high-risk clinical conditions.

Research in operations research and healthcare optimization has demonstrated that policies designed to maximize overall system efficiency may inadvertently produce such outcomes. For example, scheduling algorithms that minimize average waiting time may systematically delay complex cases requiring longer treatment times. Similarly, predictive models used in hospital readmission management may allocate resources preferentially to patients whose outcomes are easier to improve, leaving high-risk patients underserved (Bertsimas & Kallus (2020).

Another ethical challenge arises from feedback loops embedded within probabilistic decision systems. When system outputs influence future inputs, small disparities can become amplified over time. For instance, if predictive models allocate fewer resources to a particular population due to historical patterns, the resulting lack of intervention may reinforce those patterns in future data. This phenomenon, sometimes referred to as algorithmic reinforcement, can entrench inequalities even when decision rules appear neutral.

Probabilistic systems also complicate questions of accountability. Traditional models of ethical and legal responsibility assume that decision-makers can be identified and held accountable for specific actions. In stochastic systems, however, outcomes emerge from complex interactions between models, data inputs, and organizational policies. As a result, responsibility becomes distributed across multiple actors, including data scientists, healthcare administrators, regulators, and clinicians. Determining who is accountable for harm becomes difficult when no single decision point clearly caused the outcome.

Transparency and explainability present additional challenges. Many stochastic models rely on statistical optimization techniques that produce policies optimized for expected outcomes across populations. While these policies may be mathematically sound, their implications for individual patients can be difficult to interpret. Clinicians and patients may struggle to understand why certain decisions are made, particularly when decisions are influenced by probabilistic forecasts or algorithmic predictions.

Ethical governance must therefore examine system behaviour over time and across populations, including long-run state distributions, transition probabilities, and cumulative exposure to risk. The governance mechanisms for doing so are developed later in the chapter.

The discussion that follows examines how different regulatory systems approach these challenges and explores how legal and institutional frameworks can support ethical governance of probabilistic healthcare systems.

Table 1. Governance Principles for Probabilistic Healthcare Systems

Principle	Governance Objective	Implementation	Example Metric
Trajectory Accountability	Detect system-level harm	State distribution monitoring	Time in high-risk states
Ergodicity-Aware Fairness	Prevent structural inequality	Fairness constraints	Recovery probability parity
Constraint Optimization	Balance efficiency & ethics	Optimization limits	Max waiting-time disparity
Adaptive Oversight	Respond to model drift	Periodic audits	Distribution shift detection
Transparency	Improve interpretability	Simulation outputs	Policy explainability score
Legal Alignment	Ensure compliance	Ethical review	Regulatory audit compliance

COMPARATIVE REGULATORY APPROACHES TO GOVERNING PROBABILISTIC HEALTHCARE SYSTEMS

As healthcare systems increasingly rely on probabilistic modelling and algorithmic decision support, regulatory institutions around the world face the challenge of adapting governance frameworks designed for deterministic systems. Traditional health regulation typically focuses on discrete interventions—medical devices, pharmaceuticals, or clinical procedures—whose safety and effectiveness can be evaluated through controlled trials and post-market surveillance. Probabilistic decision systems, however, function differently. Their behaviour evolves over time, their outputs depend on dynamic data streams, and their outcomes emerge from repeated interactions between algorithms, clinicians, and patients.

These characteristics complicate regulatory oversight. Unlike traditional clinical technologies, stochastic decision systems cannot be evaluated solely through static performance metrics. Instead, their governance requires ongoing monitoring of system behaviour, including long-run outcome distributions, feedback loops, and adaptation to changing conditions. Several jurisdictions have begun to address these challenges, albeit through different regulatory strategies. Examining these approaches provides insight into how probabilistic healthcare systems can be governed effectively.

Global policy discussions increasingly emphasize risk-based governance frameworks for AI-enabled decision systems (Floridi et al., 2018; WHO, 2021).

The European Union: Risk-Based Governance and Algorithmic Accountability

The European Union has taken one of the most proactive approaches to regulating algorithmic systems in healthcare. Its regulatory strategy emphasizes risk-based classification, continuous oversight, and transparency requirements for high-impact technologies. While much of this framework has emerged in response to artificial intelligence, it has significant implications for probabilistic healthcare systems more broadly.

Regulation (EU) 2024/1689 (the Artificial Intelligence Act) establishes binding, risk-based obligations for AI systems. Healthcare AI that functions as a safety component of a regulated medical device, or is itself such a device, may be classified as high risk and become subject to requirements concerning risk management, data governance, technical documentation, human oversight, accuracy, robustness, and post-market monitoring (European Union, 2024).

Importantly, EU governance frameworks recognize that algorithmic systems may produce harms that are systemic rather than individual. This perspective aligns with concerns about probabilistic decision systems, where inequities may emerge gradually through repeated interactions between decision policies and population characteristics. The EU approach therefore emphasizes continuous monitoring and auditing rather than one-time approval.

The General Data Protection Regulation (GDPR) also plays a significant role in shaping algorithmic governance in healthcare. GDPR includes provisions that limit fully automated decision-making when such decisions significantly affect individuals (Voigt & Von dem Bussche, 2017). Although these provisions were not designed specifically for probabilistic healthcare systems, they establish important principles regarding transparency, accountability, and human oversight.

Taken together, EU regulatory frameworks represent an emerging model of system-level governance. Rather than focusing solely on the technical properties of algorithms, regulators evaluate the broader institutional context in which decision systems operate. This approach acknowledges that algorithmic decisions are embedded within complex socio-technical systems and that governance must address both technological and organizational factors.

The United States: Fragmented Oversight and Market-Oriented Regulation

In contrast to the EU's comprehensive regulatory approach, governance of algorithmic healthcare systems in the United States remains relatively fragmented. Multiple agencies share oversight responsibilities, including the Food and Drug Administration (FDA), the Department of Health and Human Services (HHS), and various state-level authorities.

The FDA has increasingly emphasized lifecycle management of AI-enabled device software functions. Its 2025 draft guidance recommends documentation and controls addressing the total product lifecycle, including data management, performance evaluation, transparency, and plans for managing model changes (U.S. Food and Drug Administration, 2025).

While this approach recognizes the dynamic nature of algorithmic systems, it focuses primarily on safety and performance, rather than broader ethical concerns such as distributional fairness or systemic inequity. In practice, many probabilistic decision systems used in healthcare—such as hospital scheduling algorithms or predictive analytics for population health management—fall outside traditional medical device regulation altogether.

Legal accountability in the United States often relies on tort law and malpractice frameworks, which are designed to address identifiable acts of negligence. However, probabilistic decision systems complicate this model because harms may arise from aggregate system behavior rather than specific decisions. For instance, if a scheduling algorithm consistently deprioritizes certain patient groups, responsibility may be difficult to attribute to any single actor.

Scholars have therefore argued that the U.S. regulatory system may struggle to address algorithmic harms that are structural or cumulative in nature (Cohen, 2020). Without mechanisms for evaluating long-run system outcomes, regulators may overlook inequities that emerge gradually over time.

Saudi Arabia: Hybrid Governance and Ethical Foundations in Islamic Bioethics

Saudi Arabia represents a distinct regulatory environment shaped by rapid digital transformation and strong centralized governance. In recent years, the Kingdom has invested heavily in digital health infrastructure as part of its Vision 2030 agenda, including large-scale deployment of electronic health records, national health data platforms, and AI-driven decision support systems.

The Saudi Data and Artificial Intelligence Authority (SDAIA) has developed regulatory frameworks governing data protection and responsible use of artificial intelligence. The Personal Data Protection Law (PDPL) establishes rules for collection, processing, and sharing of personal data, including health information (SDAIA, 2023). These provisions are particularly relevant for probabilistic healthcare systems that rely on large datasets to train predictive models.

Beyond technical regulation, governance of healthcare technologies in Saudi Arabia is also influenced by Islamic bioethical principles. Islamic jurisprudence emphasizes values such as justice ('adl), prevention of harm (darar), and promotion of public interest (maslahah) (Albar, 2018). These principles provide an ethical framework for evaluating emerging technologies, including probabilistic decision systems.

For example, policies that maximize overall efficiency but disproportionately harm vulnerable populations may conflict with Islamic ethical principles emphasizing fairness and protection of the weak. Similarly, probabilistic systems that obscure decision logic or reduce accountability may undermine the moral responsibility expected of healthcare institutions.

The integration of legal regulation with ethical principles provides an opportunity to develop governance models that address both technical and moral dimensions of probabilistic healthcare systems. In this context, ethical oversight becomes not merely a regulatory requirement but a broader institutional commitment.

ENFORCING TRAJECTORY-LEVEL ACCOUNTABILITY

Existing liability rules often require a claimant to identify a discrete breach and connect it causally to an individual injury. That structure is poorly suited to cumulative harms produced by repeated probabilistic allocations. A practical reform would require deploying institutions to preserve model versions, transition matrices, override logs, subgroup outcome distributions, and audit records so that cumulative patterns are legally reviewable.

The Standard of Reasoned Justification (SRJ) can be extended to stochastic systems by requiring an institution to justify the model's objective function, variables, fairness constraints, update rules, and observed long-run distributions. Failure to monitor known disparity indicators, respond to ethical tripwires, or document a defensible reason for continuing a harmful policy could support organizational negligence, regulatory enforcement, or product-liability claims, depending on the actor and jurisdiction. Courts and regulators could also permit aggregate statistical evidence to establish foreseeability and breach where harm arises cumulatively rather than from a single output.

In the European Union, these duties can connect with the AI Act's risk-management, record-keeping, human-oversight, and post-market-monitoring requirements. In the United States, similar obligations could be incorporated through FDA lifecycle controls for regulated devices, accreditation standards, contractual duties, and institutional negligence. In Saudi Arabia, PDPL duties, health-sector regulation, and the principles of justice, prevention of harm, and public interest provide a basis for requiring documented, proportionate, and auditable use of probabilistic systems.

Toward Integrated Governance of Probabilistic Healthcare Systems

Despite differences across jurisdictions, several common themes emerge from this comparative analysis. First, regulators increasingly recognize that algorithmic systems require continuous oversight rather than static approval. Probabilistic systems evolve over time, making periodic monitoring essential for detecting unintended consequences.

Second, effective governance requires attention to system-level outcomes, including long-run distributions of risk and access to care. Traditional regulatory frameworks often focus on individual decisions or technical performance metrics, but these measures may fail to capture structural inequities emerging from stochastic processes.

Third, governance must address the institutional context in which probabilistic systems operate. Algorithms do not function independently; they interact with organizational policies, clinical practices, and regulatory frameworks. Oversight mechanisms must therefore consider the broader socio-technical environment.

These insights suggest that ethical governance of probabilistic healthcare systems requires a combination of technical evaluation, institutional oversight, and ethical reflection. Regulatory frameworks must evolve to accommodate systems whose behavior cannot be fully understood through static testing alone.

The comparison across jurisdictions reveals three distinct regulatory paradigms. The European Union adopts a precautionary model emphasizing ex ante risk classification and continuous oversight of high-risk systems. The United States follows a market-oriented innovation model, relying on sector-specific regulators and post hoc liability mechanisms. Saudi Arabia represents an emerging hybrid governance model, combining centralized digital governance with ethical frameworks rooted in Islamic jurisprudence. Each approach offers partial solutions to the governance of probabilistic healthcare systems, but none yet fully addresses the trajectory-level dynamics characteristic of stochastic decision architectures.

The discussion that follows illustrates these challenges through a detailed case study of a probabilistic outbreak response model, demonstrating how non-ergodic dynamics can produce unintended harms even when individual decisions appear rational.

CASE STUDY: MARKOV-BASED OUTBREAK RESPONSE AND ETHICAL GOVERNANCE

Probabilistic models are particularly valuable during infectious disease outbreaks, when healthcare systems must allocate scarce resources under rapidly changing conditions. During such events, decision-makers face uncertainty regarding transmission dynamics, disease severity, resource availability, and patient demand. Stochastic models provide tools for representing these uncertainties and supporting adaptive decision-making.

Among these tools, Markov decision processes (MDPs) are widely used to model healthcare systems in which future states depend probabilistically on current conditions and policy choices (Ross, 2014). A hospital outbreak response system can be modelled as a Markov decision process in which patient states evolve according to probabilistic transitions and hospital administrators allocate isolation resources under capacity constraints (Ross, 2014). States may range from low-risk suspected infection to confirmed infection, recovery, or adverse outcomes.

Markov and stochastic epidemic models are widely used to analyse disease dynamics and resource allocation during outbreaks (Allen, 2017; Keeling & Rohani, 2008). While the example presented here is conceptual, it reflects operational decision environments commonly encountered in hospital infection control programs where patient isolation resources must be dynamically allocated under uncertainty.

This section illustrates how probabilistic outbreak response models can generate ethical risks when their long-run system dynamics are not carefully governed. While the case presented here is illustrative rather than empirical, it reflects modelling approaches commonly used in hospital operations research and epidemic management.

Although the state model remains illustrative, its equity concern is supported by evidence from COVID-19 crisis-allocation research. In a multicentre cohort of 95,549 intensive-care encounters, SOFA-based allocation rules overestimated mortality among Black patients relative to White patients with equivalent scores and could therefore assign Black patients lower priority under scarcity conditions (Miller et al., 2021). This finding shows how a neutral-looking transition or priority rule can generate measurable structural disadvantage.

Modelling Outbreak Response as a Markov Decision Process

Digital surveillance technologies used for public health monitoring can generate significant benefits but also raise concerns regarding privacy, proportionality, and legal accountability when deployed without adequate safeguards (Elgujja, 2020). Consider a hospital responding to an outbreak of a respiratory infection. Hospital administrators must decide how to allocate a limited number of isolation beds to incoming patients. Patients may present with varying levels of infection risk and disease severity, and their clinical conditions may evolve over time.

This decision environment can be modelled using a Markov decision process in which the system transitions between a set of discrete states representing patient risk categories. For example, patient states may include:

- S_1: Low-risk suspected infection
- S_2: Confirmed infection requiring monitoring
- S_3: Severe infection requiring intensive care
- S_4: Recovery or discharge
- S_5: Adverse outcome (e.g., clinical deterioration)

Transitions between states occur with certain probabilities determined by clinical progression, treatment availability, and healthcare capacity constraints. For instance, a patient in state S_2 may recover and move to S_4, deteriorate and move to S_3, or remain stable depending on treatment decisions and disease dynamics.

At each stage, administrators must choose actions such as:

- A_1: Immediate admission to an isolation unit
- A_2: Cohorting with other patients under infection control precautions
- A_3: Delayed admission due to resource constraints

The goal of the model is to determine the policy that maximizes expected system outcomes, such as minimizing mortality or reducing transmission within the hospital. Figure 1 illustrates the Markov state transition structure used in the outbreak response model.

Figure 1. Markov State Transition Model for Hospital Outbreak Response

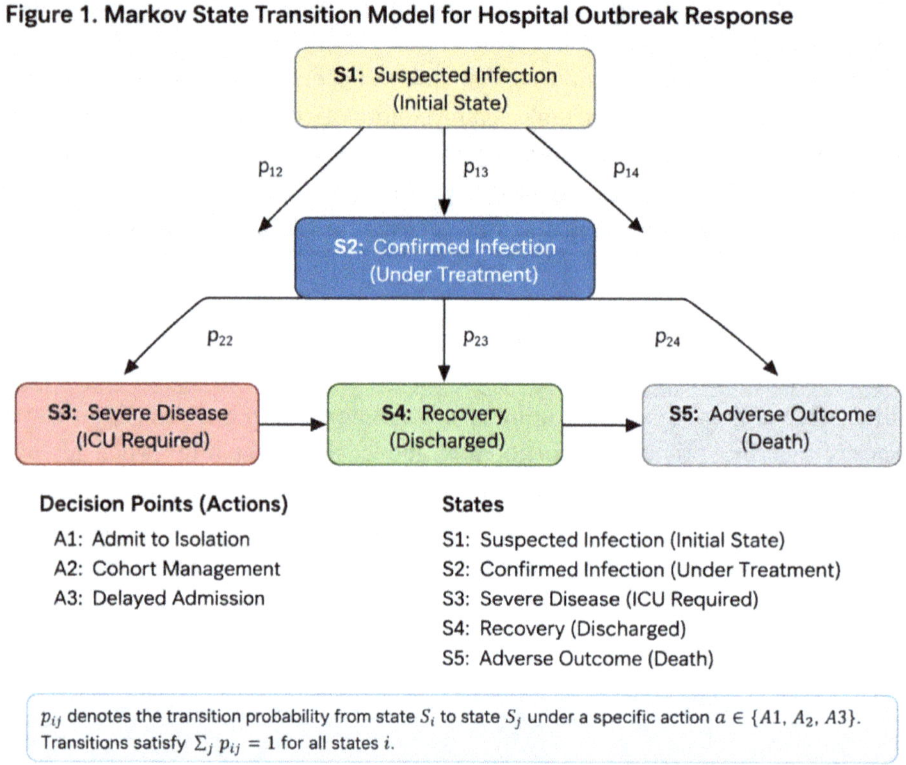

Formally, the system can be represented as a Markov decision process defined by a tuple (S, A, P, R), where S represents the set of system states, A the set of decision actions, P(s′|s,a) the transition probability from state s to s′ under action a, and R the expected reward or cost associated with each transition (Ross, 2014).

Such models can be extended with reinforcement learning or predictive analytics that update transition probabilities using real-time epidemiological data. When combined with electronic health record systems and surveillance tools, they enable adaptive policies that respond to changing outbreak conditions.

Efficiency Versus Equity in Stochastic Allocation

From a systems perspective, probabilistic allocation policies often perform better than deterministic rules. By incorporating uncertainty, stochastic models allow administrators to allocate resources dynamically based on evolving risk estimates. This approach can improve overall system efficiency and reduce the likelihood of catastrophic resource shortages during surges.

However, the objective functions used in these models typically focus on expected outcomes across the entire patient population. Policies that maximize aggregate outcomes may inadvertently create unequal risks for specific patient groups.

For example, suppose the model prioritizes admission for patients with the highest probability of survival. While this policy may minimize overall mortality, it may systematically deprioritize patients with complex comorbidities or delayed presentation to care. Over repeated iterations of the model, these patients may experience prolonged delays in treatment or reduced access to specialized care.

Because decisions are probabilistic rather than deterministic, such disparities may not appear in individual cases. Each decision may appear reasonable based on available information. Yet when viewed across many iterations of the system, a pattern of unequal outcomes may emerge.

This phenomenon illustrates the importance of evaluating probabilistic systems through trajectory-level analysis rather than isolated decisions.

Non-Ergodic Dynamics and Structural Harm

In stochastic process theory, ergodicity refers to systems in which long-run statistical properties are independent of initial conditions. In ergodic systems, time averages converge toward ensemble averages. In contrast, non-ergodic systems exhibit path dependence, meaning that early conditions or decisions may permanently shape long-term outcomes (Ross, 2014). In healthcare contexts, this implies that initial triage or allocation decisions may create trajectories that certain patients cannot easily escape, producing persistent disparities in health outcomes.

One of the most significant ethical concerns associated with probabilistic decision systems is the emergence of non-ergodic dynamics. In stochastic processes, ergodicity refers to the property that long-run averages converge across individuals regardless of their starting conditions. In an ergodic system, temporary disadvantages tend to dissipate over time.

Non-ergodic systems behave differently. In such systems, early conditions or decisions can permanently shape long-term outcomes. Certain individuals or groups may become trapped in unfavourable system states with limited probability of recovery.

In the outbreak response model described above, non-ergodicity might occur if patients who are initially assigned to delayed admission pathways have a significantly higher probability of clinical deterioration. Once these patients enter a severe disease state (S_3), their probability of recovery may decline substantially. Over time, the system may produce a stable distribution in which certain patient groups experience disproportionately high rates of adverse outcomes.

The outbreak response model described above highlights a central governance challenge in probabilistic healthcare systems: the potential conflict between efficiency-oriented optimization and equitable patient outcomes. Decision policies designed to maximize aggregate performance metrics—such as expected survival rates, throughput, or resource utilization—may inadvertently deprioritize patients whose clinical trajectories are more uncertain or resource intensive. In probabilistic systems, such optimization can systematically disadvantage particular patient groups, producing persistent disparities in recovery probabilities or waiting times across populations (Obermeyer et al., 2019). These disparities may not arise from any single decision but instead emerge cumulatively through repeated transitions across system states.

To address this challenge, governance frameworks should incorporate dynamic equity thresholds within probabilistic decision models. Rather than imposing static fairness constraints that apply uniformly across all situations, dynamic thresholds establish minimum outcome guarantees for patient subgroups while allowing optimization to occur within those bounds. Under this approach, decision systems first ensure that each subgroup maintains a minimum acceptable probability of reaching favorable health states within the model's transition dynamics. Only after these baseline equity conditions are satisfied does the system optimize aggregate performance objectives such as resource efficiency or expected survival outcomes.

This approach acknowledges that fairness and efficiency may sometimes exist in tension within algorithmic decision systems. Research on algorithmic fairness has shown that optimization processes can produce systematic trade-offs between accuracy, efficiency, and distributive equity (Kleinberg et al., 2017). By incorporating dynamic thresholds into stochastic decision policies, healthcare organizations can ensure that efficiency improvements do not occur at the expense of minimum fairness guarantees across patient groups.

Conceptually, dynamic equity thresholds resemble Pareto-constrained optimization, in which system efficiency is maximized subject to predefined fairness constraints (Bertsimas & Kallus, 2020). In stochastic healthcare systems, such constraints may be implemented by modifying transition policies or resource allocation rules so that the long-run distribution of outcomes remains within ethically acceptable bounds. For example, decision models may ensure that high-risk patient groups retain a minimum probability of transitioning to recovery states despite capacity limitations.

Embedding equity constraints directly within probabilistic decision architectures also aligns with broader ethical frameworks for responsible AI governance. Scholars in algorithmic ethics emphasize that fairness considerations should be integrated into system design rather than addressed solely through retrospective auditing (Floridi et al., 2018; Mittelstadt et al., 2016). By embedding dynamic equity thresholds within stochastic models, healthcare institutions can operationalize these principles within the mathematical structure of decision systems themselves.

In the outbreak response model described in this chapter, dynamic equity thresholds could ensure that high-risk patients retain a minimum probability of reaching the recovery state even when system capacity is constrained. Monitoring systems could then track whether observed transition probabilities fall below predefined fairness thresholds, triggering governance interventions when necessary. Through this approach, healthcare organizations can balance operational efficiency with the ethical obligation to ensure equitable access to care.

A simple sensitivity analysis can test whether the proposed safeguard is robust. The model should be rerun across plausible ranges of bed capacity, deterioration probability, and subgroup recovery rates under three policies: unconstrained optimization, a minimum recovery-probability guarantee, and a maximum waiting-time disparity constraint. Outcomes should be compared using mortality, throughput, subgroup recovery probability, time in high-risk states, and the efficiency cost of each safeguard. A constraint should be retained only where it materially reduces disparity without creating clinically unacceptable loss of overall benefit.

This outcome would not necessarily result from discriminatory rules or explicit bias. Instead, it would emerge from the interaction between probabilistic transitions, resource constraints, and optimization policies. Figure 2 presents the steady-state distribution of patients across system states under the optimized policy.

Figure 2. Long-Run Distribution of Patient Risk Across System States

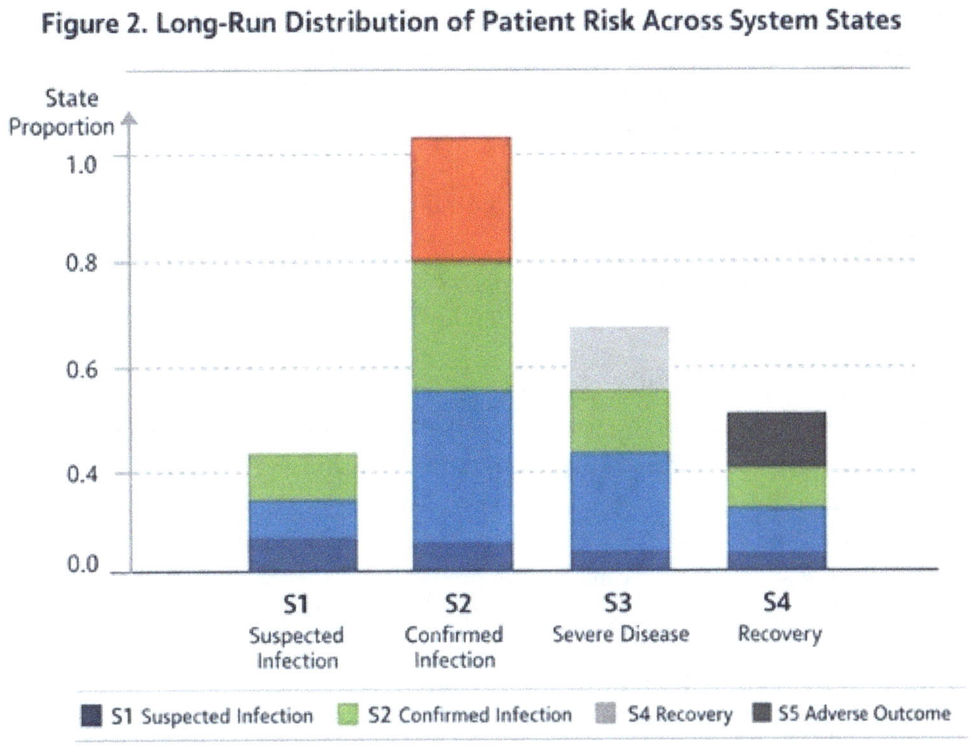

From an ethical perspective, such outcomes raise concerns about structural harm. Even though no individual decision may be unjustified, the cumulative effect of probabilistic decision policies may produce inequitable distributions of risk.

Governance Implications of Stochastic Outbreak Models

The case study illustrates why traditional oversight mechanisms are insufficient for governing probabilistic healthcare systems. Conventional approaches often focus on evaluating individual decisions or verifying that decision rules comply with clinical guidelines. However, these methods cannot detect inequities that emerge through long-run system dynamics.

Effective governance of stochastic outbreak models requires additional mechanisms, including:

- Monitoring of long-run outcome distributions across patient groups
- Simulation testing of policies under different outbreak scenarios
- Fairness constraints embedded within optimization objectives
- Regular auditing of transition probabilities to detect model drift

These findings show how individually defensible allocation decisions may generate inequity across repeated system trajectories. The following lessons translate that risk into governance requirements.

Lessons for Ethical Governance

The outbreak response case study demonstrates several broader lessons for governing probabilistic healthcare systems.

First, ethical risks in stochastic systems often arise from long-run patterns rather than individual decisions. Governance frameworks must therefore evaluate system trajectories rather than isolated events.

Second, probabilistic models must be assessed not only for efficiency but also for distributional fairness. Optimization objectives should incorporate constraints that protect vulnerable populations from persistent disadvantage.

Third, healthcare organizations must invest in analytical tools capable of detecting system-level inequities. Simulation models, predictive analytics, and real-time monitoring systems can support this form of oversight.

Finally, probabilistic systems should be governed through institutional accountability structures that bring together clinicians, data scientists, regulators, and ethicists. Effective governance requires interdisciplinary expertise capable of understanding both the mathematical properties of stochastic models and their social implications.

The design principles proposed in the following section build on these insights and provide a framework for embedding ethical governance directly into probabilistic healthcare systems.

DESIGN PRINCIPLES FOR ETHICAL GOVERNANCE OF PROBABILISTIC HEALTHCARE SYSTEMS

The preceding sections have shown that probabilistic healthcare systems introduce ethical risks that cannot be addressed through traditional governance mechanisms focused on discrete decisions or individual actors. Instead, these systems require governance frameworks capable of evaluating long-run system behaviour, distributional outcomes, and adaptive dynamics. Effective governance requires addressing both technical and sociotechnical dimensions of algorithmic decision systems (Mittelstadt et al., 2016; Selbst et al., 2019). Ethical governance must therefore move from reactive oversight toward design-oriented governance, embedding normative safeguards directly within system architecture.

Drawing on insights from stochastic modelling, comparative regulatory analysis, and bioethical theory, this section proposes six principles for governing probabilistic healthcare systems. These principles are intended to guide policymakers, healthcare administrators, and system designers in ensuring that probabilistic decision systems promote both efficiency and justice.

Trajectory-Level Accountability

Traditional models of accountability assume that decisions can be evaluated individually. In stochastic systems, however, outcomes often emerge from sequences of probabilistic transitions rather than single decisions. A policy that appears acceptable in isolation may produce inequitable outcomes when repeated across thousands of interactions. Unlike conventional algorithmic fairness approaches that evaluate decisions at a single point in time, trajectory-level governance evaluates fairness across the entire sequence of state transitions generated by probabilistic systems.

Trajectory-level accountability addresses this challenge by evaluating decision systems according to the paths they generate over time. Rather than focusing solely on point-in-time outcomes, governance mechanisms should examine how individuals and groups move through system states. This includes monitoring the frequency with which certain populations enter high-risk states, the duration they remain in those states, and the probability of recovery or improvement. Figure 3 illustrates a comparison of Decision-Level vs. Trajectory-Level Fairness in Probabilistic Healthcare Systems

Figure 3. Decision-Level vs. Trajectory-Level Fairness in Probabilistic Healthcare Systems

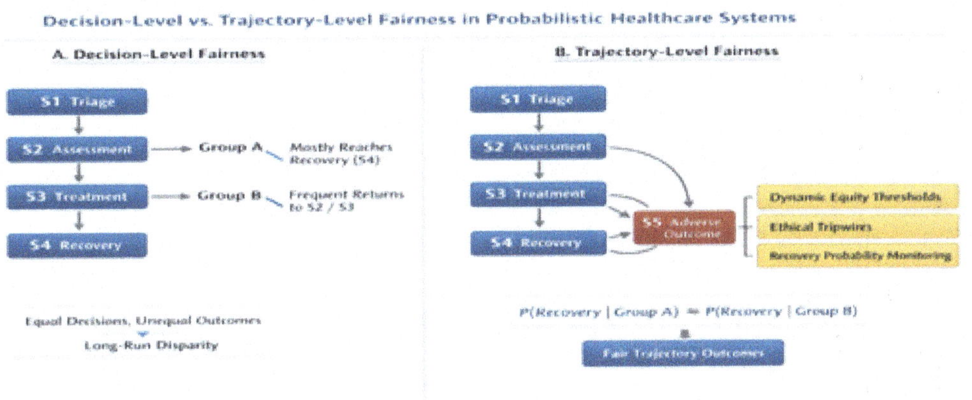

For example, in the outbreak response case described in the outbreak-response case study, trajectory-level accountability would require monitoring how frequently patients assigned to delayed admission pathways transition into severe disease states. If certain groups consistently experience prolonged exposure to high-risk conditions, governance mechanisms should trigger policy review.

From a technical perspective, trajectory-level accountability may involve analysing state transition matrices, steady-state distributions, and cumulative exposure metrics. These measures provide insight into how probabilistic policies affect populations over time.

Embedding such monitoring mechanisms aligns ethical oversight with the underlying mathematics of stochastic processes. By examining system trajectories rather than individual decisions, governance frameworks can detect structural inequities that would otherwise remain hidden.

Governance of probabilistic healthcare systems must therefore incorporate mechanisms that ensure transparency and accountability in algorithmic decision-making. Recent scholarship has emphasized that algorithmic governance must satisfy principles of reasoned justification and institutional accountability when automated systems influence rights or welfare outcomes (Elgujja, 2025a). Figure 4 shows how trajectory-level governance translates these risks into institutional oversight and accountability. Trajectory-level governance monitors system behaviour across repeated state transitions, enabling institutions to detect and mitigate structural inequities (See Table 2).

Table 2. Trajectory-Based Governance Framework

Framework level	Core components	Governance function
Stochastic system architecture	Markov decision processes; queueing systems; stochastic optimisation; adaptive learning systems	Represents uncertainty, changing system states, resource constraints, and evolving decision policies.
Ethical risk emergence	Trajectory-dependent harm; non-ergodic inequality; feedback loops; structural disadvantage	Identifies harms that develop cumulatively through repeated probabilistic transitions rather than through a single decision.
Governance principles	Trajectory-level accountability; ergodicity-aware fairness; constraint-based optimisation; adaptive oversight; transparency of system behaviour; alignment with legal and ethical norms	Translates stochastic risks into measurable ethical, legal, and operational safeguards.
Institutional implementation	Regulators; healthcare organisations; system designers and developers; accreditation bodies; workforce training	Allocates responsibility for monitoring, auditing, intervention, system redesign, and professional oversight.

Figure 4. Trajectory-Based Governance Framework for Probabilistic Healthcare Systems

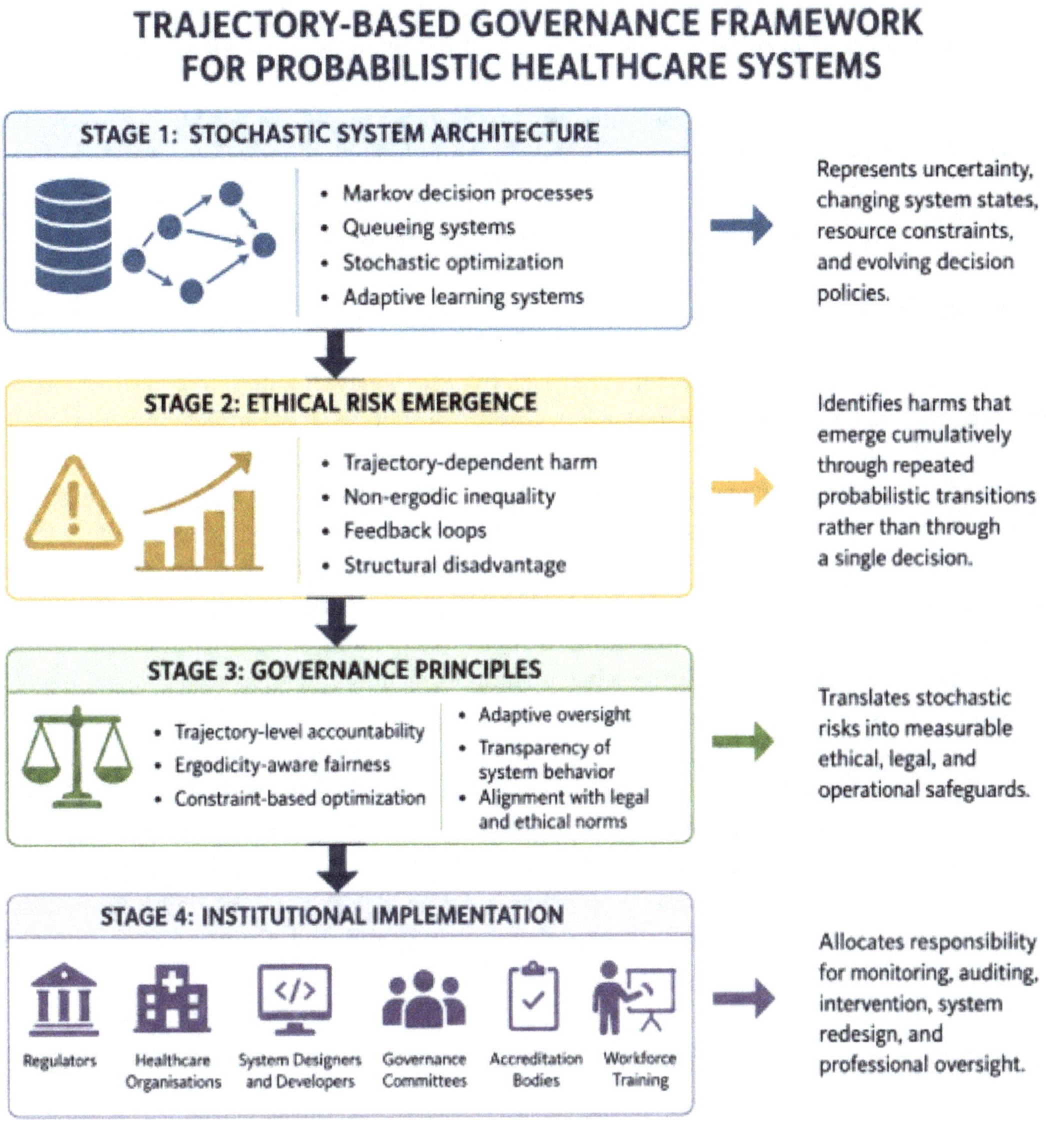

Figure 4. Trajectory-Based Governance Framework for Probabilistic Healthcare Systems

In probabilistic healthcare systems, accountability must extend beyond isolated decisions to encompass the long-run system trajectories produced by repeated probabilistic transitions. Because outcomes emerge from cumulative system behaviour rather than a single identifiable decision, traditional legal standards based on discrete acts may be insufficient for evaluating institutional responsibility. One possible approach is to apply the Standard of Reasoned Justification (SRJ) to probabilistic decision systems. Under this framework, institutions deploying algorithmic or stochastic decision tools must demonstrate that the system's design, operational parameters, and outcome distributions can be justified through transparent reasoning grounded in ethical norms and regulatory obligations (Elgujja, 2025a).

In the context of stochastic healthcare systems, the SRJ framework requires organizations to justify not only individual decision rules but also the long-run distribution of outcomes generated by those rules. If system trajectories systematically produce persistent disadvantages for certain patient groups, institutions must demonstrate that these outcomes arise from ethically defensible criteria rather than hidden biases embedded within transition probabilities or optimization parameters. By extending justification requirements to the system level, SRJ provides a governance mechanism capable of addressing the accountability gap that emerges in complex probabilistic decision environments.

Ergodicity-Aware Fairness

A related principle concerns the concept of ergodicity, which plays a central role in stochastic modelling. In an ergodic system, long-run outcomes converge across individuals regardless of initial conditions. Temporary disadvantages are eventually offset by subsequent opportunities.

Non-ergodic systems behave differently. Early conditions or decisions may permanently influence outcomes, creating persistent inequality across populations. In healthcare contexts, this may occur when certain patient groups experience systematically lower probabilities of recovery or access to treatment.

Ergodicity-aware fairness requires evaluating whether probabilistic decision systems produce persistent structural inequalities over time. Policymakers should examine whether certain groups become trapped in high-risk system states or experience disproportionately low transition probabilities toward favourable outcomes.

This analysis may involve comparing steady-state distributions across demographic groups or evaluating the expected time individuals spend in particular system states. If the system generates persistent disparities, designers may need to modify optimization objectives or introduce fairness constraints.

The importance of ergodicity-aware governance extends beyond outbreak management. Similar dynamics may occur in scheduling systems, predictive risk models, or population health management tools. Without explicit attention to ergodicity, probabilistic optimization may inadvertently institutionalize inequity.

In stochastic systems, fairness can also be evaluated through the long-run distribution of outcomes across patient groups. If a healthcare system is ergodic, the distribution of patient states converges toward a stationary distribution π, defined by the relationship $\pi = \pi P$. The stationary distribution represents the long-term proportion of patients occupying each system state. From a governance perspective, this distribution provides an important fairness indicator: if certain patient groups systematically occupy adverse states with higher probability in the long run, the system may generate structural inequities even when individual decisions appear unbiased (Ross, 2014).

Constraint-Based Optimization

Most stochastic healthcare systems are designed to optimize specific performance metrics such as minimizing mortality, reducing waiting times, or maximizing resource utilization. While these objectives are important, purely efficiency-based optimization may conflict with ethical commitments to fairness and equity.

Constraint-based optimization addresses this tension by embedding ethical requirements directly into decision models. Instead of maximizing efficiency without limits, optimization models incorporate normative constraints that restrict certain outcomes.

For example, a scheduling model may include constraints ensuring that no patient group experiences waiting times above a defined threshold. Similarly, outbreak response models may impose minimum admission probabilities for high-risk patients regardless of predicted survival outcomes.

These constraints transform ethical principles into operational parameters within stochastic models. From a governance perspective, this approach has several advantages. First, it makes ethical commitments explicit and measurable. Second, it allows designers to test how different constraints affect system performance using simulation tools. Third, it ensures that optimization processes remain aligned with broader societal values.

Research in algorithmic fairness increasingly demonstrates that fairness constraints can be incorporated into machine learning and optimization systems without eliminating efficiency gains (Bertsimas & Kallus, 2020; Kleinberg et al., 2017).

Adaptive Oversight

Probabilistic healthcare systems often evolve over time as new data become available. Machine learning models may update predictions, transition probabilities may shift as clinical practices change, and decision policies may adapt to new epidemiological conditions.

These characteristics make static governance models insufficient. Traditional regulatory frameworks often evaluate technologies at the moment of deployment, assuming that system behaviour will remain relatively stable. In probabilistic systems, however, behavior may change continuously.

Adaptive oversight addresses this challenge by establishing ongoing monitoring and review processes. Rather than approving a system once and assuming it will remain safe, regulators and healthcare organizations must continuously evaluate system performance.

Key elements of adaptive oversight may include:

- Periodic auditing of decision models
- Monitoring of outcome distributions across populations
- Real-time dashboards tracking system metrics
- Governance committees responsible for reviewing system updates

These mechanisms allow institutions to detect unintended consequences early and adjust decision policies accordingly. Adaptive oversight therefore aligns governance with the dynamic nature of probabilistic healthcare systems.

Transparency of System Behaviour

Transparency is a widely recognized principle in algorithmic governance. However, transparency in probabilistic systems requires a broader interpretation than simple disclosure of code or algorithms.

In many cases, even experts may struggle to interpret complex stochastic models. What matters for governance is not merely understanding the technical architecture of a system but understanding how the system behaves in practice.

Transparency of system behaviour therefore involves communicating key features such as:

- expected long-run outcome distributions
- probabilities of transitioning between system states
- potential trade-offs between efficiency and fairness

For clinicians and policymakers, such information may be more relevant than technical details of the algorithm itself. Visualizations, simulations, and scenario analysis tools can help decision-makers understand the implications of probabilistic policies.

Providing such transparency also enhances public trust. Patients and communities are more likely to accept algorithmic decision systems if institutions demonstrate how those systems affect access to care and health outcomes.

Alignment with Legal and Ethical Norms

Finally, probabilistic healthcare systems must operate within broader legal and ethical frameworks. Governance principles should therefore align with regulatory requirements and societal values.

As the comparative analysis demonstrates, different jurisdictions approach these issues differently. European frameworks emphasize risk-based oversight and algorithmic accountability, while U.S. regulation relies more heavily on market-based innovation and liability frameworks. Saudi Arabia combines centralized governance with ethical principles derived from Islamic jurisprudence.

Islamic bioethical traditions provide particularly relevant guidance for probabilistic healthcare governance. Concepts such as justice (‘adl), prevention of harm (darar), and promotion of public interest (maslahah) emphasize the importance of protecting vulnerable populations and ensuring equitable distribution of healthcare resources (Albar, 2018).

Embedding these principles within probabilistic decision systems reinforces the ethical foundations of healthcare institutions. It ensures that technological innovation remains aligned with moral commitments to fairness, dignity, and human welfare.

Together, these six principles provide a framework for governing probabilistic healthcare systems in ways that promote both efficiency and justice. Figure 3 illustrates how stochastic healthcare system architectures generate ethical risks through trajectory-level dynamics. Governance principles—including trajectory accountability, ergodicity-aware fairness, constraint-based optimization, and adaptive oversight—translate these risks into institutional governance mechanisms implemented by regulators, healthcare organizations, system designers, accreditation bodies, and the healthcare workforce.

POLICY AND IMPLEMENTATION IMPLICATIONS

The governance principles discussed in the preceding analysis highlight the need for institutional structures capable of overseeing probabilistic decision systems over time. While stochastic models offer powerful tools for managing uncertainty, their benefits can only be realized when supported by governance frameworks that ensure transparency, fairness, and accountability. Implementing such frameworks requires coordinated action across multiple institutional levels, including regulatory authorities, healthcare organizations, system designers, accreditation bodies, and the healthcare workforce. As illustrated in Figure 3, effective governance connects stochastic system design, ethical risk monitoring, and institutional oversight structures across regulatory and organizational domains.

This section outlines practical strategies for implementing ethical governance of probabilistic healthcare systems within these institutional domains.

Implications for Regulators

Regulatory institutions play a critical role in establishing governance frameworks for probabilistic decision systems deployed in healthcare environments. Traditional regulatory approaches often focus on discrete clinical interventions or static medical devices. However, stochastic healthcare systems operate through continuously evolving probabilistic processes whose outcomes emerge over time. As a result, regulatory oversight must move beyond one-time certification toward continuous system evaluation and adaptive governance.

One important regulatory strategy is the adoption of risk-based classification frameworks for algorithmic healthcare systems. Such approaches categorize decision systems according to the potential severity of harm they may produce and impose corresponding oversight requirements. The European Union's proposed Artificial Intelligence Act, for example, establishes regulatory obligations for high-risk AI systems, including requirements related to transparency, human oversight, and risk management (European Union, 2024). Similar risk-based regulatory approaches have been proposed in the United States for AI-enabled medical devices, where regulators emphasize post-market monitoring and lifecycle oversight (U.S. Food and Drug Administration, 2025).

For probabilistic healthcare systems specifically, regulators should also require longitudinal performance monitoring. Because harms may arise through cumulative system trajectories rather than single decisions, regulatory oversight should evaluate long-term outcome distributions across patient populations. This may involve periodic reporting of fairness metrics, transition probabilities across system states, or disparities in waiting times and treatment outcomes.

Regulatory authorities may also establish mechanisms for preventive intervention when probabilistic systems produce persistent inequities. Rather than relying solely on retrospective liability mechanisms, regulators could require healthcare organizations to demonstrate that their decision systems incorporate fairness constraints, monitoring dashboards, and human oversight mechanisms. Such approaches align with international guidance emphasizing the need for robust governance structures for artificial intelligence in healthcare (World Health Organization, 2021).

Through these strategies, regulators can ensure that probabilistic healthcare systems operate within legal frameworks that protect patient welfare while enabling technological innovation.

Implications for Healthcare Organizations

Healthcare organizations are responsible for integrating probabilistic decision systems into clinical operations. Effective governance therefore requires institutional structures capable of overseeing these systems in real-world environments. As healthcare decision-making increasingly relies on algorithmic and probabilistic models, organizations must develop governance mechanisms that ensure such systems operate within ethical, clinical, and regulatory boundaries.

Because probabilistic healthcare systems distribute decision-making across multiple actors—including system designers, administrators, and clinicians—responsibility for system outcomes cannot always be attributed to a single individual. Instead, governance frameworks must recognize that accountability in probabilistic systems is inherently distributed across the socio-technical ecosystem in which these systems operate (Mittelstadt et al., 2016; Selbst et al., 2019). In such environments, algorithmic outputs interact with clinical workflows, institutional policies, and regulatory requirements, making governance a shared institutional responsibility rather than a purely technical function.

Distributed Accountability and the Joint Responsibility Matrix

In stochastic healthcare systems, harms often arise not from individual decisions but from long-run system trajectories generated by repeated probabilistic transitions across system states (Ross, 2014; Gross et al., 2018). This creates what may be described as an accountability gap: when structural inequities emerge, it may be unclear whether responsibility lies with model designers, institutional decision-makers, or clinical users of the system.

To address this challenge, healthcare organizations should establish a Joint Responsibility Matrix that defines governance obligations across actors involved in probabilistic system design, deployment, and oversight. Rather than assigning responsibility retrospectively after harm occurs, the matrix establishes ex ante accountability structures, ensuring that monitoring and ethical oversight are clearly distributed across institutional actors. Such approaches align with emerging governance frameworks emphasizing institutional responsibility for AI systems deployed in healthcare settings (Cohen, 2020; World Health Organization, 2021).

Because probabilistic decision systems operate within institutional environments, responsibility for their outcomes cannot be attributed to a single actor. Instead, governance frameworks must allocate accountability across system designers, healthcare institutions, and clinical professionals (Elgujja, 2025a). Table 3 illustrates the distribution of governance responsibilities across key actors involved in the development, deployment, and oversight of probabilistic decision systems in healthcare. The matrix clarifies institutional accountability by defining the specific roles of technical experts, healthcare administrators, clinicians, regulators, and governance committees in ensuring that stochastic decision systems operate within ethical, legal, and operational safeguards.

Table 3. Joint Responsibility Matrix for Governance of Probabilistic Healthcare Systems

Actor	Governance Responsibility
Data scientists and system designers	Model validation, transition probability calibration, fairness constraint implementation, and detection of distribution shifts
Healthcare administrators	Monitoring outcome distributions, ensuring equitable resource allocation, and maintaining governance dashboards
Clinical leads	Exercising human-in-the-loop oversight and authorizing overrides when algorithmic recommendations conflict with clinical judgment
Regulatory authorities	Conducting external audits and ensuring compliance with legal and ethical standards
Ethics or governance committees	Reviewing fairness metrics and evaluating system impacts across patient populations

Healthcare organizations should also establish multidisciplinary governance committees responsible for reviewing system performance and recommending policy adjustments when necessary. These committees may include clinicians, data scientists, ethicists, and legal experts, ensuring that probabilistic decision systems are evaluated from both technical and ethical perspectives.

Additionally, organizations should develop monitoring dashboards that track key performance indicators related to probabilistic systems, including transition probabilities, waiting-time disparities across patient groups, and distributional outcomes across demographic categories. Continuous monitoring allows administrators to detect inequities and intervene promptly (Green, 2006; Hulshof et al., 2012).

Real-Time Governance: Monitoring and Automated Ethical Tripwires

While monitoring dashboards and governance committees provide essential oversight mechanisms, probabilistic healthcare systems may evolve more rapidly than traditional review processes can detect. Adaptive models that incorporate real-time data streams can experience model drift or distribution shift, where system behaviour gradually diverges from its original calibration as new data alter transition probabilities or decision policies. In such circumstances, periodic human review alone may be insufficient to detect emerging inequities or performance degradation (Selbst et al., 2019).

To address this challenge, healthcare organizations should incorporate automated ethical tripwires within the operational architecture of probabilistic decision systems. Ethical tripwires are predefined monitoring conditions that automatically trigger alerts or interventions when system behaviour exceeds acceptable ethical or operational thresholds. Rather than relying solely on retrospective evaluation, these mechanisms allow governance frameworks to operate proactively and continuously, aligning oversight with the real-time dynamics of adaptive healthcare systems.

Ethical tripwires may monitor several types of indicators. For example, systems may track waiting-time disparities between demographic groups, triggering alerts if the difference exceeds a predefined threshold such as 20%. Similarly, monitoring algorithms could evaluate recovery probability gaps across patient populations, flagging situations in which certain groups experience significantly lower probabilities of reaching favourable clinical states. In stochastic models, tripwires may also detect distribution shifts in state transition probabilities, indicating that the system's long-run behaviour has changed in ways that could produce unintended consequences.

When triggered, ethical tripwires can activate predefined governance responses. These responses may include temporarily suspending algorithmic updates, alerting oversight committees, or initiating automated policy reviews that examine whether system parameters should be recalibrated. In some cases, system designers may incorporate simulation tools that automatically test alternative decision policies before reactivating the algorithm.

Embedding such monitoring mechanisms aligns with broader frameworks for responsible AI governance that emphasize continuous system evaluation, risk management, and human oversight in algorithmically mediated healthcare systems (Cohen, 2020; World Health Organization, 2021). By integrating automated tripwires within probabilistic decision architectures, healthcare institutions can ensure that governance mechanisms evolve alongside the adaptive systems they are designed to supervise.

Ultimately, automated ethical tripwires represent an important complement to institutional oversight structures. Whereas governance committees and regulatory audits provide strategic supervision, real-time monitoring mechanisms enable organizations to detect emerging inequities or performance failures before they produce sustained harm. Together, these mechanisms help ensure that probabilistic healthcare systems remain aligned with ethical principles of fairness, accountability, and patient protection.

Clear escalation protocols should also be established. When monitoring systems detect persistent disparities or unexpected system behaviour, decision-makers should have procedures for reviewing and modifying decision policies. These may involve suspending algorithms, adjusting optimization parameters, or conducting simulation-based evaluations of alternative decision strategies (Ross, 2014; Gross et al., 2018).

Implications for System Designers and Developers

System designers and developers play a critical role in ensuring that probabilistic decision systems operate within ethically and legally acceptable parameters. Because stochastic healthcare systems produce outcomes through probabilistic transitions rather than deterministic rules, ethical considerations must be embedded directly within the design of system architectures.

One important approach is the use of constraint-based optimization. In such systems, ethical requirements—such as fairness constraints or minimum access guarantees—are encoded directly into optimization algorithms. Rather than maximizing efficiency alone, decision models are designed to operate within predefined ethical boundaries (Bertsimas & Kallus, 2020).

Designers should also ensure that probabilistic systems are auditable and interpretable. While stochastic models may be mathematically complex, system outputs should remain intelligible to clinicians and administrators responsible for oversight. This may involve providing explanations of how decision policies influence outcome probabilities across patient groups.

Simulation tools also play a critical role in ethical system design. By conducting scenario simulations, designers can evaluate how decision systems behave under varying conditions, including resource shortages, demand surges, or shifts in patient demographics. Such simulations allow developers to detect unintended consequences before systems are deployed in clinical environments (Ross, 2014; Gross et al., 2018).

Counterfactual Trajectory Visualizations and Interpretability

One of the principal challenges associated with probabilistic healthcare systems is the difficulty of interpreting stochastic decision models for non-technical users. Models based on Markov processes, queueing systems, or stochastic optimization often produce outcomes through complex probabilistic transitions rather than deterministic rules. While these models may be mathematically rigorous, their internal logic can remain opaque to clinicians, administrators, and patients responsible for interpreting or supervising their outputs. Without effective interpretability mechanisms, trajectory-level accountability risks becoming inaccessible to those most affected by algorithmic decisions (Mittelstadt et al., 2016; Selbst et al., 2019).

To address this challenge, healthcare decision systems should incorporate counterfactual trajectory visualizations that translate probabilistic model outputs into interpretable graphical representations. Rather than presenting clinicians with abstract probability distributions or algorithmic recommendations alone, such visualizations illustrate how different policy choices influence patient trajectories across possible health states.

For example, a decision-support interface may display the probabilities that a patient will transition to specific states within a Markov decision framework. A patient's projected trajectory might show the probability of reaching a recovery state recovery state (S_4), remaining in a treatment state treatment state (S_3), or transitioning to a deterioration state deterioration state (S_5). The interface could also generate counterfactual scenarios showing how these probabilities would change under alternative decision policies, such as earlier admission to isolation, allocation of additional resources, or different triage thresholds.

By presenting probabilistic outcomes through visual trajectories rather than numerical parameters alone, counterfactual visualizations allow clinicians to understand how algorithmic recommendations shape long-run outcomes. Such tools can improve clinical interpretability, enabling healthcare professionals to evaluate whether recommended policies align with clinical judgment and patient welfare.

Counterfactual trajectory visualizations also contribute to institutional accountability and transparency. When decision systems display how alternative policies influence outcome probabilities across patient groups, oversight committees and regulators can more easily evaluate whether algorithmic decision rules produce equitable outcomes. In this sense, visualization tools function not merely as user interfaces but as governance instruments that enable monitoring of probabilistic system behaviour.

From an ethical perspective, interpretability mechanisms are increasingly recognized as an essential component of responsible AI governance. Scholars in algorithmic ethics emphasize that decision systems must provide meaningful explanations to stakeholders affected by algorithmic outputs (Floridi et al., 2018; Mittelstadt et al., 2016). In healthcare contexts, interpretability is particularly important because clinicians retain ultimate responsibility for patient care decisions, even when assisted by algorithmic decision-support systems.

Embedding counterfactual trajectory visualizations within probabilistic decision architectures therefore represents a practical strategy for bridging the gap between technical model complexity and clinical usability. By enabling stakeholders to understand how stochastic decision policies influence patient outcomes over time, such tools help ensure that probabilistic healthcare systems remain both interpretable and ethically accountable.

Operational Deployment of Governance Controls

A healthcare organization should begin with a system inventory identifying each probabilistic tool, its clinical purpose, data sources, accountable owner, affected populations, regulatory status, and update frequency. The technical infrastructure should include version-controlled model repositories, secure event and override logs, data-quality monitoring, subgroup analytics, drift detection, simulation capability, and a dashboard linked to the electronic health record or operational data warehouse.

Oversight should sit with a multidisciplinary Probabilistic Systems Governance Committee chaired by a senior clinical or quality leader and including clinical users, data science, information security, legal, ethics, patient-safety, health-equity, and patient-representation functions. The committee should approve deployment, review validation and subgroup performance, set tripwire thresholds, authorize material model updates, and document decisions and escalation actions.

Thresholds should not be selected arbitrarily. Baselines should be established during local validation; clinically important differences should be defined with subject-matter experts; and simulation should estimate false-alert and missed-harm rates. A tripwire may combine an absolute floor, such as a minimum recovery probability, with a relative disparity threshold and a persistence rule over several review periods. Breaches should trigger graded responses: investigation, enhanced human review, recalibration, temporary suspension, and external notification where legally required.

A phased implementation is preferable: silent prospective validation, limited pilot deployment, monitored scale-up, and routine reassessment. Each phase should have predefined entry and exit criteria, rollback procedures, and evidence that clinicians understand when and how to override the system.

Workforce Development and Institutional Capacity

Effective governance of probabilistic healthcare systems also requires investments in workforce development. Healthcare professionals responsible for overseeing decision systems must possess sufficient understanding of probabilistic modelling, algorithmic governance, and ethical risk management.

Clinicians and administrators do not need to become technical experts in stochastic modelling, but they must understand the basic principles underlying probabilistic decision systems, including concepts such as state transitions, probability distributions, and long-run system behaviour. Such knowledge allows decision-makers to interpret system outputs and identify potential governance concerns.

Training programs may therefore be required to develop algorithmic literacy within healthcare organizations. Educational initiatives could include workshops on probabilistic reasoning, ethical governance of artificial intelligence, and regulatory compliance for digital health systems.

Interdisciplinary collaboration is equally important. Effective governance of probabilistic systems requires cooperation among clinicians, data scientists, ethicists, and legal experts. By developing institutional cultures that support such collaboration, healthcare organizations can ensure that probabilistic decision systems operate in ways that promote fairness, accountability, and patient welfare.

Institutionalizing Governance of Uncertainty

Collectively, the strategies described above illustrate how uncertainty can be transformed from a source of risk into a governable feature of healthcare systems. Rather than attempting to eliminate uncertainty, institutions can develop governance frameworks that monitor how probabilistic systems behave and intervene when necessary.

Such frameworks require collaboration across regulators, healthcare organizations, system designers, and the workforce. By aligning these actors around shared governance principles, healthcare systems can harness the benefits of probabilistic modelling while protecting against structural harm.

The discussion that follows concludes the chapter by reflecting on the broader implications of governing uncertainty in adaptive healthcare systems.

CONCLUSION

Healthcare systems operate within environments characterized by profound uncertainty, fluctuating patient demand, evolving disease dynamics, and constrained resources. To navigate this complexity, modern health systems increasingly rely on probabilistic decision models such as Markov processes, queueing systems, and stochastic optimization frameworks. These tools enable healthcare institutions to anticipate demand, allocate resources dynamically, and respond adaptively to changing operational conditions.

However, as this chapter has demonstrated, the adoption of probabilistic decision systems also introduces significant ethical and legal challenges. Unlike traditional clinical decision-making, where responsibility can often be traced to individual actors, stochastic systems produce outcomes through long-run system trajectories generated by repeated probabilistic transitions. In such systems, harms may emerge cumulatively across time and populations, making them difficult to detect using governance frameworks designed for discrete decisions.

This chapter therefore advances the argument that effective governance of probabilistic healthcare systems requires a shift from decision-level accountability to trajectory-level governance. By examining how stochastic models shape healthcare outcomes over time, institutions can identify structural inequities that might otherwise remain hidden within complex system dynamics. Concepts such as ergodicity, transition probabilities, and steady-state distributions provide valuable analytical tools for evaluating the long-run fairness and sustainability of healthcare decision systems.

The chapter has proposed a set of design principles for governing probabilistic healthcare systems, including trajectory-level accountability, ergodicity-aware fairness, constraint-based optimization, adaptive oversight, transparency of system behavior, and alignment with legal and ethical norms. Together, these principles translate abstract ethical commitments into operational governance mechanisms capable of addressing the challenges posed by adaptive decision systems.

The analysis has also highlighted the importance of institutional governance structures. Regulators must develop oversight frameworks capable of monitoring long-term system behaviour, healthcare organizations must implement internal monitoring and accountability mechanisms, system designers must embed ethical constraints within algorithmic architectures, and healthcare professionals must develop the knowledge required to supervise probabilistic decision tools responsibly.

Ultimately, the governance of uncertainty represents one of the defining challenges of contemporary healthcare systems. Probabilistic models offer powerful capabilities for managing complexity and improving operational efficiency, but their benefits can only be realized if they operate within transparent and ethically accountable governance structures. By reframing uncertainty as a governable feature of adaptive healthcare systems, this chapter provides a framework for integrating stochastic modelling with ethical and legal oversight.

Such integration allows healthcare institutions to harness the analytical power of probabilistic systems while preserving the foundational principles of medical practice: fairness, accountability, transparency, and the protection of patient welfare. In doing so, the chapter contributes to the broader goal of designing healthcare systems that are not only technologically advanced but also ethically resilient in the face of uncertainty.

As healthcare systems increasingly rely on probabilistic and AI-driven decision tools, developing governance frameworks capable of managing uncertainty will become an essential component of ethical and resilient healthcare system design.

DISCLOSURE OF ARTIFICIAL INTELLIGENCE USE

During the preparation and revision of this work, the author used OpenAI's ChatGPT for language refinement, structural editing, and literature organization. The author independently verified the sources, reviewed and edited the content, and takes full responsibility for the accuracy and integrity of the chapter.

REFERENCES

Albar, M. A. (2018). Islamic bioethics and healthcare decision-making. *Journal of Religion and Health*, *57*(1), 1–14. DOI: 10.1007/s10943-017-0387-3 PMID: 26160145

Allen, L. J. S. (2017). *A primer on stochastic epidemic models*. Springer., DOI: 10.1007/978-3-319-50806-1

Barocas, S., & Selbst, A. D. (2016). Big data's disparate impact. *California Law Review*, *104*(3), 671–732. DOI: 10.15779/Z38BG31

Bertsimas, D., & Dunn, J. (2017). Optimal classification trees. *Machine Learning*, *106*(7), 1039–1082. DOI: 10.1007/s10994-017-5633-9

Bertsimas, D., & Kallus, N. (2020). From predictive to prescriptive analytics. *Management Science*, *66*(3), 1025–1044. DOI: 10.1287/mnsc.2018.3253

Cohen, I. G. (2020). Regulating artificial intelligence in healthcare: Risk, trust, and governance. *Health Affairs*, *39*(7), 1135–1142. DOI: 10.1377/hlthaff.2020.00473

Elgujja, A. (2020). Impact of information technology on patient confidentiality rights: A perspective. In Cruz-Cunha, M. M. (Eds.), *Impacts of information technology on patient care and empowerment* (pp. 129–148). IGI Global., DOI: 10.4018/978-1-7998-0047-7.ch018

Elgujja, A. (2025a). *AI governance as a human right imperative: Embedding transparency, accountability, and reasoned justification in the algorithmic state. SSRN*. https://doi.org/DOI: 10.2139/ssrn.5646110

European Parliament and Council of the European Union. (2024). *Regulation (EU) 2024/1689 of the European Parliament and of the Council of 13 June 2024 laying down harmonised rules on artificial intelligence (Artificial Intelligence Act) and amending certain Union legislative acts. Official Journal of the European Union*. https://eur-lex.europa.eu/eli/reg/2024/1689/oj

Floridi, L., Cowls, J., Beltrametti, M., Chazerand, P., Chila, R., Dignum, V., Luetge, C., Madelin, R., Pagallo, U., Rossi, F., Schafer, B., Valcke, P., & Vayena, E. (2018). AI4People—An ethical framework for a good AI society. *Minds and Machines*, *28*(4), 689–707. DOI: 10.1007/s11023-018-9482-5 PMID: 30930541

Green, L. V. (2006). Queueing analysis in healthcare. In Hall, R. W. (Ed.), *Patient flow: Reducing delay in healthcare delivery* (pp. 281–307). Springer., DOI: 10.1007/978-0-387-33636-7_10

Gross, D., Shortle, J. F., Thompson, J. M., & Harris, C. M. (2018). *Fundamentals of queueing theory* (5th ed.). Wiley., DOI: 10.1002/9781119453765

Hulshof, P. J. H., Kortbeek, N., Boucherie, R. J., Hans, E. W., & Bakker, P. J. M. (2012). Taxonomic classification of planning decisions in health care. *Health Systems (Basingstoke, England)*, *1*(2), 129–175. DOI: 10.1057/hs.2012.18

Keeling, M. J., & Rohani, P. (2008). *Modeling infectious diseases in humans and animals*. Princeton University Press., DOI: 10.1515/9781400841035

Kleinberg, J., Mullainathan, S., & Raghavan, M. (2017). Inherent trade-offs in the fair determination of risk scores. In *Proceedings of the 8th Innovations in Theoretical Computer Science Conference* (Article 43). Schloss Dagstuhl–Leibniz-Zentrum für Informatik. https://doi.org/DOI: 10.4230/LIPIcs.ITCS.2017.43

Miller, W. D., Han, X., Peek, M. E., Ashana, D. C., & Parker, W. F.. (2021). Accuracy of the Sequential Organ Failure Assessment score for in-hospital mortality by race and relevance to crisis standards of care. *JAMA Network Open*, *4*(6), e2113891. DOI: 10.1001/jamanetworkopen.2021.13891 PMID: 34143190

Mittelstadt, B. D., Allo, P., Taddeo, M., Wachter, S., & Floridi, L. (2016). The ethics of algorithms: Mapping the debate. *Big Data & Society*, *3*(2), 2053951716679679. Advance online publication. DOI: 10.1177/2053951716679679

Obermeyer, Z., Powers, B., Vogeli, C., & Mullainathan, S. (2019). Dissecting racial bias in an algorithm used to manage the health of populations. *Science*, *366*(6464), 447–453. DOI: 10.1126/science.aax2342 PMID: 31649194

Rajkomar, A., Dean, J., & Kohane, I. (2019). Machine learning in medicine. *The New England Journal of Medicine*, *380*(14), 1347–1358. DOI: 10.1056/NEJMra1814259 PMID: 30943338

Ross, S. M. (2014). *Introduction to probability models* (11th ed.). Academic Press., DOI: 10.1016/C2012-0-06001-5

Saudi Data and Artificial Intelligence Authority. (2023). *Personal Data Protection Law*. https://sdaia.gov.sa/en/SDAIA/about/Documents/Personal%20Data%20English%20V2-23April2023-%20Reviewed-.pdf

Selbst, A. D., Boyd, D., Friedler, S. A., Venkatasubramanian, S., & Vertesi, J. (2019). Fairness and abstraction in sociotechnical systems. In *Proceedings of the 2019 Conference on Fairness, Accountability, and Transparency* (pp. 59–68). Association for Computing Machinery. https://doi.org/DOI: 10.1145/3287560.3287598

U.S. Food and Drug Administration. (2025). *Artificial intelligence-enabled device software functions: Lifecycle management and marketing submission recommendations—Draft guidance for industry and Food and Drug Administration staff*. https://www.fda.gov/regulatory-information/search-fda-guidance-documents/artificial-intelligence-enabled-device-software-functions-lifecycle-management-and-marketing

Voigt, P., & von dem Bussche, A. (2017). *The EU General Data Protection Regulation (GDPR): A practical guide*. Springer., DOI: 10.1007/978-3-319-57959-7

World Health Organization. (2021). *Ethics and governance of artificial intelligence for health: WHO guidance*. World Health Organization. https://www.who.int/publications/i/item/9789240029200

Compilation of References

Abràmoff, M. D., Tarver, M. E., Loyo-Berríos, N., Trujillo, S., Char, D., Obermeyer, Z., Eydelman, M., & Maisel, W. H. (2023). Considerations for addressing bias in artificial intelligence for health equity. *NPJ Digital Medicine*, *6*(1), 170. DOI: 10.1038/s41746-023-00913-9 PMID: 37700029

Aceto, G., Persico, V., & Pescapé, A. (2020). The role of information and communication technologies in healthcare: Taxonomies, perspectives, and challenges. *Journal of Network and Computer Applications*, *107*, 125–154.

Aceto, G., Persico, V., & Pescapé, A. (2024). Artificial intelligence for healthcare sustainability: Challenges, opportunities, and future directions. *Journal of Healthcare Engineering*, *2024*, 1–18.

Achiam, J., Held, D., Tamar, A., & Abbeel, P. (2017). Constrained policy optimization. In *Proceedings of the 34th International Conference on Machine Learning* (Vol. 70, pp. 22–31). PMLR.

Akarkach, M. (2026). *Inference as the exposure event: Implications for legal discovery, audit, and institutional governance. Zenodo.* DOI: 10.5281/zenodo.18993386

Alagoz, O., Hsu, H., Schaefer, A. J., & Roberts, M. S. (2010). Markov decision processes: A tool for sequential decision making under uncertainty. *Medical Decision Making*, *30*(4), 474–483. DOI: 10.1177/0272989X09353194 PMID: 20044582

Albar, M. A. (2018). Islamic bioethics and healthcare decision-making. *Journal of Religion and Health*, *57*(1), 1–14. DOI: 10.1007/s10943-017-0387-3 PMID: 26160145

Ali, H. (2022). Reinforcement learning in healthcare: Optimizing treatment strategies, dynamic resource allocation, and adaptive clinical decision-making. *International Journal of Computer Applications Technology and Research*, *11*(3), 88–104.

Ali, M. A. (2026). A broad review of AI and machine learning in healthcare informatics for predictive analytics, data analytics, and healthcare supply chain systems. *Global Trends in Science and Technology*, *43*, 43. Advance online publication. DOI: 10.70445/gtst.2.2.2026.43-63

Allen, L. J. S. (2017). *A primer on stochastic epidemic models*. Springer., DOI: 10.1007/978-3-319-50806-1

Allen, T., Manjunatha, I. G., Khoni, N. S., & Allen, A. (2026). *Noise-aware mathematical frameworks for artificial intelligence in predictive clinical decision-making: From stochastic dynamics to regulatory compliance. Zenodo.* DOI: 10.5281/zenodo.18501207

Alowais, S. A., Alghamdi, S. S., Alsuhebany, N., Alqahtani, T., Alshaya, A. I., Almohareb, S. N., Aldairem, A., Alrashed, M., Bin Saleh, K., Badreddin, H. A., Al Yami, M. S., Al Harbi, S., & Albekairy, A. M. (2023). Revolutionizing healthcare: The role of artificial intelligence in clinical practice. *BMC Medical Education, 23*(1), 689. Advance online publication. DOI: 10.1186/s12909-023-04698-z PMID: 37740191

Al-Sarayrah, A. (2024). Recent Advances and Applications of Apriori Algorithm in Exploring insights from Healthcare Data Patterns. *PatternIQ Mining, 1*(2). Advance online publication. DOI: 10.70023/piqm24123

Amutha, M. (2026). Cloud-powered intelligent ecosystems for secure healthcare analytics with artificial intelligence-driven innovation. *International Journal of Technology. Management and Humanities, 12*(1), 108–115.

Anand, A. (2025). Beyond the Epidemic Diseases Act, 1897: Rethinking India's public health laws for pandemic preparedness—Lessons from Singapore. *The Journal of Communicable Diseases, 57*(1), 33–43. DOI: 10.24321/0019.5138.202504

Anandkumar, A., Hsu, D., & Kakade, S. M. (2012). A method of moments for mixture models and hidden Markov models. In *Proceedings of the 25th Annual Conference on Learning Theory* (Vol. 23, pp. 33.1–33.34). PMLR.

Andersen, P. K., & Keiding, N. (2002). Multi-state models for event history analysis. *Statistical Methods in Medical Research, 11*(2), 91–115. DOI: 10.1191/0962280202SM276ra PMID: 12040698

Anderson, J. W., & Visweswaran, S. (2025). Algorithmic individual fairness and healthcare: A scoping review. *JAMIA Open, 8*(1), ooae149. DOI: 10.1093/jamiaopen/ooae149 PMID: 39737346

Angus, D. C., Linde-Zwirble, W. T., Lidicker, J., Clermont, G., Carcillo, J., & Pinsky, M. R. (2001). Epidemiology of severe sepsis in the United States: Analysis of incidence, outcome, and associated costs of care. *Critical Care Medicine, 29*(7), 1303–1310. DOI: 10.1097/00003246-200107000-00002 PMID: 11445675

Antoniadi, A. M., Du, Y., Guendouz, Y., Wei, L., Mazo, C., Becker, B. A., & Mooney, C. (2021). Current challenges and future opportunities for XAI in machine learning-based clinical decision support systems: A systematic review. *Applied Sciences (Basel, Switzerland), 11*(11), 5088. DOI: 10.3390/app11115088

Anupallavi, S., Ashokkumar, S. R., Premkumar, M., & Sangeetha, R. (2025). Enhanced EEG signal classification through integrated DTCWT, human learning optimization, and optimized DBN-HMM models for improved performance. *Biomedical Signal Processing and Control, 110*, 108229. DOI: 10.1016/j.bspc.2025.108229

Arora, A., Alderman, J., Palmer, J., Ganapathi, S., Laws, E., McCradden, M. D., Oakden-Rayner, L., Pfohl, S., Ghassemi, M., McKay, F., Treanor, D., Rostamzadeh, N., Mateen, B. A., Gath, J., Adebajo, A. O., Kuku, S., Matin, R., Heller, K., Sapey, E., & Liu, X. (2023). The value of standards for health datasets in artificial intelligence-based applications. *Nature Medicine, 29*(11), 2929–2938. DOI: 10.1038/s41591-023-02608-w PMID: 37884627

Ashby, W. R. (1956). *An introduction to cybernetics*. Chapman & Hall. DOI: 10.5962/bhl.title.5851

Asplin, B. R., Magid, D. J., Rhodes, K. V., Solberg, L. I., Lurie, N., & Camargo, C. A.Jr. (2003). A conceptual model of emergency department crowding. *Annals of Emergency Medicine*, *42*(2), 173–180. DOI: 10.1067/mem.2003.302 PMID: 12883504

Åström, K. J. (1965). Optimal control of Markov processes with incomplete state information. *Journal of Mathematical Analysis and Applications*, *10*(1), 174–205. DOI: 10.1016/0022-247X(65)90154-X

Aunugu, D. R., & Vathsavai, V. G. (2025). Cloud-based AI solutions for scalable and intelligent enterprise modernization. *ICCK Transactions on Emerging Topics in Artificial Intelligence*, *2*(2), 81–89. DOI: 10.62762/TETAI.2025.100106

Babu, A., & Boddu, S. B. (2024). BERT-Based Medical Chatbot: Enhancing Healthcare Communication through Natural Language Understanding. *Exploratory Research in Clinical and Social Pharmacy*, *13*, 100419. DOI: 10.1016/j.rcsop.2024.100419 PMID: 38495953

Bag, V. V., Patil, M. B., & Nagnath Kendre, S. (2024). Frequent CNN based ensembling for MRI classification for Abnormal Brain Growth detection. *Journal of Integrated Science and Technology*, *12*(3). Advance online publication. DOI: 10.62110/sciencein.jist.2024.v12.785

Balderrama, R., Peressutti, J., & Vanquez, P. (2022). Optimal control for a SIR epidemic model with limited quarantine. *Scientific Reports*, *12*(1), 12583. DOI: 10.1038/s41598-022-16619-z PMID: 35869150

Barabási, A.-L. (2016). *Network science*. Cambridge University Press.

Barabási, A.-L., & Albert, R. (1999). Emergence of scaling in random networks. *Science*, *286*(5439), 509–512. DOI: 10.1126/science.286.5439.509 PMID: 10521342

Barocas, S., & Selbst, A. D. (2016). Big data's disparate impact. *California Law Review*, *104*(3), 671–732. DOI: 10.15779/Z38BG31

Basseville, M., & Nikiforov, I. V. (1993). *Detection of abrupt changes: Theory and application*. Prentice Hall.

Bastani, O., Kim, C., & Bastani, H. (2017). Interpretability via model extraction. arXiv. https://arxiv.org/abs/1706.09773

Bates, D. W., Saria, S., Ohno-Machado, L., Shah, A., & Escobar, G. (2014). Big data in health care: Using analytics to identify and manage high-risk and high-cost patients. *Health Affairs*, *33*(7), 1123–1131. DOI: 10.1377/hlthaff.2014.0041 PMID: 25006137

Batty, M. (2018). *Digital twins*. MIT Press.

Baucum, M., & Khojandi, A. (2023). Markov decision processes: Application to treatment planning. In Pardalos, P. M., & Prokopyev, O. A. (Eds.), *Encyclopedia of optimization*. Springer., DOI: 10.1007/978-3-030-54621-2_844-1

Baum, L. E., Petrie, T., Soules, G., & Weiss, N. (1970). A maximization technique occurring in the statistical analysis of probabilistic functions of Markov chains. *Annals of Mathematical Statistics*, *41*(1), 164–171. DOI: 10.1214/aoms/1177697196

Beck, J. R., & Pauker, S. G. (1983). The Markov process in medical prognosis. *Medical Decision Making, 3*(4), 419–458. DOI: 10.1177/0272989X8300300403 PMID: 6668990

Begun, J. W., Zimmerman, B., & Dooley, K. (2003). Health care organizations as complex adaptive systems. In Mick, S. S., & Wyttenbach, M. (Eds.), *Advances in health care organization theory* (pp. 253–288). Jossey-Bass.

Bennett, C. C., & Hauser, K. (2013). Artificial intelligence framework for simulating clinical decision-making: A Markov decision process approach. *Artificial Intelligence in Medicine, 57*(1), 9–19. DOI: 10.1016/j.artmed.2012.12.003 PMID: 23287490

Berdahl, C. T., Baker, L., Mann, S., Osoba, O., & Girosi, F. (2023). Strategies to improve the impact of artificial intelligence on health equity: Scoping review. *JMIR AI, 2*, e42936. DOI: 10.2196/42936 PMID: 38875587

Bergman, R. N., Ider, Y. Z., Bowden, C. R., & Cobelli, C. (1979). Quantitative estimation of insulin sensitivity. *American Journal of Physiology. Endocrinology and Metabolism, 236*(6), E667–E677. DOI: 10.1152/ajpendo.1979.236.6.E667 PMID: 443421

Berry, D. A. (2025). Adaptive Bayesian clinical trials: The past, present, and future of clinical research. *Journal of Clinical Medicine, 14*(15), 5267. Advance online publication. DOI: 10.3390/jcm14155267 PMID: 40806890

Bertozzi, A. L., Franco, E., Mohler, G., Short, M. B., & Sledge, D. (2020). The challenges of modeling and forecasting the spread of COVID-19. *Proceedings of the National Academy of Sciences of the United States of America, 117*(29), 16732–16738. DOI: 10.1073/pnas.2006520117 PMID: 32616574

Bertsekas, D. P. (2017). *Dynamic programming and optimal control* (4th ed.). Athena Scientific.

Bertsimas, D., & Dunn, J. (2017). Optimal classification trees. *Machine Learning, 106*(7), 1039–1082. DOI: 10.1007/s10994-017-5633-9

Bertsimas, D., & Kallus, N. (2020). From predictive to prescriptive analytics. *Management Science, 66*(3), 1025–1044. DOI: 10.1287/mnsc.2018.3253

Beyan, O., Choudhury, A., van Soest, J., Kohlbacher, O., Zimmermann, L., Stenzhorn, H., Karim, M. R., Dumontier, M., Decker, S., da Silva Santos, L. O. B., & Dekker, A. (2019). Distributed analytics on sensitive medical data: The Personal Health Train. *Data Intelligence, 2*(1-2), 96–107. DOI: 10.1162/dint_a_00032

Bhandari, A. (2024). Revolutionizing Radiology With Artificial Intelligence. *Cureus*. Advance online publication. DOI: 10.7759/cureus.72646 PMID: 39474591

Bhardwaj, K., & Johari, V. (2022). COVID-19 vaccines in India: Judicial blind spots in upholding the right to health. *Socio-Legal Review, 18*(1), 119. DOI: 10.55496/EONP8082

Bhatia, M., Nagpal, M., & Jaswal, A. (2025). Adaptive therapeutics through AI-enhanced nanoscale sensors: Innovations in real-time health monitoring. In *3rd International Conference on Disruptive Technologies (ICDT)* (pp. 845–850). IEEE. DOI: 10.1109/ICDT63985.2025.10986393

Bica, I., Alaa, A. M., Lambert, C., & Van Der Schaar, M. (2021). From real-world patient data to individualized treatment effects using machine learning: Current and future methods to address underlying challenges. *Clinical Pharmacology and Therapeutics*, *109*(1), 87–100. DOI: 10.1002/cpt.1907 PMID: 32449163

Bijjargi, P. (2026). Digital human rights under the Indian Constitution: Emerging jurisprudence and policy challenges. *International Journal for Multidisciplinary Research*, *8*(1), 69665. Advance online publication. DOI: 10.36948/ijfmr.2026.v08i01.69665

Bjørnskov, C., & Voigt, S. (2021). This time is different?—On the use of emergency measures during the corona pandemic. *European Journal of Law and Economics*, *54*(1), 63–81. DOI: 10.1007/s10657-021-09706-5 PMID: 35924085

Blei, D. M., Kucukelbir, A., & McAuliffe, J. D. (2017). Variational inference: A review for statisticians. *Journal of the American Statistical Association*, *112*(518), 859–877. DOI: 10.1080/01621459.2017.1285773

Bobade, P., & Vani, M. (2020). Stress detection with machine learning and deep learning using multimodal physiological data. In *Proceedings of the International Conference on Intelligent Computing and Remote Sensing Applications (ICIRCA)* (pp. 51–57). https://doi.org/DOI: 10.1109/ICIRCA48905.2020.9183244

Bocean, C. G., & Vărzaru, A. A. (2024). Assessing social protection influence on health status in the European Union. *Frontiers in Public Health*, *12*, 1287608. DOI: 10.3389/fpubh.2024.1287608 PMID: 38528863

Borkowski, A. (2025). Multiagent AI systems in health care: Envisioning next-generation intelligence. *Federal Practitioner : for the Health Care Professionals of the VA, DoD, and PHS*, *42*(5), 188–195. DOI: 10.12788/fp.0589 PMID: 40831649

Bouderhem, R. (2026). Artificial intelligence in healthcare: Ethical challenges and promoting clinical equity and transparency. In *Handbook of Tissue Reconstruction and Regeneration* (pp. 1–29). Springer Nature Singapore. DOI: 10.1007/978-981-96-7448-0_29-1

Boutilier, C., Dean, T., & Hanks, S. (1999). Decision-theoretic planning: Structural assumptions and computational leverage. *Journal of Artificial Intelligence Research*, *11*, 1–94. DOI: 10.1613/jair.575

Brahman, K. S., & Pandey, A. (2026). AI-driven adaptive patient care framework for personalized medicine and optimized health outcomes. In *Recent advances in technology & management* (pp. 170–174). CRC Press., DOI: 10.1201/9781003768630-33

Brailsford, S. C., Harper, P. R., Patel, B., & Pitt, M. (2009). An analysis of the academic literature on simulation and modelling in healthcare. *Journal of Simulation*, *3*(3), 130–140. DOI: 10.1057/jos.2009.10

Brailsford, S. C., Lattimer, V. A., Tarnaras, P., & Turnbull, J. C. (2004). Emergency and on-demand health care: Modelling a large complex system. *The Journal of the Operational Research Society*, *55*(1), 34–42. DOI: 10.1057/palgrave.jors.2601667

Braithwaite, J., Churruca, K., Ellis, L. A., Long, J., Clay-Williams, R., Damen, N., Herkes, J., Pomare, C., & Ludlow, K. (2017). *Complexity science in healthcare: aspirations, approaches, applications and accomplishments: a white paper*. Macquarie University. https://www.mq.edu.au/research/research-centres-groups-and-facilities/healthy-people/centres/australian-institute-of-health-innovation/news-and-events/news/news/complexity-science-in-healthcare-aspirations,-approaches,-applications-and-accomplishments-a-white-paper

Briggs, A., & Sculpher, M. (1998). An introduction to Markov modelling for economic evaluation. *PharmacoEconomics, 13*(4), 397–409. PMID: 10178664

Briggs, A., Sculpher, M., & Claxton, K. (2006). *Decision modelling for health economic evaluation*. Oxford University Press. DOI: 10.1093/oso/9780198526629.001.0001

Campagner, A., Biganzoli, E. M., Balsano, C., Cereda, C., & Cabitza, F. (2025). Modeling unknowns: A vision for uncertainty-aware machine learning in healthcare. *International Journal of Medical Informatics, 203*, 106014. Advance online publication. DOI: 10.1016/j.ijmedinf.2025.106014 PMID: 40603232

Cappé, O., & Moulines, E. (2009). On-line expectation–maximization algorithm for latent data models. *Journal of the Royal Statistical Society. Series B, Statistical Methodology, 71*(3), 593–613. DOI: 10.1111/j.1467-9868.2009.00698.x

Cassandra, A. R., Littman, M. L., & Zhang, N. L. (1997). Incremental pruning: A simple, fast, exact method for partially observable Markov decision processes. In *Proceedings of the Thirteenth Conference on Uncertainty in Artificial Intelligence* (pp. 54–61). Morgan Kaufmann.

Celi, L. A., Mark, R. G., Stone, D. J., & Montgomery, R. A. (2013). "Big data" in the intensive care unit: Closing the data loop. *American Journal of Respiratory and Critical Care Medicine, 187*(11), 1157–1160. DOI: 10.1164/rccm.201212-2311ED PMID: 23725609

Chakraborty, B., & Moodie, E. E. M. (2013). *Statistical Methods for Dynamic Treatment Regimes*. Springer., DOI: 10.1007/978-1-4614-7428-9

Chalishajar, D., Kasinathan, R., Kasinathan, R., Kasinathan, D., & David, J. A. (2025). Ulam-Hyers-Rassias stability for fractional stochastic impulsive differential equations driven by time-changed Brownian motion followed by credit risk modeling. *Journal of Applied Mathematics & Computing, 71*(S1, Suppl. 1), 883–906. DOI: 10.1007/s12190-025-02497-x

Chaudhry, B., Wang, J., Wu, S., Maglione, M., Mojica, W., Roth, E., Morton, S. C., & Shekelle, P. G. (2006). Systematic review: Impact of health information technology on quality, efficiency, and costs. *Annals of Internal Medicine, 144*(10), 742–752. DOI: 10.7326/0003-4819-144-10-200605160-00125 PMID: 16702590

Chen, G., & O'Malley, A. J. (2024). Bayesian Hierarchical Network Autocorrelation Models for Estimating Direct and Indirect Effects of Peer Hospitals on Outcomes of Hospitalized Patients. Research square, rs.3.rs-4014583. https://doi.org/DOI: 10.21203/rs.3.rs-4014583/v1

Cheng, H.-T. (1988). *Algorithms for partially observable Markov decision processes* [Doctoral dissertation, University of British Columbia]. UBC Library.

Chen, J., Lowin, M., Kellner, D., Hinz, O., Adam, E. H., Ippolito, A., & Wenger-Alakmeh, K. (2023). Designing expert-augmented clinical decision support systems to predict mortality risk in ICUs. *Kunstliche Intelligenz, 37*(2-4), 227–236. DOI: 10.1007/s13218-023-00808-7

Chen, S., Liu, T., Sun, Z., Jia, J., Hang, D., & Zhang, W. (2026a). Markov Decision Process–Based Personalized Follow-Up Planning for Type 2 Diabetes: Retrospective Cohort Study. *JMIR Medical Informatics, 14*(1), e88206. DOI: 10.2196/88206 PMID: 42686193

Chen, S., Zhang, X., Liu, E., Xiong, Y., Wang, L., Gu, X., Wang, Z., Guo, J., & Luo, T. (2026b). Privacy-preserving cloud-based dermatological image processing for medical applications: A review. *Journal of Cloud Computing (Heidelberg, Germany), 15*(1), 46. Advance online publication. DOI: 10.1186/s13677-026-00886-6

Chen, Y., Clayton, E. W., Novak, L. L., Anders, S., & Malin, B. (2023). Human-centered design to address biases in artificial intelligence. *Journal of Medical Internet Research, 25*, e43251. DOI: 10.2196/43251 PMID: 36961506

Chen, Y.-X., Shih, G.-Y., Ting, H.-W., & Chien, T.-Y. (2024). Base on GAN Combined with CNN Architecture to Generate Brain Stroke CT Images. *Proceedings of the 2024 8th International Conference on Medical and Health Informatics,* 47–51. DOI: 10.1145/3673971.3674024

Chigboh, V. M., Zouo, S. J. C., & Olamijuwon, J. (2024). Health data analytics for precision medicine: A review of current practices and future directions. *International Medical Science Research Journal, 4*(11), 973–984. DOI: 10.51594/imsrj.v4i11.1732

Cho, H., Froelicher, D., Dokmai, N., Nandi, A., Sadhuka, S., Hong, M. M., & Berger, B. (2024). Privacy-enhancing technologies in biomedical data science. *Annual Review of Biomedical Data Science, 7*(1), 317–343. DOI: 10.1146/annurev-biodatasci-120423-120107 PMID: 39178425

Christensen, C. M. (1997). *The innovator's dilemma: When new technologies cause great firms to fail.* Harvard Business School Press.

Chu, A., Huber, G., McGeever, A., Veytsman, B., & Yllanes, D. (2021). A random-walk-based epidemiological model. *Scientific Reports, 11*(1), 18134. DOI: 10.1038/s41598-021-98211-5 PMID: 34588487

Churpek, M. M., Yuen, T. C., & Edelson, D. P. (2013). Risk stratification of hospitalized patients on the wards. *Chest, 143*(6), 1758–1765. DOI: 10.1378/chest.12-1605 PMID: 23732586

Çınlar, E. (2011). *Probability and stochastics*. Springer., DOI: 10.1007/978-0-387-87859-1

Clauset, A., Shalizi, C. R., & Newman, M. E. J. (2009). Power-law distributions in empirical data. *SIAM Review, 51*(4), 661–703. DOI: 10.1137/070710111

Cleynen, A., de Saporta, B., Rossini, O., Sabbadin, R., & Vernay, A. (2026). *Bridging impulse control of piecewise deterministic Markov processes and Markov decision processes: Review and open challenges.*

Cochran, J. K., & Bharti, A. (2006). Stochastic bed balancing of an obstetrics hospital. *Health Care Management Science, 9*(1), 31–45. DOI: 10.1007/s10729-006-6278-6 PMID: 16613015

Cohen, I. G. (2020). Regulating artificial intelligence in healthcare: Risk, trust, and governance. *Health Affairs*, *39*(7), 1135–1142. DOI: 10.1377/hlthaff.2020.00473

Conforti, D., Guerriero, F., & Guido, R. (2011). Optimization models for radiotherapy patient scheduling. *European Journal of Operational Research*, *210*(1), 129–138. DOI: 10.1016/j.ejor.2010.09.005

Cossette-Lefebvre, H., & Maclure, J. (2022). AI's fairness problem: Understanding wrongful discrimination in the context of automated decision-making. *AI and Ethics*, *3*(4), 1255–1269. DOI: 10.1007/s43681-022-00233-w

Crowson, M. G., Tan, J. Z. H., Dunn, J., Bhatt, J., Schneider, Z., Forger, D. B., Celi, L. A., Dorotić, M., & Malin, B. (2026). The need to develop health data transaction disclosure requirements to balance transparency, privacy, and progressive use. *The Lancet. Digital Health*, *8*(2), 100947. DOI: 10.1016/j.landig.2025.100947 PMID: 41792017

Curcin, V., Delaney, B., Alkhatib, A., Cockburn, N., Dann, O., Kostopoulou, O., Leightley, D., Maddocks, M., Modgil, S., Nirantharakumar, K., Scott, P., Wolfe, I., Zhang, K., & Friedman, C. (2025). Learning health systems provide a glide path to safe landing for AI in health. *Artificial Intelligence in Medicine*, *173*, 103346. DOI: 10.1016/j.artmed.2025.103346 PMID: 41506062

Curtis, K., Munroe, B., Fry, M., Considine, J., Tuala, E., Watts, M., Alkhouri, H., Elphick, T., Ruperto, K., Barrass, J., Balzer, S., Chisholm, B., Van, C., & Shaban, R. Z. (2021). The implementation of an emergency nursing framework (HIRAID) reduces patient deterioration: A multi-centre quasi-experimental study. *International Emergency Nursing*, *56*, 100976. DOI: 10.1016/j.ienj.2021.100976 PMID: 33882400

d'Epenoux, F. (1963). A probabilistic production and inventory problem. *Management Science*, *10*(1), 98–108. DOI: 10.1287/mnsc.10.1.98

Davis, M. H. A., & Vinter, R. B. (1985). *Stochastic modelling and control*. Chapman and Hall. DOI: 10.1007/978-94-009-4828-0

de Jong, I. P., Sburlea, A. I., & Valdenegro-Toro, M. (2026). Uncertainty quantification in machine learning for biosignal applications-a review. *Journal of Healthcare Informatics Research*, **•••**, 1–55. DOI: 10.1007/s41666-026-00249-5

Deisenroth, M. P., & Peters, J. (2012). Solving nonlinear continuous state-action-observation POMDPs for mechanical systems with Gaussian noise. In *Proceedings of the European Workshop on Reinforcement Learning*.

Dekker, S. (2011). *Drift into failure: From hunting broken components to understanding complex systems*. CRC Press.

Deming, W. E. (2000a). *Out of the crisis*. MIT Press.

Deming, W. E. (2000b). *The new economics: For industry, government, education* (2nd ed.). MIT Press.

Dempster, A. P., Laird, N. M., & Rubin, D. B. (1977). Maximum likelihood from incomplete data via the EM algorithm. *Journal of the Royal Statistical Society. Series B, Statistical Methodology*, *39*(1), 1–22. DOI: 10.1111/j.2517-6161.1977.tb01600.x

Denton, B. T. (Ed.). (2018). *Handbook of healthcare operations management* (2nd ed.). Springer., DOI: 10.1007/978-1-4614-5885-2

Domargard, A. (2026). *Standing on shifting ground: Clinical decision-making in a non-linear world. Zenodo*. DOI: 10.5281/zenodo.18221943

Donabedian, A. (1988). The quality of care: How can it be assessed? *Journal of the American Medical Association*, *260*(12), 1743–1748. DOI: 10.1001/jama.1988.03410120089033 PMID: 3045356

Doob, J. L. (1953). *Stochastic processes*. Wiley.

Doroshenkov, L., Konyshev, V. A., & Selishchev, S. (2007). Classification of human sleep stages based on EEG processing using hidden Markov models. *Medical Device Technology*, *41*(1), 24–28. DOI: 10.1007/s10527-007-0006-5 PMID: 17419342

Doshi-Velez, F., & Kim, B. (2017). Towards a rigorous science of interpretable machine learning. arXiv preprint arXiv:1702.08608.

Doucet, A., de Freitas, N., & Gordon, N. (Eds.). (2001). *Sequential Monte Carlo methods in practice*. Springer., DOI: 10.1007/978-1-4757-3437-9

Drabo, E. F., & Padula, W. V. (2023). Introduction to Markov modeling. In Bishai, D., Brenzel, L., & Padula, W. V. (Eds.), *Handbook of applied health economics in vaccines*. Oxford University Press., DOI: 10.1093/oso/9780192896087.003.0022

Drummond, M. F., Sculpher, M. J., Claxton, K., Stoddart, G. L., & Torrance, G. W. (2015). *Methods for the economic evaluation of health care programmes* (4th ed.). Oxford University Press.

Duan, M., Liu, X., Yeung, W., Hao, S., Raffa, J. D., Hu, P., Liu, C., Chen, L., Li, Z., Gao, Z., Li, T., Cao, D., Zhou, F., Zhang, Z., Zhang, Z., & Celi, L. A. (2026). Multicenter validation and updating of the ELDER-ICU model for severity assessment in elderly critical illness. *NPJ Digital Medicine*, *9*(1), 498. Advance online publication. DOI: 10.1038/s41746-026-02472-1 PMID: 41957287

Düsing, C., Cimiano, P., Rehberg, S., Scherer, C., Kaup, O., Köster, C., Hellmich, S., Herrmann, D., Meier, K. L., Claßen, S., & Borgstedt, R. (2024). Integrating federated learning for improved counterfactual explanations in clinical decision support systems for sepsis therapy. *Artificial Intelligence in Medicine*, *157*, 102982. DOI: 10.1016/j.artmed.2024.102982 PMID: 39277983

Dychiao, R. G., Nazer, L., Mlombwa, D., & Celi, L. A. (2024). Artificial intelligence and global health equity: Regulation and monitoring are needed to prevent harmful bias in AI tools. *BMJ (Clinical Research Ed.)*, *387*, e079845.

Eggleton, A. (2023). Dr Robot: Robotics and AI in healthcare. In *Research Handbook on Patient Safety and the Law* (pp. 336–368). Edward Elgar Publishing.

Elgujja, A. (2020). Impact of information technology on patient confidentiality rights: A perspective. In Cruz-Cunha, M. M. (Eds.), *Impacts of information technology on patient care and empowerment* (pp. 129–148). IGI Global., DOI: 10.4018/978-1-7998-0047-7.ch018

Elgujja, A. (2025a). *AI governance as a human right imperative: Embedding transparency, accountability, and reasoned justification in the algorithmic state. SSRN.* https://doi.org/DOI: 10.2139/ssrn.5646110

Engel, Y., Mannor, S., & Meir, R. (2003). Bayes meets Bellman: The Gaussian process approach to temporal difference learning. In *Proceedings of the 20th International Conference on Machine Learning* (pp. 154–161). AAAI Press.

Ennis, J. S., Riggan, K. A., Nguyen, N. V., Kramer, D. B., Smith, A. K., Sulmasy, D. P., Tilburt, J. C., Wolf, S. M., & DeMartino, E. S. (2023). Triage procedures for critical care resource allocation during scarcity. *JAMA Network Open*, *6*(8), e2329688. DOI: 10.1001/jamanetworkopen.2023.29688 PMID: 37642967

Eppich, W., & Reedy, G. (2022). Advancing healthcare simulation research: Innovations in theory, methodology, and method. *Advances in Simulation (London, England)*, *7*(1), 23. DOI: 10.1186/s41077-022-00219-y PMID: 35897062

Euro Health Consumer Index. (2023). *EHCI 2023 report.* Health Consumer Powerhouse.

European Commission. (2021). *Proposal for a regulation laying down harmonised rules on artificial intelligence.* AI Act.

European Parliament and Council of the European Union. (2024). *Regulation (EU) 2024/1689 of the European Parliament and of the Council of 13 June 2024 laying down harmonised rules on artificial intelligence (Artificial Intelligence Act) and amending certain Union legislative acts. Official Journal of the European Union.* https://eur-lex.europa.eu/eli/reg/2024/1689/oj

Fahim, Y. A., Hasani, I. W., Kabba, S., & Ragab, W. M. (2025). Artificial intelligence in healthcare and medicine: Clinical applications, therapeutic advances, and future perspectives. *European Journal of Medical Research*, *30*(1), 848. Advance online publication. DOI: 10.1186/s40001-025-03196-w PMID: 40988064

Farah, L., Borget, I., Martelli, N., & Vallée, A. (2024). Suitability of the current health technology assessment of innovative artificial intelligence-based medical devices: Scoping literature review. *Journal of Medical Internet Research*, *26*, e51514. DOI: 10.2196/51514 PMID: 38739911

FDA. (2021). *Artificial intelligence/machine learning (AI/ML)-based software as a medical device (SaMD) action plan.* U.S. Food and Drug Administration.

Feldstein, M. S. (1967). *Economic analysis for health service efficiency: Econometric studies of the British National Health Service.* North-Holland Publishing.

Floridi, L., Cowls, J., Beltrametti, M., Chazerand, P., Chila, R., Dignum, V., Luetge, C., Madelin, R., Pagallo, U., Rossi, F., Schafer, B., Valcke, P., & Vayena, E. (2018). AI4People—An ethical framework for a good AI society. *Minds and Machines*, *28*(4), 689–707. DOI: 10.1007/s11023-018-9482-5 PMID: 30930541

Foley, T., & Horwitz, L. I. (2025). Learning health systems. In *Cambridge University Press eBooks.* Cambridge University Press., DOI: 10.1017/9781009325912

Folkard, S., & Akerstedt, T. (2004). Trends in the risk of accidents and injuries and their implications for models of fatigue and performance. *Aviation, Space, and Environmental Medicine*, *75*(3), A161–A167. PMID: 15018280

Futoma, J., Hariharan, S., & Heller, K. (2017, July). Learning to detect sepsis with a multitask Gaussian process RNN classifier. In *International Conference on Machine Learning* (pp. 1174–1182). PMLR.

Gasmi, K., Ayadi, H., & Torjmen, M. (2024). Enhancing Medical Image Retrieval with UMLS-Integrated CNN-Based Text Indexing. *Diagnostics (Basel)*, *14*(11), 1204. DOI: 10.3390/diagnostics14111204 PMID: 38893730

Gavurova, B., Kocisova, K., & Sopko, J. (2021). Health system efficiency in OECD countries: Dynamic network DEA approach. *Health Economics Review*, *11*(1), 40. DOI: 10.1186/s13561-021-00337-9 PMID: 34642864

Gelman, A., Carlin, J. B., Stern, H. S., Dunson, D. B., Vehtari, A., & Rubin, D. B. (2013). *Bayesian data analysis* (3rd ed.). CRC Press. DOI: 10.1201/b16018

Geßler, T. (2026). *Why probabilistic AI resists auditability: From explainability to verifiable responsibility in high-risk AI systems. Zenodo.* DOI: 10.2139/ssrn.6103587

Gevorkova, E. (2025). The concept and essence of human genetic information as an object of constitutional law regulation. *Bulletin of the South Ural State University Series Law*, *25*(2), 66–73. DOI: 10.14529/law250211

Ghassemi, M., Pimentel, M. A., Naumann, T., Brennan, T., Clifton, D. A., Szolovits, P., & Feng, M. (2015). A multivariate time series modeling approach to severity of illness assessment and forecasting in ICU with sparse, heterogeneous clinical data. *Proceedings of the AAAI Conference on Artificial Intelligence*, *29*(1), 446–453. DOI: 10.1609/aaai.v29i1.9209 PMID: 27182460

Gladwell, M. (2000). *The tipping point: How little things can make a big difference.* Little, Brown and Company.

Glasserman, P. (2004). *Monte Carlo methods in financial engineering*. Springer.

Goldstein, B. A., Navar, A. M., Pencina, M. J., & Ioannidis, J. P. (2016). Opportunities and challenges in developing risk prediction models with electronic health records data: A systematic review. *Journal of the American Medical Informatics Association : JAMIA*, *24*(1), 198–208. DOI: 10.1093/jamia/ocw042 PMID: 27189013

Gouthamaan, M., Peimankar, A., Puthusserypady, S., Momeni, M., Asyari, R. A. I., Jahan, M. S., Moll, J., Wiil, U. K., & Ebrahimi, A. (2025). Explainable deep learning based techniques for ECG-based heart disease classification: A systematic literature review and future direction. *Computers in Biology and Medicine*, *199*, 111324. DOI: 10.1016/j.compbiomed.2025.111324 PMID: 41265065

Granovetter, M. (1978). Threshold models of collective behavior. *American Journal of Sociology*, *83*(6), 1420–1443. DOI: 10.1086/226707

Green, L. V. (2006). Queueing analysis in healthcare. Patient Flow: Reducing Delay in Healthcare Delivery, 281–307.

Green, L. V., Kolesar, P. J., & Soares, J. (2001). Improving the SIPP approach for staffing service systems that have cyclic demands. *Operations Research, 49*(4), 549–564. DOI: 10.1287/opre.49.4.549.11228

Gross, D., Shortle, J., Thompson, J., & Harris, C. (2018). *Fundamentals of queueing theory* (5th ed.). Wiley.

Guillaume, T. (2022). Closed form valuation of barrier options with stochastic barriers. *Annals of Operations Research, 313*(2), 1021–1050. DOI: 10.1007/s10479-020-03860-w

Gulakala, R., Markert, B., & Stoffel, M. (2023). Rapid diagnosis of Covid-19 infections by a progressively growing GAN and CNN optimisation. *Computer Methods and Programs in Biomedicine, 229*, 107262. DOI: 10.1016/j.cmpb.2022.107262 PMID: 36463675

Gul, M., & Guneri, A. F. (2015). A comprehensive review of emergency department simulation applications for normal and disaster conditions. *Computers & Industrial Engineering, 83*, 327–344. DOI: 10.1016/j.cie.2015.02.018

Gupta, D., & Denton, B. (2008). Appointment scheduling in health care: Challenges and opportunities. *IIE Transactions, 40*(9), 800–819. DOI: 10.1080/07408170802165880

Gupta, S., Gupta, P., Goel, L., & Jain, S. (2025). Enabling decentralized clinical insights: Federated learning in smart healthcare systems. In *Enabling Collaborative Health Intelligence with Federated Learning* (pp. 149–180). IGI Global. DOI: 10.4018/979-8-3373-3306-9.ch006

Gurugopinath, R., & Venugopal, B. (2024). Judicial interventions in environmental health and the right to health: A critical analysis of landmark endosulfan case in India and similar cases in USA, UK, Canada, and Australia. *Revista de Gestão Social e Ambiental, 18*(9), e07577. Advance online publication. DOI: 10.24857/rgsa.v18n9-110

Haakman, M., Cruz, L., Huijgens, H., & van Deursen, A. (2021). AI lifecycle models need to be revised. *Empirical Software Engineering, 26*(5), 95. Advance online publication. DOI: 10.1007/s10664-021-09993-1

Hafner, D., Lillicrap, T., Ba, J., & Norouzi, M. (2020). Dream to control: Learning behaviors by latent imagination. In *International Conference on Learning Representations.*

Hafner, D., Lillicrap, T., Fischer, I., Villegas, R., Ha, D., Lee, H., & Davidson, J. (2019). Learning latent dynamics for planning from pixels. In *Proceedings of the 36th International Conference on Machine Learning* (Vol. 97, pp. 2555–2565). PMLR.

Hafner, D., Pasukonis, J., Ba, J., & Lillicrap, T. (2023). Mastering diverse domains through world models. arXiv. https://arxiv.org/abs/2301.04104

Haldane, V., De Foo, C., Abdalla, S. M., Jung, A.-S., Tan, M., Wu, S., Chua, A., Verma, M., Shrestha, P., Singh, S., Perez, T., Tan, S. M., Bartos, M., Mabuchi, S., Bonk, M., McNab, C., Werner, G. K., Panjabi, R., Nordström, A., & Legido-Quigley, H. (2021). Health systems resilience in managing the COVID-19 pandemic: Lessons from 28 countries. *Nature Medicine, 27*(6), 964–980. DOI: 10.1038/s41591-021-01381-y PMID: 34002090

Hall, J. (2026). Personalized treatment response modeling from multimodal patient profiles across heterogeneous diseases, clinical interventions, and longitudinal outcomes with calibrated predictive uncertainty estimation. *International Journal of Machine Learning and Engineering*, *2*(1), 1–13.

Hall, R. W. (2013). *Patient flow: Reducing delay in healthcare delivery*. Springer. DOI: 10.1007/978-1-4614-9512-3

Hampiholi, N. (2023). Medical Imaging Enhancement with AI Models for Automatic Disease Detection and Classification Based on Medical Images. *International Journal of Engineering Applied Sciences and Technology*, *8*(5), 31–37. DOI: 10.33564/IJEAST.2023.v08i05.005

Hansen, E. A., & Feng, Z. (2000). Dynamic programming for POMDPs using a factored state representation. In *Proceedings of the Fifth International Conference on Artificial Intelligence Planning Systems* (pp. 130–139). AAAI Press.

Harutyunyan, H., Khachatrian, H., Kale, D. C., Ver Steeg, G., & Galstyan, A. (2019). Multitask learning and benchmarking with clinical time series data. *Scientific Data*, *6*(1), 96. DOI: 10.1038/s41597-019-0103-9 PMID: 31209213

Hausknecht, M., & Stone, P. (2015). Deep recurrent Q-learning for partially observable MDPs. In *AAAI Fall Symposium on Sequential Decision Making for Intelligent Agents*.

Hauskrecht, M. (2000). Value-function approximations for partially observable Markov decision processes. *Journal of Artificial Intelligence Research*, *13*, 33–94. DOI: 10.1613/jair.678

Hauskrecht, M., & Fraser, H. (2000). Planning treatment of ischemic heart disease with partially observable Markov decision processes. *Artificial Intelligence in Medicine*, *18*(3), 221–244. DOI: 10.1016/S0933-3657(99)00042-1 PMID: 10675716

Hawsawi, H. M. A., Al-Rashidi, S. A., Alghamdi, W. A. E., Alghamdi, M. A. M., Althagafi, M. E., Alsalmy, B. O., Alharthi, M. A., Alharthi, A. A., Alshawqab, A. S., Alshehri, M. M., Dosar, A. M. A., & Alhuzali, H. S. (2024). The role of health administration, social services, health informatics, and public health in driving digital transformation in healthcare systems: An integrative review. *Journal of Posthumanism*, *4*(2), 2189–2195. DOI: 10.63332/joph.v4i2.3713

He, W., Jiang, Z., Xiao, T., Xu, Z., & Li, Y. (2026). A survey on uncertainty quantification methods for deep learning. *ACM Computing Surveys*, *58*(7), 1–35. DOI: 10.1145/3786319

Hick, J. L., Hanfling, D., Burstein, J. L., DeAtley, C., Barbisch, D., Bogdan, G. M., & Cantrill, S. (2004). Health care facility and community strategies for patient care surge capacity. *Annals of Emergency Medicine*, *44*(3), 253–261. DOI: 10.1016/j.annemergmed.2004.04.011 PMID: 15332068

Higham, D. J. (2001). An algorithmic introduction to numerical simulation of stochastic differential equations. *SIAM Review*, *43*(3), 525–546. DOI: 10.1137/S0036144500378302

Hoffman, M. D., Blei, D. M., Wang, C., & Paisley, J. (2013). Stochastic variational inference. *Journal of Machine Learning Research*, *14*(1), 1303–1347.

Holdbrook, R. O., Obanla, A. K., Ani, C. P., Eboh, N. A., & Oboh, R. (2026). A comparative study of regulatory guidelines, digital pharmacovigilance, and software as a medical device across high- and low-to-middle-income countries. *Journal of Pharma Insights and Research*, *4*(2), 304–319. DOI: 10.69613/mdb50d20

Holland, J. H. (1995). *Hidden order: How adaptation builds complexity*. Addison-Wesley.

Hollnagel, E., Paries, J., Woods, D. D., & Wreathall, J. (2011). *Resilience engineering in practice: A guidebook*. Ashgate.

Holzinger, A., & Müller, H. (2021). Toward human–AI interfaces to support explainability and causability in medical AI. *Computer*, *54*(10), 78–86. DOI: 10.1109/MC.2021.3092610

Hoot, N. R., & Aronsky, D. (2008). Systematic review of emergency department crowding: Causes, effects, and solutions. *Annals of Emergency Medicine*, *52*(2), 126–136.e1. DOI: 10.1016/j.annemergmed.2008.03.014 PMID: 18433933

Houthooft, R., Chen, X., Duan, Y., Schulman, J., De Turck, F., & Abbeel, P. (2016). VIME: Variational information maximizing exploration. In *Advances in Neural Information Processing Systems* (Vol. 29, pp. 1109–1117).

Hovorka, R., Canonico, V., Chassin, L. J., Haueter, U., Massi-Benedetti, M., Federici, M. O., Pieber, T. R., Schaller, H. C., Schaupp, L., Vering, T., & Wilinska, M. E. (2004). Nonlinear model predictive control of glucose concentration in subjects with type 1 diabetes. *Physiological Measurement*, *25*(4), 905–920. DOI: 10.1088/0967-3334/25/4/010 PMID: 15382830

Howard, R. A. (1960). *Dynamic programming and Markov processes*. MIT Press.

Howard, R. A. (1971). *Dynamic probabilistic systems, Volume II: Semi-Markov and decision processes*. Wiley.

Hsu, D., Kakade, S. M., & Zhang, T. (2012). A spectral algorithm for learning hidden Markov models. *Journal of Computer and System Sciences*, *78*(5), 1460–1480. DOI: 10.1016/j.jcss.2011.12.025

Huang, Z., Zhang, J., Zhang, Y., & Shan, H. (2022). DU-GAN: Generative Adversarial Networks With Dual-Domain U-Net-Based Discriminators for Low-Dose CT Denoising. *IEEE Transactions on Instrumentation and Measurement*, *71*, 1–12. DOI: 10.1109/TIM.2021.3128703

Hüllermeier, E., & Waegeman, W. (2021). Aleatoric and epistemic uncertainty in machine learning: An introduction to concepts and methods. *Machine Learning*, *110*(3), 457–506. DOI: 10.1007/s10994-021-05946-3

Hulshof, P. J. H., Kortbeek, N., Boucherie, R. J., Hans, E. W., & Bakker, P. J. M. (2012). Taxonomic classification of planning decisions in health care. *Health Systems (Basingstoke, England)*, *1*(2), 129–175. DOI: 10.1057/hs.2012.18

Hummel, P., Braun, M., Bischoff, S., Samhammer, D., Seitz, K., Fasching, P. A., & Dabrock, P. (2024). Perspectives of patients and clinicians on big data and AI in health: A comparative empirical investigation. *AI & Society*, *39*(6), 2973–2987. DOI: 10.1007/s00146-023-01825-8

Hurley, M. E., Lang, B., Kostick, K. M., Smith, J. N., & Blumenthal-Barby, J. (2024). Patient consent and the right to notice and explanation of AI systems used in health care. *The American Journal of Bioethics*, *25*(3), 102–114. DOI: 10.1080/15265161.2024.2399828 PMID: 39288291

Igl, M., Zintgraf, L., Le, T. A., Wood, F., & Whiteson, S. (2018). Deep variational reinforcement learning for POMDPs. In *Proceedings of the 35th International Conference on Machine Learning* (Vol. 80, pp. 2117–2126). PMLR.

Ilic, A. S., Ilic, M., Stojanovic, N., & Stojanovic, D. (2026). Adaptive healthcare monitoring through drift-aware edge-cloud intelligence. *Future Internet*, *18*(3), 156. Advance online publication. DOI: 10.3390/fi18030156

Iman, R. L., & Conover, W. J. (1982). A distribution-free approach to inducing rank correlation among input variables. *Communications in Statistics. Simulation and Computation*, *11*(3), 311–334. DOI: 10.1080/03610918208812265

Insel, T. R. (2017). Digital phenotyping: Technology for a new science of behavior. *Journal of the American Medical Association*, *318*(13), 1215–1216. DOI: 10.1001/jama.2017.11295 PMID: 28973224

Institute of Medicine. (2001). *Crossing the quality chasm: A new health system for the 21st century*. National Academy Press.

Irie, K., Minar, P., Reifenberg, J., Boyle, B. M., Noe, J. D., Hyams, J. S., & Mizuno, T. (2025). Hybrid Population Pharmacokinetic–Machine Learning Modeling to Predict Infliximab Pharmacokinetics in Pediatric and Young Adult Patients with Crohn's Disease. *Clinical Pharmacokinetics*, *64*(11), 1669–1679. DOI: 10.1007/s40262-025-01564-7 PMID: 40885855

Isom, J. D., Meyn, S. P., & Braatz, R. D. (2008). Piecewise linear dynamic programming for constrained POMDPs. In *Proceedings of the 23rd AAAI Conference on Artificial Intelligence* (pp. 291–296). AAAI Press.

Iyaniwura, S. A., & Peng, Z. (2024). Asymptotic analysis and simulation of mean first passage time for active Brownian particles in 1-D. *SIAM Journal on Applied Mathematics*, *84*(2), 625–651. DOI: 10.1137/23M1593917

Izady, N., & Worthington, D. (2012). Setting staffing requirements for time-dependent queueing networks. *European Journal of Operational Research*, *219*(3), 531–540.

Jackson, C. (2011). Multi-state models for panel data: The msm package for R. *Journal of Statistical Software*, *38*(8), 1–28. DOI: 10.18637/jss.v038.i08

Jacobs, R., Smith, P. C., & Street, A. (2006). *Measuring efficiency in health care: Analytic techniques and health policy*. Cambridge University Press.

Jaidka, P., & Jain, S. (2023). Performance analysis of various deep learning techniques for brain tumor classification. *2023 International Conference on Power, Instrumentation, Energy and Control (PIECON)*, 1–6. DOI: 10.1109/PIECON56912.2023.10085796

Jain, S., & Jain, V. (2024). MRI based brain tumor segmentation with ensemble deep learning. *2024 1st International Conference on Advanced Computing and Emerging Technologies (ACET)*, 1–5.

Jain, S., Jain, V., & Chatterjee, J. M. (2025). Ensemble based brain tumor classification technique from MRI based on K fold validation approach. *Journal of Integrated Science and Technology, 13*(5), 1114. DOI: 10.62110/sciencein.jist.2025.v13.1114

Javaid, M., Haleem, A., Singh, R. P., Suman, R., & Rab, S. (2022). Significance of machine learning in healthcare: Features, pillars and applications. *Intelligent Pharmacy, 1*(1), 58–73. DOI: 10.1016/j.ipha.2022.04.001

Jellema, H. (2025). Standards of proof for future crimes and decision theory. *Quaestio facti: Revista internacional sobre razonamiento probatorio, 10*. DOI: 10.33115/udg_bib/qf.i10.23144

Jiang, L., Yang, X., Yu, C., Wu, Z., & Wang, Y. (2024). Advanced AI Framework for Enhanced Detection and Assessment of Abdominal Trauma: Integrating 3D Segmentation with 2D CNN and RNN Models. 2024 *3rd International Conference on Robotics, Artificial Intelligence and Intelligent Control (RAIIC)*, 337–340. DOI: 10.1109/RAIIC61787.2024.10671250

Jiang, N., & Li, L. (2016). Doubly robust off-policy value evaluation for reinforcement learning. In *Proceedings of the 33rd International Conference on Machine Learning* (Vol. 48, pp. 652–661). PMLR.

Johnson, A. E. W., Pollard, T. J., Shen, L., Lehman, L. H., Feng, M., Ghassemi, M., Moody, B., Szolovits, P., Anthony Celi, L., & Mark, R. G. (2016). MIMIC-III, a freely accessible critical care database. *Scientific Data, 3*(1), 160035. DOI: 10.1038/sdata.2016.35 PMID: 27219127

Johnson, A., Pollard, T., & Mark, R. (2016b). *MIMIC-III Clinical Database Demo (version 1.4)*. PhysioNet.

Josephs, T. (2020). Patterns of mortality in children presenting to a tertiary paediatric emergency unit in Sub-Saharan Africa: A cross-sectional study.

Joshi, P. B., & Wamankar, Y. (2025). Algorithmic policing and due process in cybercrime investigations: A constitutional analysis under Articles 14, 19 and 21 of the Indian Constitution. *ShodhSamajik Journal of Social Studies, 2*(2), 153–167. DOI: 10.29121/ShodhSamajik.v2.i2.2025.57

Junior, A. A., Ndayizigamiye, P., Bokaba, T., & Idemudia, E. C. (2025). Resilient healthcare systems through AI-powered cloud computing: Perspectives on resource allocation. In *Proceedings of the 58th Hawaii International Conference on System Sciences* (pp. 3310–3319).

Jun, J. B., Jacobson, S. H., & Swisher, J. R. (1999). Application of discrete-event simulation in healthcare clinics. *The Journal of the Operational Research Society, 50*(2), 109–123. DOI: 10.1057/palgrave.jors.2600669

Kabir, H. M., Khosravi, A., Hosen, M. A., & Nahavandi, S. (2024). Neural network-based uncertainty quantification: A survey on methods and applications. *IEEE Access : Practical Innovations, Open Solutions, 12*, 33540–33556. DOI: 10.1109/ACCESS.2024.3372345

Kaelbling, L. P., Littman, M. L., & Cassandra, A. R. (1998). Planning and acting in partially observable stochastic domains. *Artificial Intelligence, 101*(1–2), 99–134. DOI: 10.1016/S0004-3702(98)00023-X

Kalman, R. E. (1960). A new approach to linear filtering and prediction problems. *Journal of Basic Engineering, 82*(1), 35–45. DOI: 10.1115/1.3662552

Kansagara, D., Englander, H., Salanitro, A., Kagen, D., Theobald, C., Freeman, M., & Kripalani, S. (2011). Risk prediction models for hospital readmission: A systematic review. *Journal of the American Medical Association, 306*(15), 1688–1698. DOI: 10.1001/jama.2011.1515 PMID: 22009101

Kaplan, E. H., Craft, D. L., & Wein, L. M. (2002). Emergency response to a smallpox attack: The case for mass vaccination. *Proceedings of the National Academy of Sciences of the United States of America, 99*(16), 10935–10940. DOI: 10.1073/pnas.162282799 PMID: 12118122

Karthika, P., & Premkumar, M. (2026). An in-depth exploration of CNN-based deep learning models in cervical carcinoma analysis. *Advances in Biomarker Sciences and Technology, 8*, 19–33. DOI: 10.1016/j.abst.2025.11.007

Karthikeyan, N. K., & Ali, S. S., & R, V. S. (2024). Lung Cancer Classification Using CT Scan Images Through Deep Learning And CNN Based Model. 2024 *International Conference on Advances in Data Engineering and Intelligent Computing Systems (ADICS)*, 01–05. DOI: 10.1109/ADICS58448.2024.10533528

Kaul, V., Enslin, S., & Gross, S. A. (2023). History of artificial intelligence in medicine. *Gastrointestinal Endoscopy, 97*(5), 807–812. PMID: 32565184

Kaur, S., & Kaur, S.Ms. Navjot KaurMrs. Rajinder Kaur. (2025). Article 21: A lifeline to new rights in a progressive society. *International Journal on Science and Technology, 16*(2), 4692. Advance online publication. DOI: 10.71097/IJSAT.v16.i2.4692

Kee, K. A. L., Hashim, J. H., & Tan, S. S. L. (2024). The adoption of advanced healthcare technologies in the private healthcare industry: Case of IHH Healthcare Berhad, Malaysia. *Jesselton Journal of Educators and Scholars, 1*(1), 46–67. DOI: 10.68440/3009-0881.1005

Keeling, M. J., & Rohani, P. (2008). *Modeling infectious diseases in humans and animals*. Princeton University Press., DOI: 10.1515/9781400841035

Kendall, A., & Gal, Y. (2017). What uncertainties do we need in Bayesian deep learning for computer vision? *Advances in Neural Information Processing Systems, 30*, 5574–5584.

Kermack, W. O., & McKendrick, A. G. (1927). A contribution to the mathematical theory of epidemics. *Proceedings of the Royal Society of London. Series A, Containing Papers of a Mathematical and Physical Character, 115*(772), 700–721. DOI: 10.1098/rspa.1927.0118

Ketcheson, D. I. (2021). Optimal control of an SIR epidemic through finite-time non-pharmaceutical intervention. *Journal of Mathematical Biology, 83*(1), 7. DOI: 10.1007/s00285-021-01628-9 PMID: 34176029

Khalifa, M., & Albadawy, M. (2024). AI in diagnostic imaging: Revolutionising accuracy and efficiency. *Computer Methods and Programs in Biomedicine Update, 5*, 100146. DOI: 10.1016/j.cmpbup.2024.100146

Khan, Q. W. (2024). Exploring Markov decision processes: A comprehensive survey of optimization applications and techniques. *IgMin Research, 2*(7), 508–517. DOI: 10.61927/igmin210

Khetarpal, K., Riemer, M., Rish, I., & Precup, D. (2022). Towards continual reinforcement learning: A review and perspectives. *Journal of Artificial Intelligence Research, 75*, 1401–1476. DOI: 10.1613/jair.1.13673

Killian, T. W., Konidaris, G., & Doshi-Velez, F. (2017). Robust and efficient transfer learning with hidden parameter Markov decision processes. In *Advances in Neural Information Processing Systems* (Vol. 30, pp. 6250–6261). DOI: 10.1609/aaai.v31i1.11065

Kim, D., Lee, J., Lee, K.-E., & Sung, T.-K. (2011). Point-based value iteration for constrained POMDPs. In *Proceedings of the 22nd International Joint Conference on Artificial Intelligence* (pp. 1968–1974). AAAI Press.

Kim, M. J., Prieto-Merino, D., Nicholas, J., Allen, L., Burton, M. J., Bastawrous, A., & Macleod, D. (2025). Evidence-based approaches to quality improvement: A narrative review of integrating Bayesian adaptive trials into health services. *Journal of Evaluation in Clinical Practice*, *31*(5), e70197. Advance online publication. DOI: 10.1111/jep.70197 PMID: 40618403

Kim, S. C., & Horowitz, I. (2002). Scheduling hospital services: The efficacy of elective-surgery quotas. *Omega*, *30*(5), 335–346. DOI: 10.1016/S0305-0483(02)00050-6

Kim, S. Y., Kim, D. H., Kim, M. J., Ko, H. J., & Jeong, O. R. (2024). XAI-based clinical decision support systems: A systematic review. *Applied Sciences (Basel, Switzerland)*, *14*(15), 6638. DOI: 10.3390/app14156638

Kim, S., Breen, J., Dudkina, E., Poloni, F., & Crisostomi, E. (2023). On the effectiveness of random walks for modeling epidemics on networks. *PLoS One*, *18*(1), e0280277. DOI: 10.1371/journal.pone.0280277 PMID: 36626406

Kleinberg, J., Mullainathan, S., & Raghavan, M. (2017). Inherent trade-offs in the fair determination of risk scores. In *Proceedings of the 8th Innovations in Theoretical Computer Science Conference* (Article 43). Schloss Dagstuhl–Leibniz-Zentrum für Informatik. https://doi.org/DOI: 10.4230/LIPIcs.ITCS.2017.43

Kloeden, P. E., & Platen, E. (1992). *Numerical solution of stochastic differential equations*. Springer.

Kloeden, P. E., & Platen, E. (1992). *Numerical Solution of Stochastic Differential Equations*. Springer. DOI: 10.1007/978-3-662-12616-5

Kocsis, L., & Szepesvári, C. (2006). Bandit based Monte-Carlo planning. In *European Conference on Machine Learning* (pp. 282–293). Springer. DOI: 10.1007/11871842_29

Kolker, A. (2008). Process modelling of emergency department patient flow: Effect of patient length of stay on ED diversion. *Journal of Medical Systems*, *32*(5), 389–401. DOI: 10.1007/s10916-008-9144-x PMID: 18814495

Komorowski, M., Celi, L. A., Badawi, O., Gordon, A. C., & Faisal, A. A. (2018). The artificial intelligence clinician learns optimal treatment strategies for sepsis in intensive care. *Nature Medicine*, *24*(11), 1716–1720. DOI: 10.1038/s41591-018-0213-5 PMID: 30349085

Koppolu, H. K. R. (2025). *The intersection of data, artificial intelligence, and healthcare: Creating predictive and personalized care models* (pp. 128–143). DOI: 10.70593/978-93-49910-67-6_8

Koppolu, H. K. R., Recharla, M., & Chakilam, C. (2022). Revolutionising patient care with AI and cloud computing: A framework for scalable and predictive healthcare solutions. *International Journal of Scientific and Engineering Research*, *11*(12), 1457–1472.

Kulkarni, V. G. (2011). *Modeling and analysis of stochastic systems* (2nd ed.). CRC Press.

Kuramoto, Y. (1984). *Chemical oscillations, waves, and turbulence.* Springer. DOI: 10.1007/978-3-642-69689-3

Kurniawati, H., Hsu, D., & Lee, W. S. (2008). SARSOP: Efficient point-based POMDP planning by approximating optimally reachable belief spaces. In *Proceedings of Robotics: Science and Systems IV.* DOI: 10.15607/RSS.2008.IV.009

Kushwaha, G. (2026). *From Gian Kaur to living wills: The changing landscape of euthanasia law in India. Zenodo.* DOI: 10.5281/zenodo.19152320

Lai, T. L. (2001). Sequential analysis: Some classical problems and new challenges. *Statistica Sinica, 11*(2), 303–408.

Lakshmi, C., & Iyer, S. A. (2013). Application of queueing theory in health care: A literature review. *Operations Research for Health Care, 2*(1–2), 25–39.

Lampropoulos, G., Garzón, J., Misra, S., & Siakas, K. (2024). The role of artificial intelligence of things in achieving sustainable development goals: State of the art. *Sensors (Basel), 24*(4), 1091. DOI: 10.3390/s24041091 PMID: 38400249

Langer, C. (2024). Decision-making power and responsibility in an automated administration. *Discover Artificial Intelligence, 4*(1), 59. Advance online publication. DOI: 10.1007/s44163-024-00152-1

Lee, J., Hauskrecht, M., & Cooper, G. F. (2018). Monte-Carlo tree search for constrained POMDPs. In *Advances in Neural Information Processing Systems* (Vol. 31, pp. 7934–7943).

Lee, S. A., Jain, S., Chen, A., Ono, K., Biswas, A., Rudas, Á., Fang, J., & Chiang, J. N. (2025). Clinical decision support using pseudo-notes from multiple streams of EHR data. *NPJ Digital Medicine, 8*(1), 394. DOI: 10.1038/s41746-025-01777-x PMID: 40604255

Lefebvre, M. (2024). A first-passage-place problem for integrated diffusion processes. *Journal of Applied Probability, 61*(1), 55–67. DOI: 10.1017/jpr.2023.19

Lekadir, K., Frangi, A. F., Porras, A. R., Glocker, B., Cintas, C., & Langlotz, C. P.. (2025). FUTURE-AI: International consensus guideline for trustworthy and deployable artificial intelligence in healthcare. *BMJ (Clinical Research Ed.), 388*, e081554. DOI: 10.1136/bmj-2024-081554 PMID: 39909534

Levy, M. M., Evans, L. E., & Rhodes, A. (2018). The Surviving Sepsis Campaign Bundle: 2018 update. *Critical Care Medicine, 46*(6), 997–1000. DOI: 10.1097/CCM.0000000000003119 PMID: 29767636

Lind, Y. (2023). Pandemocracy in Europe: Power, parliaments and people in times of COVID-19. *The American Journal of Comparative Law, 71*(2), 491–494. DOI: 10.1093/ajcl/avad025

Li, S. (2024). SIR epidemic model with general nonlinear incidence rate and Lévy jumps. *Mathematics, 12*(2), 215. DOI: 10.3390/math12020215

Little, R. J. A., & Rubin, D. B. (2019). *Statistical analysis with missing data* (3rd ed.). Wiley., DOI: 10.1002/9781119482260

Litvak, E., & Long, M. C. (2000). Cost and quality under managed care: Irreconcilable differences? *The American Journal of Managed Care*, *6*(3), 305–312. PMID: 10977431

Litvak, E., Long, M. C., Cooper, A. B., & McManus, M. L. (2001). Emergency department diversion: Causes and solutions. *Academic Emergency Medicine*, *8*(11), 1108–1110. PMID: 11691678

Liu, Q., Li, L., Tang, Z., & Zhou, D. (2018). Breaking the curse of horizon: Infinite-horizon off-policy estimation. In *Advances in Neural Information Processing Systems* (Vol. 31, pp. 5356–5366).

Liu, S., McCoy, A. B., Peterson, J. F., Lasko, T. A., Sittig, D. F., Nelson, S. D., Andrews, J., Patterson, L., Cobb, C. M., Mulherin, D., Morton, C. T., & Wright, A. (2024). Leveraging explainable artificial intelligence to optimize clinical decision support. *Journal of the American Medical Informatics Association : JAMIA*, *31*(4), 968–974. DOI: 10.1093/jamia/ocae019 PMID: 38383050

Lock, D., de Londras, F., & Hidalgo, P. G. (2023). Delegated legislation in the pandemic: Further limits of a constitutional bargain revealed. *Legal Studies*, *43*(4), 695–733. DOI: 10.1017/lst.2023.25

Lopes, F. P. (2026). *From human-in-the-loop to institutional oversight of judicial decision support systems*. Tilburg University Research Portal. https://research.tilburguniversity.edu/en/publications/e1f1c14a-464b-473b-b7fb-e517ea3cc100

Lorenz, E. N. (1963). Deterministic nonperiodic flow. *Journal of the Atmospheric Sciences*, *20*(2), 130–141. DOI: 10.1175/1520-0469(1963)020<0130:DNF>2.0.CO;2

Lovejoy, W. S. (1991). A survey of algorithmic methods for partially observed Markov decision processes. *Annals of Operations Research*, *28*(1), 47–65. DOI: 10.1007/BF02055574

Lundberg, S. M., & Lee, S.-I. (2017). A unified approach to interpreting model predictions. In *Advances in Neural Information Processing Systems* (pp. 4765–4774).

Lyu, G. (2025). Data-driven decision making in patient management: A systematic review. *BMC Medical Informatics and Decision Making*, *25*(1), 239. DOI: 10.1186/s12911-025-03072-x PMID: 40598137

Madani, O., Hanks, S., & Condon, A. (1999). On the undecidability of probabilistic planning and infinite-horizon partially observable Markov decision problems. In *Proceedings of the 16th National Conference on Artificial Intelligence* (pp. 541–548). AAAI Press.

Madani, O., Hanks, S., & Condon, A. (2003). On the undecidability of probabilistic planning and related stochastic optimization problems. *Artificial Intelligence*, *147*(1–2), 5–34. DOI: 10.1016/S0004-3702(02)00378-8

Madej, M., Sąsiadek, M., & Witt, M. (2021). Genetic testing—Whether to allow complete freedom? Direct to consumer tests versus genetic tests for medical purposes. *Journal of Applied Genetics*, *63*(1), 119–126. DOI: 10.1007/s13353-021-00670-z PMID: 34826052

Mahendra, R. R., Cahya, D. A., Ningsih, N., Kurniawan, L. S., & Judijanto, L. (2025). Critique of the concept of efficiency in public health management: A qualitative review of social justice-based health policy. *Health Leadership and Quality of Life*, *4*, 762. DOI: 10.56294/hl2025762

Marcus, S. I., Fernández-Gaucherand, E., Hernández-Hernández, D., Coraluppi, S., & Fard, P. (1997). Risk sensitive Markov decision processes. In Byrnes, C. I., Datta, B. N., Martin, C. F., & Gilliam, D. S. (Eds.), *Systems and control in the twenty-first century* (pp. 263–279). Birkhäuser., DOI: 10.1007/978-1-4612-4120-1_14

Martin, R. (2026). Possibilistic inferential models: A review. *Journal of the American Statistical Association, 121*(553), 807–826. DOI: 10.1080/01621459.2025.2606127

Matsuyama, E., Watanabe, H., & Takahashi, N. (2024). Performance Comparison of Vision Transformer- and CNN-Based Image Classification Using Cross Entropy: A Preliminary Application to Lung Cancer Discrimination from CT Images. *Journal of Biomedical Science and Engineering, 17*(09), 157–170. DOI: 10.4236/jbise.2024.179012

Mazzolo, A. (2024). First-passage time distribution of a Brownian motion: Two unexpected journeys. *Stochastic Analysis and Applications, 42*(4), 753–766. DOI: 10.1080/07362994.2024.2378327

McCullum, L., Webb, T., Huq, S., Fuentes, D., Court, L., & Ludmir, E. B. (2024). Markov models for clinical decision-making in radiation oncology: A systematic review. *Journal of Medical Imaging and Radiation Oncology, 68*(4), 417–428. DOI: 10.1111/1754-9485.13656 PMID: 38766899

McMahan, B., Moore, E., Ramage, D., Hampson, S., & Arcas, B. A. y. (2017). Communication-efficient learning of deep networks from decentralized data. In *Proceedings of the International Conference on Artificial Intelligence and Statistics* (pp. 1273–1282).

Meier, L. J. (2022). Systemising triage: COVID-19 guidelines and their underlying theories of distributive justice. *Medicine, Health Care, and Philosophy, 25*(4), 703–714. DOI: 10.1007/s11019-022-10101-3 PMID: 35796935

Miche, M., Strippoli, M. F., Preisig, M., & Lieb, R. (2024). Evaluating the clinical utility of an easily applicable prediction model of suicide attempts, newly developed and validated with a general community sample of adults. *BMC Psychiatry, 24*(1), 217. DOI: 10.1186/s12888-024-05647-w PMID: 38509477

Miller, W. D., Han, X., Peek, M. E., Ashana, D. C., & Parker, W. F.. (2021). Accuracy of the Sequential Organ Failure Assessment score for in-hospital mortality by race and relevance to crisis standards of care. *JAMA Network Open, 4*(6), e2113891. DOI: 10.1001/jamanetworkopen.2021.13891 PMID: 34143190

Miotto, R., Wang, F., Wang, S., Jiang, X., & Dudley, J. T. (2018). Deep learning for healthcare: Review, opportunities and challenges. *Briefings in Bioinformatics, 19*(6), 1236–1246. DOI: 10.1093/bib/bbx044 PMID: 28481991

Mishra, A., Naik, B. N., Kumar, S., & Agarwal, N. (2022). Covid-19: Catalyst for a comprehensive law to combat potential pandemics in India. *Indian Journal of Medical Ethics, 7*(3), 231–236. DOI: 10.20529/IJME.2022.039 PMID: 35699302

Mittelstadt, B. (2022). Protecting health privacy through reasonable inferences. *The American Journal of Bioethics, 22*(7), 65–68. DOI: 10.1080/15265161.2022.2075980 PMID: 35737503

Mittelstadt, B. D., Allo, P., Taddeo, M., Wachter, S., & Floridi, L. (2016). The ethics of algorithms: Mapping the debate. *Big Data & Society*, *3*(2), 2053951716679679. Advance online publication. DOI: 10.1177/2053951716679679

Mnih, V., Kavukcuoglu, K., Silver, D., Rusu, A. A., Veness, J., Bellemare, M. G., Graves, A., Riedmiller, M., Fidjeland, A. K., Ostrovski, G., Petersen, S., Beattie, C., Sadik, A., Antonoglou, I., King, H., Kumaran, D., Wierstra, D., Legg, S., & Hassabis, D. (2015). Human-level control through deep reinforcement learning. *Nature*, *518*(7540), 529–533. DOI: 10.1038/nature14236 PMID: 25719670

Mohammed, M. A., Worthington, P., & Woodall, W. H. (2001). Plotting basic control charts: Tutorial notes for healthcare practitioners. *Journal of Quality in Clinical Practice*, *21*(1), 14–19.

Mohammed, S. Y., Jumaah, N. S., Abbas, E. H., Ali, H. M., & Aljanabi, M. (2024). Healthcare intelligence and decision making: Big data's role in predictive analytics for clinical decision-making. *Mesopotamian Journal of Big Data*, *2024*, 223–229. DOI: 10.58496/MJBD/2024/016

Mohr, D. C., Zhang, M., & Schueller, S. M. (2017). Personal sensing: Understanding mental health using ubiquitous sensors and machine learning. *Annual Review of Clinical Psychology*, *13*(1), 23–47. DOI: 10.1146/annurev-clinpsy-032816-044949 PMID: 28375728

Molbæk-Steensig, H., & Scheinin, M. (2025). Human rights and artificial intelligence in healthcare-related settings: A grammar of human rights approach. *European Journal of Health Law*, *32*(2), 139–164. DOI: 10.1163/15718093-bja10146 PMID: 40368349

Monahan, G. E. (1982). A survey of partially observable Markov decision processes: Theory, models, and algorithms. *Management Science*, *28*(1), 1–16. DOI: 10.1287/mnsc.28.1.1

Monks, T., Currie, C. S. M., Onggo, B. S., Robinson, S., Kunc, M., & Taylor, S. J. E. (2019). Strengthening the reporting of empirical simulation studies: Introducing the STRESS guidelines. *Journal of Simulation*, *13*(1), 55–67. DOI: 10.1080/17477778.2018.1442155

Mooney, P. T. (n.d.). Chest X-ray pneumonia [Dataset]. Kaggle. https://www.kaggle.com/datasets/paultimothymooney/chest-xray-pneumonia

Motamed, S., Rogalla, P., & Khalvati, F. (2021). Data augmentation using Generative Adversarial Networks (GANs) for GAN-based detection of Pneumonia and COVID-19 in chest X-ray images. *Informatics in Medicine Unlocked*, *27*, 100779. DOI: 10.1016/j.imu.2021.100779 PMID: 34841040

Moustakides, G. V. (1986). Optimal stopping times for detecting changes in distributions. *Annals of Statistics*, *14*(4), 1379–1387.

Mukherjee, S. P. (2025). Balancing liberty and legality: The expanding horizon of the doctrine of proportionality in Indian administrative law after Puttaswamy. *International Journal on Science and Technology*, *16*(4), 9423. Advance online publication. DOI: 10.71097/IJSAT.v16.i4.9423

Murphy, K. P. (2002). *Dynamic Bayesian networks: Representation, inference and learning* [Doctoral dissertation, University of California, Berkeley]. UC Berkeley Library.

Murtozalikhon. (n.d.). Brain tumor multimodal image CT and MRI [Dataset]. Kaggle. https://www.kaggle.com/datasets/murtozalikhon/brain-tumor-multimodal-image-ct-and-mri

Nachum, O., Chow, Y., Dai, B., & Li, L. (2019). DualDICE: Behavior-agnostic estimation of discounted stationary distribution corrections. In *Advances in Neural Information Processing Systems* (Vol. 32, pp. 2318–2328).

Naimi, A. I., Cole, S. R., & Kennedy, E. H. (2017). An introduction to g methods. *International Journal of Epidemiology*, *46*(2), 756–762. PMID: 28039382

Najjar, R. (2023). Redefining Radiology: A Review of Artificial Intelligence Integration in Medical Imaging. *Diagnostics (Basel)*, *13*(17), 2760. DOI: 10.3390/diagnostics13172760 PMID: 37685300

Nale, G. S. (2025). Right to speedy trial: A critical study. *Indian Journal of Legal Review*, *5*(13), 678. DOI: 10.65393/OWJF3694

Namkoong, H., Keramati, R., Yadlowsky, S., & Brunskill, E. (2020). Off-policy policy evaluation for sequential decisions under unobserved confounding. In *Advances in Neural Information Processing Systems* (Vol. 33, pp. 18819–18831).

Narla, S., Valivarthi, D. T., & Peddi, S. (2020). Cloud computing with artificial intelligence techniques: GWO-DBN hybrid algorithms for enhanced disease prediction in healthcare systems. *Journal of Current Science & Humanities*, *8*(1), 14–30.

Nawaz, A.Dr. Ali Nawaz. (2025). Cloud computing and edge computing: Converging technologies for real-time data processing. *Multidisciplinary Research in Computing Information Systems*, *5*(3), 157–179. DOI: 10.71465/mrcis93

Nayak, K. (2025). Adaptive multi-cloud AI architectures for predictive healthcare analytics and cybersecurity automation. *International Journal of Science. Resources and Technology*, *8*(6), 15359–15368.

Nazar, M., Alam, M., Yafi, E., & Mazliham, M. (2021). *A systematic review of human–computer interaction and explainable artificial intelligence in healthcare with artificial intelligence techniques*. IEEE., DOI: 10.1109/ACCESS.2021.3127881

Nemati, S., Holder, A., Razmi, F., Stanley, M. D., Clifford, G. D., & Buchman, T. G. (2018). An interpretable machine learning model for accurate prediction of sepsis in the ICU. *Critical Care Medicine*, *46*(4), 547–553. DOI: 10.1097/CCM.0000000000002936 PMID: 29286945

Ng, A. Y., & Jordan, M. (2000). PEGASUS: A policy search method for large MDPs and POMDPs. In *Proceedings of the Sixteenth Conference on Uncertainty in Artificial Intelligence* (pp. 406–415). Morgan Kaufmann.

NIST. (2023). *Artificial intelligence risk management framework (AI RMF 1.0)*. National Institute of Standards and Technology.

Niu, S., Yin, Q., Ma, J., Song, Y., Xu, Y., Bai, L., Pan, W., & Yang, X. (2024). Enhancing healthcare decision support through explainable AI models for risk prediction. *Decision Support Systems*, *181*, 114228. DOI: 10.1016/j.dss.2024.114228

Norheim, O. F., Abi-Rached, J. M., Bright, L. K., Bærøe, K., Ferraz, O. L. M., Gloppen, S., & Voorhoeve, A. (2020). Difficult trade-offs in response to COVID-19: The case for open and inclusive decision making. *Nature Medicine*, *27*(1), 10–13. DOI: 10.1038/s41591-020-01204-6 PMID: 33340033

Obermeyer, Z., & Emanuel, E. J. (2016). Predicting the future—Big data, machine learning, and clinical medicine. *The New England Journal of Medicine, 375*(13), 1216–1219. DOI: 10.1056/NEJMp1606181 PMID: 27682033

Obermeyer, Z., Powers, B., Vogeli, C., & Mullainathan, S. (2019). Dissecting racial bias in an algorithm used to manage the health of populations. *Science, 366*(6464), 447–453. DOI: 10.1126/science.aax2342 PMID: 31649194

OECD (2024). Health at a glance 2024: OECD indicators. OECD Publishing. DOI: 10.1787/9789264055896-ko

OECD. (2021). *Recommendation of the Council on artificial intelligence.* OECD.

OECD. (2024).*Health at a glance 2024: OECD indicators.* OECD Publishing.https://doi.org/DOI: 10.1787/19991312

Okabe, Y., & Shudo, A. (2022). Spread of variants of epidemic disease based on the microscopic numerical simulations on networks. *Scientific Reports, 12*(1), 523. DOI: 10.1038/s41598-021-04520-0 PMID: 35017624

Øksendal, B. (2003). *Stochastic differential equations: An introduction with applications* (6th ed.). Springer., DOI: 10.1007/978-3-642-14394-6

Osband, I., Russo, D., & Van Roy, B. (2013). (More) efficient reinforcement learning via posterior sampling. In *Advances in Neural Information Processing Systems* (Vol. 26, pp. 3003–3011).

Osband, I., Van Roy, B., Russo, D. J., & Wen, Z. (2019). Deep exploration via randomized value functions. *Journal of Machine Learning Research, 20*(124), 1–62.

Öztürk, Ş., Alhudhaif, A., & Polat, K.ÖZTÜRK. (2021). Attention-based end-to-end CNN framework for content-based X-ray image retrieval. *Turkish Journal of Electrical Engineering and Computer Sciences, 29*(SI-1), 2680–2693. DOI: 10.3906/elk-2105-242

Page, E. S. (1954). Continuous inspection schemes. *Biometrika, 41*(1–2), 100–115. DOI: 10.1093/biomet/41.1-2.100

Paina, L., & Peters, D. H. (2012). Understanding pathways for scaling up health services through the lens of complex adaptive systems. *Health Policy and Planning, 27*(5), 365–373. DOI: 10.1093/heapol/czr054 PMID: 21821667

Pal, J. (2025). Assessing India's readiness for public health emergencies: Governance, policy, and executive powers. *International Journal for Multidisciplinary Research, 7*(6), 61769. Advance online publication. DOI: 10.36948/ijfmr.2025.v07i06.61769

Pandey, A., & Singh, R. (2025). Article 14 and social justice: A constitutional mandate for an egalitarian society. *International Journal of Research Publication and Reviews, 6*(8), 3723–3729. DOI: 10.55248/gengpi.6.0825.3087

Pang, G., & Szlitzer, M. (2026). Governing AI in operations: Ethical risks, accountability mechanisms, and responsible digital operations. *AI and Ethics*, *6*(4), 338. Advance online publication. DOI: 10.1007/s43681-026-01191-3

Papadimitriou, C. H., & Tsitsiklis, J. N. (1987). The complexity of Markov decision processes. *Mathematics of Operations Research*, *12*(3), 441–450. DOI: 10.1287/moor.12.3.441

Papadopoulou, E., Exarchos, T. P., Jenko, S., Krepelkova, K., & Namorado, J. (2025). Artificial intelligence (AI) in health systems: Introducing a 'Do Good' approach. *AI and Ethics*, *5*(6), 6339–6357. DOI: 10.1007/s43681-025-00757-x

Parycek, P., Schmid, V., & Novak, A.-S. (2023). Artificial intelligence (AI) and automation in administrative procedures: Potentials, limitations, and framework conditions. *Journal of the Knowledge Economy*, *15*(2), 8390–8415. DOI: 10.1007/s13132-023-01433-3

Paul, P. K. (2026). Demystifying Digital Healthcare Systems: Aspects of Emerging Technologies, Initiatives, Opportunities and Issues—The Indian Context. *International Journal of Information Science and Computing*, *12*(2), 259–265.

Paul, P. K., Bandyopadhyay, A., Kayyali, M., Das, N., Chatterjee, R., & Sharma, S. K. (2025). Integrating Big Data and AI in nutrition: Current trends and future directions. [IJRQEH]. *International Journal of Reliable and Quality E-Healthcare*, *14*(1), 1–22. DOI: 10.4018/IJRQEH.372690

Paul, P. K., Pradhan, U., Jena, S. K., Bommali, T., Kayyali, M., & Saavedra, R. (2024). Emerging Healthcare Systems with AI based Medicine, EHRs, VHAs, & Precision Healthcare: A Scientific Study. *International Journal of Applied Science and Engineering*, *12*(2), 133–151. DOI: 10.30954/2322-0465.2.2024.3

Peel, J. K., Whiteley, J., Stuart-McEwan, T., Waddell, T. K., Selzner, M., Litvak, E., & Keshavjee, S. (2025). Improving timely transplantation while reducing cancellation of scheduled surgery. *The Journal of Thoracic and Cardiovascular Surgery*. PMID: 41205904

Pillai, A. S. (2021). Utilizing deep learning in medical image analysis for enhanced diagnostic accuracy and patient care: Challenges, opportunities, and ethical implications. *Journal of Deep Learning in Genomic Data Analysis*, *1*(1), 1–17.

Pineau, J., Gordon, G., & Thrun, S. (2003). Point-based value iteration: An anytime algorithm for POMDPs. In *Proceedings of the 18th International Joint Conference on Artificial Intelligence (IJCAI 2003)* (pp. 1025–1032).

Pineau, J., Gordon, G., & Thrun, S. (2003). Point-based value iteration: An anytime algorithm for POMDPs. In *Proceedings of the 18th International Joint Conference on Artificial Intelligence* (pp. 1025–1030). Morgan Kaufmann.

Pineau, J., Gordon, G., & Thrun, S. (2006). Anytime point-based approximations for large POMDPs. *Journal of Artificial Intelligence Research*, *27*, 335–380. DOI: 10.1613/jair.2078

Plsek, P. E., & Greenhalgh, T. (2001). The challenge of complexity in health care. *BMJ (Clinical Research Ed.)*, *323*(7313), 625–628. DOI: 10.1136/bmj.323.7313.625 PMID: 11557716

Porter, M. E. (1985). *Competitive advantage: Creating and sustaining superior performance*. Free Press.

Powell, W. B. (2011). *Approximate dynamic programming: Solving the curses of dimensionality* (2nd ed.). Wiley., DOI: 10.1002/9781118029176

Prayitno, S., Shyu, C.-R., Putra, K. T., Chen, H.-C., Tsai, Y.-Y., Hossain, K. S. M. T., Jiang, W., & Shae, Z.-Y. (2021). A systematic review of federated learning in the healthcare area: From the perspective of data properties and applications. *Applied Sciences (Basel, Switzerland)*, *11*(23), 11191. DOI: 10.3390/app112311191

Precup, D., Sutton, R. S., & Singh, S. (2000). Eligibility traces for off-policy policy evaluation. In *Proceedings of the 17th International Conference on Machine Learning* (pp. 759–766). Morgan Kaufmann.

Puterman, M. L. (2014). *Markov decision processes: Discrete stochastic dynamic programming*. Wiley., DOI: 10.1002/9780470316887

Qi, J., Zhou, Q., Lyu, L., Yang, Q., & Wang, S. (2021). Federated reinforcement learning: Techniques, applications, and open challenges. arXiv. https://arxiv.org/abs/2108.11887

Rabiee, P. (2026). Artificial intelligence in healthcare systems of low- and middle-income countries: Opportunities, challenges, and pathways to ethical integration. In Malawana, J., Arjomandi Rad, A., Vardanyan, R., & Miller, G. (Eds.), *Artificial intelligence in healthcare and biomedical visualization* (pp. 157–170). Springer Nature Switzerland., DOI: 10.1007/978-3-032-06520-9_9

Rabiner, L. R. (1989). A tutorial on hidden Markov models and selected applications in speech recognition. *Proceedings of the IEEE*, *77*(2), 257–286. DOI: 10.1109/5.18626

Raghupathi, W., & Raghupathi, V. (2014). Big data analytics in healthcare: Promise and potential. *Health Information Science and Systems*, *2*(1), 3. DOI: 10.1186/2047-2501-2-3 PMID: 25825667

Rajabi, E., & Etminani, K. (2021). Towards a knowledge graph-based explainable decision support system in healthcare. *Studies in Health Technology and Informatics*, *281*, 502–503. DOI: 10.3233/SHTI210215 PMID: 34042621

Rajkomar, A., Dean, J., & Kohane, I. (2019). Machine learning in medicine. *The New England Journal of Medicine*, *380*(14), 1347–1358. DOI: 10.1056/NEJMra1814259 PMID: 30943338

Rasmy, L., Xiang, Y., Xie, Z., Tao, C., Zhi, D., & Zeng, J. (2021). Med-BERT: Pretrained contextualized embeddings on large-scale structured electronic health records for disease prediction. *npj. Digital Medicine*, *4*(1), 86. DOI: 10.1038/s41746-021-00455-y PMID: 34017034

Ravasz, E., & Barabási, A.-L. (2003). Hierarchical organization in complex networks. *Physical Review. E*, *67*(2), 026112. Advance online publication. DOI: 10.1103/PhysRevE.67.026112 PMID: 12636753

Ray, A., Achiam, J., & Amodei, D. (2019). *Benchmarking safe exploration in deep reinforcement learning* [Technical report]. OpenAI.

Raza, A., Ahmed, N., & Shahid, N. (2024). Stochastic delayed analysis of coronavirus model through efficient computational method. *Scientific Reports*, *14*(1), 21170. DOI: 10.1038/s41598-024-70089-z PMID: 39256433

Raza, A., & Shafique, U. (2024). Mathematical modeling and dynamics of gonorrhoea epidemic within stochastic fractional delay differential equations. *Modeling Earth Systems and Environment, 10*, 5939–5959. DOI: 10.1007/s40808-024-02124-x

Reddy, S. (2024). Global harmonization of artificial intelligence-enabled software as a medical device regulation: Addressing challenges and unifying standards. *Mayo Clinic Proceedings. Digital Health, 3*(1), 100191. DOI: 10.1016/j.mcpdig.2024.100191 PMID: 40207007

Reshi, A. A., Rustam, F., Mehmood, A., Alhossan, A., Alrabiah, Z., Ahmad, A., Alsuwailem, H., & Choi, G. S. (2021). An Efficient CNN Model for COVID-19 Disease Detection Based on X-Ray *Image Classification. Complexity, 2021*(1). Portico. .DOI: 10.1155/2021/6621607

Revathy, G., Dinesh, L., Sathish, P., & Selvan, S. T. (2026). Support systems: Revolutionizing patient care in Industry 6.0: Integrating cloud computing and IoT for enhanced patient care. In *Generative AI revolution: Transforming healthcare and life sciences towards sustainable development in Industry 6.0* (p. 73).

Reza, A. W., Hossain, M. S., Wardiful, M. A., Farzana, M., Ahmad, S., Alam, F., Nandi, R. N., & Siddique, N. (2022). A CNN-Based Strategy to Classify MRI-Based Brain Tumors Using Deep Convolutional Network. *Applied Sciences (Basel, Switzerland), 13*(1), 312. DOI: 10.3390/app13010312

Ribeiro, M. T., Singh, S., & Guestrin, C. (2016). Why should I trust you?: Explaining the predictions of any classifier. In *Proceedings of the ACM SIGKDD International Conference on Knowledge Discovery and Data Mining* (pp. 1135–1144). DOI: 10.1145/2939672.2939778

Rieke, N., Hancox, J., Li, W., Milletarì, F., Roth, H. R., Albarqouni, S., Bakas, S., Galtier, M. N., Landman, B. A., Maier-Hein, K., Ourselin, S., Sheller, M., Summers, R. M., Trask, A., Xu, D., Baust, M., & Cardoso, M. J. (2020). The future of digital health with federated learning. *npj. Digital Medicine, 3*(1), 119. DOI: 10.1038/s41746-020-00323-1 PMID: 33015372

Ristevski, B., & Chen, M. (2018). Big data analytics in medicine and healthcare. *Journal of Integrative Bioinformatics, 15*(3), 20170030. DOI: 10.1515/jib-2017-0030 PMID: 29746254

Ross, S. M. (2014). *Introduction to probability models*. Academic Press.

Ross, S., Pineau, J., Chaib-draa, B., & Kreitmann, P. (2011). A Bayesian approach for learning and planning in partially observable Markov decision processes. *Journal of Machine Learning Research, 12*, 1729–1770.

Rucinski, K. B., Knight, J., Willis, K., Wang, L., Rao, A., Roach, M. A., Phaswana-Mafuya, N., Bao, L., Thiam, S., Arimi, P., Mishra, S., & Baral, S. (2024). Challenges and opportunities in big data science to address health inequities and focus the HIV response. *Current HIV/AIDS Reports, 21*(4), 208–219. DOI: 10.1007/s11904-024-00702-3 PMID: 38916675

Sadanandan, B. (2026). Multimodal deep learning for early prediction of patient deterioration in the ICU: Integrating time-series EHR data with clinical notes. arXiv. https://arxiv.org/abs/2603.14719

Sahoo, S., Mishra, S., Panda, B., Bhoi, A. K., & Barsocchi, P. (2023). An Augmented Modulated Deep Learning Based Intelligent Predictive Model for Brain Tumor Detection Using GAN Ensemble. *Sensors (Basel)*, *23*(15), 6930. DOI: 10.3390/s23156930 PMID: 37571713

Saleh, M., Awad, O. R. D., Bizun, H. K. M., & Oufi, M. R. H. (2025). Advanced statistical techniques in healthcare: Innovations in data analysis and decision making. In *Bright Sky Publications eBooks*. DOI: 10.62906/bs.book.293

Sangeetha, R., Premkumar, M., Ashokkumar, S. R., Mohanbabu, G., Anupallavi, S., & Gloria Jeyaraj, J. P. (2026). The digital technologies in healthcare: Navigating the digital transformation with security and operational efficiencies. In *BioMed Bots Assurance*. CRC Press., DOI: 10.1201/9781003561309-13

Sathpathy, S., Kant, S., Sood, R., Tyagi, M., Dwivedi, S., & Gupta, S. K. (2023). Impact of application of queuing theory on operational efficiency of patient registration. *Medical Journal, Armed Forces India*, *79*(3), 300–308. DOI: 10.1016/j.mjafi.2021.06.028 PMID: 37193519

Sato, K., & Sawaki, K. (2024). An optimal policy for lockdown periods in a pandemic based on the stochastic SIR model with time delay. In Nakamura, S., Sawaki, K., & Nakagawa, T. (Eds.), *Probability and statistical models in operations research, computer and management sciences*. Springer., DOI: 10.1007/978-3-031-64597-6_2

Saudi Data and Artificial Intelligence Authority. (2023). *Personal Data Protection Law*. https://sdaia.gov.sa/en/SDAIA/about/Documents/Personal%20Data%20English%20V2-23April2023-%20Reviewed-.pdf

Schaefer, A. J., Bailey, M. D., Shechter, S. M., & Roberts, M. S. (2005). Modeling medical treatment using Markov decision processes. In Brandeau, M. L., Sainfort, F., & Pierskalla, W. P. (Eds.), *Operations research and health care* (pp. 593–612). Springer., DOI: 10.1007/1-4020-8066-2_23

Schelling, T. C. (1971). Dynamic models of segregation. *The Journal of Mathematical Sociology*, *1*(2), 143–186. DOI: 10.1080/0022250X.1971.9989794

Schulman, J., Wolski, F., Dhariwal, P., Radford, A., & Klimov, O. (2017). Proximal policy optimization algorithms. *arXiv:1707.06347.*

Selbst, A. D., Boyd, D., Friedler, S. A., Venkatasubramanian, S., & Vertesi, J. (2019). Fairness and abstraction in sociotechnical systems. In *Proceedings of the 2019 Conference on Fairness, Accountability, and Transparency* (pp. 59–68). Association for Computing Machinery. https://doi.org/DOI: 10.1145/3287560.3287598

Sendak, M. P. (2019). Machine learning in health care: A critical appraisal of challenges and opportunities. *EGEMS (Washington, DC)*, *7*(1), 1. DOI: 10.5334/egems.287 PMID: 30705919

Sendak, M. P., D'Arcy, J., Kashyap, S., Gao, M., Nichols, M., Corey, K., & Balu, S. (2020). A path for translation of machine learning products into healthcare delivery. *EMJ Innovations*, *10*, 19–00172.

Shafer, G., Shen, A., Vereshchagin, N., & Vovk, V. (2011). Test martingales, Bayes factors and p-values. *Statistical Science*, *26*(1), 84–101.

Shah, N. H., Milstein, A., & Bagley, S. C. (2019). Making machine learning models clinically useful. *Journal of the American Medical Association, 322*(14), 1351–1352. DOI: 10.1001/jama.2019.10306 PMID: 31393527

Shah, P. M., Ullah, H., Ullah, R., Shah, D., Wang, Y., Islam, S. U., Gani, A., & Rodrigues, J. J. (2022). DC-GAN-based synthetic X-ray images augmentation for increasing the performance of EfficientNet for COVID-19 detection. *Expert Systems: International Journal of Knowledge Engineering and Neural Networks, 39*(3), e12823. DOI: 10.1111/exsy.12823 PMID: 34898799

Shaik, T., Tao, X., Higgins, N., Li, L., Gururajan, R., & Zhou, X.. (2023). Remote Patient Monitoring Using Artificial Intelligence: Current State, Applications, and Challenges. *Wiley Interdisciplinary Reviews. Data Mining and Knowledge Discovery, 13*, e1485. DOI: 10.1002/widm.1485

Sharma, S. (2023). Artificial intelligence for fracture diagnosis in orthopedic X-rays: Current developments and future potential. *SICOT-J, 9*, 21. DOI: 10.1051/sicotj/2023018 PMID: 37409882

Sheller, M. J., Edwards, B., Reina, G. A., Martin, J., Pati, S., Kotrotsou, A., Milchenko, M., Xu, W., Marcus, D., Colen, R. R., & Bakas, S. (2020). Federated learning in medicine: Facilitating multi-institutional collaborations without sharing patient data. *Scientific Reports, 10*(1), 12598. DOI: 10.1038/s41598-020-69250-1 PMID: 32724046

Shickel, B., Tighe, P. J., Bihorac, A., & Rashidi, P. (2017). Deep EHR: A survey of recent advances in deep learning techniques for electronic health record (EHR) analysis. *IEEE Journal of Biomedical and Health Informatics, 22*(5), 1589–1604. DOI: 10.1109/JBHI.2017.2767063 PMID: 29989977

Shin, D.-H., Lee, D.-J., Son, Y.-H., & Kam, T.-E. (2026). Treatment stitching with Schrödinger bridge for enhancing offline reinforcement learning in adaptive treatment strategies. *Proceedings of the AAAI Conference on Artificial Intelligence, 40*(21), 17697–17705. DOI: 10.1609/aaai.v40i21.38826

Shiryaev, A. N. (2007). *Optimal stopping rules*. Springer.

Siebert, U., Alagoz, O., Bayoumi, A. M., Jahn, B., Owens, D. K., Cohen, D. J., & Kuntz, K. M. (2012). State-transition modeling: A report of the ISPOR-SMDM modeling good research practices task force—3. *Medical Decision Making, 32*(5), 690–700. DOI: 10.1177/0272989X12455463 PMID: 22990084

Silver, D., & Veness, J. (2010). Monte-Carlo planning in large POMDPs. In *Advances in Neural Information Processing Systems* (Vol. 23, pp. 2164–2172).

Silver, D., Huang, A., Maddison, C. J., Guez, A., Sifre, L., van den Driessche, G., Schrittwieser, J., Antonoglou, I., Panneershelvam, V., Lanctot, M., Dieleman, S., Grewe, D., Nham, J., Kalchbrenner, N., Sutskever, I., Lillicrap, T., Leach, M., Kavukcuoglu, K., Graepel, T., & Hassabis, D. (2016). Mastering the game of Go with deep neural networks and tree search. *Nature, 529*(7587), 484–489. DOI: 10.1038/nature16961 PMID: 26819042

Silverman, B. W. (1986). *Density estimation for statistics and data analysis*. Chapman and Hall.

Simpkin, A. L., & Armstrong, K. (2019). Communicating uncertainty in the diagnosis of rare conditions. *Medical Decision Making, 39*(2), 167–174. DOI: 10.1177/0272989X19827517

Simpson, M. J., & Plank, M. J. (2025). Inference and prediction for stochastic models of biological populations undergoing migration and proliferation. *Journal of the Royal Society, Interface*, *22*(231), 20250536. DOI: 10.1098/rsif.2025.0536 PMID: 41151767

Singer, M., Deutschman, C. S., Seymour, C. W., Shankar-Hari, M., Annane, D., Bauer, M., Bellomo, R., Bernard, G. R., Chiche, J.-D., Coopersmith, C. M., Hotchkiss, R. S., Levy, M. M., Marshall, J. C., Martin, G. S., Opal, S. M., Rubenfeld, G. D., van der Poll, T., Vincent, J.-L., & Angus, D. C. (2016). The Third International Consensus Definitions for Sepsis and Septic Shock (Sepsis-3). *Journal of the American Medical Association*, *315*(8), 801–810. DOI: 10.1001/jama.2016.0287 PMID: 26903338

Singh, K. (2023). Artificial intelligence & cloud in healthcare: Analysing challenges and solutions within regulatory boundaries. *SSRG International Journal of Computer Science and Engineering*, *10*(9), 1–9.

Singh, P., Singh, S., Mishra, A., Tripathi, R., & Bhatt, D. (2024). Multimodality treatment planning using the Markov decision process: A comprehensive study of applications and challenges. *Research on Biomedical Engineering*, *40*(2), 435–450. DOI: 10.1007/s42600-024-00349-4

Sittig, D. F., & Singh, H. (2010). A new sociotechnical model for studying health information technology in complex adaptive healthcare systems. *Quality & Safety in Health Care*, *19*(Suppl 3), i68–i74. DOI: 10.1136/qshc.2010.042085 PMID: 20959322

Skaletska, Z. S. (2026). International legal regulation of medical algorithms: Challenges and prospects for control of artificial intelligence in healthcare. *Uzhhorod National University Herald Series Law*, *5*(92), 250–257. DOI: 10.24144/2307-3322.2025.92.5.34

Smallwood, R. D., & Sondik, E. J. (1973). The optimal control of partially observable Markov processes over a finite horizon. *Operations Research*, *21*(5), 1071–1088. DOI: 10.1287/opre.21.5.1071

Smith, R. C. (2014). *Uncertainty quantification: Theory, implementation, and applications*. SIAM., DOI: 10.1137/1.9781611973228

Smith, T., & Simmons, R. (2004). Heuristic search value iteration for POMDPs. In *Proceedings of the 20th Conference on Uncertainty in Artificial Intelligence* (pp. 520–527). AUAI Press.

Smith, T., & Simmons, R. (2005). Point-based POMDP algorithms: Improved analysis and implementation. In *Proceedings of the 21st Conference on Uncertainty in Artificial Intelligence* (pp. 542–549). AUAI Press.

Sondik, E. J. (1971). *The optimal control of partially observable Markov processes* [Doctoral dissertation, Stanford University]. Stanford Digital Repository.

Sonnenberg, F. A., & Beck, J. R. (1993). Markov models in medical decision making: A practical guide. *Medical Decision Making*, *13*(4), 322–338. DOI: 10.1177/0272989X9301300409 PMID: 8246705

Spanos, S., Dammery, G., Pagano, L., Ellis, L. A., Fisher, G., Smith, C. L., Foo, D., & Braithwaite, J. (2024). Learning health systems on the front lines to strengthen care against future pandemics and climate change: A rapid review. *BMC Health Services Research*, *24*(1), 829. Advance online publication. DOI: 10.1186/s12913-024-11295-3 PMID: 39039551

Srinivasan, S. (2022). The vaccine mandates judgment: Some reflections. *Indian Journal of Medical Ethics, 8*(2), 134–140. DOI: 10.20529/IJME.2022.056 PMID: 36880474

Srivatsa, S. S. (2026). Epistemic uncertainty in clinical machine learning: Sources, detection, and mitigation. *JVS-Vascular Insights*. Advance online publication. DOI: 10.1016/j.jvsvi.2026.100492

Steimle, L. N., & Denton, B. T. (2021). Markov decision processes for screening and treatment of chronic diseases. In Boros, E., McLay, L., & Tiwari, A. (Eds.), *Markov decision processes in practice* (pp. 189–222). Springer., DOI: 10.1007/978-3-030-18500-8_7

Steiner, S. H., Cook, R. J., Farewell, V. T., & Treasure, T. (2000). Monitoring surgical performance using risk-adjusted CUSUM charts. *Biostatistics (Oxford, England), 1*(4), 441–452. PMID: 12933566

Sterman, J. D. (2000). *Business dynamics: Systems thinking and modeling for a complex world*. McGraw-Hill.

Stooke, A., Achiam, J., & Abbeel, P. (2020). Responsive safety in reinforcement learning by PID Lagrangian methods. In *Proceedings of the 37th International Conference on Machine Learning* (Vol. 119, pp. 9133–9143). PMLR.

Sutton, R. S., & Barto, A. G. (2018). *Reinforcement learning: An introduction* (2nd ed.). MIT Press.

Tamba, H. (2026). *The institutional production of causation: Predictive classification and the governance of human behaviour. Zenodo*. DOI: 10.2139/ssrn.6412758

Tao, F., Zhang, H., Liu, A., & Nee, A. Y. C. (2019). Digital twin in industry: State-of-the-art. *IEEE Transactions on Industrial Informatics, 15*(4), 2405–2415. DOI: 10.1109/TII.2018.2873186

Tennenholtz, G., Mannor, S., & Shalit, U. (2020). Off-policy evaluation in partially observable environments. In *Proceedings of the 34th AAAI Conference on Artificial Intelligence* (Vol. 34, pp. 10276–10283). DOI: 10.1609/aaai.v34i06.6590

Tessler, C., Mankowitz, D. J., & Mannor, S. (2019). Reward constrained policy optimization. In *International Conference on Learning Representations*.

Theocharous, G., Murphy, K., & Kaelbling, L. P. (2004). Representing hierarchical POMDPs as DBNs for multi-scale robot localization. In *Proceedings of the 2004 IEEE International Conference on Robotics and Automation* (Vol. 1, pp. 1045–1051). IEEE. DOI: 10.1109/ROBOT.2004.1307288

Thille, P., Tobin, A., Evans, J. M., Katz, A., & Russell, G. M. (2024). Evolving through multiple, co-existing pressures to change: A case study of self-organization in primary care during the COVID-19 pandemic in Canada. *BMC Primary Care, 25*(1), 285. DOI: 10.1186/s12875-024-02520-3 PMID: 39103760

Thrun, S., Burgard, W., & Fox, D. (2005). *Probabilistic robotics*. MIT Press.

Tiwari, A., Hannan, S. A., Pinnamaneni, R., Al-Ansari, A. R. M., El-Ebiary, Y. A. B., Prema, S., Manikandan, R., & Vidalón, J. L. J. (2023). Optimized Ensemble of Hybrid RNN-GAN Models for Accurate and Automated Lung Tumour Detection from CT Images. *International Journal of Advanced Computer Science and Applications, 14*(7). Advance online publication. DOI: 10.14569/IJACSA.2023.0140769

Topol, E. (2019). *Deep medicine: How artificial intelligence can make healthcare human again*. Basic Books.

Topol, E. J. (2019). High-performance medicine: The convergence of human and artificial intelligence. *Nature Medicine*, *25*(1), 44–56. DOI: 10.1038/s41591-018-0300-7 PMID: 30617339

Tracey, P. (2025). *The atomization of vulnerability: An ethnographic investigation of quantification and automation in Philadelphia's homeless services coordinated entry system*. Deep Blue. DOI: 10.7302/27071

Treacy, M., & Wiersema, F. (1995). *The discipline of market leaders: Choose your customers, narrow your focus, dominate your market*. Addison-Wesley.

U.S. Food and Drug Administration. (2025). *Artificial intelligence-enabled device software functions: Lifecycle management and marketing submission recommendations—Draft guidance for industry and Food and Drug Administration staff*. https://www.fda.gov/regulatory-information/search-fda-guidance-documents/artificial-intelligence-enabled-device-software-functions-lifecycle-management-and-marketing

Upadhyay, U., Sudarshan, V. P., & Awate, S. P. (2021). Uncertainty-aware GAN with Adaptive Loss for Robust MRI Image Enhancement. 2021 *IEEE/CVF International Conference on Computer Vision Workshops (ICCVW)*, 3248–3257. DOI: 10.1109/ICCVW54120.2021.00364

Vaswani, A., Shazeer, N., & Parmar, N.. (2017). Attention Is All You Need. *Advances in Neural Information Processing Systems*, *30*. Advance online publication. DOI: 10.48550/arXiv.1706.03762

Vedder, A., & Spajić, D. (2023). Moral autonomy of patients and legal barriers to a possible duty of health related data sharing. *Ethics and Information Technology*, *25*(1), 23. Advance online publication. DOI: 10.1007/s10676-023-09697-8

Velmovitsky, P. E., Bevilacqua, T., Alencar, P., Cowan, D., & Morita, P. P. (2021). Convergence of precision medicine and public health into precision public health: Toward a big data perspective. *Frontiers in Public Health*, *9*, 561873. DOI: 10.3389/fpubh.2021.561873 PMID: 33889555

Venigandla, K. (2022). Integrating RPA with AI and ML for enhanced diagnostic accuracy in healthcare. *Power System Technology*, *46*(4), 33–42.

Venigandla, K., & Tatikonda, V. M. (2021). Improving diagnostic imaging analysis with RPA and deep learning technologies. *Power System Technology*, *45*(4), 237–249.

Verma, A., Murali, V., Singh, R., Kohli, P., & Chaudhuri, S. (2018). Programmatically interpretable reinforcement learning. In *Proceedings of the 35th International Conference on Machine Learning* (Vol. 80, pp. 5045–5054). PMLR.

Voeneky, S., Burgard, W., Tallinn, J., Misselhorn, C., Thoma, J., Durt, C., Risse, M., Burri, T., Schmidt, T., Shen, W., Metzinger, T., Zittrain, J., Wendehorst, C., von Hein, J., Hinsch, W., von Ungern-Sternberg, A., Poscher, R., & Paal, B. P. (2022). *The Cambridge handbook of responsible artificial intelligence*. Cambridge University Press., DOI: 10.1017/9781009207898

Vogelmeier, C. F., Criner, G. J., Martinez, F. J., Anzueto, A., Barnes, P. J., Bourbeau, J., Celli, B. R., Chen, R., Decramer, M., Fabbri, L. M., Frith, P., Halpin, D. M. G., López Varela, M. V., Nishimura, M., Roche, N., Rodriguez-Roisin, R., Sin, D. D., Singh, D., Stockley, R., & Agustí, A. (2017). Global strategy for the diagnosis, management, and prevention of chronic obstructive lung disease 2017 report: GOLD executive summary. *American Journal of Respiratory and Critical Care Medicine, 195*(5), 557–582. DOI: 10.1164/rccm.201701-0218PP PMID: 28128970

Voigt, P., & von dem Bussche, A. (2017). *The EU General Data Protection Regulation (GDPR): A practical guide*. Springer., DOI: 10.1007/978-3-319-57959-7

Volf, P., & Kouřím, T. (2022). A model of discrete random walk with history-dependent transition probabilities. *Communications in Statistics. Theory and Methods, 52*(12), 4241–4256. DOI: 10.1080/03610926.2021.2004425

Wang, Y., Yang, N., & Li, J. (2025). GAN-Based Architecture for Low-dose Computed Tomography Imaging Denoising. *Proceedings of the 2nd International Conference on Machine Learning and Automation, CONF-MLA* 2024, November 21, 2024, Adana, Turkey. DOI: 10.4108/eai.21-11-2024.2354627

Wang, T., & Li, J. (2025). Transient analysis of patient flow in hospitals: A dynamic queueing network approach. *IISE Transactions on Healthcare Systems Engineering, 15*(4), 336–353. Advance online publication. DOI: 10.1080/24725579.2025.2562131

Watts, D. J., & Strogatz, S. H. (1998). Collective dynamics of 'small-world' networks. *Nature, 393*(6684), 440–442. DOI: 10.1038/30918 PMID: 9623998

Weldon, M. N., Thomas, G., & Skidmore, L. (2024). Establishing a future-proof framework for AI regulation: Balancing ethics, transparency, and innovation. *Tennessee Journal of Business Law, 25*(2), 2–24.

Welzel, C., Cotte, F., Wekenborg, M., Vasey, B., McCulloch, P., & Gilbert, S. (2023). Holistic human-serving digitization of health care needs integrated automated system-level assessment tools. *Journal of Medical Internet Research, 25*, e50158. DOI: 10.2196/50158 PMID: 38117545

Whitt, W. (1991). The pointwise stationary approximation for Mt/Mt/s queues is asymptotically correct as the rates increase. *Management Science, 37*(3), 307–314. DOI: 10.1287/mnsc.37.3.307

WHO. (2021). *Ethics and governance of artificial intelligence for health*. World Health Organization.

Widlas-Klimsiak, K. (2025). The ECtHR and mental health jurisprudence: Progressive interpretation or doctrinal stagnation? *Prawo i Więź, 59*(6), 8. Advance online publication. DOI: 10.36128/w78k2k58

Wiens, J., Saria, S., Sendak, M., Ghassemi, M., Liu, V. X., Doshi-Velez, F., Jung, K., Heller, K., Kale, D., Saeed, M., Ossorio, P. N., Thadaney-Israni, S., & Goldenberg, A. (2019). Do no harm: A roadmap for responsible machine learning for health care. *Nature Medicine, 25*(9), 1337–1340. DOI: 10.1038/s41591-019-0548-6 PMID: 31427808

Wilden, R., Garbuio, M., Angeli, F., & Mascia, D. (Eds.). (2018). *Healthcare entrepreneurship*. Routledge. DOI: 10.4324/9781315157993

Williams, D. (1991). *Probability with martingales*. Cambridge University Press.

Woodall, W. H. (2006). The use of control charts in healthcare and public-health surveillance. *Journal of Quality Technology*, *38*(2), 89–104.

World Health Organization. (2021). *Ethics and governance of artificial intelligence for health: WHO guidance*. World Health Organization. https://www.who.int/publications/i/item/9789240029200

Worthington, D. (1987). Queueing models for hospital waiting lists. *The Journal of the Operational Research Society*, *38*(5), 413–422. DOI: 10.1057/jors.1987.69 PMID: 10282336

Xu, J., Xiao, Y., Wang, W. H., Ning, Y., Shenkman, E. A., Bian, J., & Wang, F. (2022). Algorithmic fairness in computational medicine. *EBioMedicine*, *84*, 104250. DOI: 10.1016/j.ebiom.2022.104250 PMID: 36084616

Xu, Y., Sun, X., & Hu, H. (2022). Extinction and stationary distribution of a stochastic SIQR epidemic model with demographics and non-monotone incidence rate on scale-free networks. *Journal of Applied Mathematics & Computing*, *68*(5), 3367–3395. DOI: 10.1007/s12190-021-01645-3 PMID: 34840543

Yancy, C. W., Jessup, M., Bozkurt, B., Butler, J., Casey, D. E.Jr, Colvin, M. M., Drazner, M. H., Filippatos, G. S., Fonarow, G. C., Givertz, M. M., Hollenberg, S. M., Lindenfeld, J., Masoudi, F. A., McBride, P. E., Peterson, P. N., Stevenson, L. W., & Westlake, C. (2017). 2017 ACC/AHA/HFSA focused update of the 2013 ACCF/AHA guideline for the management of heart failure. *Journal of the American College of Cardiology*, *70*(6), 776–803. DOI: 10.1016/j.jacc.2017.04.025 PMID: 28461007

Yang, Y., Zhang, H., Gichoya, J. W., Katabi, D., & Ghassemi, M. (2024). The limits of fair medical imaging AI in real-world generalization. *Nature Medicine*, *30*(10), 2838–2848. DOI: 10.1038/s41591-024-03113-4 PMID: 38942996

Ye, N., Somani, A., Hsu, D., & Lee, W. S. (2017). DESPOT: Online POMDP planning with regularization. *Journal of Artificial Intelligence Research*, *58*, 231–266. DOI: 10.1613/jair.5328

Yu, C., Liu, J., Nemati, S., & Yin, G. (2019). Reinforcement learning in healthcare: A survey. *ACM Computing Surveys*, *55*(1), 1–36. DOI: 10.1145/3477600

Yu, Y., Liao, J., Ma, D., & Zhu, W. (2024). Measuring the COVID-19 treatment efficiency in OECD countries: A multiplicative network DEA approach. *INFOR*, *62*(3), 419–448. DOI: 10.1080/03155986.2024.2337978

Zhang, N. L., & Liu, W. (1996). *Planning in stochastic domains: Problem characteristics and approximation* (Tech. Rep. HKUST-CS96-31). Department of Computer Science, Hong Kong University of Science and Technology.

Zhang, G., Li, Z., & Din, A. (2022). A stochastic SIQR epidemic model with Lévy jumps and three-time delays. *Applied Mathematics and Computation*, *431*, 127329. DOI: 10.1016/j.amc.2022.127329 PMID: 35784101

Zheng, H., Zhu, J., Xie, W., & Zhong, J. (2021). Reinforcement learning assisted oxygen therapy for COVID-19 patients under intensive care. *BMC Medical Informatics and Decision Making*, *21*(1), 350. DOI: 10.1186/s12911-021-01712-6 PMID: 34920724

About the Contributors

Anastasius Moumtzoglou is a thought leader pioneering a post-Deming, human-centric paradigm for healthcare quality. His research merges quality theory with e-health and complexity science to create new scientific disciplines. He proposes frameworks that view healthcare as a complex adaptive system, where patients are co-producers and technology enables holistic care. His work aims to reshape healthcare for the digital age, moving beyond obsolete industrial models.

***

Tanusree Chakraborty is a Ph.D. in Applied Psychology from the University of Calcutta, with specialization in Organizational Psychology, and holds an MBA (HR) and PGDHRM. With over 23 years of experience in academia, research, training, and consulting, she is currently Associate Professor, Great Lakes Institute of Management, Channai, India. An ex-Research Fellow of the Indian Council of Medical Research (ICMR), her research spans organizational behavior, leadership, workplace well-being, HRM, and management education. She has authored over 80 publications and presented more than 110 papers at international conferences, receiving several Best Paper Awards. She has edited and authored multiple scholarly books with leading publishers and serves as a reviewer, editor, and academic mentor. Her research and consulting work has impacted numerous public and private sector organizations across India.

Suchismita Das is a PhD CIS Scholar in the Department of Computer and Information Science (CIS), Raiganj University, West Bengal, India- 733134. She is doing her research work in Computer and Information Science in the area of Cloud Computing and Green Computing. She has obtained BCA Degree from RUC under North Bengal University, India. She has completed M.Sc. in Computer and Information Science, Department of Computer and Information Science, Raiganj University, West Bengal, India. She secured 1st position in his MSc in Computer and Information Science exam. She has research interests in Information Science centric Cloud Computing & Green Computing, Cloud-based Information Systems, Environmental Systems, Social Informatics and Emerging ICTs, among others. She has presented some of his research papersat various national and International Events, Conferences, and Symposia. Some of her works are associated with New Delhi Publishers (India), IGI Global (USA), Elsevier (Netherlands, UK), Bentham Science (Singapore), Springer (Singapore), CRC Press, T&F (USA).

R Deepa is an Assistant Professor in the Department of Computing Technologies at SRM Institute of Science and Technology, Chennai, India. She earned her B.E. degree in 2006 from Anjalai Ammal Mahalingam Engineering College, completed her M.Tech. in 2011 and Ph.D. in 2023 from Sathyabama Institute of Science and Technology. With more than a decade of teaching and research experience, including service at St. Joseph's College of

Engineering from 2011 to 2023, she joined SRMIST as an Assistant Professor in 2023. Her research interests include Natural Language Processing (NLP), Computer Vision, and Information Systems, and she has contributed to numerous journal articles, conference proceedings, and book chapters in these areas.

Abba Elgujja is a healthcare law scholar and infection prevention specialist affiliated with King Saud University Medical City, Riyadh, and Al-Ansar University, Nigeria. His research focuses on healthcare governance, AI regulation, digital health ethics, and the legal dimensions of infection prevention and public health systems. He has published widely on algorithmic accountability, health data governance, and constitutional aspects of health regulation, and contributes interdisciplinary scholarship bridging law, ethics, and healthcare system design.

Saravanan Elumalai is a technology professional associated with the Digital Engineering – Next Generation business unit at L&T Technology Services (LTTS), a global engineering research and development company specializing in digital transformation, product engineering, and advanced technology solutions. In his role, he contributes to the development and implementation of next-generation digital engineering initiatives, leveraging emerging technologies such as artificial intelligence, cloud computing, Industry 4.0, and intelligent automation to address complex business challenges. His expertise aligns with LTTS's focus on delivering innovative engineering solutions across diverse industries, including mobility, sustainability, healthcare, and high-tech sectors. Through his professional work, Mr. Saravanan Elumalai supports organizations in accelerating digital innovation, enhancing operational efficiency, and driving technology-led business growth.

Gangotri Ganguly is an Assistant Professor in the Department of Information Technology and Systems at EIILM-Kolkata, West Bengal, India. She has 14 years of academic experience. She has completed her B.Tech (CSE) and M.Tech (CSE) from West Bengal University of Technology (WBUT). She is currently pursuing her Ph.D. in CIS under guidance of Dr. P.K. Paul from the Department of Computer and Information Science at Raiganj University, India – 733134. She has published a number of research papers in International Journals. She also has participated and presented papers at various national and international conferences. Her research interests include Artificial Intelligence, AI applications, Ethical concerns of AI & Technology and emerging ICT.

Deepak Gupta is a distinguished academician with over 20 years of teaching experience and expertise in Computer Science and Engineering. He holds a Ph.D. in Computer Engineering and has an extensive research portfolio, including many international journal papers, multiple conference proceedings, and several books. His research interests span machine learning, artificial intelligence, and data mining. Currently, Dr. Gupta serves as an Associate Professor and Head of Department of CSE (Emerging Branches) at ITM Gwalior, MP, India. He has also contributed significantly to the field through patents and copyrights and actively engages as a reviewer, conference chair and editor.

Rajiv Gurugopinath is an Assistant Professor of Law at Ramaiah College of Law (Autonomous), Bengaluru, and is also enrolled as an advocate with the Karnataka State Bar Council. He began his academic journey with a B.A. LL.B. degree from B.M.S. College of Law, Bengaluru, and went on to complete his Master of Laws (LL.M.) in Constitutional and Administrative Law from University Law College, Bangalore University, where he authored a thesis on "Constitutional Implications of the

Appointment of Judges of the Higher Judiciary in India – A Critical Evaluation." He further pursued a Master of Business Laws (M.B.L.) at the National Law School of India University, Bengaluru. Dr. Gurugopinath earned his doctorate from the School of Law, Vel Tech Rangarajan Dr. Sagunthala R&D Institute of Science and Technology, Chennai, with his research focusing on "Right to Health – A Study on the Legal Framework and Its Implementation with Special Reference to Bangalore Urban District." An active academic and practitioner, he has presented and published widely in national and international conferences, delivered invited lectures, judged moot courts and legal events, and engaged as a resource person

Sachin Jain is working as an Associate Professor in the Department of Computer Science and Engineering at Ajay Kumar Garg Engineering College, Ghaziabad. He completed his B.Tech in Computer Science and Engineering in 2007 from UPTU, Lucknow and M.Tech in Computer Science and Engineering in 2010 from GGSIPU, Delhi. He has completed his Ph.D in Computer Science and Engineering from Sharda University Greater Noida in 2025. He is a UGC-NET qualified teacher and has total 16 years of teaching experience. His research interests lie in Artificial Intelligence, Deep Learning and Machine Learning. He has published more than 35 research papers in International SCIE, ESCI and SCOPUS Journals and Conference proceedings. Dr. Jain has also published more than 25 patents for his work.

Manoj K is an Assistant Professor in the Department of Statistics at Manonmaniam Sundaranar University, Tamil Nadu, India. He has several years of teaching and research experience in statistics. His research interests include outlier detection methods, biostatistics, time series analysis, and stochastic modeling, with applications to healthcare and biomedical data. He has published research papers and book chapters in peer-reviewed journals and edited volumes and is actively involved in interdisciplinary research applying statistical methods to real-world healthcare and social science problems.

Ramya Krishnappa is an accomplished legal academic and Assistant Professor of Law at School of Law, CHRIST University, Bengaluru. A member of the Karnataka State Bar Council, she graduated with a B.A. LL.B. from B.M.S. College of Law, Bengaluru. She went on to pursue her Master of Laws (LL.M.) in Constitutional and Administrative Law at KLE's Law College, Bengaluru, where she was awarded a Gold Medal for academic excellence. Her doctoral research was undertaken at Christ University, Bengaluru, where she earned a Ph.D. in Law on the theme "Study on the Legal Framework and Working of Panchayat Institutions with Special Reference to Mandya District." Her scholarship reflects a deep commitment to grassroots governance and constitutional development. With over eight years of combined teaching, research, and practice experience, Dr. Krishnappa has established herself as a dedicated educator who prioritizes interactive learning, critical analysis, and student engagement. She is passionate about mentoring young law students, advancing legal research, and contributing meaningfully to both academia and practice.

Premkumar M., M.E., Ph.D., is a Professor and Head of the Department of Artificial Intelligence and Data Science at SSM Institute of Engineering and Technology, Dindigul, Tamil Nadu, India. He is an Anna University recognized Ph.D. supervisor and holds a doctoral degree in Information and Communication Engineering from Anna University, Chennai. His research interests include Artificial Intelligence, Data Science, Deep Learning, Cyber security, Wireless Sensor Networks, Internet of Things,

Healthcare, and Smart Agriculture. He has authored and co-authored research articles and book chapters in various emerging areas of intelligent computing and AI-driven applications.

Senthil Kumar M., M.E., is an Assistant Professor in the Department of Electronics and Communication Engineering at Theni Kammavar Sangam College of Technology, Theni, Tamil Nadu, India. He has an academic background in VLSI and has a strong interest in the design and development of advanced electronic and embedded systems. His research interests include Internet of Things (IoT), Embedded Systems, Micro controllers, and VLSI, with a focus on emerging IoT-based technologies and intelligent systems.

Karthika P., M.E., is an Assistant Professor in the Department of Electronics and Communication Engineering at SSM Institute of Engineering and Technology, Dindigul, Tamil Nadu, India. She is currently pursuing her Ph.D. in the area of Image Processing and Machine Learning. Her research interests include Artificial Intelligence, Machine Learning, Deep Learning, Medical Image Processing, Computer Vision, and Healthcare Applications.

Rohit Pal is a distinguished academic leader, educator, and researcher based in Kolkata, widely recognized for his interdisciplinary expertise in life sciences, sustainability, leadership, and education management. He is pursuing Post-Doctoral Research at Lincoln University College, Malaysia, further strengthening his research contributions in sustainability, education, and interdisciplinary studies. He currently serves as the Head of Department for Biological and Environmental Sciences at the RICE-Adamas Group, Kolkata and also associated with the School of Professional Studies at Adamas University. His academic journey is marked by a Professional Doctorate in Education Management from European International University, Paris, France, an MBA in Human Resource Management, and an M.Sc. in Life Sciences from Presidency University, Kolkata. A dedicated advocate for environmental literacy and transformative education, Dr. Pal's research explores the intersection of leadership, sustainability, and emerging educational paradigms. His commitment to innovative pedagogy earned him the prestigious Excellence in Science Teaching Award at the Asian Education Conclave 2023. Beyond the classroom, he is a prolific author of several books on leadership and human resource development, with numerous scholarly contributions indexed across international journals and academic platforms like Google Scholar, Scopus, Researchgate etc. As a National Geographic Society Certified Educator, a UGC-NET qualified academic, and a WBSET qualified professional, Dr. Pal continues to bridge the gap between traditional science education and modern professional learning through research, mentorship, and academic leadership.

Dimitris Papakyriakou is a PhD Candidate at the Hellenic Mediterranean University, specializing in Big Data Analytics and Data Mining (Edge Computing) in high-performance computing (HPC) systems, with recent research on benchmarking, parallel processing, and neural network workloads on Raspberry Pi clusters. He holds an MSc in European Studies and an MBA in Telecoms from the Athens University of Economics and Business, and a BSc in Electronic Engineering. With over 25 years of professional experience in telecom and cloud services, he has served as AI/ML Business Analyst, Technical Product Manager, and Project Manager at Deutsche Telekom, Cosmote, and WIND, leading large-scale innovation, cloud, and VAS infrastructure projects. His expertise spans AI/ML, MLOps, cloud platforms, benchmarking, and data science, supported by international certifications (e.g., SAFe 5

Practitioner, HarvardX) and a strong record of scientific publications. He is proficient in English and Greek, with a passion for technology leadership, training, and applied research in advanced engineering environments.

Dhanshri Parihar is working as Assistant Professor in the department of CSE(AI&ML) Krishna Institute of Engineering & Technilogy, Ghaziabad(U.P). She has completed B.Tech and M.Tech in CSE from Himachal Pradesh University.Currently pursuing a PhD in computer Science and Engineering from Galgotias University Greater Noida (U.P). She has over 11 plus years of academic experience. Her area of interest includes Cyber Security, Machine Learning and Deep Learning.

Prantosh Paul holds prestigious and unique D.Sc. (Doctor of Science) in Information Science and Technology (IST) & D.Tech. (Doctor of Technology) in Agricultural Informatics & Management degree from Azteca University, Mexico under Dr. Agustin Yoh International Postdoctoral Fellowship (DAYIPF) Program. Dr. Paul perhaps the first person globally who holds DSc in Infornation Science & Technology and DTech in Agricultural Informatics. He also hold PhD in IST from IIEST Shibpur, Post Doctoral Fellow Certificate (PDFC) Program in Environmental Informatics. He holds degrees like M.Tech. (by Research), MS (by Research) in addition to M.Sc. (Double). He is working as Asst. Professor (IST) & Executive Director (MCIS Program), at Dept. of Computer & Information Sciences, and additionally Information Scientist Position at Raiganj University, West Bengal, India. Significantly He is also holds many National and International designations and position such as Honorary Professor, Logos University International, Louisiana, USA, Chief Advisor (Innovative Program & Research Planning), Srinivas University, Mangalore, India. He has credited over 35 Books in diverse areas of interdisciplinary Information Science. He holds 400+ research/review and policy papers, Members in more than 150+ Journals and 250+ Int. Conf. Membership, organization and holds more than a dozen of Awards.

Shivansu Sachan is Pursuing Ph.D. in Management, a Master's holder from Integral University, Lucknow, Bachelor's from IHM, Lucknow. Academic and professional accomplishments of 6 years with renowned organizations and institutes. His Teaching Career has been very satisfying and have continuously upgraded the skills and knowledge by attending many courses and training programs, seminars, conferences organized by different organizations and also delivered many lectures as a Hospitality sector. He is working as an Assistant Professor at Chhatrapati Shahu ji Maharaj University Kanpur .

Neyyila Saibabu is an Associate Professor and Dean of the School of Postgraduate Studies (SPGS) and the School of Arts, Management and Social Sciences (SAMSS) at Skyline University Nigeria. He holds an M.Com and an MBA from Andhra University, a PGDIM from Pondicherry University, and a Ph.D. from Acharya Nagarjuna University, India. His teaching and research expertise includes Accounting, Finance, Economics, Banking, Marketing, Entrepreneurship, and Management. He has taught undergraduate, postgraduate, and doctoral courses and supervised research projects. Dr. Neyyila has published over 25 research articles in reputed national and international journals, presented papers at conferences, authored 27 academic books, and holds three patents. He qualified for the Andhra Pradesh State Eligibility Test (APSET) in both Commerce and Management. He is a member of ISTE, IFERP, IAA, and IOASD. His research interests include accounting, finance, fintech, entrepreneurship, sustainability, economic development, and higher education.

Aastha Sharma completed her B.Tech. from the College of Engineering Roorkee (UTU) in 2019 and earned her M.Tech. (AKTU) in 2024. Her research interests include Blockchain Technology, Machine Learning, Artificial Intelligence, and emerging intelligent systems. She has published several research articles in IEEE, springer international, and national conferences, as well as reputed journals. Additionally, she has contributed book chapters with renowned publishers (IEEE,Taylor & Francis) and holds patents in cutting-edge technological domains, reflecting her commitment to innovation and interdisciplinary research.

Divya Sharma is working as an Assistant Professor in the Department of Electronics and Communication Engineering at Ajay Kumar Garg Engineering College, Ghaziabad. She received her Ph.D. in Electronics and Communication Engineering from the National Institute of Technical Teachers' Training & Research (NITTTR), Chandigarh, in collaboration with Panjab University, in 2023. She also holds an M.E. degree in Electronics and Communication Engineering from NITTTR Chandigarh/Panjab University, awarded in 2013. She completed her B.Tech. in Electronics and Communication Engineering from UPTU, Lucknow, in 2008. She has over 14 years of teaching experience and has guided B.Tech. and M.Tech. students in various engineering projects. Her research interests include perovskite solar cells, photovoltaic devices, semiconductor devices, VLSI, wireless sensor networks, and emerging materials and technologies. She has published more than 50 research papers in international SCIE, ESCI, and Scopus-indexed journals and conference proceedings and has published five patents. She is a member of The Institution of Engineers (India) (M-1724562) and Life Member of the Indian Society for Technical Education (ISTE) (LM 108122).

Noorjahan Siddiqui holds a Master's degree in Statistics and Data Analytics, with a strong interest in statistical analysis and data-driven research.

Madhawa Surendar is a Professor in the Department of Computer Science at Garden City University, Bengaluru. He holds a Ph.D., M.Tech., and B.E. in Computer Science and Engineering, and is an IEEE Senior Member. He brings over 17 years of industry experience along with more than 7 years in academia and research. His expertise spans Artificial Intelligence, Internet of Things (IoT), Embedded Systems, and Applied Machine Learning, with a strong focus on real-world and industry-driven applications. His research interests include healthcare analytics, smart systems, digital twins, and edge intelligence. He has contributed to interdisciplinary research areas such as federated learning and intelligent monitoring systems. He actively mentors postgraduate students and supervises research in emerging technology domains. Dr. Surendar has published and reviewed research papers in reputed journals and conferences and serves as a certified peer reviewer. He is actively involved in academic collaborations, conference organization, and curriculum development aligned with current technological advancements.

M Thalaimalaichamy currently serves as an Assistant Professor in the Department of ECE (Electronics and Communication Engineering) at SASTRA Deemed University. He has 18 years of academic experience and 2 years of industry experience, which helps him combine strong teaching foundations with practical industry exposure. In terms of his educational background (highest degree to lowest degree), he is currently pursuing a Ph.D. in Wireless Sensor Networks (WSN). His completed degrees include M.E (Communication Systems), followed by B.E in ECE, and earlier, Diploma in ECE. This academic progression has strengthened his expertise in both communication systems and wireless sensing technologies. His research and publication activities focus on Machine Learning and Deep Learning, with significant interest in Wireless Sensor Networks (WSN), Wireless Networks, and the Internet of Things (IoT). Through these areas, he works on developing solutions relevant to modern wireless and IoT-based system requirements. Along with teaching and research, he actively contributes to the academic ecosystem through conference organization, participation in FDPs (Faculty Development Programs), and involvement in workshops that support skill development and knowledge sharing among students and faculty. Further, he serves as a reviewer for Springer Nature journals and reviews for Scopus-indexed journals, contributing to academic quality and peer-review processes.

Egamberdiyev Farmankul Tursunkulovich is a Doctor of Economics, Professor, and Advisor to the Rector on Scientific Affairs and Innovation at Alfraganus University, Tashkent, Uzbekistan. He is a distinguished academic and research leader with extensive experience in economics, scientific development, and innovation management. His work focuses on strengthening research capacity, promoting innovation-oriented academic strategies, and advancing institutional excellence in higher education. He plays a significant role in guiding scientific policy, supporting interdisciplinary research, and fostering collaboration between academia and practical sectors. His academic interests include economic development, innovation systems, research management, and strategic advancement in higher education institutions. As a senior academic advisor, he contributes to shaping research priorities, enhancing scholarly productivity, and encouraging a culture of innovation within the university. Through his leadership, teaching, and scholarly engagement, Dr. Egamberdiyev continues to support the growth of academic quality, scientific achievement, and institutional recognition at both national and international levels.

Manoj Deva Yeddu is an Assistant Professor in the Department of Commerce and Management Studies at Adikavi Nannaya University, Andhra Pradesh, India. He holds an MBA, APSET, and pursuing Ph.D. in Management. His research focuses on Rural entrepreneurship, MSMEs, innovation, entrepreneurial finance, family business, IoT, Business Informatics and sustainable development. He has published research articles in reputed national and international journals and has contributed chapters to internationally recognized edited books. He is the author of patents in innovation and human-centered design for social entrepreneurship and actively engages in interdisciplinary research. Recently, he has strengthened his global academic profile through international collaborative research with scholars from the Diesis Foundation and European Union and other countries, along with academic interactions in Vietnam. His work is dedicated to promoting innovation, entrepreneurship education, and inclusive socio-economic development through impactful teaching, research, and international collaboration.

Index

K

L

M

O

P

Q

R

S

U

www.ingramcontent.com/pod-product-compliance
Lightning Source LLC
LaVergne TN
LVHW062029101126
852251LV00005B/65
9798337397054